M Schmidt RN

INFECTION
CONTROL
an integrated approach

INFECTION
CONTROL
an integrated approach

Edited by

KAREN J. AXNICK, R.N., B.S.

Director,
Care Review/Risk Management Program,
Stanford University Medical Center,
Stanford, California

MARY YARBROUGH, R.N., M.S.

Director of Nursing,
O'Connor Hospital,
San Jose, California

With 9 contributors

Illustrated

The C. V. Mosby Company
ST. LOUIS   TORONTO   1984

MOSBY

A TRADITION OF PUBLISHING EXCELLENCE

Editor: **Barbara Norwitz**
Assistant editor: **Bess Arends**
Manuscript editor: **Linda L. Duncan**
Design: **Jeanne Bush**
Production: **Barbara Merritt, Teresa Breckwoldt, Carol O'Leary**

The C.V. Mosby Company
11830 Westline Industrial Drive
St. Louis, Missouri 63146

Library of Congress Cataloging in Publication Data
Main entry under title:

Infection control, an integrated approach.

Includes index.
1. Communicable diseases—Nursing. 2. Nosocomial
infections—Prevention. 3. Asepsis and antisepsis.
I. Axnick, Karen J. II. Yarbrough, Mary.
[DNLM: 1. Infection—Prevention and control.   WC 195 I43]
RT95.I533 1984   614.4'4   82-24933
ISBN 0-8016-0411-7

AC/VH/VH 9 8 7 6 5 4 3 2 1   02/C/234

CONTRIBUTORS

Karen J. Axnick, R.N., B.S.
Director, Care Review/Risk Management Program, Stanford University Medical Center, Stanford, California

Trisha Barrett, R.N., B.S.N.
Infection Control Nurse, Alta Bates Hospital, Berkeley, California

Cheryl Cox, R.N., B.S.
Coordinator, Hospital Quality Improvement; Clinical Supervisor, Infection Control, Inter-Community Hospital, Covina, California

Lu Ann W. Darling, Ed. D.
Independent Consultant, Lu Ann Darling & Associates, Los Angeles, California

Ramona Hodges, R.N., B.S.
Clinical Coordinator, Neurosurgical Unit, O'Connor Hospital, San Jose, California

Marguerite Jackson, R.N., M.S.
Coordinator, Infection Control Team, University of California Medical Center; Assistant Clinical Professor of Community Medicine, University of California School of Medicine, San Diego, California

Jane DeGroot-Kosolcharoen, R.N., M.S.
Infection Control Nurse, William S. Middleton Memorial Veterans Hospital; Lecturer, University of Wisconsin School of Nursing, Madison, Wisconsin

Elad Levinson, L.C.S.W.
Manager, Human Resources Development, Stanford University Hospital; President, Levinson Associates; Stress Management Consultant, Palo Alto, California

Patricia Lynch, R.N.
Infection Control Coordinator, St. Cabrini Hospital, Seattle, Washington

Frances Arnold Weaver, B.A.
Private Consultant, F.A.W. Media Design, Racine, Wisconsin

Mary Yarbrough, R.N., M.S.
Director of Nursing, O'Connor Hospital, San Jose, California

To
Larry, Bill, and Kyle

PREFACE

As one surveys the art and science of infection control practice, it is easy to focus on a spectrum of individual theories and knowledge: epidemiology, microbiology, sanitation and disinfection, biostatistics, infectious diseases, diagnostic and treatment modalities, education, consultation, and research. The *process* of infection control, that vital link between theory and practice, can too easily be overlooked. This text, therefore, highlights the process of integrating scientific information and transforming this knowledge into pragmatic approaches to behavioral change. The content is divided into three parts: the role development theory and model for the infection control practitioner (ICP), the prerequisite skills for program development, and the body of knowledge with particular attention devoted to differentiating between the "hard" and the "soft" scientific data bases.

The role of the ICP has evolved into a hybrid clinical role. The practitioner must not only have knowledge of infection control but also have the ability to influence employees' practice at every level in the health care setting. The ICP must also be able to function within the structure and influence the bureaucracy of the health care setting.

The ICP role offers the opportunity for personal and professional growth because of its evolvement in an atmosphere of unparalleled freedom. This freedom for creativity in role performance is sometimes perceived as a barrier; that is, ICPs want exact answers for how to do this job of infection control. Initially ICPs viewed knowledge of epidemiology, microbiology, and infectious diseases as the key to performing the role. However, practitioners soon learned that the ability to work *through* other people to change practice required more than this type of knowledge. They then began to integrate information from the behavioral sciences into the practice of infection control, with the understanding that only if they can influence other health care providers to value what they themselves value and to practice within the knowledge available about the control and prevention of infections can they truly establish consistent changes within the health care setting.

We have written this book in an effort to address this synthesis of ideas from the behavioral and technological sciences. Infection control is built on areas of highly specialized knowledge. Although the theories and information presented are intended for direct application by the ICP, we cannot give the "right" or "wrong" way to practice infection control. We can only present information that comes from the experience of ICPs and suggest that this experience can be helpful to others faced with the same responsibilities.

Karen J. Axnick
Mary Yarbrough

CONTENTS

1 KAREN J. AXNICK

A historical perspective

Modern hospital epidemiology has become a specialized field with its own unique problems, literature, and techniques.

R.N. Haley*

Association for Practitioners of Infection Control (APIC) The national professional organization of nurses and other health care workers who work in the field of infection control.

infection control program A program implemented for the development of systems within a hospital that will provide a high level of patient care through the surveillance, prevention, and control of nosocomial infections.

Two decades ago a new role emerged in the health care team, that of the infection control practitioner (ICP). Since that time, the clinical specialty of hospital epidemiology has become a major influence on the provision of quality patient care. Assessing the origin of this movement from the vantage point of the present provides insight into and perspective on the current status of the role; more importantly, it stimulates planning for future direction in role development.

In the 1950s pandemics of staphylococcal disease sharply focused the attention of all health care providers on the problem of nosocomial infections. This development occurred within a changing sociological environment that contributed to both endemic and epidemic disease. After World War II there was a proliferation of hospitals, which resulted in a shift from home care to institutional care; for example, hospital obstetrical deliveries increased dramatically. Concomitantly, increasing access to health care (viewed as a "right," not a privilege) and new medical advances dependent on science and technology ultimately created a hospital milieu that reemphasized the need for basic aseptic practices.

In 1959 an innovative response to this need was formulated in Great Britain. Gardner et al.[6] described a "new scheme of infection control" that employed the services of an infection control sister (nurse). The basic responsibilities of this full-time position included (1) documenting the incidence of infection, (2) advising on preventive measures, and (3) assessing the efficacy of these interventions.

*From Infect. Control 1:21-32, 1980.

1

Four years later, at Stanford University Hospital, Kay Wenzel[10] pioneered the role of the infection control nurse (ICN) in the United States. Envisioned as the central figure of the hospital's infection control program, the ICN had several primary functions: surveillance of infections, supervision of isolation techniques, education of staff, and advisement of the infection control committee. The ultimate goal of the program was to increase the level of patient care by reducing the risk of hospital-acquired infection.

Within a year, Shirley Streeter[9] was appointed to a similar position at the Research and Education Hospitals in Chicago. From the efforts of these two women to carve out a new professional role, the movement slowly and steadily gained momentum.

INFECTION CONTROL PROGRAMS

Strong, nationally based advocates of comprehensive infection control programs also emerged. The American Hospital Association (AHA), the National Communicable Disease Center (now the Centers for Disease Control, or CDC), and the Joint Commission on Accreditation of Hositals (JCAH) all expressed concern for the development of systems within hospitals to ensure a high level of patient care through the surveillance, prevention, and control of nosocomial infections.

Initially, surveillance, or casefinding, was heavily emphasized. This focus reflected the prevailing need to characterize the nature and incidence of nosocomial infections. However, it was soon apparent that documentation of numbers and types of infections did not achieve the objectives for prevention and control. Effective control required a balance between surveillance, educational, and consultative activities. Thus, as interest and concern escalated over the estimated 5% of patients affected by nosocomial disease,[1] infection control programs increased in size and complexity.

By the mid-1970s, health care professionals were beginning to question the efficacy and efficiency of the myriad activities involved with infection control. Although it is perhaps easy to enumerate the tasks of infection control programs, the tangible benefits are more elusive. Two deficiencies can be noted. Cost-benefit analyses are foreign to most infection control programs. Next, most accepted infection control practices have evolved as logical and reasonable extrapolations from scanty data and anecdotal experience rather than from scientifically designed, prospective studies. Eickhoff[4] succinctly summarizes this dilemma:

> Taken individually, each of the recommended infection control activities may have some intrinsic merit or rationale. Viewed collectively, it is frankly appalling and wholly devoid of any indication of relative importance or priority. The reason for this dilemma relates directly to our central failure, that is, the absence of any substantive body of data from which to rationally deduce a set of priorities in hospital infection control. Nor is there acceptable scientific

evidence to suggest that the entire program, if carried out as recommended, would reduce nosocomial infections.

Haley et al.[3] have recently completed a comprehensive study that addresses infection control programs. The Study on the Efficacy of Nosocomial Infection Control, known as the SENIC Project, was undertaken in early 1974. Data were collected by questionnaire to assess the contemporary structure of infection control programs, as well as by retrospective chart review to assess the incidence of nosocomial infections for the period between 1970 and 1976. Designed to address the question "What, if any, components of infection control programs achieve a reduction in infection rates?" the SENIC Project has thus far provided descriptive information on roles and functions of practitioners. Yet to be analyzed and published are the specific findings on efficacy of practices.

INFECTION CONTROL PRACTITIONER

The veil of ambiguity surrounding the value of infection control programs has also characterized the role development process of practitioners of the art and science of hospital infection control. In the realm of the program this ambiguity clouds intelligent decision making concerning the functions and practices within the hospital. In the context of the role it prevents clarity in identifying the qualifications required for individuals to supervise or coordinate these efforts. Thus the role development process for the ICP is complicated by a lack of clear role definition and role preparation.

As mentioned previously, the original women appointed to these positions were called infection control nurses because they had a clinical nursing background. This trend continued, as demonstrated by the SENIC Project; for the period 1976 to 1977, 94% of these positions were filled by registered nurses.[5]

Although this trend may be interpreted as an implicit endorsement of the specialized clinical knowledge base nurses bring to this role, others have argued for a broader definition of practice. McGuckin[7] has suggested that the clinical laboratory professional offers a background rich in basic sciences, clinical laboratory theory and practices, pathogenesis of infectious diseases, and research design and thus may be better qualified.

Deliberately choosing a broad approach to the role, the Association for Practitioners of Infection Control (APIC), established in 1972, coined the title *infection control practitioner*. Furthermore, in a 1978 position paper, the APIC membership (composed of 79% nurses)[11] outlined eight different areas of prerequisite knowledge and asserted that "while this expertise may be most readily acquired through a degree program, it may also be gained through nondegree courses or experience. Those persons currently active in the field who have demonstrated proficiency through their work activities shall be considered to have the necessary qualifications."[8]

Yarbrough[10] summarizes the three critical issues facing infection control practitioners. First, there is a need for adequate educational preparation. No longer can practitioners expect on-the-job training or workshops to suffice as preparation for this complex role. Second, all health care professionals must assume responsibility and be held accountable for effective application of infection control principles in their practice. Finally, research is needed to develop the "substantive body" of knowledge that will result in eliminating costly, yet ineffective, infection control methods.

CURRENT RESPONSES TO NEEDS

In recognition of the dynamic nature of the practitioner role and the internal and external pressures for competency, two major educational efforts are underway. APIC has undertaken defining standards of practice that will become the basis for curriculum development and a certification process. The content not only acknowledges the traditional areas of epidemiology, microbiology, statistics, and patient care practice but also expands the knowledge base to include communication, management, and educational theories. This ambitious project will add much to the definition of the role, but it is limited in its ability to assess effective *practice* within the institution.

In a more pragmatic vein the CDC has developed and piloted a new course that stresses management skills for the ICP. The design format is criterion based. Small groups of students work with instructional materials both independently and in groups under the direction of a course manager. The course will be marketed through schools of public health.

The CDC has also responded to a third concern. To assist practitioners in setting priorities and in making intelligent decisions, expert panels have reviewed and categorized the guidelines for patient care and infection control practice[2]:

Category I Measures that are strongly supported by clinical studies or are viewed as useful by a majority of the experts

Category II Measures that may not be generalized to the field but that are supported by highly suggestive studies reported by institutions; measures with a strong theoretical rationale despite inadequate study

Category III Measures that have been proposed but lack either supporting clinical data or strong theoretical bases

This systematic analysis of infection control practices has several benefits. First, it will develop a more critical mind-set for practitioners to use in assessing the value of current and future recommendations. In addition, the tertiary rating will also identify those areas that are vulnerable to scientific scrutiny and will perhaps stimulate needed research.

FUTURE DIRECTIONS FOR PRACTITIONERS

The prevailing health care market faces two major threats to its ability to provide care: spiraling costs and diminishing resources. Every aspect of hospital service is being carefully evaluated by administrators who are increasingly concerned with providing quality care at minimal cost. Pressures are mounting from both public and private sectors for hospitals to demonstrate fiscal restraint without compromising care. In this milieu it is imperative that the ICP adopt a flexible stance to maintain usefulness and relevancy. Clinical expertise, a vital cornerstone in establishing credibility in this role, must now be coupled with a broader base of management skills. Practitioners must be able to assess institutional needs from the administrator's perspective and translate infection control activities into proposals and systems that gain priority by stressing quality and economy. One active approach is to initiate an integration or collaboration of infection control activities with related services, such as risk management, quality assurance, and utilization review. The survival of the ICP role in this time of economic crisis will depend on individual and collective efforts to anticipate needs and to develop creative solutions.

SUMMARY

Significant forces both internal and external to the infection control field have molded the role of the ICP. Without a well-defined model and a standardized educational preparation, the role has evolved in the past 20 years to become a major influence in developing quality-of-care systems. The great challenge facing practitioners in the next decade will be the establishment of a clear definition of role function and the development of a scientific knowledge foundation which to base and evaluate practice. Professional survival and growth will depend on the practitioner's ability to creatively respond in a changing health care environment.

REFERENCES

1. Bennett, J.V., et al.: Current national patterns: United States, Proceedings of the International Conference on Nosocomial Infections, Atlanta, Aug. 3-6, 1970, Centers for Disease Control, Chicago, 1971, American Hospital Association, pp. 42-49.
2. Centers for Disease Control: Guidelines for the prevention and control of nosocomial infections, Washington, D.C., 1981, U.S. Department of Health and Human Services, Public Health Service.
3. Eickhoff, T.C.: General comments on the study on the efficacy of nosocomial infection control (SENIC Project), Am. J. Epidemiol. 111:465-469, 1980.
4. Eickhoff, T.C.: Nosocomial infections—a 1980 review: progress, priorities, and prognosis, Am. J. Med. 70:381-388, 1981.
5. Emori, T.G., Haley, R.W., and Stanley, R.C.: The infection control nurse in U.S. hospitals, 1976-1977: characteristics of the position and its occupant, Am. J. Epidemiol. 111:592-607, 1980.
6. Gardner, A.M.N., et al.: The infection control sister, Lancet 2:710-711, 1962.
7. McGuckin, M.: Clinical correlations: infection control, Am. J. Med.Technol. 44:315, 1978.
8. Position paper: A.P.I.C. Journal 6:9, 1978.
9. Streeter, S., Dunn, H., and Lepper, M.: Hospital infection—a necessary risk? Am. J. Nurs. 67:526-533, 1967.
10. Wenzel, K.S.: The role of the infection control nurse, Nurs. Clin. North Am. 5:89-98, 1970.
11. Yarbrough, M.G.: Training needs of the infection control nurse, Ann. Intern. Med. 89:815-817, 1978.

PART ONE

Role development process

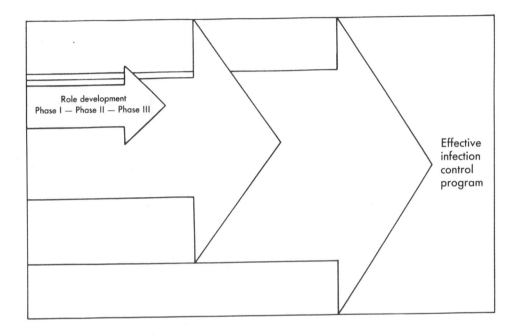

Role development
Phase I — Phase II — Phase III

Effective
infection
control
program

This section of the book presents a theoretical framework based on role theory. It provides a review of basic concepts of role theory necessary for the reader to relate to the role development model. It is not intended to provide an in-depth background in role theory.

The role development model structures the activities of role enactment (how the job is done). It is based on extensive field research conducted by Oda at the University of California School of Nursing in San Francisco. Oda has observed and supervised many students within the Masters of Nursing program as they apply nursing knowledge in a variety of clinical settings. From this work she has identified a three-phase role development model. This model defines a specific order for implementing a specialized nursing role, and when adhered to, it seems to facilitate successful role enactment.

The first phase is *role identification*, which focuses on clarifying the purpose and objective of the role. The second phase, *role transition*, encompasses the implementation phase of the infection control practitioner's job. The third phase is *role confirmation*, which verifies that the role is recognized by others.

Role theory

role Acceptance by an individual to play a particular part as defined by organizational needs.

role confirmation phase Achieved when co-workers have identified a particular person as performing a particular role.

role development process As described by Oda, this process consists of three phases: role dentification, role transition, and role confirmation.

role identification phase Clarification of the purpose and objectives of the role in which the key influence is the practitioner's own philosophy of practice.

role transition phase Activities include accurate identification of the role boundaries, skilled communications with others, and responsibilities as a consultant.

The infection control practitioner (ICP) functions within a complex organizational structure that responds to both internal and external demands for maintaining smooth operations. Each component within the organization views its function as a priority and places demands on the organization to accomplish its goals. Resources such as money, people and support, supplies, and equipment are allocated by the organization based on how it perceives the importance of demands and establishes priorities for distribution. The ICP competes with this structure and has the responsibility to represent the needs of the infection control program to obtain the resources necessary to maintain program viability, effectiveness, and growth.

Without a systematic approach to this process, it is easy to get "lost" and become frustrated in the job. Statements such as "No support is given" and "No one cares" typify the feelings expressed by ICPs struggling to maintain and/or develop their program. The concepts of role theory and a role development framework can be useful in describing a process that can provide a structured approach to accomplishing program goals within the hospital system.

KEY IDEA: The role development process provides direction

Such an organized approach offers both direction and purpose to ICPs who will use the concepts. By understanding themselves and by constantly examining and evaluating their interactions within the environment, they can focus their energies to produce maximal effectiveness.

Oda[3] presents a conceptual model for developing specialized roles, such as the ICP role. The model integrates the concepts of role theory into a structured process that gives direction to the ICP, may strengthen the successful implementation of the ICP's role, and thereby strengthen the overall success of the infection control program.

ROLE THEORY CONCEPTS

I will review some of the major elements of role theory to help the reader understand the role development model.

An organization requires its employees to perform a wide variety of functions to accomplish its goals. Effective performance demands that these functions be assigned to specific positions and that these positions be filled by individuals who have a clear idea of what they are to do. These defined responsibility sets are called *roles*.

Sarbin[5] defines role as a "metaphor intended to denote that conduct [what a person does] adheres to certain positions [a person's job] rather than to the individual [a person's self-concept]."

KEY IDEA: Role and identity: an important distinction [2]

The distinction Sarbin identifies between role and self-identity is critical. Society places strong emphasis on identifying people by the work that they perform. When a person is introduced to someone else, the typical conversation progresses something like this: "Hello, my name is Mary." The other person responds, "Hello, I'm Karen." "It's nice to meet you, Karen," Mary says. "What do you do for a living?" This conversation illustrates how people use occupations to categorize each other and to direct the type of communication that will ensue.

If people identify themselves through their work roles, they may define themselves through their work: "I work, therefore I am."[4]

In role theory people are not synonymous with their work role. They separate themselves from behaviors required in the role. What they are—their self-identity, self-esteem, and personal values—may be expressed through many roles but may be none of the roles themselves. If a person accepts a role, such as the ICP role, that person agrees to perform certain behaviors outlined in a job description; however, the individual may not agree to modify self-identity to value all of the role expectations. A person may "act" one way in the role, even though she may not personally want to or need to. In role theory "all the world's a stage," and a person "performs" the "part" assigned by the job description. With this perspective in mind, it is much less threatening to receive feedback about performance. When feedback informs the ICP that she is not performing within her role, the feedback is perceived as positive. It is helping the ICP achieve behavior necessary for the role. When the ICP can hear criticism without being threatened by it, the comments can be examined with an open mind, not a closed, defensive mind, and they can be applied for self-improvement if they are, in fact, useful.

The important point is that the ICP should not perceive criticism as specific, direct criticism of her self-identity; her "self" is not wholly involved. The criticism is of how she is performing the behaviors within the role. The criticism is directed to the ICP's ability to perform the role expectations outlined in the job description. The criticism is a reality; that is the ICP can choose how to perceive it. Criticism cannot be changed, but the way it is interpreted can be. If the criticism is directed to the ICPs role performance, she separates her role from her self-identity and places distance between herself as a person and herself as a person functioning in a role. The ICP chooses to use the feedback in a constructive way because it helps her see her behavior as others view it, and she can modify her behavior, if she chooses, to meet the role objectives. It is important to remember that the ICP is only performing the expectations of the job successfully if others perceive she is doing so. Therefore what others have to say about the ICP's performance is necessary for her to validate her own performance.

A role, then, is defined by organizational needs and requires certain conduct by people occupying each particular role. It is not the specific conduct of an individual in isolation but how others perceive the conduct and the results achieved through interaction (social behavior) that establishes the success of the role.

KEY IDEA: The ICP role is only as successful as others perceive it to be

---

OVERT SOCIAL BEHAVIOR

This basic orientation to role theory helps to focus discussion on social behavior and role behavior that is appropriate and convincing. Sarbin[5] describes three critical questions to ask that give insight to social behavior and consequent inferences:

- Is the conduct appropriate to the position?
- Is the enactment proper?
- Is the enactment convincing?

Answers to these questions require that judgments be made about observable behavior, both by those observing the behavior external to the performer (others) and by the performer (the ICP).

Is the conduct appropriate to the position?

Role expectations are composed of the rights, privileges, duties, and obligations of any occupant of the role. The conduct expected of anyone occupying the role of ICP will be relatively constant within an organization.

It is imperative that the ICP discuss and clarify the rights, privileges, duties, and obligations associated with the role to ensure that her conduct will be appropriate to the position.

Is the enactment proper?

In role enactment an individual is expected to behave in a predictable way; more importantly, however, the individual is expected to behave as others expect. In short, role expectations are specifications for adherence to group norms. The feedback the ICP receives from co-workers about her behavior many times reflects how the group sees her "fitting in with the routine" and "the way we do things," "following channels," or "not rocking the boat." This feedback carries values of "good" and "bad" and needs to be examined by the ICP so that she can accomplish her role within the existing structure. If others view the ICP as "bad," her influence will be weak. The ICP needs to work within the system as much as possible to keep her influence strong.

Is the enactment convincing?

The ICP will be evaluated according to specific expectations associated with the enactment of her role. Among these are expectations that she is what she claims to be—she has a knowledge base needed by an ICP; that she is committed to and involved in her role—not too much, not too little; and that her role behavior is expected to occur at the proper time and proper place—she can give appropriate instruction to the isolation of a patient with a draining wound infection.

Because total performance is measured by the results achieved through interaction with others, the ICP will need to organize her behavior according to feedback. Feedback is *positive* and helpful because it relates to the ICP how others perceive her ability to perform the role. It gives the ICP information to base decisions on. The ICP has the responsibility to examine the feedback and modify her behavior as she feels it is appropriate.

MULTIPLE ROLES

An ICP functions in different roles; she may be a parent, spouse, employee, consumer, and provider. For each role assumed the ICP has different behaviors and priorities to meet different expectations. For example, as a provider of health services, the ICP is concerned about total performance. How many wound infections have occurred within the surgical service? The ICP's priority is to establish baseline infection rates for the surgical service and to monitor deviations from this baseline. The ICP exhibits behaviors of surveillance over a large area, uses an expert knowledge base to determine appropriate deviations, and consults to correct any inappropriate deviations. However, if the ICP were to become the consumer of surgical services in this same setting, she might find that she cares only about *her* surgical wound. The ICP's attention and behavior would center on using all available resources to care for herself. She is the same individual, but her focus would be entirely different. Within the same set of circumstances the ICP may behave differently, depending on the role she occupies—provider (ICP) or consumer (patient).

For ICPs, many different subroles are required. Those that will be addressed specifically in this book include consultant, educator, manager, epidemiologist, and researcher.

The ability of the ICP to recognize the overt behavior required and expected for each subrole and to demonstrate expected behaviors will increase her effectiveness in implementing each role. The ICP develops the ability to exhibit different behaviors in different roles through experience. It may be helpful to imagine that each individual has a repertoire of behaviors to draw from in any given situation. Through the process of trial and error, the ICP learns which behaviors produce the desired results, based on feedack. As ICPs learn new behaviors that are useful, she places them in her repertoire.

KEY IDEA: The ability to spontaneously exhibit behaviors appropriate to the subrole influences how successfully multiple roles are performed

---

I have worked with ICPs who have identified behaviors that they feel are not useful to them, and they have struggled to eliminate these behaviors. They have found that this is an extremely difficult, if not impossible, task.

My suggestion is that the ICP simply recognize undesirable behaviors as one *choice* she has in her repertoire. The ICP should not spend a lot of time trying to eliminate the undesirable behavior. Instead, she should spend time developing other more desirable behaviors that will expand her "operating repertoire." For example, the ICP may have new information relevant to clinical practice that she wishes to share with the nursing staff members. Her expectation is that they will change their behavior based on this new information. Although the ICP has many managerial functions, in this instance it would be inappropriate to approach staff members as *their* line manager. If the ICP's immediate approach is to "tell the staff to change" without working through the line manager, she would be operating in the wrong subrole for the situation. A more appropriate subrole is that of consultant. Instead of telling members to initiate a change, the ICP might ask for a meeting with the appropriate line manager to determine a mutually agreeable approach to the change she is seeking. As a result of this discussion, the ICP might then move into another subrole—the educator role—to share the new information in conjunction with the line manager setting the new behavioral expectation with the staff.

The ICP has the responsibility of choosing which behavior will fit with each situation she finds herself in, in any of the subroles involved with being an ICP. As new experience is obtained through a variety of role enactments, the repertoire will be expanded. The more behaviors the ICP maintains in her repertoire, the better prepared she will be to meet the demands of the social expectations within the health care setting specific to her role.

The ability to identify and enact appropriate behavior for specific situations can be developed and used instinctively. Developing skills can be likened to learning to drive a car. Initially, each behavior must be identified, dissected, analyzed, synthesized, and integrated on a conscious level; that is, a driver puts the clutch in, shifts the gear, steps on the gas, and lets out the clutch. However, with systematic practice, this process becomes unconscious and automatic, allowing the brain to concentrate on how the skill is intended to be used in the specific situation. Once the mechanics of driving a car are mastered, a person can look for traffic signals, listen to the radio, and carry on a conversation, all at the same time. Developing behaviors requires a systematic, critical analysis of social interactions, both successful and unsuccessful. ICPs should select and practice behaviors that work and avoid those that do not. This process will be reviewed in detail in the second phase of the role development model.

ROLE CONFLICT

Goode[1] defines several reasons why people may experience role conflict:
- People devote more time and attention to one role or subrole than they feel they should.
- People devote more time and attention to one role or subrole than others feel is necessary.
- People are required to perform behaviors that conflict with their own values or with the behaviors and values of others.

In role conflict people can experience stress, worry, pressure, and vague feelings of uneasiness. It is important to resolve the situation. When role conflict is allowed to continue, it may dissipate available energy for role performance, decrease job satisfaction, and ultimately decrease general satisfaction with life (see Chapter 6).

To identify role conflict, the ICP first needs to understand her own internal demands, expectations, and needs. In doing this she may discover that the conflict exists because of her own perceptions. For example, the ICP may feel that she needs to spend too much time in her work role to accomplish expected objectives; thus she does not have enough time and energy for her family.

The conflict may originate from external sources. The ICP may have dual responsibilities in her position. It is not uncommon for an ICP to be in that position part-time and to have part-time supervision responsibilities. In the ICP position there are staff responsibilities, whereas in the supervision position there are line responsibilities.

Although both types of conflicts may have different origins, they need to be resolved to ensure that all energies are directed toward role performance.

ROLE AMBIGUITY

When role definition is not clear, that is, when all parties are not agreeing and understanding the exact behaviors expected, role ambiguity occurs. To the extent that role expectations are unclear, behavior will be less readily predictable. This is especially critical when a supervisor has one set of expectations and the ICP has another. The necessity of expending a great deal of time and effort on trying to predict others' behavior decreases the time available to spend on task activity. Ambiguity is significantly related to tension and dissatisfaction with one's job, leading to a sense of futility and loss of self-confidence.

ROLE OVERLOAD

Role overload is the outcome of role conflict. This occurs when the roles expected of an individual are legitimate and compatible but combine to create demands that are impossible to satisfy. The ICP may have a clear understanding that her job is to perform total surveillance for a 2500-bed institution, provide in-service time once a month to all departments, complete all reports to the infection control committee and the hospital administration by the third Thursday of each month, publish an article at least every year, and perform house supervision once a month. However, it is also clear that this is impossible to do. The required task in this example will pile up to the point that the ICP responsible for them cannot accomplish them. The ICP will be forced to set up priorities to handle the tasks, thereby delaying dealing with some of the demands made, or try to accomplish parts of all tasks, doing none of them well.

SUCCESSIVE ROLES

Successive roles are roles that naturally evolve. For example the ICP was first a student, then a student nurse, then a practitioner, and then an ICP. A review of ICPs' experiences indicates that there is a natural evolution of the ICP role. First, ICPs were data gatherers, then educators, epidemiologists, consultants, managers of programs, and finally researchers. Each role phase is built on the experience and knowledge of the previous phase. Because of successive roles, it is natural to feel a need for "changing" behaviors periodically within the ICP role. There seems to be a natural time span for new practitioners to announce their intentions to do more than surveillance or for experienced practitioners to become more influential in the organizational hierarchy. These times of change should be expected and viewed as normal. Dissatisfaction with a current level of behavior often leads to positive growth and can lead to a more rewarding sphere of operating. Many times, these periods elicit reactions such as "Something's wrong with me" and "I should get out of this job." Perhaps with understanding, evaluation of stressful times will be perceived as a growth crisis leading to the next successive role. The Chinese character for crisis means "dangerous opportunity." When the ICP encounters a "dangerous opportunity," she needs to mobilize her energies to make the most of the situation.

It should be stressed that moving to a higher order of role behaviors cannot occur at the expense of critical behaviors necessary for the total program to function. For example, wanting to do more than surveillance does not mean abandoning surveillance; rather, through negotiations with her supervisor to ensure minimal role conflict and role ambiguity, the ICP establishes a mutually agreeable program for surveillance that allows time for expanding her role.

ROLE DEVELOPMENT PROCESS

Oda[3] devised the role development model by observing many nurses entering a variety of specialized roles, recording their activities, relating their activities to success and failure, and identifying the most successful order of behavior occurrences. Based on these observations, she defined role development in three phases: role identification, role transition, and role confirmation (Fig. 2-1).

Role identification

The identification phase involves clarifying the purpose and objective of the role. The ICP needs to know what is to be accomplished within the role and how to begin to make it happen. The key influence in this phase is the ICP's own philosophy of practice. As the ICP clarifies the hospital's expectations of her within the role, she will be able to analyze how these expectations fit with her philosophy of practice and, ultimately, if she accepts the role, how she will develop it.

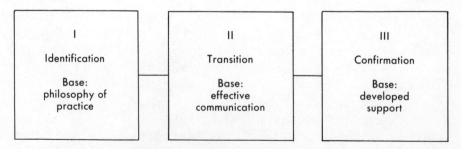

FIG. 2-1. Role development process: resocialization between self and role. (Modified from Oda, D.: Nurs. Outlook **25:**374-377, 1977.)

Role transition

The activities within the role transition phase include (1) accurate identification of the boundaries of the role, (2) skillful communications with others for gathering and giving information, and (3) responsibilities as a consultant. As new information and ideas develop, ICPs need to be perceptively knowledgeable to modify their approach and thus maximize their impact and efficiency.

Role confirmation

The third phase of role development is role confirmation. When co-workers in the hospital identify a particular person as the ICP, that person has actualized this phase of role development. The ability to understand the expectations of the role and to demonstrate behaviors other health care providers expect from the role will directly influence how effectively the ICP is perceived in and identified with the role.

SUMMARY

Even though the role development model has been separated into three distinct parts, in actuality each phase blends into the next. There may not only be constant movement from one phase to another but also simultaneous involvement in different phases for different activities required in the role. As ICPs develop the ability to recognize which phase they are operating within, or which phase they should be planning for, the movement will be more purposeful for them and the results more predictable.

Each of the three phases of role development will be discussed in detail to allow for greater understanding of the skill and knowledge necessary for successful role development.

REFERENCES

1. Goode, W.J.: A theory of role strain, Am. Sociol. Rev. **25**:483-496, 1969.
2. Hartwig, M.S.: Role and identity: an important distinction, Nurs. Outlook **20**:665-669, 1972.
3. Oda, D.: Specialized role development: a three phase process, Nurs. Outlook **25**:374-377, 1977.
4. Rohrlick, J.B.: Work and love: the critical balance, New York, 1980, Summit Books.
5. Sarbin, T.R.: Role theory. In Lindzey, G., editor: Handbook of social psychology, vol 1, Reading, Mass., 1954, Addison-Wesley Publishing Co., Inc.

SUGGESTED READINGS

Gross, N., Mason, W.S., and McEachern, A.W.: Explorations in role analysis, New York, 1958, John Wiley & Sons, Inc.
Hadley, B.J.: The dynamic interactionist concept of roles, J. Nurs. Educ. **6**:5-10+, April 1967.
Lindesmith, A., and Strauss, A.: Roles, role behavior, and social structure. In Lindesmith, A., and Strauss, A., editors: Social psychology, ed 3, New York, 1968, Holt, Rinehart & Winston.
Neiman, L.J., and Hughes, J.W.: The problem of the concept of role—a re-survey of the literature, Social Forces **30**:141-149, Dec. 1951.
Sargent, S.: Concepts of role and ego in contemporary psychology. In Rohrer, J.H., and Sherif, M., editors: Social psychology at the crossroads, New York, 1951, Harper & Brothers.

3 MARY YARBROUGH

Role development: phase 1

entree A means of obtaining entry into a particular professional world.

negotiation To deal or bargain with another or others; to arrange for or bring about by discussion and settlement of terms; to manage, transact, or conduct.

value A learned belief so thoroughly internalized that it colors the action and thoughts of an individual; what a person considers important and relevant influences what is observed and how it is perceived.

values clarification A technique for clarifying values, developed by Louis Raths; a process designed to give an individual the opportunity to find meaning and significance in personal values.

The primary focus of the identification phase of role development is the establishment of mutual consensus about specific role expectations and limitations. It is equally useful when a person is entering a new role or changing the parameters of an established role. The identification phase is a natural beginning step for role development because it involves a review of credentials, both the employer's and the ICP's, and a mutual discussion of role expectations.

The time set apart for the identification phase should be used to discuss expectations about the work environment, expected performance, necessary or desired qualifications, expected rewards, and plans for orientation. During this process, both parties, the ICP and her employer (or prospective employer), will attempt to identify areas of agreement and disagreement and develop consensus about the role that is mutually satisfactory.

Each of these areas is vital to explore *before* the ICP makes a decision to accept a role or change a role. A thorough discussion will minimize confusion about the role and/or capabilities to perform the role for both parties and will give the ICP the best information on which to base her decision to accept or change the role.

Planning and preparation before a scheduled meeting is necessary to ensure that the ICP does, in fact, accomplish review and resolution of each issue. The process of gaining access to an organization or employer for this type of discussion is called entree.[10]

ENTREE

Entree is defined as "a way of obtaining access."[10] This may refer to initial access to an organization, such as a job interview, as well as access that may be sought as a role changes in focus, scope, and/or content. Entree is a continuous process of establishing and nourishing relationships for the purpose of access. The first relationship that must be established as an ICP enters a new job is between the ICP and her employer (or potential employer, as will be implied throughout this chapter). To prepare for the initial meeting the ICP should be aware that she is requesting that specific time be devoted to her—her needs, desires, and development—and that she has a responsibility to direct the conversation to ensure that she has covered her agenda. The ICP also has a responsibility to give the employer enough information about the item(s) she wishes to discuss so that she can be prepared to discuss each item in depth. When both parties are prepared, the time is constructively spent. Conversely this type of meeting can be unproductive when either or both parties are not prepared. How the ICP presents information will give the employer insight into her abilities to plan, articulate her viewpoint, and use time, both her time and the time of others. If the ICP seems disorganized, she may leave an impression of being generally disorganized; if the ICP uses aggressive behavior during the session, she may leave an impression of being generally aggressive. The ICP needs to develop a presentation that helps the employer concentrate on the information she is presenting rather than react to her style or technique of presentation. This allows energy to be used to clarify misunderstandings, confusion, and/or conflicts, rather than to be used to react to the ICP's behavior.

Entree means that the ICP must risk disclosure and potential rejection. I have heard ICPs say, "I never ask" or "They'd only say no." However, the ICP needs support and help in implementing her role and in successfully navigating the infection control program. Without appropriate entree, access to certain areas of the hospital can be blocked, or cooperation can be withheld. Entree provides the ICP with an arena for gathering support, encouragement, and a critical review of her plans and proposals. It provides a setting for mutual goal setting and collaboration, and when conducted appropriately, it will provide a safe environment for testing ideas and developing mutual respect and trust. Trust can be built from disclosure. If the ICP is willing to reveal her true feelings, concerns, and expectations, the employer will be more willing to respond with equal candor.[6] This type of disclosure can begin at a professional level. Discussion of such things as the ICP's beliefs and values about nursing and her impressions of her strengths and weaknesses in personal practice are all topics that will promote an environment for disclosure from the employer. The ICP may feel that this type of risk is not necessary, or is too "risky," but she needs to consider the greater risk taken when she changes the program or role significantly without consent from the supervisor. I believe the greatest risk is taken when program changes or role changes are made based on "assumptions" that an ICP has made but has not clarified. The clearer the ICP is about what she wishes to accomplish and how, the more supportive the employer can be in working within the system to help accomplish these goal(s).

PREPARING FOR ENTREE

To prepare for an initial entree session such as a job interview, the ICP should prepare a statement about herself, her work experience, and topics she would like to discuss during the interview session. This is usually done in the form of a resume. The resume introduces the ICP to the potential employer and should contain the following information:

- Name
- Valid license information
- Educational preparation
- Work experience
- Publications
- Awards and honors
- Philosophy of work practice statement (beliefs, work values, and personal values are outlined)

The resume should be prepared to ensure that the ICP's skills and accomplishments can be identified from the information presented. One method of outlining both professional and technical skills is described by Bolles[1] in *The Three Boxes of Life*. He suggests that skills be listed in three categories*:

Functional skills	Work content skills	Self-management skills
What kinds of actions are you good at that help you do your job well? Examples: Self-analyzing Goal setting Planning	What special knowledge do you have for doing this job well? Examples: Infectious diseases Epidemiology Adult Education Theory	What types of personal characteristics do you have that make you good for the role? Examples: Work independently Self-discipline Extrovert

If the ICP identifies her abilities in these categories for each role she has had in her professional experience, she can demonstrate her strengths, show how her skills have progressed with experience, and be able to forecast her abilities in the position she is discussing. The ICP should carefully and clearly outline the skills she possesses that demonstrate her abilities to perform within the role she is interviewing for.

If the ICP is planning for entree within the identification phase in a continuing work situation, she should prepare her information for discussion in much the same way. The ICP should describe the area she wishes to discuss and her reasons for requesting the discussion. For example, the ICP may wish to alter her responsibility on the infection control committee from being a passive member (no vote) to being an active member (vote). The ICP might prepare a statement of the problem, as she sees it, and list all the reasons she feels the change needs to be made:

*From Bolles, R.N.: The three boxes of life, Berkeley, Calif., 1978, Ten Speed Press.

Problem statement: Because I cannot vote, I do not have formal representation on the infection control committee.

Proposed change: Change the medical staff bylaws to include the ICP as a voting member of the committee.

Benefits of change:

1. Formal recognition of the ICP role and its valid input into decision making
2. Increased influence of the ICP in decision making
3. Public statement of support by the medical staff and hospital administration for the ICP role
4. Supportive information of poor decisions that the ICP could have influenced with her vote had she been a voting member

The ICP should be prepared to discuss both the strengths and weaknesses of her proposal and defend the request or decision. It is important to be prepared to discuss the pros and cons of the recommendation. If the ICP is prepared, this type of discussion will usually strengthen her position, since she will have maximal information on all aspects of the topic being discussed.

In both types of entree discussions it is necessary that the ICP is clear about her values and can articulate her personal and professional philosophy. The ICP's values influence her entire concept of reality, including why she works, what she wants to achieve, and how she measures success for herself. Her values will influence how she prepares for entree sessions, what she chooses to discuss, and what she is willing to accept, compromise, or reject.[5]

KEY IDEA: The ICP needs to have a thorough understanding of her philosophy of practice and value system to accomplish meaningful discussion during the identification phase

---

VALUE

"A value is a learned belief so thoroughly internalized that it colors the actions and thoughts of the individual and produces a strong emotional and intellectual response when anything counters it."[8] In any situation, and especially in the identification phase of role development, the ICP determines what she considers important and relevant based on her personal and professional values. In addition, what she considers important and relevant influences what she observes and how she perceives what she observes.

KEY IDEA: Reality is constant, but it will seem different to everyone because of individual value systems

---

For example, the ICP may have been taught the importance of handwashing before attending to the next patient to reduce the spread of infection. If she internalizes this concept as a value, she will always wash her hands after seeing each patient, even when handwashing is inconvenient. However, if she internalizes that handwashing is important only in certain circumstances, such as when her hands are very dirty, she will only wash her hands when she judges that this circumstance exists. Those who value handwashing will wash their hands; those who value handwashing only in certain circumstances will only wash their hands under those circumstances. Those who value handwashing all the time will most likely perceive those who wash their hands under certain circumstances as "sloppy." Those who value handwashing in certain circumstances will most likely perceive those who wash their hands all the time as "fastidious."

KEY IDEA: Values are learned through observations and actions[5]

One person may consider death to be the worst that can happen to an individual, whereas another person involved in the same situation may feel that living with a severe handicap is a worse alternative when there is a choice to be made.

Learning values through observations

Through observing situations and the responses they elicit, the ICP will develop values based on situations (what she observes) and response (what happened). This process develops in infancy and continues throughout life. Learning begins in the family setting and is extended through the educational setting, religious affiliations, social encounters, and work settings. An example of this type of learning follows:

Situation: The ICP observes departments quoting the Joint Commission on the Accreditation of Hospitals (JCAH) as a reason for making a proposed change.
Response I: Departments using JCAH as a reason for their request get positive response to their request, whereas those who do not use JCAH do not get their request approved.

The ICP is likely to value JCAH requirements and use them whenever possible to ensure that her request is granted.

Response II: Departments that use JCAH do not get listened to any more than departments that do not use JCAH requirements.

If this is the response the ICP sees repeatedly, she will be likely to ignore JCAH as a justification to support her request.

Learning values through actions

The ICP also learns values through experience. An example of this type of learning follows:

Situation: The ICP confronts the chief of surgery about the increased wound infection rate.

Response I: The chief of surgery reminds the ICP that she is "just" a nurse; she cannot identify an infection because that is a diagnosis, and she cannot diagnose because she is "just" a nurse. He then threatens to report the ICP to the hospital adminstrator for her insubordination.

If this is the ICP's experience over a period of time with physicians at various levels, she may choose not to value discussions with physicians and will avoid such opportunities.

Response II: The chief of surgery reviews the increased wound infection rate with the ICP and works with her in developing a plan of action for correction.

If this is the ICP's experience over a period of time with physicians at various levels, she may choose to value decision making with physicians.

The ICP's learned value system is complex, beginning with values learned from her parents and expanded through her association with friends, teachers, and family.

The ICP's philosophy of professional practice is influenced by her personal value system, the values she learned in nursing training, and by her professional experience. The ICP's philosophy of practice for nursing has been continually refined, extended, and adjusted to the present time and will continue to be dynamic throughout her professional life. These professional values form standards for direction and purpose in her work performance and are the foundation for decisions she makes throughout her work experience.

Because the ICP may not always be aware of her values, there is a method, *values clarification*,[7] that can be used to help her determine the content and power of her own set of values. This method is not concerned with what the specific values are; rather it is a process to help the ICP become aware of what her values are.

Confusion about personal values is reflected by a confused relationship with self and society and is reflected in behavior. Being a victim,[2] being angry,[4] and being disinterested may all indicate unclear values. There are many techniques to help clarify values. One of the most popular is based on the work of Raths,[9] who has identified three criteria that can be used to identify a value:

1. *Choosing*—Freely choosing with full knowledge of the consequences
2. *Prizing*—Being satisfied with the choice and personally and publicly sharing the satisfaction
3. *Acting*—Incorporating the choice into consistent behaviors

Anything that does not meet all three criteria is a *value indicator*. A value indicator indicates that a value is in the process of "becoming." Value indicators include goals or purposes: aspirations and attitudes; and interests, feelings, beliefs, worries, problems, and obstacles.

To clarify values requires that the ICP identify all the beliefs, purposes, goals, objectives, worries, aspirations, and standards that she believes. Once these have been written down, they should be reviewed against the three criteria of a value: choosing, prizing, acting. The ICP should ask herself if she has chosen each one freely, if she personally and publicly shares satisfaction with the concept, and if she incorporates it into her behaviors consistently.

The less people understand about their values, the more confused their lives are. In discussions with many ICPs, I have seen the frustrations with their roles emerge. It was interesting to learn from a significant number that there was a common conflict: they did not value the same behaviors in the role as their employers did. ICPs wanted to have a totally integrated program within the hospital; employers wanted to get by JCAH. It is even more interesting that ICPs had an understanding that the value difference existed but believed that through their performance (doing a great job) they could convince their employers to change value and role expectations to match those of the ICPs. None of the ICPs had a formal plan for changing this value difference either through observation or performance. They just "knew" that if they did a good job, someone would notice, and the change would somehow come about.

People who have clarified their values will perform zestful, independent, consistent, and decisive acts, with courage to say what has to be said and do what needs to be done. Values provide meaning and practical guidance. As ICPs become more aware of their values through value clarification, they will gain the ability to be more consistent and to exhibit more personal control. They will be aware that their value systems are dynamic and can change based on their observations and experience. ICPs will also be aware that others' values are also dynamic and can change based on their observations and experience. This knowledge will be very useful in planning change strategies that may involve value conflict and will give direction for and insight into useful ways to resolve such conflicts.

An example of the valuing process is freely choosing to be an ICP. The choice is made after other career alternatives have been considered, with no pressure from external sources. The ICP publicly discusses her choice and prizes it both personally (feeling good about the job) and publicly. In addition, the ICP demonstrates consistent behaviors within the role (not moving in and out of roles).

An example of a philosophy of practice statement based on clarified values might be, "I believe the ICP has unique skills and knowledge that support independent decision making." In this example it is obvious that a nurse with such a basic philosophy would undoubtedly have trouble if she accepted a role that allowed no independent decision making.

Phase I of the role development model requires that these types of value conflicts be identified, discussed, and resolved, not ignored or handled in isolation. The ICP should be able to negotiate a resolution to these conflicts without violating any critical areas of her philosophy of practice. Because negotiation is a critical skill for initial entree sessions and for continuing entree, it is worth discussing in detail.

NEGOTIATIONS

"Negotiation is a field of knowledge and endeavor that focuses on gaining the favor of people from whom we want things. It is the use of information, time, and power to affect behavior within a 'web of tension.' "[3] Cohen also states that the effective type of negotiation requires a person to find out what the other side really wants and show them a way to get it, at the same time getting what the individual wants. To accomplish this a working knowledge of the three primary elements in negotiation is needed:

- Information
- Power
- Time

Information

The typical perception the ICP has as she thinks of herself in a negotiation process is that "they" have more information than she does. The term "they" refers to whatever group is perceived as having the ability to block or interfere with an individual's goals. The reality is that many times the area the ICP is concerned with (a high priority to her) is not a high priority to the other party. If the ICP gathers all the facts surrounding the situation, she may be in an advantageous position. In gathering information the ICP will be shaping attitudes, establishing relationships, and developing expectations. Good listening skills are critical in understanding what is being said and what is being omitted.

For example, the ICP may want to negotiate a change in her position in the organization structure from reporting to the director of nursing to reporting to the hospital administrator. To discuss this issue the ICP would collect information about what the philosophy of the organizational structure within the hospital is, how other hospitals place the ICP within their organization, and why they have done so. She might gather information about how those she works with directly would be influenced by such a change and what the overall ramifications of this move would mean to the infection control program and to her personally. By asking these types of questions, the ICP gets others to begin thinking about what she is thinking about. This approach can be nonthreatening, because the ICP is just asking, not acting. If the ICP prepares in this way, it is unlikely that "they" will have more information than she does.

Power

The second assumption the ICP might have is that "they" have more power and authority than she does. However, she needs to realize that she has plenty of power, based on the definition that power is the capacity to get things done. This power is demonstrated in the ICP's ability to do the following:
- Plan options
- Not be intimidated
- Mix courage with common sense and take risks
- Get others committed (people support what they help to create)
- Learn to share the risk with others
- Have an expert knowledge base
- Demonstrate energy and willingness to accomplish purpose (people have the energy and time to do the things they want to do)
- See the situation objectively

Power is in the eye of the beholder, and as the ICP demonstrates the behaviors outlined previously, she will be perceived by others as being powerful. To follow the example of changing the organizational position of the ICP, there are many ways that the ICP can be perceived as powerful:

1. *Planning options.* The ICP can develop several options for reporting to the hospital administrator.
2. *Choosing not to be intimidated.* It is important to remember that "no" is a reaction, not a position. The ICP should not become personally involved. She is in a role, and she is proposing a change that will improve her ability to function.
3. *Taking risks.* The ICP is already taking a risk by raising the request, but she can support the proposal with facts.
4. *Getting others committed.* One of the side benefits of gathering information is that the ICP has started people thinking about her proposal. As she gets more information she can keep everyone informed of the findings.
5. *Sharing the risks with others.* In the quest for information the ICP may discover others interested in revising the organizational structure. The ICP should encourage them to raise their questions at the same time she is.
6. *Acquiring an expert knowledge base.* Here the ICP is unique because she may be the only ICP, or one of a very few in her organization. She alone can speak to the advantage this change will give her.
7. *Demonstrating energy.* The ICP should be diligent. She should keep gathering information and presenting it in different ways.

8. *Seeing the situation objectively.* The ICP is in a role, and this change is proposed to make the role more productive. She cares about the proposed change, but she *should not care too much.* It is not a personal issue. Her attitude will conserve her energy to accomplish her goal.

Time

The third assumption an ICP might have is that "they" do not have the same time constraints and restriction deadlines as she does. Patience is a key quality in negotiation. When the ICP does not know what to do, it is best to do nothing. Circumstances change over time, and change needs time to be accepted. The ICP should not push because she might solidify an opposing position unnecessarily. She has all the time there is and should use time to influence, gather more information, and examine her position. She should not use time to belittle others. It is not a good tactic for the ICP to make herself look "good" by denigrating others.

KEY IDEA: A win-win outcome of negotiations is accomplished by shifting the focus of negotiations from defeating each other to defeating the problem through a mutually beneficial outcome. The most desirable outcome of negotiations is a win-win situation. The primary focus for both parties is to both win.

Win-win. In a win-win negotiation outcome both parties feel that the decision is beneficial to them. The issues are specifically identified, and both parties are clear about what they want. Energy is focused on problem solving instead of personalizing the issues through blaming and fault finding.

Other types of negotiation outcomes will be described only because the ICP may be involved in these types of situations and will need to be able to recognize them. Once these are recognized, the ICP should make every effort to turn them into a win-win resolution.

Win-lose. Winning at all cost is called the win-lose situation. The ramification is often long term, because the loser(s) does not forget. The victory may haunt the ICP in future negotiations. It is the "win the battle, lose the war" technique.

Lose-lose. Neither side gets what they want in a lose-lose situation. It is extremely destructive and has no beneficial outcomes. It is the "well if I can't get what I want, neither will you" technique.

Specific items that need to be negotiated during the identification phase are salary, job expectations, orientation (both initial and during the first 6 months while the ICP adjusts to the role), organizational placement, resources available (e.g., money, equipment, office space, secretarial help), and educational benefits.

The ICP's first step in negotiation is to have her information as complete as possible for each one of the items she is concerned about. She wants to find out what the other party (employer or prospective employer) wants *without giving away what she wants*. She does this by questioning, suggesting options, and listening to both verbal and nonverbal replies.

The ICP must use her power by being nondefensive, proposing options, getting commitments to the more obvious issues, being diligent, and by not being judgmental. When options are discussed that the ICP is willing to settle with, then she should confirm that portion of the negotiation and move on to other issues.

Patience. The ICP should use her time to achieve the things she really wants. It is better for her to leave a meeting and reschedule another than to settle for a decision that she is not comfortable with. Once she has left the meeting she will have time to gather more information, develop new strategies, and be prepared to negotiate further. The ICP is worth every minute she spends on herself, so she should be patient. I would suggest that the ICP settle salary last. Once she has resolved all the other issues, she has established a rapport with the employer. Because the employer has now invested time in the ICP, it will be difficult not to settle the issue of salary. Once a service has been rendered, it is never as valuable as it was before being rendered. Once the ICP has accepted the position, she will lose a great deal of negotiating power. The ICP should spend the time up front to get the things she really wants before accepting the position.

During this negotiation phase it is important to listen and understand how the employer views the role and the requests. The ICP should ask the employer to review the job description with her and explain how the required skills outlined are interpreted. The employer should be asked to list the three major accomplishments desired from the role. The organizational placement of the role and the reasons for the placement should be outlined.

The ICP should verify that she understands the following:
1. What is to be accomplished.
2. The resources available.
3. Time frame for accomplishing the tasks outlined (is the ICP to have the hospital ready for JCAH, and is JCAH coming next week?).
4. Parameters on what services are appropriate for the infection control program; what services are possible, acceptable, or required?
5. Has the ICP negotiated a reasonable orientation period, both initial and long term? During orientation the ICP will need a reliable, extensive and intensive overview of the hospital. She will need time to become familiar with the social, professional, and psychological personality of the hospital environment. She will want to meet the people and become familiar with their positions and their impact on the operation of the hospital. The ICP will need to learn the ebb and flow of people, goods, services,

and communication. She will need to identify both the formal and informal systems for knowing what is going on.

   a. Has the ICP negotiated a formal introduction to each of the departments by the employer to ensure that each department recognizes the power and authority of her role?

   b. If the ICP or employer feels that she needs to gain additional competencies to perform within the role, has she outlined a plan and commitment to obtain these?

   c. Has the ICP negotiated specific job description changes and/or organizational changes with a time frame for implementation?

   d. Has the ICP established a time frame for written goals and objectives to be written for both her role and for the infection control program?

SUMMARY

The identification phase of role development focuses on establishing mutual consensus between an employee and employer regarding role expectations and limitations. Because there may be a negotiation process to arrive at the consensus, the ICP needs to have a clear understanding of her own expectations, philosophy of professional practice, and values. Agreement on mutual expectations diminishes ambiguity about the role function of the ICP for both parties and provides a consistent direction for the ICP. By clarifying each of these issues during the identification phase, the ICP will minimize the chances of getting herself in a position of being all things to all people and will have a defined role that is within the boundaries of her practice.

REFERENCES

1. Bolles, R.N.: The three boxes of life, Berkeley, Calif., 1978, Ten Speed Press.
2. Bunning, R.L.: Victims, persecutors and reservers, Superv. Nurse **10:**13-17, Nov. 1979.
3. Cohen, H.: You can negotiate anything, Secaucus, N.J., 1980, Lyle Stuart, Inc.
4. Duldt, B.W.: Anger: an alienating communication hazard for nurses, Nurs. Outlook **29:**640-644, 1981.
5. Ford, J.A.G., Trygstad-Durland, L.N., and Nelms, B.C.: Applied decision making for nurses, St. Louis, 1979, The C.V. Mosby Co.
6. Gabarro, J., and Kotter, J.P.: Managing your boss, Harvard Bus. Rev. pp. 92-100, Jan.-Feb. 1979.
7. Kirschenbaum, H.: Clarifying values clarification: some theoretical issues and review research, Group Organizational Stud. **1:**99-114, 1976.
8. McNally, J.M.: Values: part I, Superv. Nurse **11:**27-30, May 1980.
9. Raths, L.E., Harmin, M., and Simon, S.B.: Values and teaching, Columbus, Ohio, 1966, Charles E. Merrill Publishing Co.
10. Schatzman, L., and Strauss, A.L.: Field research, Methods of Social Science Series, Englewood Cliffs, N.J., 1973, Prentice-Hall, Inc.

Role development: phase 2

The Role Developer must take the initiative in exchanging information in various ways, keep the process active, and monitor the direction and level of progress. Success in a new role is not merely a matter of expertise; it calls for the nurse to articulate her role and secure the collaboration of her co-workers in implementing it.

Dorothy Oda*

---

basic communication pattern The basic pattern of communication consists of a sender, a message, and a receiver.
communication The process of sharing information whereby one person sends a message to another with the conscious intent of receiving a response.
listening An active skill requiring attention to what is being said and what is not being said, while matching the nonverbal messages and understanding the total message.
role transition The phase of actually performing the role.

ROLE TRANSITION

Once the infection control practitioner (ICP) has decided that she wants to perform the activities necessary to accomplish the mutually agreed role functions in phase 1 of role development and has accepted the position, she moves into phase 2, role transition. This is the phase most people begin in, that is, the phase of actually enacting the role. The goal in this phase is to develop the role to fit within specific staff and institutional needs.[7]

The primary foundation necessary in this phase is the ability to communicate, both sending and receiving messages. The ICP needs to gather information about her role performance, develop the ability to validate data collected, and modify her approach based on this information.

> KEY IDEA: Communication and listening skills are the foundation for enacting the ICP role

COMMUNICATION

Communication is the process of sharing information whereby one person sends a message to another with the conscious intent of evoking a response.

*Reprinted from Nurs. Outlook **25**:375, 1977. Copyrighted by the American Journal of Nursing Company.

Although communication skills are discussed at length in Chapter 9, some basic concepts important for communication will be reviewed in this chapter:
- Observation of and listening to others
- Sending clear messages
- Willingness to consider ideas that may alter previous beliefs

Basic communication pattern

The basic pattern of communication consists of a sender, a message, and a receiver (Fig. 4-1).

The sender sends a message that has credibility and is understandable, and the receiver, through feedback, verifies that the same message the sender intended was heard. Chartier[2] points out "two faulty assumptions (in communication) are 'you' always know what 'I' mean, and 'I' should always know what 'you' mean." It is only through clear message content and constant feedback to confirm that the message was received as sent that clear communication has occurred.

The message the sender gives has several components:
- The intention of the message
- The idea
- The feelings of the sender

The receiver also has the same components to contend with in receiving the message. These components make the matter of communicating very complex. Words are used as symbols to send a message. They are neutral and only take on meaning through the perceptions and experience people attach to them. They comprise one component of the total communication process. The larger component consists of the feelings and body language expressed with the words. In many instances the nonverbal aspects of communication communicate more than the words themselves. It is not that words are unimportant but that they are only a portion of the messages sent and received. Nonverbal messages account for approximately two thirds of communication. Albertie[1] describes some basic body language techniques used in daily communication. As these are reviewed, physical presentation methods should also be considered, with close attention paid to nonverbal cues that may act as a barrier to clear interpretation.

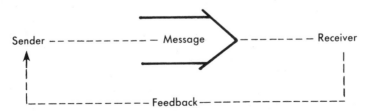

FIG. 4-1. The basic pattern of communication requires a sender, message, and receiver.

Eye contact. By looking directly at the person she is speaking with, the ICP demonstrates interest and sincerity. The look indicates that she is directing her remarks to that person. An aggressive stare can be perceived as an overpowering gesture, whereas looking away or down indicates a lack of self-confidence or disinterest.

Body posture. The ICP increases the impact of her message by facing a person or leaning toward a person instead of away. Moving her body forward demonstrates interest. A straight, erect posture demonstrates confidence in the message, whereas a slumped posture indicates a passive attitude. A stance with the arms held open indicates honesty and invites trust, but a stance with closed arms and tightly clenched hands indicates a closed, noncommunicative attitude.

Gestures. Gestures, to a point, give added interest and emphasis to a message. Overly enthusiastic gestures, however, can be distracting. Most important, gestures should be congruous with the message intended.

Facial expressions. The effective use of facial expressions requires that the expression match the message. Expressing anger while smiling will not give a clear message to the receiver.

Voice tone, inflection, and volume. A level, well-modulated conversational statement is convincing, interesting, and generally attention getting. The ICP needs to review how these nonverbal methods of communication are used. She should watch herself in the mirror and examine the messages she sends with her posture, facial gestures, and other expressions. If she identifies any traits she feels could be improved on to more effectively communicate the message, she has taken the first step in improving communication skills. The ICP should practice the behaviors she would like to change in front of a mirror, especially practicing matching body language with the message she wants to send.

Listening skills

Listening is an active skill, requiring attention to what is being said and what is not being said, while matching the nonverbal messages and filtering out personal assumptions and biases to end up with the "total" message. Darling[4] developed a model that represents the "active listening" process (Fig. 4-2).

The major barrier to mutual interpersonal communication is the natural tendency to judge, evaluate, or approve or disapprove of the statement of the other person. A person either judges by thinking "for" the other person, explaining what that individual "ought" or "should" do, or may judge by guessing why the other person is doing certain things. Rogers[8] explains that when the listener concentrates on the situation, the tendency is to think "for" the sender. When the listener concentrates on the sender, the tendency is to think "about" the sender and guess "why" that person is responding to the situation in certain ways. Only by concentrating on the feelings expressed, both verbally

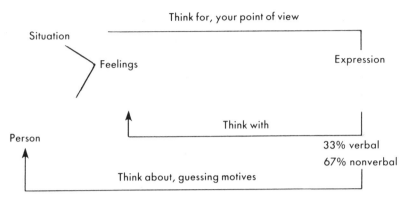

FIG. 4-2. Active listening model.

and nonverbally, and the situation can the listener think "with" the sender and the total message of the sender be understood. Chartier[2] states that the receiver's psychological frame of reference must be understood. The psychological framework refers to the individual's values, attitudes, perceptions, and assumptions—all the details that make the individual unique. By knowing how the sender perceives the message, the listener can employ the appropriate interpersonal skills to keep communications open.

KEY IDEA: The only person the ICP can control is herself

The ICP achieves her role by working through and with other people. The ICP's role is typically a staff position within the organizational structure; that is, the authority delegated to this specialized position has no direct line supervision or control over health care personnel (no "hire or fire" authority). The line of power is achieved by *influencing* the staff through written policies or procedures, in-service education, and consultation. To accomplish this the ICP needs to have an understanding of self-control, the ability to influence others, and a mechanism to evaluate performance on an ongoing basis.

Self-control. Claus and Bailey[3] describe three components necessary for self-control and explain the way they influence a person's ability to function in a role, such as the ICP role:
- Strength (the things that can be done)
- Energy (the willingness to do)
- Action (doing)

Strength is based on a strong self-concept within the reality of a person's abilities. The ICP does not make the difference; she *is* the difference. For the ICP to be aware of her abilities, she needs to identify both her strengths and weaknesses. A detailed method for this will be outlined later in this chapter under "Field Notes."

Energy is dynamic and is observed by others through what the ICP does. Her enthusiasm and drive not only direct her own activities but also can influence the activities of others. A positive attitude is the result of the ICP having clear values and being well prepared, with the confidence that she has the skills to adapt her behavior to handle the situation. Through energy the ICP is able to get others excited about her ideas, beliefs, and professional concerns.

With strength and energy, the next step is to *act*. There is an old saying that states, "What you *do* speaks so loudly, I cannot hear what you say." As I pointed out in phase I, one of the ways to be a powerful person is to be willing to act.

KEY IDEA: Power is defined as the ability to get things done

The following situation will illustrate how the ICP's action can influence the actions of others:

> *Situation:* Dr. Jones has refused to place a baby with possible meningitis (etiology unknown) in isolation. Hospital policy states that these types of babies must be placed in isolation until the disease has been properly identified and treated.

The obvious solution is for Dr. Jones to change his mind and isolate the baby. However, the ICP's problem is that she does not control Dr. Jones. She only controls herself. It will do no good for her to focus her strength, energy, and action on blaming Dr. Jones for not complying with the policy. Instead, the ICP should look at *herself* and concentrate on how *she* can change *her* approach, information, and or communication to *influence* Dr. Jones.

Through the communication process responses are elicited. To discover why Dr. Jones is acting the way he is, the ICP should ask herself, "Is there something about the way I communicate information that may be causing his response?" If so, she can now change the way her information is sent, and this change will automatically influence Dr. Jones to respond differently. For example, the ICP may be approaching Dr. Jones this way:

> *Verbal message:* Dr. Jones, the infection control committee has established a policy that requires babies with this disease to be isolated.
> *Nonverbal message:* The expressions the ICP uses include eyes narrowed and glaring and hands clenched or finger pointing. Her mouth is drawn tightly, and she is speaking with a strained deliberate voice. Dr. Jones may be hearing, "I am ordering you to isolate."

By changing the approach, the ICP can influence Dr. Jones. What might happen if the message was changed in the following way?

> *Verbal message:* Can you give me more information about your patient? I would like to understand your thinking about the problem of isolating this baby.
>
> *Nonverbal message:* The ICP has a puzzled tone of voice and has a concerned, open, accepting expression on her face. The ICP might also choose a time away from the immediate situation to discuss this with Dr. Jones.

Most important, the ICP must be willing to *listen* to Dr. Jones, hearing both his verbal and nonverbal message. She must view herself as the party to change and not give that responsibility away to another. As she changes, others will change in response. If the ICP waits for others to change, she has lost control in the situation.

Influencing others. In addition to the three components of personal control, Claus and Bailey[3] describe three power bases that provide the ICP with power:

> *Personal power base:* This emphasizes a strong self-concept that enables the ICP to accept the responsibility for her own personal and professional growth.
>
> *Social power base:* This entails allowing others to participate in making decisions through cooperation and interaction, and it promotes the attitude of "you and me" instead of "you versus me."
>
> *Organization power base:* The ICP's position within the organization is as a staff member. As she develops her role, she needs to develop programs that are not dependent on her presence or constant participation for implementation; rather, she should maximize the participation of others. By using situations to teach skills or enable others to discover their ability to solve the situation for themselves, she is empowering them with skills that will work for them throughout their lives.

Willingness to change a viewpoint. When conflicts exist within an organization, there is a definite negative impact. Communication decreases, decisions tend to be made on the basis of emotions and not facts, boundaries become rigid, and in general there is a decrease in trust. When the ICP experiences differences in viewpoints with others, resolution is facilitated through an objective review of the situation. The more removed from the basis of the conflict, the easier it is to be objective. However, it is important that the ICP resolve conflicts that involve her. A technique to gain an objective perspective for conflict resolution involves identifying the cause of the conflict, identifying areas of agreement, developing a plan of action, implementing the plan, and evaluating.[5,6]

Identifying causes of conflict. Conflict can originate over differences in values, facts, stated goals and objectives, or methods of operations. The ways of identifying conflict may include testing for perceptions, asking for clarification, determining what assumptions are being made about conflict, and deciding which are valid or invalid. To identify areas of conflict, the ICP should use active listening skills to check for understanding of the conflict as others perceive it. It may even be helpful for the ICP to list the information and validate her information through feedback. She wants to confirm that she has accurately heard the other party's viewpoint.

Identifying areas of agreement. The ICP should examine the information she has collected and search for areas that are compatible with her view. By beginning with areas of agreement, the ICP can establish a solid base for resolving areas of disagreement. This technique gets the other person involved, and, as discussed previously, that person's active involvement increases the commitment to making the outcome successful.

Developing a plan of action. The skills needed to develop a plan of action are the same as those involved in the negotiation process. Alternatives that give both parties what they want should be developed.

Implementing and evaluating. The agreed resolution should be put into action. By keeping communication open, that is, remaining nonjudgmental and open, the ICP will have a strong influence on resolving the conflict.

Evaluation

Schatzman and Strauss[9] have developed a technique for helping ICPs examine their own behavior, allowing them to analyze themselves and identify areas they may wish to change. The technique is termed *field notes* and uses a process of discovering personal skills, strengths, and weaknesses through a systematic self-examination. It consists of keeping detailed notes on each significant interaction that occurs during the performance of a role.

KEY IDEA: Field notes provide a systematic self-examination of personal behavior

---

Keeping field notes is one of those activities similar to learning to drive a car; it is jerky, cumbersome, and time consuming at first, but with practice, it becomes a smooth, automatic activity. Field notes are used to make discoveries through self-examination of situations that occur within the reality and context of the work environment, that is, observing events in their natural situation.

There are three types of information the ICP needs to record in field notes. First, an accurate account of the event should be placed in the first column, labeled "Event." The recorded information should contain what happened, who was involved, what everyone said, where they said it, why they said it, and any other facts that exist about the situation as the ICP perceives it. Because of the detailed nature of this recording, it is necessary to record the facts as close to the time of the event as possible.

Second, the ICP needs to record her feelings about the event in the second column, labeled "Feelings." This too needs to be as specific as possible. The ICP may have many different levels of feelings through the interaction and should try to capture each and record it, correlating the feelings with what was actually happening. This is directed at separating the factual event—reality—from the ICP's perceptions and feelings about the event—her reality. Because accuracy is critical, these recordings should also be made as close to the time of the event as possible.

The third column, "Theoretical Application," is used to record the ICP's analysis of the situation. This column will help the ICP identify and record trends or patterns in the way she handle's herself and reacts in different situations. The usefulness of this column will depend directly on the ICP's ability to write productive notes about her experience and make these types of deductions.

In the example of Dr. Jones, the following field note might be generated:

Event	Feelings	Theoretical application
8:00 AM, 8/1 Dr. Jones admitted a 3-week-old baby with R/O meningitis, etiology unknown. The nurse called me and said Dr. Jones did not want to isolate the baby because he thought the infection was of viral etiology. I went to the unit and talked with Dr. Jones immediately and told him the ICC said all babies with meningitis of unknown etiology *must* be isolated at least 24 hours.	I can't believe that people are so slack! Why can't the head nurse handle this problem? I'm feeling really used by everyone. I'm so angry with this physician. He always does this. He doesn't care about any patient but his own. He has no respect for rules and regulations. I hate working with him. His patients never do well anyway. I'm just going to tell him the rules.	

This example can be expanded to include another incident that occurs on the same day. A head nurse reports to the ICP that a staff nurse is refusing to follow isolation procedures. The ICP discusses the incident with the staff nurse, who confirms that it is true. She states that she does not believe isolation

is really that necessary because none of the physicians are observing the precautions. The ICP's field note for this incident might read as follows:

Event	Feelings	Theoretical application
Nurse Brown was seen not observing isolation and was reported to me by her head nurse. I went to the unit and talked with her, explaining it was her responsibility to observe the hospital policy of isolation, regardless of what others are doing. She stated that it was obviously not necessary, since the physician was not doing it, and he knows more about isolation than I do. I told her that she must follow through with isolation or we would be personally liable if any patient got infected from this patient. She stated she did not have time to do unnecessary things and would do what she could.	I can't believe that people are so slack. Why can't the head nurse handle this problem? I'm feeling really used by everyone. These people are professionals, so why should I have to tell them what to do? I have better things to do with my time. I get so discouraged. I tell people what to do and share current information, but they just do what they want.	

Now that these incidents are recorded, the ICP has captured the situation,
her feelings, and her impressions for future examination. It is not necessary to
analyze the notes immediately. It may, in fact, be more beneficial to put them
away for a few days. When the ICP does finally take time to review them, she
will be examining them almost as a third party would. She is removed from the
situation because she has allowed time to pass. The ICP becomes a critical
reviewer of her own actions.

The expected outcome from analyzing field notes is to identify trends or
patterns of behavior that are not necessarily apparent.

The third column might read as follows:

Event	Feelings	Theoretical application
Nurse Brown was seen not observing isolation and was reported to me by her head nurse. I went to the unit and talked with her, explaining it was her responsibility to observe the hospital policy of isolation, regardless of what others are doing. She stated that it was obviously not necessary, since the physician was not doing it, and he knows more about isolation than I do. I told her that she must follow through with isolation or we would be personally liable if any patient got infected from this patient. She stated she did not have time to do unnecessary things and would do what she could.	I can't believe that people are so slack. Why can't the head nurse handle this problem? I'm feeling really used by everyone. These people are professionals, so why should I have to tell them what to do? I have better things to do with my time. I get so discouraged. I tell people what to do and share current information, but they just do what they want.	When I'm angry I respond by telling nurses to give me the problem, and I take it. Why am I angry? The head nurse gives me the problem, and I take it. I own the IC program; others are not responsible. I am discouraged. I might want to get help in developing responsibilities and clear communication.

Should future notes also demonstrate these same types of behaviors, the ICP has established a trend. If this trend is one she feels is useful, the field notes have helped her identify that she has it, and therefore she can use it more consciously in the future. If the field notes reveal a trend that the ICP does not feel is useful, she can set about developing different behaviors to expand her options available for choosing behaviors in the future. The trend itself is not the ultimate focus of analysis. The ultimate benefit is knowledge that the trend exists. Once the ICP has knowledge of its existence, she then has the ability to use it, not use it, and/or develop options around trend behaviors. The ICP can use it instead of allowing it to use her.

In this example, the ICP might want to develop additional skills of confrontation, clear communication, and not accepting responsibility for the actions of others. Through identifying her own needs through field notes, she can now be self-directive in seeking opportunities for developing new behaviors to manage these types of problems.

Field notes give insight about the ICP and enable her to see herself "up close and personal." Seeing the event in writing is different from thinking about it. Once the ICP has identified areas she wishes to change or expand, she will be self-directed in seeking help.

Field notes are also an evaluation tool to provide feedback to the ICP when she experiments with new behaviors. As the ICP records events in which she has exhibited new skills, she will have direct feedback about what did and did not work and can use this information to base choices on for future directions of growth.

Field notes help the ICP to practice gathering information and to develop the ability to use valid data to modify her approach. The record is private and can contain all information she wishes to examine. Writing down the experience also releases some of the frustration caused by the experience.

> **KEY IDEA: The ICP's priorities may be different from those of other health care workers**

ICPs many times feel that situations are urgent or important and are discouraged when others on the health team do not act with mutual urgency. This may be a problem of priorities. If the ICP could hear from others about the tasks and activities that are filling their day, she might even agree that her priorities would not necessarily be their priorities.

For example, the ICP has found a resistant *Serratia* organism growing in the urine of a patient in the intensive care unit. She wants this patient isolated to prevent the spread of this organism. The ICP speaks to the head nurse of the intensive care unit, but she seems unconcerned. However, when the ICP learns that two patients who have undergone recent heart surgery are both bleeding and must be returned to the operating room, and a patient is coming into the unit who needs an external pacemaker immediately, it becomes easier to understand the head nurse's "unconcern."

I believe that one of the primary responsibilities of the ICP is to help, as much as possible, other health professionals fit her expectations into their priorities of daily activities. In the previous example, the ICP might choose to explain that her concern is even more critical because of the type of patient in the unit. To demonstrate her level of concern, the ICP may choose to stay and help get the situation resolved. The ICP should offer to coordinate the move of the patient with the *Serratia* infection. The ICP can involve the housekeeping staff members in this phase and ask for their help in pushing the bed. Her message is, "I understand your priorities. Mine is also critical. Let's work together to get this resolved." This type of commitment, concern, and demon-strated belief in what she is doing gives a strong message that she values what she is saying. By focusing on the situation and not on the people, the ICP uses her strength, energy, and ability in successfully managing the situation. The other staff involved in this type of situation will also see the ICP as having true concern for patient safety.

SUMMARY

Phase 2 of role development involves the process of enacting the role to fit within the specific staff and institutional needs. Because the process is inter-active, effective communication skills are essential for the ICP to be successful. Communication skills are used to influence the behavior of others to move toward the expected level of performance needed for an effective infection control program.

A useful method for the ICP to record and analyze the effectiveness of her communication skills in influencing others is through field notes. As the ICP reviews and interprets the information in field notes, she will have information that can suggest ways to improve her effectiveness in her role.

REFERENCES

1. Albertie, R.E., and Emmons, M.L.: Stand up, speak out, talk back: the key to self-assertive behavior, New York, 1975, Pocket Books.
2. Chartier, M..: Clarity of expression in interpersonal communication, J. Nurs. Adm. 11:42-46, July 1981.
3. Claus, K.E., and Bailey, J.T.: Power and influence in health care, St. Louis, 1977, The C.V. Mosby Co.
4. Darling, L.A.: Unpublished material.
5. Marriner, A.: Conflict theory, Superv. Nurse 10:12-16, April 1979.
6. Marriner, A.: Conflict resolution, Superv. Nurse 10:46-54, May 1979.
7. Oda, D.S.: Specialized role development: a three-phase process, Nurs. Outlook 25:374-377, 1977.
8. Rogers, C.: Dealing with psychological tensions, J. Appl. Behav. Sci. 1(1):6-25, 1965.
9. Schatzman, L., and Strauss, A.L.: Field research, Prentice-Hall Methods of Social Science Series, Englewood Cliffs, N.J., 1973, Prentice-Hall Inc.

5 KAREN J. AXNICK

Role development: phase 3

Success is the promise that is never kept.
Satisfaction happens only in the present. Now.

*Tom Jackson**

---

as if psychology People's mythical or fairy tale orientation to their world.
feedback system An essential process in the evaluation of the degree of congruence
  between the hospital and the infection control practitioner's expectations as defined
  in phase 1 and in the implementation of the program activities in phase 2.
networking A process that links individual members in an expanding communication
  system for the giving and receiving of information.

The third phase of the developmental model is role confirmation.[7] The practitioner has realized this objective when the hospital staff recognizes her as the
infection control practitioner (ICP) and provides feedback that her services are
valued and appropriately used. It is important for the ICP to distinguish between feedback that validates her in a personal sense (i.e., approval of her
personality) and feedback that validates her behavior in fulfilling the ICP role.
Although personal confirmation is an integral part of role success, it is of
limited value in the assessment of the ICP's performance. It is possible to be
well liked and still fail at developing and implementing an infection control
program that meets patient and staff needs. Conversely, there will be situations
in which the ICP will be required to take a firm, yet unpopular, stand in her role
to ensure standards of excellence in services and practice. Therefore, to the
extent that she is able to maintain a clear, objective, and distinct view of her
self-worth and the role, she will be able to function optimally for both personal
satisfaction and fulfillment of institutional expectations.

> **KEY IDEA: Assessing confirmation is an ICP responsibility**

PSYCHOLOGY OF AS IF

Vaihinger,[10] a social psychologist, notes that individuals often build careers
(a succession of roles) on false or unrealistic truisms; he coined the phrase "the

psychology of as if" to denote people's mythical or fairy tale orientation to their world.

To varying degrees, people describe their experiences through a filter of attitudes, beliefs, and values. "Reality" is not an accurate, objective view of people and situations but is more a projection of personal perceptual patterns that exist only in their minds. These perceptual patterns, based on past experiences, are valuable in providing some order and predictability to existence. However, a danger exists when people do not check out these perceptual patterns with others and act "as if" there is agreement between individual world views.

"The psychology of as if" infiltrates role development when an ICP is basing goals and choices on what she thinks *should be* rather than realistically assessing the physical, social, and psychological environment. For example, the infection control committee chairman at the ICP's hospital is board certified in internal medicine but has no background in infectious disease or epidemiology. Operating under the "psychology of as if," the ICP approaches this physician for assistance in problems and questions with the expectation of receiving reliable guidance. When the physician is unable to provide answers and, in fact, expresses discomfort at being expected to fulfill this role, the ICP becomes frustrated at a perceived lack of support and disinterest. What has occurred is that she has effectively created a situation in which she feels dissatisfied and could easily be locked into a viewpoint that limits her options. One alternative approach is for the ICP to view the physician in a collegial role rather than as the authority figure. By jointly identifying role boundaries and responsibilities, the ICP can maximally use the skills and attributes of the physician and learn to make decisions together based on researching the literature, consulting other hospitals, and assessing the specific needs of the institution. If the ICP accepts responsibility for accurately identifying the situation and modifies her behavior accordingly, the outcome has a positive sustaining effect on her role and the program.

FEEDBACK SYSTEMS

The goal of the role development process is for the ICP to create a work environment that supports her personal satisfaction and professional growth through the fulfillment of the institution's expectations and needs. Creating such an environment requires the ICP to assume responsibility for the establishment of feedback systems.

The meaning of the word *responsibility* necessitates further exploration. In American culture responsibility often carries a negative connotation; it is perceived as a burden. In contrast, the two root words, response and ability, convey the capacity to accurately assess a situation or relationship and to behave in a mature, constructive manner. Responsibility bestows the ICP with the power to generate options, determine the scope of her practice, and develop a solid base of support for her role.

In the role confirmation phase the ICP is responsible for seeking feedback from all levels of hospital staff, assessing the validity of the responses, integrating the variety of viewpoints, and using relevant information to guide further role development. Feedback is essential to evaluate the degree of congruence between the hospital and ICP expectations identified in phase 1 and to implement the program activities in phase 2.

The dynamic nature of infection control and health care does not permit a static approach to role development. The ICP role will never be established "once and for all," even when the ICP is satisfied with the feedback. Change is the byword of society. For the hospital, change is reflected in shrinking financial bases, modified regulations and laws, altered patient populations, shifting staff needs, and technological advances. For the ICP, change is manifested by the aforementioned pressures on the hospital, coupled with the natural evolution of increasing personal knowledge and skills.

Change has become the rule rather than the exception in people's lives. In relationship to successful role development, change presents two choices: the ICP can resist it or flow with it. To resist is to relinquish power; the ICP is "at effect" rather than "at cause" of change. Paradoxically, the more control (resistance) she attempts to exercise to maintain the status quo, the more she *loses* control over the change process. By flowing with change and acting in the present, the ICP has the ability to influence the process. This latter approach involves risking the security and comfort of the past for an unknown future outcome.

Role-oriented feedback is critical to participating actively in the present to determine the future direction of the role. Often the ICP will label feedback as critical (negative) or complimentary (positive). These labels obstruct the true value of feedback. All role-oriented feedback is neutral, for it is feedback about how others view the ICP's performance. If she perceives criticism as an attack on her personal identity or value, then she may become mired in self-doubt and choose to become a "victim" of the hospital system. Similarly, the absence of feedback is a sure path to obsolescence, since the ICP role is evolving in a vacuum and prevents her from responding to the changing hospital milieu.

The energy and ability of the ICP to respond to the challenge of fulfilling hospital needs in her role are directly contingent on others' recognition of her contribution (external feedback) and her job satisfaction (internal feedback). Actually, the "myth" that good work is always rewarded is a truth contingent on two factors that influence the ICP's responsibility for role confirmation. First, internal satisfaction, or reward inherent in the process of work is more sustaining for mature adults than external validation through the organizational hierarchy. Second, tangible evidence of the ICP's program and her skills should be created and marketed to foster the evolution of her role and, subsequently, her own growth and development.

KEY IDEA: Role confirmation is process oriented

ATTITUDINAL CHANGES

A variety of methods are available to the ICP to enhance job satisfaction and role confirmation. The first step, however, is an attitudinal change. Role confirmation is *process* rather than *task* oriented. Role development is actually a series of interactions and accomplishments that provide direction and focus to creativity. People are easily coaxed, based on past experience and cultural expectations, into believing that success is equated only with the accomplishment of task-specific goals. In role confirmation the success or failure of individual activities is *not* the central issue. Two questions require affirmative answers from the ICP:

- Am I recognized as the ICP?
- Is my support sought appropriately within the limits of my assigned responsibility?

This aspect of role confirmation is often difficult for the ICP to accept. People are programmed to identify self-worth and satisfaction with the outcome of their efforts. This view ignores the learning value of the process of problem solving and places inordinate emphasis on subjective value judgments (i.e., labeling the outcome "success" or "failure"). In society, satisfaction with work is an emotional state associated with a *mastery* of skills or tasks.[9] A broader definition of work, which includes the concept of role development, is "the skillful organization, manipulation, and control of external and internal environments to achieve a desired goal most efficiently and effectively."[9]

The "internal environment" encompasses the growth and development inherent in each person in an assumed role. Essentially, the ICP's work may be viewed as "a formal opportunity to solve problems" and, in this process, to discover talents and skills that then prepare the ICP for solving larger, more complex problems.[2] Her efforts, in this context of work, are never wasted or viewed as failures. Feedback, in this context of role confirmation, is never superfluous or a personal attack on her worth or integrity. The ICP's efforts and the resultant feedback form a matrix from which she can make choices for future goals and activities.

Accomplishments serve as guideposts in role confirmation. If an infection control program is successful in its achievement of goals (e.g., surveillance, educational, or consultative activities), it provides concrete evidence that the ICP role is recognized and supported by the organization. Evaluation or assessment parameters are important to both role and program confirmation. These parameters are, again, the ICP's responsibility to build into the role confirmation process.

ASSESSMENT PARAMETERS

Assessment parameters for role confirmation can be divided into three broad categories: organizational, social, and personal.

Organizational parameters

Communication is the foundation for developing a strong base of support. Marketing of the ICP role and the program is crucial in a hospital environment where all services and departments are competing for funding in a climate of limited fiscal resources. It is particularly important for the ICP to demonstrate competence and service in her role. Since infection control is primarily a *preventive* service, it is difficult to demonstrate the financial impact of the program. The cost of an epidemic that never occurred because of an ICP's intervention cannot be quantified.

Methods to demonstrate the abilities and the scope of the ICP's services draw on a variety of skills outlined in greater detail in Part Two of this book.

Managerial skills. The ICP's ability to systematically identify, plan, organize, and control resources to accomplish goals and solve problems must be documented. This is no time for the ICP to be shy or display false modesty. An assertive stance is important for role confirmation.

Written reports are a formal means to document accomplishments and enhance credibility and visibility in the role. Individual reports are appropriate for outbreak investigations (e.g., a cluster of staphylococcal infections in the newborn nursery), product evaluation (e.g., investigation and trial of disposable isolation equipment), and special projects (e.g., planning and implementing a rubella screening program for employees). These reports are excellent marketing tools and should include the following:

- A problem statement
- Objectives
- Methodology
- Key people involved
- Outcome or results
- Recommendations

The Joint Commission on Accreditation of Hospitals requires written reports from the infection control committee to the medical board of the hospital.[3] These reports should not only document the committee's activities and recommendations but also should highlight the program's accomplishments.

A program report, prepared at regular intervals and submitted to the administration, is a strong advocacy tool for the ICP role. The format and frequency of these reports may already be determined by the institution. If not, two approaches that have proven helpful to other ICPs follow:

1. Keeping monthly personal reports that are collated quarterly for distribution to the infection control committee chairman and supervisor. (See Fig. 5-1 for a suggested format.) An annual report with assessment of goals and objectives can be culled from these.

2. Using action plans as a formal system of organizing and assessing goals and objectives. In this format (Fig. 5-2) each objective or task is broken down into simpler steps with a time frame assigned to each. This approach, although more time consuming, has three advantages: (a) writing a report (for the individual project or for the annual program evaluation) is simplified, (b) the format documents the planning process and enables the ICP to identify specific tasks or procedures that enhanced or inhibited the project, and (c) the detailed nature of the plan allows the ICP to demonstrate to herself and others progress on tasks that often seem overwhelmingly large in scope or lengthy in nature.

In addition, newsletters are also an excellent means of creating awareness of the ICP role. If the ICP is unable to initiate a separate infection control issue, then she might arrange to "piggyback" on existing publications in the hospital; providing a regular, featured column in the hospital, nursing, and medical staff newsletters is positive involvement in role confirmation.

Oral presentations are also helpful in documenting accomplishments, particularly when these presentations are reflected in minutes of the meetings. For example, if the ICP documented that a modification of IV care by changing administration sets every 48 hours rather than 24 hours has resulted in a large cost savings with no demonstrable increase in infections related to IV use, this information should be presented to the infection control committee, quality assurance committee, and the nursing department.

Educational skills. Educational skills address three levels of activity:

- Developing and maintaining the discipline and means to keep the ICP's knowledge base current
- Sharing knowledge and facilitating communication of "state of the art" information to members of the hospital staff
- Providing and promoting patient and family educational materials and sessions relevant to the program

These steps provide avenues for role confirmation as staff members associate the ICP with expertise in infection control issues.

Epidemiological skills. The ability to conduct a systematic investigation and to resolve a problem offers challenges for the individual's growth and learning and provides a vehicle to enhance role confirmation. The ICP's objec-

MONTHLY REPORT

Surveillance and care review activities:

Educational activities:

Consultative activities:

Unusual events and activities:

Personal growth and development activities:

Assessment of objectives:

Comments:

Name _____

Date _____

FIG. 5-1. Infection control report.

INFECTION CONTROL

Action plan

Problem statement:

Objective	Approval date:	Department/service:
	Start date:	Responsible person for objective:
	Completion date:	Participants:
	Review date:	
Criteria for achievement:	Evaluation methods:	
	Monitoring methods:	

Actions	Resources	Responsibility	Dates		Progress
			Target	Completed	

FIG. 5-2. Action plan.

tivity and creativity, often needed in the heat of an emotionally charged atmosphere, lead others to identify her as a positive resource they can rely on in both crises and normal hospital operations for infection control issues.

In summary, the goal of the organizational component is to market the ICP's role through official channels and to broaden the base of support for her role within the hospital's hierarchy.

Social parameters

Although it is imperative to establish channels within the organizational structure to disseminate information about the ICP role, a complementary and vital link in communication is the creation of a system for feedback to occur. Feedback comes through relationships with people.

The hospital environment is a complex matrix of social relationships, which, in itself, forms a small society complete with implicit and explicit rules of acceptable behaviors. If there is any doubt about the validity of this statement, the ICP should test it in her own environment. As an ICP, what is an "acceptable" approach for a nurse to inform a physician that his patient, who is in a five-bed ward, requires isolation in a single room? At the infection control committee meetings, do members who are not physicians have equal say in patient care issues?

Within this cultural microcosm, it is not necessary for the ICP to act on her observations, to try to modify the system, or to change another person's behavior, but it is important to the success of the role to become a student of the formal and informal sociopolitical system of the institution.

KEY IDEA: Survival in this milieu requires formation of a network of support

---

Networking. Networking, the operative word of the 1980s, is a concept, a technique, and a process.[11] Simply defined, it is a system of interconnected and cooperative individuals. In actual operation, networking is a process that links individual members in an expanding communication system for the giving and receiving of information, advice, and moral support in professional career development.[11]

A support network should not be confused with friendship.[8] Although friends often participate in the same network, or friendships emerge from the supportive structure, the purposes of the two social interactions are different. Friendships address the personal needs of individuals, often providing emotional support in all aspects of a person's life. As Kleinman[5] points out, networks, in the context of role development, are professional relationships that offer a means (1) to facilitate communication, (2) to share support, information, and technical assistance, (3) to use and enhance activities, and (4) to increase visibility.

Networks are particularly important for ICP role confirmation. Because this position is often unique within the organization, there are few mentors or role models readily available to the ICP. This uniqueness of the ICP role poses a paradox: it provides the opportunity for freedom and creativity juxtaposed with a sense of isolation and frustration. Networking can ease the latter feeling by providing support. The resulting sense of mastery reduces the feelings of vulnerability and powerlessness, while enhancing the ability to cope with crisis and initiation of change.[6]

The astute ICP will actively develop networks internal and external to the institution. Internal support systems can be created through contact with other "one-of-a-kind" people or individuals who share similar role responsibilities, such as the clinical specialist. Outside the institution, networks can consist of individuals with similar responsibilities (local and national Association for Practitioners of Infection Control contacts), interweaving professional commitments (nursing administrators, quality assurance coordinators, publishers) and different, but complementary, pursuits (business womens' groups). It is important to remember that these networks should foster professional enhancement; liking or disliking individuals personally is not critical for development of the network. All network resources are positive in role development.

Establishing networks takes time and energy, but the reward is a strong base of support. To participate in a network, open communication is vital. One way of encouraging communication is self-disclosure,[4] the willingness to risk sharing concrete feelings and reactions to the immediate situation. It is based on trust and honesty.

Feedback outside of networks, but within the institution, also requires initiation through self-disclosure and other communication skills. Channels for such communication often travel across traditional hierarchical lines of reporting relationships and are commonly referred to as the "grapevine." As an ICP, the best policy is to listen and use the information after assessing the reliability of the source of the information to others and never add gossip to the system. Accessibility to this often valuable resource, like networking, is dependent on personal integrity.

Power base. Power is another social aspect of role confirmation. Is the ICP viewed by others as a powerful person in her role? Claus and Bailey[1] describe power as flowing from personal, social, and organizational bases. However, power arising from all three bases manifests itself in social interactions in role development. The ICP's strength in her role arises from the ability to empower others. Simply, this means that her role is to support others to act. Each interaction the ICP has with a staff nurse that increases the latter's knowledge of and decision-making ability in infection control issues empowers that nurse to act as an independent clinician. Far from robbing the ICP of status or control, this type of interaction liberates the ICP to progress into other areas in her own role exploration.

Personal parameters

The personal aspect of role confirmation depends on the ICP's own value system. All people have different perceptions of knowing when they feel valued and when they value what they are doing. Rohrlich[9] identifies several motivating forces for why people work:

- A sense of self (identity)
- A feeling of security
- Competence, power, and self-respect

People will put varying importance on any one factor, but together they form a complex psychological milieu within which they measure satisfaction or dissatisfaction with a role. One way for the ICP to assess the health of her feedback system for her role is to ask herself periodically what happens when she does an average job, a mediocre job, or a great job.

If she answers, "Not much difference," she needs to either establish or rejuvenate her communication system. It is also important for the ICP to identify specific outcomes, based on her own values, that she perceives as a means of providing validation that in her role she is a valued, contributing member of the hospital staff. Once the ICP has identified these outcomes or "rewards," then she can develop strategies to make them happen. The responsibility for choosing and seeking these rewards lies with the ICP. Some examples of possible personal role confirmation outcomes follow:

Autonomy—The freedom of the ICP to set her own hours and plan her own goals

Salary—A salary reasonably comparable to that of other ICPs and similar responsible positions within the hospital

Office space—A private, pleasant environment in which to work

Department head status—Access to memoranda; meetings of the middle management level

Clerical support (or expansion of staff)—To facilitate efficacy and efficiency of the program and her time

Collegial relationship with physicians—Few nurses command the respect that the ICP enjoys based on a credible knowledge base and joint decision making in the consultative role

Inclusion in other work groups—The ICP's services are requested because of her skills and expertise with appropriate departmental groups

As mentioned previously, the external environment is only one portion of this vital feedback loop. Self-assessment, the internal check of success, will increase the ICP's awareness of behaviors that "work," that is, produce the results she wants. For example, if the ICP leaves the hospital feeling happy, energetic, and satisfied that she had a "good" day, she should take a few moments to analyze how she is feeling, what happened, and with whom she was interacting. The ICP should identify the specific elements that made her feel successful so she can consciously seek or build them into future projects or interactions.

Similarly, the ICP can review tasks, situations, or relationships that left her feeling unfulfilled, lacking energy, or even depressed. It is important to remain objective in this process; it is not meant to be an exercise in projecting blame onto others or rationalizing behavior. The ICP should ask herself, "How can I turn this problem into a learning opportunity?" She can identify what did not "work" and move on with the knowledge that she has a new insight for handling future problems.

A powerful means of monitoring progress is through the use of field notes mentioned in phase II. As the ICP becomes more skilled in her ability to observe her behavior, she will not need to rely on this retrospective writing technique of field notes and can concurrently monitor her interactions with others as they happen.

Personal growth and fulfillment are key factors in determining the evolution of an individual's role. The creative tension between the expectations of the ICP and hospital needs is the driving force in the dynamics of role development. As needs are satisfied, new ones emerge, leading the ICP back to phase 1, role negotiation, and phase 2, role implementation. Her awareness that she is not her role keeps this process fluid and exciting to benefit both her and the institution.

SUMMARY

The third phase of role development, role confirmation, is built on a strong base of support for the ICP and the infection control program. Active feedback systems are vital for the ICP to assess the acceptance of her role and the use of her skills and services. The responsibility for monitoring role confirmation lies with the ICP and includes evaluating the external and internal environment, personal satisfaction, and degree of congruence between practice and values.

REFERENCES

1. Claus, K.E., and Bailey, J.T.: Power and influence in health care: a new approach to leadership, St. Louis, 1977, The C.V. Mosby Co.
2. Jackson, T.: Guerilla tactics in the job market, New York, 1978, Bantam Books, Inc.
3. Joint Commission on Accreditation of Hospitals: Accreditation manual for hospitals, Chicago, 1982, The Commission.
4. Jourard, S.M.: The transparent self, rev. ed., New York, 1971, D. Van Nostrand Co.
5. Kleinman, C.: Women's networks, New York, 1980, Ballantine Books, Inc.
6. Norbeck, J.S.: Social support: a model for clinical research application, Adv. Nurs. Sci. **3:**43-59, July 1981.
7. Oda, D.S.: Specialized role development: a three phase process, Nurs. Outlook **25:**374-377, 1977.
8. Richard, K.M.: Executive sweets versus executive suites, unpublished paper, 1979.
9. Rohrlich, J.B.: Work and love: the crucial balance, New York, 1980, Summit Books.
10. Weiler, N.W.: Reality and career planning, Reading, Mass., 1977, Addison-Wesley Publishing Co., Inc.
11. Welch, M.S.: Networking, New York, 1980, Harcourt Brace Jovanovich, Inc.

6 ELAD LEVINSON

Stress management

attitude A habit of thinking, as in opinions, judgments, beliefs, biases, and prejudices.

paradigm A framework of thought; a scheme for understanding and explaining certain aspects of reality.

paradigm shift A distinctly new way of thinking about an old problem, issue, or situation; usually involves a powerful new insight.

stress Any emotional, physical, social, economic, or other factor that requires a response or change.

transformation A forming over or restructuring; a transformed substance takes on a different nature or character.

The word stress is enough to elevate one's blood pressure ten points, for it brings to mind for most health practitioners the experience of too many wanting and needing too much from too few. This chapter will discuss, in the context of the practice of infection control, what stress is and how to manage it. In addition, the scope will include strategies for dealing with stress on three levels that interface within a hospital or clinic setting: the individual, the interpersonal, and the organizational.

Stress is the factor that determines both the quantity and quality of one's work. Simply, stress is the bottom line for all productivity and for the product (illness) with which the infection control practitioner (ICP) copes. Stress is both the context of infection control (the background that all activity takes place within) and the content ("nuts and bolts") of the job.

HISTORICAL ROOTS OF STRESS THEORY[7]

Stress theory emerged from a powerfully reinforced paradigm: the industrial age. The result of the paradigm of the 1800s and mid-1900s was that people were viewed as expendable, as objects, or as reducible to scientific scrutiny and were thus sometimes quantified out of existence.

The experience of Americans, when articulating their inner perception of the results of the paradigm, is, "I am powerless, a cog in a wheel, an unimportant or insignificant noncontributor, and a statistic." The paradigm or world view that many people grew up with left them with these attitudes of powerlessness, and many consider this factor to be at the root of the national problems of drug addiction, crime, and violence.

In the following sections the factors of the development of stress theory will be discussed.

54

Biomedical model

The biomedical model has evolved over the last several centuries of Western civilization. The world view of the medical model is rational, scientific, or mechanistic. Emphasizing analysis, action, and achievement, it has helped make the world much more livable. Medical practice reflects this method of thought.

Since Descartes' time, philosophy, translated into behavioral terms in medicine, has separated the mind and body into a mechanical operation and its components.

The paradox of this thought process is that on the one hand, it has produced remarkable achievements in treating pathological conditions, and on the other hand, it robs individuals of responsibility and the power to heal themselves.

Biomedical scientists believed that once they could identify the disease, virus, or bacteria and synthesize the appropriate drug, all disease could be eradicated. Even mental illness and abnormal interpersonal relationships could be repaired by healing the malfunctioning portion of the mind or body.

The explanatory power and the real achievements of the biochemical model tended over time to narrow the perspective of those who used it. It limited their paradigm for healing to technology, knowledge, and science. In the process of explaining disease in these terms the importance of social, economic, and environmental causes of illness and health were lost.

Because of the mind-body split so prevalent in Western medicine, individuals were denied access to an approach that would integrate the ill person's self-regulating ability to heal through his own efforts.

The focus of health very slowly but inexorably has moved from the individual experiencing the pain or illness to the physician or medical establishment. Over 50% of those who go to a physician do so for reassurance or simple knowledge that common sense would dictate. The net result of the medical model is a sense of powerlessness. It is a prime contributor to the importance of stress theory. Individual powerlessness and lack of experience in self-health care coupled with the universal problem of mounting health care costs have contributed to a crisis that reflects the country's need to shift to a new paradigm.

Psychological context

The second factor that has contributed to the roots of stress theory might be termed the psychological world view that people have grown up with. People have been deeply influenced by a perception inherent in both freudian and behavioristic schools of thought: that human behavior is habitual, is determined by age 5, or is no more grand than instincts allow.

The behaviorists claim that most of human behavior is based on stimulus and response; that is, if a certain input is applied the outcome can be predicted. The behaviorists intentionally neglect dealing with the interior of the human being, that is, the emotions, thoughts, and feelings that dwell within the "black box." The "black box" is their term for anything that is not directly observable by scientific and analytical thought and experience.

Freudian psychology, although delving into the unconscious and acknowledging that the unconscious and subconscious have an impact on behavior, left another largely deterministic viewpoint for observing human behavior. In freudian terms people are who they are by 5 years of age, and what their lives are about is making do with their already existing world view, no matter how faulty it may be. Freudians believe that if people can figure out or understand why they are the way they are, it will free them to move forth in more positive directions.

The net results of both schools of psychology is that they leave out the magnificence, mystery, and potential of individuals to transform and grow far beyond their conditioned roots.

Sociocultural context

The third factor that has contributed to the paradigm or world view that stress theory was born into is the sociocultural context or backdrop. Simply stated, there have been three major aspects to the sociocultural perspective. The first aspect is an oversupply in the labor force, caused by the baby boom of the 1950s and early 1960s. This led to a point of view that human beings were expendable and that the supply would always be replenished.

Second, individual concerns took precedence over social concerns. Rugged individualism and the expansionistic ethic of a capitalistic society promoted overevaluation of the individual's desires and devaluation of social conscience and concerns.

The third force impinging on the sociocultural perspective is the dominant theme of religious dogmas that dictate that personal suffering is essential to strengthening character and that the kingdom to be sought is heavenly rather than earthly. This philosophy allowed injustice and exploitation to be commonplace. This religious perspective allowed many to nobly or needlessly suffer in horrendous conditions while holding onto hope of better worlds to follow.

Philosophical context

The fourth factor leading to stress theory is the set of philosophical beliefs held by Westerners.

Since the time of Aristotle, the dominant force in Western philosophy has been to explain the universe. The current conception of a cause and effect universe depicts a series of actions and reactions being generated on a massive scale, leading to a predictable future. Descartes' statement "I think, therefore I am" heralded the much vaunted explorations into the mind as the source of life, explanation, knowledge, and well-being. Rational philosophy left enough unexplained (special cases); hence cracks in the logic of mind over matter, body, or universe became the rule rather than the exception.

The most significant drawback to cartesian philosophy and aristotelian cause and effect reality is that both eliminate or mask human potential. Thanks to the new physics and the psychology and philosophies that have contributed to the new physics, people have a transforming world view: the mind is recognized as only a small part of the total human being and is the doorway for individuals to expand their vision of what is possible.

Physics context

The physics of the pre–stress theory paradigm was newtonian, mechanistic, scientific, and objective. People were taught that the universe was a grand clockwork that would be and could be explained on at least a macrocosmic level.[12]

The major trend in pre–Einstein physics was that the objective scientist could "know" the universe. This led to an excessive, predominant logic that viewed knowledge as everything and explanation its tool. It also elevated the physicist-scientist to the level of priest or seer and left the ordinary person powerless, as in the reductionist world view of the medical model.

Management theory context

The final factor of the paradigm is the management theory of the past 50 years. Before 1927 there was no management science. Management science began with Mayo's now famous study[6] of the Western Electric Company. Mayo found that money was not the only, or even necessarily the most significant, motivation for workers. Most managers had assumed that money was the only motivation. In this study it was found that demands and needs of workers were a prime consideration.

Before this study there were two schools of management, the autocratic and the laissez-faire. The autocratic, "old boy," or "big stick" approach was typified by the once dominant theme "What's good for the organization is good for the employee." The laissez-faire attitude, although a contrast in style to the autocratic approach, was not a contrast in form. The same attitudes were inherent in both, and what looked like diametrically opposed pairs were in fact two expressions of the same attitude. In neither case did they develop human resources. In neither case was there an assumption that an individual's needs are an important consideration for employees. In neither case did they take into account stimulating and intentionally building a positive climate in the workplace. Production was the only value considered.

STRESS THEORY

Stress theory is an idea so radical that it has taken almost 50 years to have an impact on mainstream medical thought; it is a paradigm shift "extraordinaire" as a method for and a conveyance to personal and organizational health and achievement.

Against the backdrop of these schools of thought, a quiet transformation has been evolving, one that returns to people their personal power and their ability to see creative solutions in the midst of national declining productivity and strength.

It is very important to realize that the aforementioned world views are held by most people and are reflected in such areas as science, the supervisor in a person's first job, sermons on Sunday morning, and the care provided by health care professionals.

All of these forces, when taken in total, leave people with positions, points of view, world views, attitudes, opinions, and beliefs about who they are, why they are here, what the world is like, and what others are like.

The basis of stress management is transformation. Transformation takes the already existing paradigm and views it in a whole new way. The essence of this transformation may be summed up as a shift from people thinking that they are who they have been conditioned to believe they are, to being able and willing to observe the self-imposed limitations that come from the old points of view. In other words, I am not my past; my past is in me, and I am capable of transcending or reaching beyond my past by becoming aware of it.

DEFINING STRESS

It is common, no matter how sophisticated the audience is, to attribute stress to pressure, tension, deadlines, anxiety, or a supervisor who does not communicate well. These are all examples not of stress but what stress looks and feels like when it has accumulated beyond the point of comfort or biological syntony. The word that is used to categorize these occurrences is *distress.*

Stress is a nonspecific response that the body and mind makes to any and all stimuli.[10] The body-mind[4] is the way I will describe the human organism. The conjugation of body and mind suggests a split between heart and intellect and feelings and rationality; this is misleading, since the body-mind responds as one unit to all stress. When the mind is conversing with the body, as it does so frequently, the body is registering an analogous response; conversely, if the body experiences fear or joy, the mind, at the same time, is having thoughts that correspond to the quality of sensations.

Stress is the body-mind's responsiveness to everyday life. In fact, Selye,[10] the father of the stress theory, says, "Stress is the wear and tear of everyday life." Selye says that stress is "everyday life," not the special circumstances of trying to learn a new job or the overwhelming pressures of being a single mother who also has a career. Stress is life. As the basis for health, as well as illness, stress is basic to all life processes; without stress there would be no breathing, procreation, or self-preservation:

It is vital to make a distinction between injurious and noninjurious stress responses. Obviously, not all stress can or should be avoided. A normal adaptive stress reaction occurs when the source of stress is identifiable and clear. When this particular challenge is met, an individual returns to a level of normal functioning relatively quickly. However, when the source of stress is ambiguous, undefined or prolonged or when several sources exist simultaneously, the individual does not return to a normal mental and physiological baseline as rapidly.*

Awareness and management of stress is essential to the infection control practitioner (ICP) for several reasons. The ambiguity and uniqueness of this emerging role creates stress. The ICP is constantly facing a multiplicity of pressures, often of long duration. The pressure may or may not abate when the function of the position is learned because other components of the ICP's environment are also adjusting and adapting to the role of ICP.

In addition to the ICP's special stress, there is added the input of the stress of health care professions:

A preliminary National Institute for Occupational Safety and Health (NIOSH) Report of 130 job classifications identified 40 of them as being high-stress jobs. A review of health clinic data among a variety of organizations in Tennessee identified 10 jobs as involving the highest incidences of reported stress disorders.†

Nursing and health care technicians placed fourth within the top ten. The evidence suggests that the ICP's personal and professional success or failure may ultimately be connected to how she manages everyday stress.

STRESS RESPONSE

Distress, not stress, is the problem; distress is an accumulation of normal stress beyond an individual's personal limits. The method for avoiding distress is a three-stage plan: (1) awareness, (2) attitude, and (3) action.

Awareness

Awareness refers both to becoming aware of one's response to stress and understanding the nature of the stress response:

According to Selye, the stress response or General Adaptation Syndrome (G.A.S.) passes through three phases: alarm, resistance, and exhaustion. The alarm phase is the first and most dramatic response to a stressor. At that point the entire body's stress mechanism is mobilized and the stressor has a generalized effect of psychophysiological functioning.*

---

*Excerpted from the book MIND AS HEALER, MIND AS SLAYER: A Holistic Approach To Preventing Stress Disorders by Kenneth R. Pelletier. Copyright © 1977 by Kenneth R. Pelletier. Reprinted by permission of DELACORTE PRESS/SEYMOUR LAWRENCE.
†From Albrecht, K.: Stress and the manager: making it work for you, Englewood Cliffs, N.J., 1979, Prentice-Hall, Inc., p. 43.

An example from the daily life of the ICP illustrates this concept. A person has been a very competent floor nurse, working with patients daily and administering clinical care, and she is asked to become an ICP. She finds herself literally a clinical practitioner one day and a teacher and manager the next. In addition, the ICP's hospital staff is not familiar with the role of ICP, so she has the dual responsibility of learning a new role and knowledge base and of teaching the other members of her environment how to relate to this new, ambiguous position. Also, the possibility that she may be unknowingly infringing on individuals who are experiencing some competitiveness toward her and the new position can lead to an example of the "alarm" stage of the GAS.

If the ICP could examine the microscopic processes going on inside her body, she would find an assortment of happenings. The sympathetic nervous system activates a chemical orchestra of hormones. The hypothalamus triggers the pituitary gland, which releases adrenocorticotropic hormone (ACTH) into the bloodstream. When the ACTH reaches the adrenal glands, there is an increased output of adrenaline, along with a family of related hormones called corticoids. Subsequently, muscle tone quickly increases and the liver immediately initiates conversion of stored glycogen into glucose. Breathing becomes more rapid and intense, increasing the amount of oxygen in the blood. The pupils of the eye dilate. Clearly the stress reaction is a coordinated chemical mobilization of the entire body to meet the requirements of a perceived threat.

As Shakespeare wrote, "Ay, there's the rub." The physical body does not know the difference between an actual threat to its physical integrity (e.g., an impending car crash) and a perceived threat to self-esteem. In fact, the alarm stage may be triggered off equally by a conflict-laden encounter or a car swerving into a driver's lane.

If a supervisor or colleague chooses to berate the ICP in front of others, her natural impulse will probably be the desire to run or to attack. However, social conditioning dictates that it is not appropriate to the situation to fight or run. Ironically, the body knows nothing of the rational decision-making process. It merely takes the trigger signal from the brain and sets off the standard chain of automatic chemical events called the stress response.

Actually the stress response is not an off-on phenomenon but rather a continuing process that varies in the level of intensity. While a person is asleep or very calm and relaxed, daydreaming for example, the internal activation level will be at a minimum. If a person decides to get up and move from the chair, the activation level will increase.

To carry this observation further, exercise produces the same activation of the sympathetic nervous system as is produced by the fear situation described earlier.

Selye[10] describes the stress response as "nonspecific"; he means that the response pattern is independent of the actual stressor. Although each stressor (heat, cold, bacteria, physical injury, or an externally perceived threat) produces its own specific changes in the body, they all produce additional nonspecific effects:

> From the point of view of its stress producing or stressor activity, it is immaterial whether the agent or situation we face is pleasant or unpleasant. . . . It is difficult to see how such essentially different things as cold, heat, drugs, hormones, sorrow and joy could provide an identical biochemical reaction in the body. Nevertheless, this is the case.*

As noted previously, the stress response is a three-stage reaction. The alarm stage is the initial mobilization stage of the overall process by which the body meets that challenge of an internal or external stressor. After some time, such as the initial period of sickness caused by infection, the alarm reaction subsides, and the stage of resistance ensues. During this stage, the body's resistance capability actually increases, and the battle for survival is on.

However, if the body does not win the battle (i.e., the person cannot escape from the threat), or if the body's chemical processes cannot overcome the infection, then the resistance level progressively weakens, and the stage of exhaustion sets in.

The stage of exhaustion does not occur once in a person's lifetime. As many ICPs note, it may be a daily process that leaves them physically and mentally exhausted each day after work.

The important fact to underline is that the stress response can be triggered by real or perceived threats. A perceived threat may be a situation, person, or event that is seen by the individual as a potential threat to the self-esteem or ego. If the individual is not aware of responding to another person, place, or event with the alarm reaction, it is likely that the alarm stage will continue unabated, and the person will move naturally into the stage of resistance. The body is fighting off an *imagined* threat, and yet the body's responses are the same, as if the threat were an acute attack of bacteria. The logical progression of the stress response is that the body-mind breaks down in a state of exhaustion as long as the challenge is not acted on in an appropriate way.

The most successful way to cope with the stresses of the ICP role is to become aware of the stress triggers that may excite the alarm reaction's initial response. In other words, if the ICP is aware from the very onset that her position is demanding, she is more likely to become aware of the automatic physiological reactions in the alarm stage before they continue into the downward spiral that terminates in exhaustion.

One concrete way to develop this awareness is to become proficient in reading the symptoms or signs of alarm. The ICP should become alert to the

*From Selye, H.: The stress of life, rev. ed., New York, 1975, McGraw-Hill, Inc.

desire to fight or run. She should be aware of the physiological warnings: pulse and blood pressure rising, perspiring, muscles tensing for action, hands clenching, and rapid and shallow breathing. By observing her own psychological and physiological telltale signs of alarm, the ICP may be able to counterbalance them by slowing her breathing down and loosening, relaxing, and softening the muscles that have become tensed. More will be said about counteracting the alarm stage in the section on positive stresses.

Attitude: the source of action

The second aspect of stress management is awareness of attitude. Selye[10] states that stress is neither positive nor negative; it just exist. How one interprets stress determines the body's response. In the context of a situation, if the ICP perceives a person as a threat, then she reacts with "flight" or "fight"; if that very same person is seen as an ally, the alarm reaction is not triggered. Emotionally, developing the role of ICP is potentially both fear producing and challenging. The body, however, does not know the difference between excitement and fear, except in the attitude of the observer.

Two specific examples of how the attitude can limit perception follow:

1. "One man's meat is another man's poison." Simply stated, this means that the way in which a person looks at something will have a profound impact on the results.
2. Attitude is the source of action. To know why people act as they do, one must realize that behavior is founded on decisions, attitudes, beliefs, notions, and opinion. These attitudes are based on past experience. Since children do not discriminate in deciding which culturally conditioned beliefs are appropriate to life support, they may adopt ones that are injurious. For example, competitive behavior in inappropriate situations may be counterproductive. The net result is that numerous values and beliefs are stored that may or may not be helpful to health, creativity, and personal satisfaction.

If a stressor is considered positive, then the body has a tendency to be enhanced in vitality as a result of it. If that very same stressor is out of the "comfort zone," then it will have a tendency to lower body defenses.

The role of the ICP can be viewed from a variety of personal viewpoints. If the position was assigned but the ICP has little personal interest in the role, she may express her frustration by becoming ill. Conversely, she may have desired, work for, and now enjoys the excitement of this challenging and demanding new position, but even with the positive attitude, she may become exhausted because excitement, challenge, or growth places demands on adaptation energies. The major difference is that if the ICP has intentionally sought the stress of being an ICP, her ability to rebound and grow is more likely than if her attitude is one of passively accepting a position about which she feels ambiguous or negative.

In professional and personal roles it is clear that an individual can only adjust one day at a time. For that reason, starting with this reading, the ICP must become a more alert observer of her attitude toward her work. Some ways to work with attitudes appear in the following sections.

If the ICP experiences negative feelings about her job, she is probably in a state of distress. The ICP should take an inventory of her basic stress needs. Is she too hungry, angry, lonely, or tired? Table 6-1 is a chart for taking an inventory of personal needs. The ICP should see which square she can identify with and give it a try. The way she uses the chart is to read each square. The squares are a combination of a state of consciousness (e.g., being hungry, angry, lonely, or tired) and an aspect of the totality (e.g., the mental, emotional) of self. So each square is a composite of the two (e.g., spiritually hungry or emotionally angry).

If the ICP finds that she identifies with more than one of the squares, she should pick one that she can do something about immediately. For example, the ICP may be spiritually hungry and emotionally lonely. It may be more appropriate for her to sit for 15 minutes and meditate and then go out and find someone with whom to relate. "First things first."

Acting "as if" personal needs counted

The third A in this triad of A's is action. Acting on one's own behalf is the cornerstone of preventive health care; ICPs have a responsibility to model behaviors that lead to and maintain well-being. As the National Institute of Occupational Safety and Health (NIOSH) study states, ICPs are also among the most distressed professionals. When the strains and pressures of becoming an ICP are added to the study's findings, it is clear that only intentional planning to care for one's own health is reasonable.

Selye[10] has given ICP a tremendous gift of information and philosophy about stress theory. He states that because people's perceptions are so much at the heart of the positive and negative effects of stress, it is essential for them to become responsible for how they adapt and perceive their lives. Therefore, for the ICP, it is doubly important to carry an attitude of intending to adapt positively to each new situation.

The most powerful personal or individual obstacles to self-care on the part of the ICP are attitudes that are unconscious and subconscious. These attitudes can usually only be visible by the results seen in daily life. For example, how many times has an ICP thought about or started an exercise or weight loss program or tried to stop smoking but given up because of various reasons? How many minutes a day does the ICP spend relaxing consciously and intentionally? If she is not taking a minimum of 30 minutes per day, there is little or no chance to release stored up stress.

It is important to remember that stress is not negative. Stored up negative effects are not what is being talked about. Positive, challenging activity is just

TABLE 6-1. Inventory of personal needs

States of consciousness	Mental	Emotional	Physical	Spiritual
Hungry	Symptoms: Mental laziness; don't want to think about yourself or life goals; would rather be watching television Remedy: Take junior college course (not for credit): forget about competition; try new hobby; run; walk; go to a stimulating lecture; think about it	Symptoms: Craving companionship; feeling isolated and withdrawn; you want physical contact, not words; you want feelings, not ideas Remedy: See if you are willing to communicate your feelings to others; give from yourself to people who need it	Symptoms: Lightheadedness, dizziness, hunger pangs, and irritable feelings; craving for sugar or something sweet Remedy: Eat something good for you, such as protein found in nuts, fish, cheese, and yogurt; eat raw vegetables and fruit	Symptoms: Boredom; easily upset; a sense of missing something; lack of peace of mind; a sense of needing help from a power greater than yourself Remedy: Meditate; examine your religious beliefs and find a new spiritual contact
Angry	Symptoms: Thinking over and over about something someone did to you; fantasizing about yelling at someone or hitting someone Remedy: Realize your anger comes from you because you're not happy with yourself; use angry energy to run an extra mile, dance at a disco, or walk three miles	Symptoms: Rage; irritation; annoyance; cynicism; sarcasm; biting remarks Remedy: Cry; yell where you'll be safe; run fast; talk it out with friend; be real and own up to it	Symptoms: Burning in hands; flushing of face; butterflies in stomach; heat in solar plexus spreading to face and extremities Remedy: Get it out in a constructive way; hit a punching bag, walk a long way; dance; go to the ocean and yell at the waves; cry; scream; hit pillows	Symptoms: A clear sense that something is a moral outrage; a conflict in your internal values Remedy: Communicate your point of view while allowing others their own; don't criticize; just accept what you are feeling

Lonely	Symptoms: Sense of isolation; no one to bounce ideas off; haven't had a good discussion in awhile Remedy: Go to a group meeting and participate; learn something new every day, and share it with someone; read a book, and tell someone about it; go to class, group, or study session where you can converse	Symptoms: "I'd rather be alone" even when you know you need a friend; choosing television as a friend; emptiness inside; sense of dreariness about life Remedy: Risk a bit and talk about it with an objective listener; be with people you like; attend self-help groups like AA where you will feel safe enough to speak up	Symptoms: Need to be touched, caressed, or stroked Remedy: Everyone needs to be touched; get a straight massage from a registered masseur/ masseuse; trade a foot massage with a friend; find a friend and ask to be held; take a hot bath; cry it out	Symptoms: A sense of being out of touch with nature and with the flow of life; loneliness of spirit; emptiness of heart Remedy: Go to the country and sit quietly; listen to inspiring music; meditate; reconnect with a spiritual group of your choice; act "as if" a higher power runs the universe
Tired	Symptoms: Feeling overstimulated; too much input; not able to sleep because ideas keep running through your mind Remedy: Keep it simple; slow down; listen to a record; get your mind off ideas; run or dance	Symptoms: "I'm drained, worn out, and I can't cope with. . . ." Remedy: Rest; be alone; go to the ocean; do something fun and simple; quit mulling it over; let yourself be distracted by something entertaining	Symptoms: Aches and pains; fatigue; boredom; drowsiness; yawning a lot; "I don't want to do anything, nothing seems good to me" Remedy: Take a hot bath or sauna; sleep; nap; do deep relaxation; rest for 10 to 15 minutes	Symptoms: Feeling like you have to do it all alone; need for a new energy to fill your body and life Remedy: Meditate; do deep relaxation and concentrate on nature; help a friend; volunteer time with senior citizens or children

as taxing. All adaptation requires an energy expenditure. Thirty minutes per day of intentional relaxation is essential to the release, rebounding, and relaxation of the physical system. When a person begins to consider doing activities that produce positive stress, the natural resistance to change is stimulated. It is often noted by busy professionals that taking 30 minutes a day to relax seems an impossible challenge.

One case history of an ICP will illustrate the obstacles often faced in scheduling time for relaxation.

> Louise is a 28-year-old nurse who has been assigned the position of ICP in a large midwestern teaching hospital. Louise is extremely responsible in her new position and has actively sought out and participated in infection control programs to develop her expertise. Even with her educational efforts, Louis has felt a vague sense of anxiety about her competency. This feeling arose when she assumed the new role of ICP. As she states, "Even though I try very hard, I'm still sure someone is going to question my proficiency." For Louise this vague, ambiguous stress has put a tremendous unconscious burden on her ability to adapt. In addition, Louise has a husband and two young children who are important in her life. She states, "When I first heard of the idea of taking 30 minutes per day for myself, I said, 'Sure, if they make a 24½-hour day.' My typical day starts at 5:30 with feeding the children, then waking Gary, my husband, at 6:30, and finally rushing to be at work at 7:30. I ask you, where am I going to squeeze time in?"

The direct result of Louise's conflict was that her body responded with an assortment of aches and pains, and she thus required sick leave days.

Part of the problem for Louise resides in a common work ethic. The ICP caught up in the work ethic is enmeshed in a spiraling, escalating cycle of "work harder, not smarter." In other words, she unconsciously is so caught up in having to get all the jobs and roles done to her entire satisfaction that there is no time or space for leisure, rest, or relaxation. As a direct result, her rationality is seriously impaired, and there is a tendency to work longer hours, with more mistakes. In fact, the work pressure and family pressure syndrome that is so common among ICPs can literally lead to serious illness, loss of a good position, divorce, or possibly death. Some people work themselves or a good relationship to death. The high incidence of stress-related illnesses that the NIOSH study showed is not an accident of statistics. This is the time for the ICP to reconsider and reevaluate her willingness to intentionally plan relaxation time.

The consequences of stress accumulating and being stored as distress are severe. Much research points to a link between personality and illness:

> Subtle psychological changes initiate subtle neurophysiological changes which in turn create further aberrations of the psychological processes in a negative closed-loop system which ultimately predisposes the individual toward the development of severe organic pathology later in life.*

*Excerpted from the book MIND AS HEALER, MIND AS SLAYER: A Holistic Approach To Preventing Stress Disorders by Kenneth R. Pelletier. Copyright © 1977 by Kenneth R. Pelletier. Reprinted by permission of DELACORTE PRESS/SEYMOUR LAWRENCE.

Furthermore, Selye[10] states that 90% of all illness is stress related.

A comprehensive study of the relationship between personality and illness is that of Friedman, Rosenman, and their colleagues in the formulation of type A and type B behavior in coronary heart disease:

> Over years of observation, using questionnaires and personal interviews to assist them, Friedman and Rosenman developed a detailed profile of that Type A personality and his less-stressed Type B counterpart. They attribute the inordinate degree of Type A behavior in the U.S. to a legacy of the Puritan ethic and the evolution of our economic system, since both encourage competition, achievement and the acquisition of material wealth.*

They suggest that in the personality attitudes of the type A individual are predictable. These include an excessive competitive drive, coupled with a chronic, continual sense of time urgency to meet ever present deadlines.

A composite profile of the cancer patient has been derived from many researchers. Typically a cancer victim has suffered a severe emotional disturbance in early childhood, or up to age 15. For example, reacting to divorce, death, separation, or chronic friction between parents, the child may experience a great sense of loss, loneliness, anxiety, and rejection. This loss may lead to an attitude that fosters behavior that symbolically tries to regain the lost parent. The need to please a parent, teacher, boyfriend or girlfriend, spouse, and boss may exclude the natural expression of negative or conflictual emotions. Later in life, cancer victims are described by their friends, family, and co-workers as too good to be true: "This 'too-good-to-be-true' trait can assume an almost martyr-like quality, that many cancer researchers speculate masks a chronic low-key depression."[8] As Voth of the Menninger clinic clearly sums up:

> We know that the ability to handle life's vicissitudes is tied to childhood experience. Research shows that individuals who experience loss in the years before adolescence are especially pregnable to loss later. The child does not know how to mourn, or is taught to be "a good boy or girl" and not to mourn. Grief gets frozen within him, then losses later in life reawaken painful memories and the person is confronted with a double loss.†

Six key points summarize the nature of stress:
1. Stress is life; it is the adaptation of the organism to all stimuli regardless of positive or negative characteristics.
2. Stress accumulates through a process of adaptation called the general adaptation syndrome (GAS).[10]
3. The GAS is initiated by a perceived stressor being a threat to the person viewing it. In other words, as Flip Wilson's character Geraldine so eloquently stated, "What you see is what you get."

*Excerpted from the book MIND AS HEALER, MIND AS SLAYER: A Holistic Approach To Preventing Stress Disorders by Kenneth R. Pelletier. Copyright © 1977 by Kenneth R. Pelletier. Reprinted by permission of DELACORTE PRESS/SEYMOUR LAWRENCE.
†From Moneysworth, May 26, 1975.

4. The cycle of alarm–resistance–exhaustion continues unabated, taxing the immune systems' adaptation and energy if the individual does not consciously intervene.
5. The most successful interventions in stopping the GAS from taking its course are relaxation and self-awareness.
6. Conscious, intentional relaxation and self-awareness can either keep the alarm stage from being initiated or bring the response back to a baseline calm before reaching its accumulated end product, exhaustion.

In the next section the issues of individual, interpersonal, and organizational stress will be examined in more depth.

MANAGING STRESS FOR PRODUCTIVITY AND SATISFACTION
Coping with individual stress

Seven methods are highlighted for the ICP in this examination of practical means to convert stress on an individual basis.

Deep relaxation. Deep relaxation training can be traced many thousands of years to the science of yoga. In the *Patanjali Sutras*, an ancient text of philosophy and medicine, many references are given in styles and techniques for physical, emotional, and mental relaxation. In a branch of yoga called Hatha yoga, toe-to-head relaxation (in the "corpse pose," or supine position) is employed after each posture and/or at the end of the entire set of *asanas*, or postures.

The importance of mentally imagining oneself "going through" each portion of the body, intentionally relaxing and softening each separate part, is essential.

Deep breathing. There is nothing that a person can do that a deep breath will not make better. The ICP will probably notice that if she pays attention to her breathing right now, it is probably shallow and involves only the upper portion of her lungs. More often than not, if the ICP observes herself she will find that she and her colleagues and patients are using about one quarter of their lung capacity. Generally, people are underoxygenated. One test of this is for the ICP to take a dozen long, full deep breaths. As she breathes, she should inhale through her nostrils until she feels she cannot take in any more air. When she exhales she should do the same, expelling the air through her mouth. After doing this is there a feeling of lightheadedness, dizziness, or sleepiness? Has she yawned as a result of oxygenating the body? Any or all of these signs point to chronic underoxygenation. A yawn signals that the body is trying to throw off carbon dioxide and return to homeostasis. A few hints about deep breathing follow:

1. The ICP can put up signs around her home, office, and car that say "Take a breath," or simply "breathe."
2. She can take a 5-minute oxygen break every hour, outside if possible, to

clear her head of the cobwebs that accumulate just by doing her stressful job.

3. The ICP can skip lunch or a coffee break, seek a place where she will not be interrupted (e.g., a meditation room in the hospital, car, bathroom), and practice deep relaxation and deep breathing.

4. If the ICP is in a meeting and feels anxious, she can breath slowly and deeply. No one will notice. The other people are so caught up in their own distress, it is not likely they would notice anyone breathing slowly and deeply.

5. Instead of getting nervous or tense in traffic, the ICP can calm herself by relaxing the tension in the shoulders, jaw, arms, and chest and breathe slowly and deeply.

Exercise. Exercise typifies positive stress. Positive stresses are always known by their results. Selye[10] calls them *eustress*, or good stress. A eustress is an activity, event, situation, or relationship that makes a person feel more alive, vital, joyous, or relaxed *after* the encounter. The key word is *after*. Most people assume that for something to be positive, it must be fun or enjoyable while doing it. Exercise is certainly not fun. It can be downright boring, or at least repetitious. The key is that after doing exercise, the ICP's body thanks her. The benefits may not be seen immediately. The ICP may have to delay gratification of seeing gains in her physical conditioning for day or weeks. The visible benefits are usually proportionate to the number of years since the last regular exercise program. If the ICP has not exercised regularly for 10 years, it will be a while before she sees any visible gains. That should not get in the way though. It is guaranteed that if she works on an aerobic program or exercise three to four times per week for 15 to 20 minutes per day at her exercise heart rate,[3] she will be doing cardiovascular fitness conditioning. Exercise is a Catch-22 for most of health care practitioners. They know it is good for them and feel guilty not doing it. The guilt reinforces negative self-esteem, which lowers the energy they have for starting a program of positive stress.

Some suggestions for getting started in an exercise program follow:

1. The ICP should consult a physician for approval before starting. Ask what type, how much, and what limits current health will allow in the realm of exercise.

2. The ICP can start exercising anywhere, but she should *start*. She can begin with moderate exercise, such as walking, and work up to more strenuous activity.

3. If the ICP knows she is unlikely to exercise alone, she could do it with others in a sponsored exercise class or an aerobic dance or yoga course.

4. Above all, the program should be enjoyable. Exercising with music is one way to make it more fun and go faster. One nurse in a stress course illustrated this point. She was in her sixties and looked much younger,

so her program visibly demonstrated its success. She said, "For the last fifteen years, I've been exercising a half hour per morning. I didn't have much motivation to get going on this, so I looked around for a way to get started. I realized that I love John Phillip Sousa marches and I bought a record and have been marching around my living room-bedroom for the last fifteen years for one-half hour per morning. I pull the shades down, because I wouldn't want the neighbors to know." As funny as it sounds, the woman has been successful in maintaining a high level of well-being through her creativity. Whatever it takes, everyone should exercise.

Time management. It is true that time is the only variable that is constant for everyone. All people have 24 hours available in a day. From that point, every-thing else with respect to time is subjective. Time is an experience that must be addressed intentionally. Intentionally means "with a carefully formulated plan of action." This experience that most ICPs have is that there is never enough time.

Porat[9] has dealt with the issue of time in a remarkable way. In going beyond traditional time management concepts to the essence of managing time, the essential question is "for what end purpose?" Do people organize and plan their waking hours only to have more time to do more work? Porat suggests that *quality* time, or that time people plan just for themselves to nurture their physical, emotional, and mental selves, is essential to time management. This process is "creative procrastination, the planned, deliberate gift of prime time to yourself each day to do what gives you greatest satisfaction including not doing anything, if that is your choice."[9] For someone who has as much respon-sibility as the ICP it is essential to schedule enough time to renew oneself.

For those who feel guilty or in conflict over managing to find time for creative procrastination, Selye[10] has some words of wisdom. He states that the purpose of life is to be of use, or essential to other human beings. Certainly the ICP is useful in her role and her organizational setting. To fulfill that purpose she must have something valuable to give. What she has to offer is time, energy, information, and her own being. The quality of all of these is seriously im-paired when she is distressed. Selye[10] advises that to be of service and to do the best, people must be selfish enough to take care of personal needs daily. He calls this paradox "altruistic egoism": Being selfish to be of service.

Meditation. The term meditation refers both to a specific practice of a disci-pline associated or affiliated with a religious or spiritual organization and to a state of conscious alertness, present whenever someone is concentrating on a single task, event, person, or situation.

Christianity, Judaism, and all of the Eastern spiritual groups have some form of organized, structured experiences that produce "mindfulness." To be mindful means simply to be as alert and aware as one is capable of being at any given moment. Meditation produces an internal alertness, which in turn allows the individual to view rationally and objectively his own and others' behavior and reactions. Meditation also produces external acuity. There are numerous studies that clearly demonstrate that meditation increases responsiveness, productivity, proficiency, and intellectual discrimination.

Developing a meditative discipline toward work means giving complete attention to each discrete aspect of the day's activities. The Western cultural view, in contrast, is often more concern with speed, efficiency, and quantity than it is with care, effectiveness, and quality. Product becomes more important than process. To translate this concept of meditation into practice, the ICP should recall a situation in which the time and energy required to get several tasks accomplished created a conflict for her. Perhaps she needed to finish a report for the infection control committee and also received a telephone call about a potential infection problem in the nursery. The usual response is that neither problem is done well. If the ICP chooses to respond to the nursery problem, the report deadline is looming in her mind and clouding ability to finish the report. The nursery problem is still present. A meditative approach would allow her to sequentially address problems. Contrary to the myths present in society, meditation does not produce introversion, apathy, a lack of ambition, cults, or passivity. In fact, in one study, Carrington[2] suggested people who mediated were more productive than others within the groups studied.

The other aspect of meditation being explored is the physiological effect of meditation. As the studies of transcendental meditation suggest, meditation (all forms, including transcendental meditation, Zen, Mantra meditation, and yoga) produces (1) lowered heart rate and blood pressure, (2) reduced stress and tension, and (3) decreased addictive behavior to cigarettes, alcohol, coffee, and food.[1] Carrington[2] concludes after exhaustive research on the varieties of meditation forms that mantra meditation is the most successful for the Western mind.

Humor. The next stress management tool for individual self-care is humor. Simonton,[11] in his book *Getting Well Again*, states that a significant contributing factor to the recovery of a terminally ill cancer patient is his prescription of 1 hour of fun each day. Cousins' masterpiece, *Anatomy of an Illness as Perceived by the Patient*,[3a] illustrates how the conscious intentional use of laughter-producing agents had a significant healing effect on Cousins' "terminal" condition.

The idea of taking time to have fun runs counter to the American cultural work ethic. Many people have lost the ability to laugh. In hospital settings there is an unconscious, subterranean attitude that laughter is inappropriate in a hospital. In fact, through research at the University of California, Los Angeles, it has been documented that laughter produces endorphins, which aid and abet the healing process and give relief from some pain.

My suggestion to the ICP is to develop a good sense of humor. Humor can be likened to the oil on a duck's back. As it rains, the oil is a protective waterproofing. Humor can assist the ICP to keep cheerful in the midst of suffering and pain. This is not to suggest that she is expected to be blasé or uncaring. The point is that a smile can foster more good health than dour expressions in her repertoire.

If there is little laughter in the ICP's life, she may be one of the millions who are suffering from humoristic nervosa. This condition is typified by a drooping in the corners of the mouth, a loss of sparkle in the eyes, no sense of humor toward children's activities, an inability to laugh at oneself, a tight chest, rigidly held in stomach (precluding belly laughs), and a general attitude that life is SERIOUS. The only remedy for the condition is to view movies, read books, and listen to records that are comic in nature. Large doses of the Marx Brothers, Woody Allen, Lily Tomlin, and Laurel and Hardy are recommended.

On a somewhat more serious note, it is clear that without a sense of humor, life is really drudgery. Many have not laughed in so long that they must learn to flex their laughter muscles again. To that end, the ICP should schedule opportunities to participate with people in events and situations likely to bring back the joy of life.

Coping with stress on an interpersonal level

If the ICP observes communication on a day-to-day basis, she can note that interpersonal communication improves measurably as individuals become responsible for intentional skill building in sending and receiving messages. Training is the bedrock for developing skills. If the ICP takes courses in how to listen or send messages, supervise, or team build, the ability to put these skills into practice will depend on whether she is also accountable for the 75% of communication that is nonverbal. Success of communication depends on the individuals involved, taking into consideration the nonverbal aspect of communication.

The space that surrounds all communication is the context or background of the words. In other words, the stress that has been described as an ability to respond to life's stimuli is also the context of communication. A few vignettes may illustrate the point. When the ICP gets up on the wrong side of bed and feels grumpy or tired, she has a tendency to find others who have also gotten up on the same wrong side. The ICP has someone to commiserate with. If she is upset and another person is not, she has the tendency to make the other person feel upset after interaction with her distress level. Often the ability to assist others is blocked by the personal distress felt because of overwork, deadlines, or sickness.

Stress is the determinant for whether communication is sent successfully or listened to effectively. It is all too common for an ICP to give instructions to a co-worker or family member and see that he is preoccupied. The faraway look reflects an overload of information, noise, and projects going through his mind. The remedy for preoccupation is any one of the seven suggested stress management techniques just discussed.

To improve communication, the ICP should take care of her basic stress needs. If she is calm, relaxed, refreshed, and full of energy, she will be much less likely to growl at a communication from someone else or add her own distress to her messages. It is as if the words she sends, when she is tired or hungry, are coated with the flavor of her tiredness. The experience the receiver has when picking up the communication is clouded by the coating. Often the receiver's reaction will be to the nonverbal distress. That is why the ICP as a communicator may get back more than she intended; she may be receiving a response pattern that is largely distress generated and not directed personally toward her.

Suggestions for handling interpersonal stress. These suggestions are not meant to be an exhaustive examination of the theory of communication. They are simply ways to apply the stress theory to interpersonal dynamics.

1. Before any important meeting or conference, the ICP should take 20 minutes to "go through" her body and relax the hot spots of tension, paying special attention to the shoulders, jaws, face, and neck. In addition to relaxing the tension, she should breathe slowly and deeply through the nose, if possible, and out through the mouth. She may want to count slowly to four or five as she inhales and then exhales.

2. The ICP must be aware of any tendency to blame herself or others for problems. Adding blame or responsibility adds insult to injury. The ICP should try and remain rational about problems. More times than not, when a problem emerges, it is not hers personally to work out but rather a problem that must be shared by all concerned. It is all too common for health care professionals, especially women, to take problems on as if they had personally been the target for the blame. Rational problem solving among managers or a specific subgroup is always preferable to burdening oneself. The group's intelligence and problem-solving ability is usually greater than any single perspective.

3. The ICP should make eye contact with the people she is trying to reach. By making eye contact, she adds a dimension of humanness to any interaction. In addition, she gains a measure of control because the person who seeks eye contact is usually the one perceived as the most in charge interpersonally. The third plus for making eye contact is that the ICP knows, with greater certainty, whether her message was received.

4. Speech should be clear and articulate. Some ICPs have real trouble marketing their in-service education programs because their communication is halting, uncertain, and filled with garbled words, soft-spoken unintelligible phrases, or swallowed endings to sentences. Before the ICP speaks, she should take time to be clear about what she intends to get across. She should not expect to automatically become a public speaker because her position requires it. A great percentage of ICPs started out organizationally in staff or administrative positions, and it is not a part of

their skills to be polished lecturers or effective managers. Courses such as "Toastmasters," junior college speech courses, or Dale Carnegie's classes for effective public speaking are extremely valuable. The message the ICP has for the hospital staff is valuable, so her own inexperience should not get in the way of getting it to the ones who can do something with it.

5. The ICP's physical presentation should reflect what she is attempting to be. Like it or not, people do judge on the basis of first impressions, and the first impression often lasts beyond the initial encounter. Careful use of clothing, makeup, jewelry, posture, hairstyling, and accessories is a great aid to being believable as a competent ICP. If the ICP wants others to view her as competent, authoritative, and certain, she must present herself that way. The ICP should ask herself, "What in my physical presentation may be a barrier to others seeing me as competent?" Although the ICP can never be totally responsible for others' judgments about, opinions of, or attitudes toward her, it is true that she can elicit positive evaluations by intentional attention to detail in her physical presentation.

6. The ICP should learn to listen with her full attention. If she is preoccupied and cannot listen, she should excuse herself and make another appointment to handle whatever is not finished. She will earn the goodwill of others more quickly by being a good "ear" than by any other method I know. She should make eye contact when someone is talking to her and *intend* to be really attentive. Quite often she can transform negative feelings about or distraction to her goals being accomplished, just by listening with full attention and letting the other party know she heard and valued what they said.

In addition to these six suggestions, the ICP might consider taking courses in communication skills, management, training, and supervisory skill building, and other classes or seminars that will increase her effectiveness. It is essential to remain open to feedback. To be open means that the ICP should take stock of the skills both interpersonally and organizationally that she has and that she lacks. To know where improvement is required and to have the willingness to go out and obtain the information and knowledge is the sign of an enlightened person.

Coping with organizational stress

The third level in which stress occurs and must be dealt with is the organizational level.

Although organizations are composed of individuals, there is a function of group dynamics that changes the effects significantly from one-on-one interaction.

For the most part, hospitals are disease management industries rather than health maintenance or primary prevention-oriented institutions. The modus operandi of most hospitals is management by crisis. It is a rare health organization that considers management training or skill development as an integral part of the skills necessary for survival within the system. It is even rarer for the hospital administration to be run by consistent goals or management by objectives (MBO).

The consequence of these facts is that decisions are made by very few and interpreted in a downhill, unidirectional flow of communication. In addition, there is little or no input from staff, and when input is offered, it is primarily ignored. The ambience of most hospitals runs quite contrary to stress management principles.

Because of a lack of administrative direction by objectives, middle management (both line and staff positions) is often left with tremendous accountability and little authority to carry out the responsibilities.

Another obstacle of organizational climate may include a "personality" that permeates the decision-making process of the entire hospital. For example, many hospitals qualify as a type A (personality) work environment. Typical of this organizational way of operating is a constant overflow of projects, structural improvements, fund raising, management turnover, and systems reappraisals, all in the name of efficiency. In fact, to the middle manager or supervisor, the experience is quite the opposite. All the efforts appear to confuse and impede the ability of personnel to get the job done. There is a further sense of time urgency, coupled by a sense that all deadlines are top priorities. Often it seems that dollars and quantity of care are more important than patients and the quality of good patient care.

The type A organizational climate can create role conflict for the ICP. An incongruence emerges between her philosophy of infection control (i.e., prevention of nosocomial infections) and the behavioral expectations demanded by the environment (i.e., the crisis intervention approach to problem solving). In a type A organization the ICP is less likely to fulfill the role as educator consultant and is more likely to be involved in crisis resolution. It is important that the ICP be aware of the organizational structure and climate she works in to know what realities her efforts are going to face.

There is an attitude in many hospitals that no matter what a health care worker does it will never be enough. Nurse clinicians, therapists, and physicians are well experienced with this attitude because disease management provokes the attitude of "too little for too many." In the way most hospitals are structured the physician is responsible for the recovery and health of the patient. This is contrary to the actual fact: the patient is an equal partner in the recovery and health process.

When patients are treated as if they are responsible for their health, the burden of getting people well shifts, and the load lightens for the health care professional.

If the ICP is working within a system that covertly or overtly assumes that the physician and nurse are exclusively responsible for the patients' health, then the consequences are that (1) she will probably share in the sense of being overworked or burdened by the patients' conditions, and (2) her efforts at health education will be unsupported by the physician and most administrators.

An additional organizational stressor is the unique role of the ICP literally being "one-of-a-kind." Not only will the ICP be required to have a substantial knowledge base of infection control but also she must understand that she will probably be "carving out her own niche." To create this role in any organization is both an exciting and challenging task.

The ICP should remember one thing over all others as she develops her role: health care professionals are often very bureaucratic and territorial. When the ICP makes a place for herself, she is entering an existing system of relationships and territories.

These major points are worth remembering:

1. Being a pioneer is both challenging and anxiety producting. The physical body does not know the difference between excitement and fear. Even though the ICP may be highly motivated and enjoying her work, it is cause for adjustment and adaptation. Her immune system is under pressure to cope with the efforts, however enjoyable.

   In addition, since the ICP is entering into what others perceive as their areas of responsibility, she may feel under scrutiny and, at times under attack. The body's natural reaction to self-esteem being under observation is a constant state of alarm. The alarm may be well controlled (in fact, the only person who may know this is the ICP), but the body is still going through the alarm whether it is visible to others or not. As I said earlier, if the ICP does not relax and allow the body to rebound from the alarm stage, the general adaptation syndrome continues uninterruptedly through the stage of resistance into exhaustion. A sure sign that this is occurring will be if the ICP is exhausted, drained, or irritable at the end of the day. Therefore the ICP should take care of herself; she is the only one who will or who can.

2. The resistance the ICP encounters to entry within the hospital system is generally not personal. *She is not the target!* Individuals resist change and the ICP is the symbol of that change.

3. If and when the ICP does take innuendos or outright challenges to her authority personally, she should "own up" to it. She should find a "safe" person who is objective and not personally involved with the results of her problem and clear it from her mind. The ICP and the "safe" person can discuss solutions to the problem. The ICP should not attempt to

resolve conflict with the involved individuals *until* she is objective and rational (as compared to being in a feeling or emotional mode of functioning).

4. The ICP must be alert as to who is safe and appropriate to share feelings with. She should avoid being self-disclosing or emotionally vulnerable with those who can use her feelings against her. This is not to suggest that she should be guarded or automatically defensive around co-workers. It is appropriate, however, to be discriminating in divulging hopes and fears. Some people are defensive about their real or imagined position being threatened by "the new kid on the block." A network of support can include colleagues in similar roles within the institution, fellow ICPs at other hospitals, or someone outside the work setting completely.

5. It is important to be aware of the fact that a large percent of ICPs are women and that women managers have a tendency to blame themselves when things go wrong. In contrast, male managers have a tendency to view co-workers or the system as the reason things did not work. If the ICP is the type of person who first looks to herself for fault or blame, she should beware. Being responsible to the point of it becoming a weight or burden is not healthy.

   A new way of defining responsibility is, "What did I do that didn't work and what can I do about it?" Being responsible also means not taking on others' responsibility for the breakdown. To be responsible means to objectively discriminate who owns the problem and when involvement is appropriate to the situation.

6. It is vital for the ICP to be authoritative, even when she does not feel that way. The way the ICP can be authoritative is to know the material, information, and data so thoroughly that she trusts herself to be certain. This will minimize others discounting her because she will be unlikely to allow it. In addition, having a thorough knowledge base will eliminate the tendency of physicians to discount all other health care personnel as less professional or competent. Then the ICP can act "as if" she knows what she is doing. This is not to suggest that the ICP be unteachable or close minded; rather, when it is time for the ICP to make a decision and stand by it, but she does not feel sure, she should act as if she knew what she were doing. Through the repetition of actions that are unfamliar and anxiety provoking, she will gain comfort, alacrity, and excellence. In the meanwhile, she is building a base of support and trust with co-workers. For that reason, the ICP must present herself with authority.

7. It is important for the ICP to know her co-workers and their staff. She should not assume that "they" are the enemy. It is necessary and appropriate to assess others' strengths and weaknesses. Everyone has idiosyn-

crasies, and some can be obstacles to projects being completed or communication occurring.

In one instance an ICP had been trying to get a procedure approved by her immediate supervisor for over 6 weeks. He kept sending it back to her with comments such as "incomplete," "not enough research," or "not ready yet." In her frustration she was responding in an irrational manner to his communications. Instead of asking him directly what he meant by his responses, she assumed that it was a personal affront and that she was incompetent in his eyes. Finally, she decided to ask him what he meant by his rejections. She discovered that her supervisor was also relatively new to the management staff and was concerned for his own position. He knew he would have to sell the idea to his immediate superior, and he was delaying the confrontation as long as possible. He told her that he was not sure how much supporting research he would need to feel comfortable about presenting her project. She offered her support to him, and they mutually agreed on a timetable and deadline to present the project together to his supervisor.

The ICP should find people within the organization who have common sense, look for down-to-earth insights in co-workers' personalities, and learn to interview them.

It is appropriate and necessary for the ICP to have some insight into how her colleagues see her and her newly emerging position. She may, in addition, be able to find ways to encourage the support and goodwill of even the most "difficult" people, by learning which approaches work and which do not from individual to individual. The ICP is increasing her repertoire of role behaviors with each encounter in a relationship.

SUMMARY

This chapter has been a means to demonstrate how the stress theory can aid and abet the ICP in delivering high quality service in the ICP role. Selye[10] states that the greatest way to be successful is to be needed by others. The ICP is a very necessary part of the hospital setting. She brings a perspective that adds importance to disease prevention efforts. She is also in an objective position of somone who travels through the hospital setting and can observe, record, and suggest ways for organizational effectiveness in patient care.

These final observations can make a significant difference in the ICP's ability to contribute to the well-being of others.

First, the ICP should use *all aspects of problem solving*. She should gather information from reliable sources, talk to co-workers who may view the problem from a different angle, and read the literature pertinent to the problem. In addition, she should use her intuitive capacity, which comes from reflection and from actively contemplating the issues.

Second, the ICP should *take care of herself*. Selye[10] states that for people to be most productive in their lives they must use "altruistic egoism." To paraphrase, if the ICP's motivation is to assist others and contribute to their lives, then she must have something to give. For example, a dear, trustworthy friend asks to borrow $500 but the ICP is without extra funds. Her intent is to give but there is nothing left to give. In the same way, if a client, friend, or family member comes, needing support or time and the ICP is distressed, she will not be able to give that person her best quality time and energy.

Third, the ICP must *take a rational approach to her own blocks to learning and necessary change.* She should train herself to be willing to question her own input to problems or conflicts. There are those times when ICPs get in the way of their progress because they may be reacting in an inappropriate or dysfunctional manner. Is there any attitudinal mindset that is preventing the ICP from hearing information relevant to the problem or solution?

Fourth, the ICP should *develop a sense of humor about her learning process.* In my first contact for a stress seminar, I started at a very prestigious, highly professional medical clinic. I was going to lecture on this particular day on how to focus attention so that concentration is improved. On the morning of the lecture, I walked out of my home with a pair of my underwear attached to my briefcase. I had shut my briefcase on them and not noticed. I had been in such a rush to get to the lecture in which I was going to demonstrate efficient concentration that I had neglected to notice the appendage growing out of my briefcase. I discovered my jockey shorts just in time to laugh and think, "Isn't this a great illustration of how well stress management works!"

Fifth, the ICP should *enjoy the ride.* She should set concrete goals and know where she wants to be professionally and personally. It is important that the ICP acknowledge herself for achieving them. She must rationally think through the setbacks but above *all* else enjoy the process. The secret of niche carving is that the niche was always there. It is not a matter of force or manipulation. Space in the organization is assured. What the ICP has to do is claim it. How she does that and what she does once she is there is important. The end product of role development includes the entire learning process. The ICP's ability to know that she is choosing how and what she is doing from moment to moment makes the ride much less bumpy.

Sixth, the ICP must learn to *take it one day at a time.* She can only live one day at a time and should do what she can today toward developing her knowledge base, self-awareness, and well-being. The future will reflect the integrity she has devoted to today's efforts.

Seventh, Selye[10] offers some good advice for the ICP: *"Fight for your highest attainable aim, but never put up resistance in vain."* Concretely, this means to be willing to discover, set, and obtain the highest ideals, goals, and values. When the ICP cannot go any further, think any more creatively, or lead another person in the direction she desires, she should not fight it. That same energy should be placed in a new channel that brings positive returns on the investment.

REFERENCES

1. Albrecht, K.: Stress and the manager: making it work for you, Englewood Cliffs, N.J., 1979, Prentice-Hall, Inc.
2. Carrington, P.: Freedom in meditation, Garden City, N.Y., 1978, Doubleday & Co., Inc.
3. Cooper, K.H.: The new aerobics, New York, 1975, Bantam Books, Inc.
3a. Cousins, N.: Anatomy of an illness as perceived by the patient, Boston, 1980, G.K. Hall & Co.
4. Dychtwald, K.: Bodymind, New York, 1977, Jove Publications, Inc.
5. Friedman, M., and Rosenman, R.H.: Type A behavior and your heart, New York, 1974, Fawcett Books.
6. Kinzer, N.S.: Stress and the American woman, New York, 1979, Ballantine Books, Inc.
7. Levinson, E.: Stress management to increase productivity, Palo Alto, Calif., 1981, Productivity Specialists.
8. Pelletier, K.R.: Mind as healer, mind as slayer, New York, 1977, Dell Publishing Co., Inc.
9. Porat, F.: Creative procrastination: organizing your own life, New York, 1980, Harper & Row, Publishers, Inc.
10. Selye, H.: The stress of life, rev. ed., New York, 1975, McGraw-Hill, Inc.
11. Simonton, O.C., Matthews-Simonton, S., and Creighton, J.: Getting well again, Los Angeles, 1978, J.P. Tarcher, Inc.
12. Toben, B.: Space, time, and beyond, New York, 1975, E.P. Dutton & Co., Inc.

SUGGESTED READINGS

Benson, H.: The relaxation response, New York, 1975, William Morrow & Co., Inc.
Davidson, J.: The physiology of meditation and mystical states of consciousness, Perspect. Biol. Med. **19:**345-379, 1976.
Farquhar, J.W.: The American way of life need not be hazardous to your health, New York, 1978, W.W. Norton & Co., Inc.
Hastings, A.C., Fadiman, J., Gordon, J.S., editors: Health for the whole person: the complete guide to holistic medicine, Boulder, Colo., 1980, Westview Press.
LeShan, L.: How to meditate, New York, 1974, Bantam Books, Inc.
Maslow, A.: Toward a psychology of being, New York, 1968, Van Nostrand Reinhold Co.
Moneysworth, May 26, 1975.
Pelletier, K.R.: Holistic medicine: from stress to optimum health, New York, 1979, Delacorte Press.
Selye, H.: Stress without distress, New York, 1974, J.B. Lippincott Co.
Shapiro, D., and Walsh, R.: Meditation: self-regulation strategy and altered state of consciousness, New York, Aldine Publishing Co. (In press.)

PART TWO

Skills

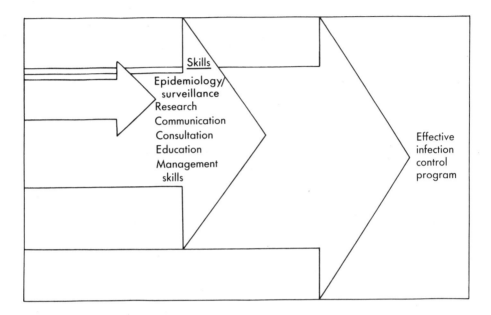

It is obvious that the infection control practitioner (ICP) accomplishes the job by using skills, both specific to infection control, such as epidemiology and surveillance, and universal, such as communication, management principles, consultative skills, research, and education.

In this section of the book each of these skills is illustrated, with specific examples provided for application to the unique role of ICP. Each of these areas is a book in itself. We have identified content that we have found *most* useful in practicing infection control. The reader is encouraged to use these chapters as beginnings. The more the reader develops these skills with effective application, the more effective the reader will be in the role of ICP.

7

PATRICIA LYNCH

Epidemiology and surveillance

epidemiology The study of the occurrence, distribution, and causes of disease in humans.
National Nosocomial Infection Study (NNIS) A large collaborative data pool organized and coordinated by the Hospital Infections Program of the Centers for Disease Control.
nosocomial infection An infection acquired during hospitalization.
surveillance "The systematic collection of pertinent data, the orderly consolidation and current evaluation of the data, and the prompt dissemination of the data to those who need it."[12]

Nosocomial infections represent a major hazard of hospitalization, the effects of which are felt by the infected patient, the family, and the economy. In countries where nosocomial infections are perceived to be a serious threat there is a trend toward developing infection control programs in hospitals.

In the United States support for such programs was initially derived from humanitarian concern. Long before accreditation required such action, some hospitals voluntarily supported innovative infection control programs financially and administratively. Subsequently, federal financial support could be withheld from hospitals failing to meet accreditation standards, which came to include specific recommendations for the infection control program.

One element of the federally mandated programs that was also felt to be important by voluntary programs was surveillance for nosocomial infections. Surveillance has been defined in several ways. The philosophy of the Centers for Disease Control (CDC),[12] as expressed by Langmuir, is that "surveillance is the systematic collection of pertinent data, the orderly consolidation and current evaluation of the data, and the prompt dissemination of the data to those who need it."

Moore[12] provides a second definition of surveillance: "monitoring of the patients, combined with monitoring procedures and practices in order to detect and eliminate factors which have been or may become determinants of infection."

Both definitions share the notion of systematically collecting, recording, and analyzing information about patients with infections to institute proper preventive and control procedures. Problems arise when one attempts to determine exactly how much time must be spent surveying, how much information must be recorded routinely, how extensive the analysis must be, and what control measures are really indicated by the data. In other words, how does a hospital get maximal benefit from surveillance?

The major purpose and benefits of the surveillance aspects of infection control programs today follow:

1. *To establish a system to evaluate the incidence of nosocomial infections and the factors that influence their development.* The system must be sufficiently sensitive in detecting nosocomial infections to determine a baseline rate with some validity. It must also be efficient enough to permit prompt recognition of changes from that baseline. Furthermore, the system should be specific for nosocomial infections, differentiating them from community-acquired infections and from noninfectious conditions. The time spent collecting and recording data should not be disproportionate to the value derived from the analysis, or the program will be placing too much emphasis on counting infections rather than preventing them.

2. *To identify hospital practices that may result in nosocomial infections.* Some practices can be clearly identified as unsafe without the need for further documentation of resulting infection, but some practices require quite a bit of scrutiny before a danger is recognized. For example, for years hospital employees have been diligently cleaning the urinary meatus of every catheterized patient two or three times daily with an antiseptic and then applying antiseptic ointment to the area. The recommendation to perform this time-consuming, costly, and rather personal procedure was based on the premise, unsupported by research, that some bacteria might be prevented from traveling up the catheter and causing infection. It became a standard of "good" practice until some investigators measured the effect by comparing two populations, one of which received the practice as described and the other of which did not. The investigators concluded that "rather than showing significant benefits, the treated groups frequently displayed higher rates of bacteriuria."[7] By performing such studies, investigators can measure the efficacy of infection control activities that have not been based on actual data.

3. *To meet national and local accreditation standards.*

4. *To use an epidemiological approach to evaluate infections and other events.* Epidemiology is a method or discipline for studying events or conditions in populations to understand them better and/or to determine causal relationships between risk factors and outcomes. Infectious diseases have long been characterized by epidemiologists, and nosocomial infection control is a logical extension of that experience.

   Other hospital events may benefit from epidemiological evaluation, but few hospital committees have become as proficient in epidemiological methods as infection control committees. Noninfectious events that lend themselves well to epidemiological analysis include surgical complications, major medication errors, health care planning for the future, and a host of other possibilities. For example, Trunet et al.[26] have recently published an article analyzing the role of iatrogenic complications as a precursor to admission to the intensive care unit of a hospital in France. The point is that unless information is collected systematically and then recorded and analyzed epidemiologically, relationships between certain events are never understood well enough for corrective or preventive measures to be applied.

5. *To provide direction for the infection control committee.* Control measures, strategy for continuing education emphasis, and other program objectives can be related to data generated from infection surveillance. When substantiated by such data, these program objectives will be more readily accepted by the committee and the hospital than if presented on the basis of theory alone or studies done elsewhere.

The intent of this chapter is to describe elements of surveillance and epidemiology and their practical applications in a hospital infection control program. It is written for the infection control practitioner (ICP) seeking to establish an effective program for the surveillance and prevention of nosocomial infections.

ESTABLISHING A SYSTEM OF SURVEILLANCE

The scope of surveillance is best determined by the ICP and the members of the infection control committee meeting together to discuss goals. The objectives for the program must be realistic for the particular hospital in terms of time available and other priorities. The purposes and uses of the collected, tabulated, and analyzed data should also be determined before a routine is established; it is more difficult to discontinue collection of information than it is to refrain from collecting it in the first place.

Comprehensive surveillance

In some hospitals, particularly those with fewer than 10,000 discharges annually, surveillance of all patients all of the time is a reasonable method to determine the baseline rates of infection. In larger or more complex medical centers the cost in personnel time for such a program may exceed the benefit. In such cases surveillance may focus on a specific, limited population for a specified period of time and then focus on another target group. In this way baseline data can be accumulated gradually for the entire hospital.

An advantage of total hospital surveillance is that the ICP and the infection control program become visible to all hospital employees; the employees will become more conscious of infection control, and the ICP will become acquainted with all of the nursing units, clinical departments, and services and with their unique potential for preventing infection risk. By determining the usual or baseline rates of infections, the infection control program will be able to recognize significant changes more readily. These rate changes may indicate that more specific information about the cases is needed to determine if the infections may be potentially preventable and if corrective measures are necessary.

The advantages of comprehensive hospital surveillance are balanced by disadvantages, chiefly the time necessary to perform the work. If surveillance regularly occupies most of the ICP's time, the program might be better served by focusing only on high-risk areas or specific types of infections. Prevention of infection problems should be the goal of the infection control program; surveillance is a tool to detect the problems.

The National Nosocomial Infections Study (NNIS)[15] is a large collaborative data pool organized and coordinated by the Hospital Infection Program of the CDC. The hospitals that participate range from small community nonteaching facilities to large tertiary centers. All participant hospitals perform comprehensive surveillance using somewhat similar methods and the same definitions and classifications of infection. Enormous amounts of data are generated that can provide a comparison base for hospitals willing to use the same methods and definitions. (NNIS will be referred to again later in the chapter.)

Selective surveillance

Comprehensive surveillance may not be suitable or cost effective for all hospitals because the disadvantages outweigh the advantages. Usually, limited surveillance programs monitor specific services in which patients may be at increased risk of infection, specific sites of infection that produce increased risk of patient morbidity, or specific departments in which high-risk patients receive care.

Some of the rationale for limiting routine monitoring is apparent in the results of the Study of the Efficacy of Nosocomial Infection Control (SENIC Project). Haley et al.[20] reported that in a stratified random sample of 169,526 adult patients from 338 hospitals, 71% of the nosocomial infections occurred in patients who had undergone surgery, and the risk of infection was increased significantly by other invasive procedures. Although pneumonia was the third most common nosocomial infection, preceded by urinary tract and surgical wound infections, it was the infection most frequently associated with patient death.

If much of the ICP's time is spent on routine surveillance, she may want to explore using one of the innovative methods described in the literature, which, by limiting the target population being monitored, attempt to get maximal information about serious or potentially preventable infections with minimal expense and effort. The ICP will want to select a method that is compatible with the infection control committee's objectives.

Prevalence surveys. Prevalence surveys for nosocomial infections are used to count all infections existing at a specific point in time, that is, cases with new onset and old cases. The number of infections prevailing in the hospital on a given day will usually exceed the number of cases with new onset; thus the prevalence rate will be higher than the incidence rate. If the ICP wishes to compare her hospital's infection rate with those of other hospitals, it is necessary for her to compare incidence rates with incidence rates and prevalence rates with prevalence rates. There are few published studies of nosocomial infections measured by prevalence survey, compared to the number of studies published that report incidence rates.

Prevalence surveys are particularly useful for determining the number of patients with specific risk factors present, such as urinary catheters. These data are often difficult to obtain, unless the ICP surveys the hospital and counts the patients.

Prevalence surveys may be quite tedious to perform because of the amount of chart review that must be completed in a short period of time. Latham et al.[22] describe the use of prevalence surveys in acute and chronic care facilities, and Britt et al.[8] reported on their experience with prevalence surveys in a group of small hospitals. The CDC[14] developed a protocol for performing prevalence surveys in hospitals, which has been used for years by the Hospital Infections Program. (The protocol can be obtained free of charge from the CDC.)[14]

Surveillance by service. Haley et al.[20] reported in the SENIC summary that 71% of all infections occurred in surgical patients, although surgical patients constituted only 42% of the patients in the study. Cruse and Foord[18] discussed their experience with surveillance of a surgical service, reporting on 62,939 patients with surgical wounds. The NNIS[15] reports on surgical infections in detail, so there is a comparison base available if the ICP selects this method for use in her hospital.

There may be an additional benefit in focusing surveillance on patients who have surgical procedures because many of their infections are potentially preventable, whereas many of the infections in patients on the medical services represent a failure of host defenses and may not be preventable.

Periodically performed comprehensive surveillance. Chelgren and LaForce[17] initially described performing comprehensive surveillance for 1 month and bacteremia monitoring for 2 months out of each quarter. Many ICPs have adapted this method in their hospitals. Some ICPs do comprehensive surveillance 1 month and monitor bacteremias the next month, believing that they are less likely to overlook an important trend or the beginning of an outbreak if comprehensive surveillance is reduced by half rather than by two thirds. The data obtained will still be comparable to other comprehensive surveillance reports because the definitions and methods are the same. The difference is the time interval during which comprehensive surveillance is performed.

If the ICP plans to monitor bacteremias, it is essential to determine that blood cultures are obtained in the hospital with enough frequency to be an indicator of sepsis.

Threshold method of detecting epidemics. McGuckin and Abrutyn[24] developed a system for detecting outbreaks of nosocomial infection from the laboratory rather than by performing comprehensive surveillance. This is an important distinction, since an epidemic detection system will not provide information about endemic levels of infection. If an infection control program has already generated information about endemic levels of infection and the ICP has already implemented and evaluated methods of reducing the endemic infection levels, she may not need to continue monitoring, except to detect unusual infections or outbreaks. The threshold method consists of calculating the expected number of different microbial isolates, based on past experience, and comparing the findings with the present experience. Investigations are performed when the number of isolates rises above the predicted threshold. For this system to be practical it is essential that enough nosocomial infections be cultured to accurately represent infection experience in a hospital.

Formulating objectives

Having considered the advantages and disadvantages of different surveillance systems, the ICP and the infection control committee should formulate definite long- and short-range objectives for the program. The following questions should be considered:

1. How long is comprehensive surveillance necessary?
2. If surveillance detects rates of infection that seem unacceptably high to the committee, how will the committee approach the situation?
3. How will the data be analyzed and by whom?
4. Will the surveillance be retrospective or concurrent?
5. Who will receive summaries and evaluations of the data?
6. Are the definitions of infection and the methods of collecting the data acceptable to most of the physicians?
7. How can the committee ensure that surveillance data are accurate enough to stand challenge? Validity is essential for credibility.
8. What will the procedure be for epidemic investigation?
9. What regularly collected information will the committee evaluate?

This is not an exhaustive list; undoubtedly other questions will arise during discussion. The members of the committee will be committed to aspects of the program they understand clearly, value, and play a part in developing, so the process is as important as the outcome. If the ICP is leading the discussion, she should review Chapter 9 on communication and role development and Chapter 8 on research before proceeding.

For illustration, a mythical infection control committee at Community Memorial Hospital, a 300-bed acute care teaching facility, has arrived at the following objectives:

1. The infection control committee will perform comprehensive, current surveillance of nosocomial infections for 1 year. If the time necessary exceeds half the ICP's available time, routine data collection will be discontinued in the units where the patients are at lowest risk for infection.

2. The committee will use the CDC's "Guidelines for Determining Presence and Classification of Nosocomial Infection"[13] as the definition base, publicizing these definitions at the medical staff section meetings. The committee will request that the medical records department become familiar with the definitions.

3. Monthly the committee will evaluate infections by site, service, pathogen, attending physician, and nursing ward and then compare these rates of infection by site, service, and pathogen to those reported by NNIS hospitals. When Community Memorial Hospital's rates differ from NNIS hospital rates substantially, the differences will be analyzed.

4. Summaries and evaluations of the data will be distributed to members of the infection committee and executive committee, staff section chiefs, and nursing department supervisors.

5. The ICP and a designated physician will review pertinent patient data until they agree on a diagnosis of infection by site in each patient approximately 90% of the time.

6. The efficiency of detection of the surveillance system will be evaluated by a prevalence study three times during the year.

7. When the circumstances of some nosocomial infections seem to warrant scrutiny, the investigation will be conducted by the ICP and the designated physician.

8. When the data suggest that the number of infections could be reduced, the committee will initiate or support a program to accomplish this.

With surveillance objectives this precise, the ICP can proceed.

METHODS

The first three objectives relate to data collection. The committee wishes to evaluate the incidence of nosocomial infection in all hospital patients. The number of new events, in this case nosocomial infections, in a particular population over a designated time period is termed *incidence*. By contrast, *prevalence* is a cross-sectional measure in which the total number of events, both old and new, is determined in the same population at a given point in time. Both methods measure the quantity of the event in the population, but incidence reflects new onset better, whereas prevalence weighs the total amount (incidence plus duration). Ongoing surveillance for nosocomial infections provides incidence data. Incidence may be expressed numerically as a rate:

$$\frac{\text{Number of new cases of disease}}{\text{Population at risk during specified time}}$$

Incidence rates for nosocomial infections are calculated as follows:

$$\frac{\text{Number of nosocomial infections}}{\text{Population at risk during specified time}}$$

The *numerator* in the equation is the number of infections that occurred, and the denominator is the number of persons exposed to the risk during a known period of time. In this case the risk factor is hospitalization. When converted to a rate, a calculation of the likelihood of occurrence of the event, the numerator is divided by the denominator and multiplied by whatever multiple of 10 permits the answer to be expressed as a whole number. In hospitals, incidence rates for nosocomial infection commonly use 100 as a rate base and are expressed as percents. The term *attack rate* is often used in place of incidence rate (different rate bases may be used in other calculations):

$$\frac{\text{Numerator}}{\text{Denominator}} \times 100 = x$$

$$\frac{13 \text{ infections}}{532 \text{ patients}} \times 100 = 2.4\%$$

Denominator population

The denominator selected should reflect the number of patients actually at risk; for instance, the denominator for surgical infections should be the patients who experienced a surgical procedure. The denominator may be either the number of admissions or number of discharges, whichever is more readily obtained, but the base should be used consistently. The denominator should include all patients, including those who expire, and may usually be obtained from the medical record department. The use of patient days as a denominator will provide valuable information, but so few hospitals use this denominator that comparison of rates would be difficult.

Patients have increased risk of developing infection after exposure to events that are more specific than simply being "in the hospital." Rates should be calculated to reflect these risks. The ICP will probably want to know the rate of infection for various services, such as gynecology or general surgery. To ensure that such denominators are valid it is essential that the diagnosis be the basis for determining the service classification and that the definitions of service be used consistently. Many record departments use Thompson and Hayden's service classification guide,[25] an excellent source for this purpose. Unfortunately, some hospitals use the specialty of the attending physician as the basis for determining the service classification. This practice results in the same diagnosis being classified in various ways: a female with low back pain admitted by an internist could be classified as "medical service," by an orthopedist as "orthopedics," by a neurosurgeon as "neurosurgery," and by a gynecologist as "gynecology," even though the disease and treatment were identical. This inconsistency should be corrected, particularly in smaller hospitals where six or seven misclassified patients could substantially affect the denominator. If the medical record department is unable to improve the accuracy of service classification, the ICP will have to use broad classifications.

Service classifications are more precise in identifying populations at risk than simply looking at the whole hospital, and the use of other denominators may narrow the focus even more. For example, the ICP might consider the case of a hospitalized patient who develops pneumonia. He is one of 1500 patients discharged in the month. He was one of 800 patients on the medical service. He was one of 100 patients cared for in the medical intensive care unit, and he was one of 30 patients who received mechanical ventilation. In this case, knowledge of the service does not describe risk well, except to clarify that the pneumonia was unrelated to surgery or anesthesia. Special denominators describe risk more precisely and are often useful in situations such as this. However, such denominators may be difficult to obtain, depending on what the risk factor is and how accurately certain records are maintained.

Numerators

The numerator is the number of nosocomial infections, defined as infections that were not present or incubating on admission to the hospital. This definition includes all nosocomial infections, whether caused by endogenous or exogenous agents or whether classified as preventable or nonpreventable. Using the number of infections rather than the number of patients as the numerator will reflect multiple infections in single patients. "Guidelines for Determining the Presence and Classification of Nosocomial Infections" is published by the CDC[13] as part of the "Outline for Surveillance and Control of Nosocomial Infections."

The site definitions the ICP's infection committee chooses should have some of the same characteristics as the surveillance system, that is, sensitivity, specificity, and consistency of application.

Austin and Werner[1] define sensitivity as the ability to identify and include all positive cases or other specified deviations; specificity is the ability of the definition to exclude all negative cases. The definitions should identify a specific infection accurately with measurable criteria. For example, if urinary tract infection is defined as the presence of dysuria and frequency, patients with bladder and urethral irritation will be mixed with those who have real urinary tract infections.

The definition must be sensitive enough to encompass most, if not all, of the situations it seeks to define. Using the same example, if urinary tract infection is defined as the presence of more than 100,000 colonies of a recognized pathogen in a patient with a previously negative culture, only patients who have been cultured at least twice will be considered; the definition is insensitive to the majority of urinary tract infections because few are cultured twice.

Consistency of application means that one is actually able to apply the definitions to all cases. If groups of patients are excluded, such as patients who were not cultured, the inconsistency will alter the statistics. It is worth emphasizing again that the committee must approve the definitions, make them acceptable to the majority of physicians, and distinguish between infection and colonization.

Clinical judgment

Applying the definitions accurately to the patient charts being reviewed is difficult for most inexperienced ICPs. The problem is that nurses and laboratory technicians receive little supervised practice assessing patient conditions and validating their judgments with a more experienced person; hence well-developed clinical judgment is often lacking. Because of this lack of experience in making assessments and having that assessment scrutinized and challenged, many health care workers are uncomfortable exposing themselves to the risk of being wrong.

The fact still remains that the ICP does have to develop good clinical judgment in the area of nosocomial infections. Without it, infections will be defined inaccurately, the infection control committee statistics will be invalid, and the ICP will be a poor technical resource for the staff and employees.

The ICP should begin to improve her clinical judgment by working with a physician or an experienced ICP until her classification of infection, using any patient's chart, agrees with the advisor consistently. The advisor need not be the chairman of the committee; however, the advisor should be someone who is competent, who the ICP is comfortable with, and who will agree to spend time with the ICP reviewing charts until proficiency is achieved. The ICP should present the case, including the classification of the infection and any control measures she would recommend, before the advisor's opinion is delivered. Experienced ICPs moving to a new hospital may find it necessary to go through the same process to be sure that they and the advisors agree on application of the definitions.

Community-acquired infections

In the objectives developed by Community Memorial Hospital it was decided to collect data on nosocomial infections only. This is not to say that the ICP should not be aware of patients with community-acquired infections and see that proper precautions are taken, but there is little value in collecting, recording, and analyzing data. The ICP may be responsible for reporting some of these infections to the local health department, and, if so, this should be specified in the job description for the ICP.

Sources of information

Generally it has been found that relying on physicians and nurses to notify the ICP about patient infections yields substantial underreporting. In all hospitals, large and small, it is essential that the ICP actively seek out the information rather than wait for it to come to her. This is time consuming, so the system for gathering the information should be as efficient as possible, relying on the best sources of information in the hospital and spending little time with unproductive sources.

Microbiology laboratory. In most hospitals the microbiology laboratory is one of the best sources; this is true in teaching centers where potential sites of infection are cultured at least once and often more frequently, and it is also true in smaller facilities where cultures are less common.

In the microbiology laboratory the ICP should share whatever clinical data she may have about patients whose specimens are being analyzed; the laboratory receives sparse information about patients, and this process can influence the quality of the workup. Sometimes the laboratory would like to know the patient diagnosis, the suspected infection, whether the patient was receiving antimicrobial therapy, and the urgency of the situation.

From the microbiologist or laboratory technician, the ICP hopes to learn about significant isolates already identified, interesting workups (particularly if they involve pathogens with a potential for cross infection), and isolates with unusual characteristics.

Some of this information may be available in the microbiology log book, if one is kept. If the ICP is unfamiliar with methods of identification or the significance of various isolates, this deficiency can be corrected by individual study and by working with and observing the microbiologist for awhile. An ICP who understands the importance of adequate specimens and the elements of identification, including the value of Gram stains of clinical material will gladden the hearts of the microbiology staff.[23] Because all patients with clinical infections will not be cultured in the average hospital, sources other than the laboratory will be necessary for more complete surveillance information.

Nursing stations. Patients are cared for on the nursing units, and it is essential that the ICP become familiar with patient care practices. Again, the ICP has information of value to nursing personnel and often requires information from them. Nurses receive laboratory reports they are occasionally unable to interpret. They lose track of what potential infections are being investigated in which patients, and they sometimes fail to initiate precautions or discontinue them promptly. If the ICP helps nurses address these problems regularly, the latter will be more willing to take time to discuss their patients and nursing practices.

Potential infections can be detected efficiently in most hospitals by checking the Kardex or a similar condensed record of the drugs and treatments received by a patient. The ICP should note the use of antimicrobial agents, infection precautions, or antiinfective treatments, such as wound irrigations. The ICP should review the charts of these patients swiftly and spend little or no time on charts with none of these indications.

The ease with which an ICP can evaluate clinical information depends a great deal on her experience and familiarity with common nursing practices, particularly those that involve invasive procedures or maintenance of indwelling urinary, pulmonary, or intravascular devices. If this is an area that the ICP needs to improve, reading nursing procedure books and spending some time working and observing care on a busy unit, such as an ICU, will help. Examining the nursing change of shift report or reading the written report prepared for nurse administrators can also be a valuable source of patient information.

In most hospitals nursing and laboratory services provide the best and most consistent information. There are articles describing experience with either one as the major source. Following are other good sources in the hospital:

1. *Personal contacts.* Informal verbal reports from nurses and physicians will increase as the ICP becomes identified with the infection control program.
2. *Radiology.* The radiology department may be a good source of information about patients with chest x-ray film suggestive of pneumonia, empyema, or tuberculosis.
3. *Pathology.* Information about autopsied patients who had infections is available from the pathology department; some of these infections may need follow-up among contacts, such as a patient with tuberculosis diagnosed at autopsy.
4. *Pharmacy.* The pharmacy generally is familiar with patients who are receiving newly prescribed antimicrobial agents or unusual treatment programs. In community hospitals the pharmacy also knows the prescribing patterns of many of the physicians.
5. *Medical records.* Medical records departments have the completed chart information; in some hospitals the ICP may find that physicians' notes are too sparse to constitute documentation until the chart is completed. Medical records personnel who are familiar with the definitions the ICP uses may identify infections in the charts they are reviewing and bring this information to the ICP's attention.

6. *Employee health.* Employee health service personnel should observe infections among employees that may be nosocomial and notify the ICP. The service should also inform the ICP of tuberculin conversions, employees with infections that have potential for widespread or patient morbidity, and the results of exposure follow-up in employees.

Discharged patients. As the length of hospital stay is reduced, more infections will first become apparent in patients who have been discharged. In some groups, such as normal newborns, uncomplicated obstetrical patients, and patients undergoing short-stay surgical procedures, infections will most often become apparent after discharge. Recently Burns and Dippe[9] reported that in their study 53% of surgical wound infections initially became apparent after the patients were discharged.

Outpatient clinics are an excellent source of postdischarge infection information if patients receive most of their follow-up care there. The ICP's interest in receiving information on nosocomial infections will be readily accepted, and the cooperation of the clinic staff will be gained if they understand why the information is needed. They need to be told the value of investigating sources of similar infections and their role in making information about the infections available. Even clinically minor infections may contribute valuable epidemiological information if a specific infection problem is being investigated.

In community hospitals patients may return to their private physicians or to the local emergency department when infections manifest. The emergency department log book may provide clues to nosocomial infections if the presenting complaints are recorded accurately. If surgeons and their office staff are acquainted with the potential benefits of having postdischarge nosocomial infection data available to the infection control program, they will frequently provide outstanding cooperation.

Visiting nurses may be seeing patients at home after their discharge from the hospital. If the local visiting nurse agency understands the value of information on nosocomial infections in discharged patients, and if it is easy for them to report the data, they will probably do so.

Information to collect routinely

The amount of information that can be routinely analyzed profitably is fairly small, so it is a good idea to collect and record only that information. Useful data include the patient's name, age, and sex; identifying number; service; nursing station; date of onset of the infection; site of the infection; pathogens isolated; antibiogram of pathogens; physician most responsible for direct care; and death of patient when infection contributed.

Additional information that is used in some institutions includes date of admission; prophylactic antimicrobial agents; antimicrobial agents used therapeutically; surgical procedures and the date performed; other predisposing factors, such as urinary catheters or respiratory therapy; host factors, such as diabetes, malignancy, or immunosuppression; and other comments.

Records

Most ICPs record their initial impressions in a workbook, on worksheets, or on plain or preprinted index cards before transcribing the final information to a line listing, margin punch card, or computer. Line listings display the information in a simple format, but when large numbers of infections are recorded, data retrieval becomes difficult, and the advantages of a sortable system become apparent. There are prepunched cards commercially available at reasonable cost (McBee, Indecks). The rapid technological advancement and price decreases in programmable small business computers make these devices practical for many hospitals. The ICP should investigate a variety of methods for data storage and retrieval.

A point to remember is that each unproductive chart reviewed, that is, a chart in which the patient does not have a nosocomial infection, lowers the total efficiency of the infection control program because it takes time away from more valuable activities. One way the ICP can determine the effectiveness of the surveillance system is to count the number of charts reviewed each month, and the number of nosocomial infections in the same month, and calculate a ratio from this. If the ICP finds that 10 charts are reviewed for each infection detected, the ratio is 1:10; in other words, 90% of the chart review time is unproductive, leaving a large margin for improvement.

Some programs continue to generate statistical data without examining the cost or the value of the information. In the previous example surveillance with a 1:10 ratio is very expensive. If the hospital has 20 infections a month, the ICP reviews 300 charts. At a cost of 5 minutes per chart, the time spent is 23 hours, 2.3 hours of which are productive. At the salary the average ICP earns, the financial impact quickly becomes apparent. Any method that will reduce the amount of time spent in unproductive chart review has value, and several articles describe innovative methods.[17,22,24,27]

Starting points

Cultures. In most teaching hospitals the frequency of culturing exceeds that of community hospitals, and there will be abundant microbiological data available. A surveillance system in which the chart of each patient with a "positive culture" is reviewed will result in much unproductive review time in a hospital in which culturing is extensive. In community hospitals, however, the microbiology laboratory is the most consistently reliable initial source of information about nosocomial infections.

Kardex. In a community hospital the frequency of culturing may be lower, and the ICP will rely on supplemental information sources. Wenzel et al.[27] describe a surveillance system that relies on Kardex review done weekly to detect patients likely to have infections. Their method is almost as reliable as the traditional multiple source method in their situation. Obviously this is only successful when the Kardex is kept up-to-date.

Pharmacy. In a hospital where antimicrobial use is restricted the pharmacy is a good starting point. The ICP should attempt to learn of patients started on antimicrobial therapy after 72 hours of hospitalization. If antimicrobial agents are widely used for unclear reasons, this system will not be effective.

EPIDEMIOLOGY
Analyzing routine surveillance data

Epidemiology is defined in various ways, but the word derivation is clear: *logia* means study or knowledge; *demos* means people; and *epi* means upon or to. Epidemiology is the knowledge of events that happen to people or the understanding of the ecology of those events. Historically, epidemiology has been concerned with infectious disease occurrence in the population, although chronic disease epidemiology is also a focus of many public health and research programs.

The ICP strives to understand the occurrence and distribution of nosocomial infections in the hospital population. By observing the infected and the uninfected in relation to each other, to the environment, and to the practices in their care, the ICP should be able to determine why certain infections developed and what can be done to prevent or control them.

Epidemiological methods

Epidemiological methods are descriptive, analytical, and experimental. The ICP will most often be using elements of descriptive epidemiology but will have need for knowledge of analytical and experimental methods also.[1,16,19] (See Chapter 8 for a classification of epidemiological approaches.)

Descriptive epidemiology observes "what" happened to "whom," "when," and "where." In the hospital setting it is concerned with determining incidence rates of nosocomial infections in the various subpopulations of the hospital. When descriptive epidemiology is expanded from the study of "who, what, when, and where" to address a determination of "how and why," it becomes analytical epidemiology. Experimental epidemiology seeks to answer questions about causality by manipulating risk factors or variables to change the outcomes.

Elements of descriptive epidemiology

Descriptive information can be "two-way tabulated" easily. Analyzing incidence by site of infection and medical service, or by site of infection and pathogen isolated, are examples of two-way tabulations. For analysis of three or more variables a computer is almost essential simply because of the mechanics involved.

A summary of the infections occurring in a month, which is normally prepared for the infection committee members and other interested persons, is an example of graphic display using descriptive epidemiology. The nosocomial infection summary on pp. 99-100 has much information, but it lacks visual appeal, and it is confusing. In addition, one month is a small sample in the life of the hospital, and there may not be enough infections (numerators) or patients (denominators) in a given group, such as the urology service, to analyze with any validity. The ICP should beware of drawing conclusions from scant information.

Statistical tables may answer several questions:
- How many infections occurred at each site?
- How many of each pathogen-site combinations occurred?
- How does the number of infections by site compare with those of other hospitals or to a standard (e.g., NNIS reports)?

The ICP reviewing a large number of sites and pathogens may want to convert the raw numbers to a percentage of the total.

Comparing rates

The ICP may wish to compare the hospital rates with those of another hospital. NNIS figures are ideal for this, since the pool of data from the participating hospitals is very large and the example hospital, Community Memorial, is a community teaching hospital. The NNIS hospitals use CDC definitions, and they perform total hospital surveillance in a manner similar to that described for Community Memorial. NNIS data are published twice a year and contain statistical information and detailed review articles on some aspects of infection control. The reports are available from the CDC.[15] NNIS reports the incidence of infection by site, service, and pathogen and also calculates what percentage of the total is represented by each kind of infection. This last item can be very helpful if the ICP suspects that the hospital's endemic rates are higher than another hospital's (or all hospitals') but an epidemic is not apparent.

Haley et al.[20] reported on the frequency of nosocomial infection at the four major sites in a stratified random sample of 169,526 adult, general medical and surgical patients. They determined that of all nosocomial infections identified in the study, 53% were urinary tract infections, 28% were surgical wound infections, 13% were pneumonias, and 6% were bacteremias. The ICP may wish to compare the experience at her hospital with that described in this study. A pie graph would draw attention to the difference between the ICP's hospital and the reported study (Fig. 7-1). The ICP and the committee can then see clearly how their experience differs from others or from that cited in the literature.

Nosocomial infection summary

Hospital discharges _____   _____ Month/year

Number of infections _____

_____ Rate   _____ Previous month

Service	Discharge	Infection	Rate	Urinary tract infection	Pulmonary	Surgical wounds	Other
Medicine							
General surgery							
Orthopedics							
Urology							
Gynecology							
Surgical specialty							
Pediatrics							
Obstetrics							
Newborn							

Sites and pathogens for nosocomial infections

Pathogens	Blood	Urinary tract	Upper respiratory tract	Lower respiratory tract	Gastro-intestinal	Burns	Surgical wounds	Gynecological	Other	Total
Candida species										
Escherichia coli										
Enterobacter species										
Enterococcus species										
Klebsiella species										

Continued.

Nosocomial infection summary—cont'd

Sites and pathogens for nosocomial infections

Pathogens	Blood	Urinary tract	Upper respiratory tract	Lower respiratory tract	Gastro-intestinal	Burns	Surgical wounds	Gynecological	Other	Total
Proteus indole +										
Proteus mirabilis										
Pseudomonas aeruginosa										
Other Pseudomonas species										
Serratia species										
Coagulase-negative staphylococci										
Coagulase-positive staphylococci										
Group A streptococci										
Gamma streptococci										
Streptococcus pneumoniae										
No pathogen										
No culture										
Total										

Total surgical procedures _____
Total surgical wound infections _____
Percent of patients developing wound infection _____

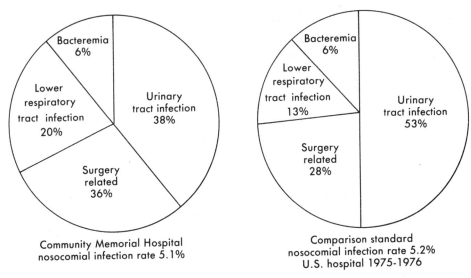

FIG. 7-1. Pie graphs comparing sites of infection as a percentage of the total. The comparison standard can come from the same facility or from another source, such as summaries of data reported by the National Nosocomial Infection Study. (Based on data from Haley, R., et al.: Am. J. Med. **70:**947-959, 1981.)

If the ICP at Community Memorial Hospital has developed an efficient system for gathering data, for recording it so that it can be retrieved when needed, for summarizing it, and for identifying the epidemiology of nosocomial infections in the hospital, there should still be sufficient time for her to put this surveillance data to work. The remaining infection control committee objectives from Community Memorial involve using the data.

Prevalence

Infection committee objective number six was to perform a prevalence survey at 4-month intervals. Prevalence refers to that which prevails at a point or period in time, in this case the sum of patients with nosocomial infection regardless of the time of onset. Because all charts of the survey population will be reviewed rather than just those with indications of infections, it can be assumed that the prevalence survey would be 100% efficient in detecting the information it seeks.

Some uses for prevalence studies follow:

1. The infections detected by the surveillance system (numerator) can be compared with the number of infections detected by the prevalence survey (denominator), and a rate of efficiency of detection can be developed. The charts of those patients with infections found on the prevalence survey but missed by the surveillance system can be reviewed. It is not

necessary for every infection to be detected by the surveillance system, but a representative sample should be. For example, if the prevalence survey found 100 infections, and the surveillance system found 80 of those infections, the system is 80% effective. If the missed infections are major, such as fatal uncultured pneumonia or suppurative phlebitis, the ICP should find a method of detecting those infections; if the infections are minor or already well represented in the surveillance data, the ICP may just let them go by.

2. It is reasonably easy to audit the use of antimicrobial agents, including the apparent indication for use, by prevalence survey. One can determine what percentage of patients received antimicrobial agents, how many drugs were prescribed, how many patients received multiple agents, and whether they were prescribed for therapeutic or prophylactic reasons.

3. Special procedure denominators, such as the number of patients with IVs or Foley catheters, can be gathered in this way if records are not available elsewhere.

4. Compliance with certain procedures can be evaluated if the records permit. If hospital policy states that peripheral IV sites are to be changed every 72 hours, the charts can be audited to see what percentage of patients have IVs for periods exceeding that recommendation.

The prevalence survey is a tool with some remarkable advantages for an infection control program. Of course there are a few disadvantages:

1. Few papers have been published recounting experience with prevalence data. For small community hospitals, the article by Britt et al.[8] is excellent.

2. The shorter the duration of the disease or event being audited, the more likely it is to be missed in a single prevalence survey.

3. Chart review is repetitive and boring. In community hospitals an estimate of 5 to 7 minutes review time per chart is reasonable. As the charts become more complex the review time increases, and occasionally a single large chart will take nearly an hour.

4. Prevalence surveys may not give the ICP a clear picture of incidence.

Once the ICP is familiar with the techniques, subjects that can best be examined by prevalence survey will become apparent and the practice may become firmly established with the infection committee and other quality review committees. Once the hospital is familiar with the technique, other departments may request assistance in designing prevalence surveys for their own needs or ask the ICP to audit "just one little thing" for them. It certainly furthers good public relations to comply whenever possible. However, the hospital gets maximal benefit if personnel from other departments learn to design and perform their own prevalence surveys.

A method for performing a prevalence study

1. Select the population. The charts of the population the ICP selects should take less than 2 days to review. In a large hospital, the ICP should survey units where patients are at greatest risk of acquiring infections, such as ICUs and surgical services or units where the endemic rates are believed to be excessive. She should try to schedule the review when the census is representative of usual experience. This will vary in the ICP's hospital; for example, if she wishes to review surgical services where the average length of stay is 6 days, with most operations performed early in the week, she should do the prevalence survey on a Friday or Saturday, not on Monday when most of the patients are newly admitted. The review should be done at a time of day when the charts are accessible, perhaps at night or in the evening.

2. Design worksheets so that the information may be summarized easily. The final summary should be able to be condensed to one page. Even interested readers appreciate conciseness, and those less interested will rarely read beyond one page.

3. Determine precisely what information to record for all patients. Some possibilities follow:
   a. Service classification
   b. Nursing unit
   c. Antimicrobial therapy classified as prophylactic if begun before surgery and discontinued within 48 hours; therapeutic if the drug is to treat an existing or suspected infection; or unclassified if the use does not meet either criterion
   d. Age of patient
   e. Culture performed
   f. Presence of predisposing factors such as Foley catheters and IVs

4. Determine the information to record for patients with infection apparent in the chart. Possibilities include the following:
   a. Name
   b. Service classification
   c. Nursing unit
   d. Age and sex
   e. Date of onset of the infection
   f. Site of the infection (with a new line for each infection)
   g. Status of the infection (current or inactive)
   h. Whether the infection is community acquired or nosocomial
   i. Culture results, including no culture and no pathogen isolated
   j. Antimicrobial use as described in number 3
   k. Admitting diagnosis
   l. Surgical procedures performed
   m. Any additional risk factors or special information

5. Conduct the survey. The ICP should then gather up her worksheets and go to the nursing unit. With the supervising nurse, the ICP can determine the number of patients on the unit by going over the daily census or the ward temperature sheet. The ICP may record by checking off names from the master list as she goes along. However, she should not attempt to track down charts of patients in surgery or other places. The ICP should record carefully and explain what she is doing to the nurses and physicians who are interested.

6. If the ICP is going to calculate the efficiency of detection by the surveillance system, she must save all of her worksheets, copies of the daily census, and anything else she might need. She should check the worksheets to be sure they are complete and then put the whole project out of her mind while she returns to her usual activities. She should try to resist the temptation to rush around doing supersurveillance or to copy on her surveillance forms all of the infections she detected on the prevalence survey. It is valuable to know how efficiently the normal surveillance system is at detecting infections. If the infections found on the prevalence survey are added to the surveillance figures, the surveillance system is not really being measured.

7. Complete the summaries and preparing the report. The CDC[14] has an excellent publication, "Prevalence Survey for Nosocomial Infections," which can be obtained without charge. The worksheets and summaries can be reproduced without infringing on a copyright. The forms probably will need to be changed a bit to fit specific needs, but the material in the publication is very helpful.

8. Calculate efficiency. When enough time has elapsed that usual surveillance methods have had a reasonable opportunity to detect all of the nosocomial infections that were present on the day of the prevalence survey, surveillance efficiency of detection can be calculated. This is done by comparing the number of individual infections present on prevalence survey (denominator) with those detected by surveillance (numerator). Efficiency of detection reported by participants in the Comprehensive Hospital Infection Project (CHIP), a federally funded study conducted from 1969 to 1971, often exceeded 80%, but that level is not always necessary, as long as the surveillance detects most infections consistently and does not have any major "blind spots." In addition to calculating the rate of efficiency of detection, the ICP should review the charts of patients missed by surveillance to see why they were not detected and determine whether a new source of information is necessary to fill the gap.

Economy of time and ease of performance makes the prevalence survey a valuable tool, one that is probably greatly underutilized in most infection control programs. It is an effective means of measuring total numbers of infections present, gathering information on specific denominators that may not be accessible by any other method, and evaluating a variety of practices. Performed frequently enough, prevalence surveys can be an efficient form of surveillance. Some hospitals are presently conducting routine surveillance by prevalence surveys performed every month.

The eighth objective developed by the infection control committee at Community Memorial Hospital involved initiating or supporting programs to reduce the incidence of nosocomial infections at specific sites or in target populations. Fig. 7-1 demonstrates the differences between the Community Memorial Hospital and SENIC summaries in the percentage of infections at specific sites. The infection control committee should consider whether a program to reduce the incidence of nosocomial pneumonia and surgical wound infections at Community Memorial would be productive. The hospital benefits when programs to change patient care practices can be developed in response to specific needs demonstrated by the data.

The infection control committee at Community Memorial also regularly reviews nosocomial infections by service and by pathogen and compares the results with a reference base. The committee also monitors the infection rates of patients of individual physicians and may compare them with the average rate or a reference base. The prevalence surveys review frequency of antimicrobial use and the apparent indications for use and may measure a variety of risk factors of the hospital. The purpose of examining any of these features is to identify those that might be improved and then to initiate and maintain efforts by the personnel and staff involved to anchor that improvement.

Epidemic investigations

Principles. Infection committee objective number seven at Community Memorial Hospital involved investigating potential epidemic situations. Surveillance is performed to determine the incidence of nosocomial infections so that the endemic or usual baseline can be recognized and deviations can be identified. An epidemic can be defined as an increase in incidence above the usual or expected level. When the ICP maintains records that clearly identify the site, pathogen, and date of onset of most nosocomial infections, the ability to distinguish between outbreaks and usual level of occurrence is greatly enhanced. Even with vigilant surveillance and good bookkeeping it is still difficult to make the distinction; therefore the ICP and the infection control physician must be familiar with some techniques for epidemic investigation. When a serious outbreak occurs, the pressure to solve the problem is considerable, and both the physician and ICP will wish they had practiced investigative techniques when the pressure was less.

Practice can be obtained by reviewing reports of investigations conducted by others and by diligently investigating every possible outbreak in the hospital. The ICP should start with book work if she has not conducted an investigation on her own. The problem investigations detailed in the back of the book *Epidemiology for the Infection Control Nurse*[3] provide excellent practice. No book can provide perfect recipe for conducting every investigation, and even skilled investigators occasionally are unsuccessful. Two factors that will influence success are the care with which the investigation is planned and the skills (practice) the investigators have.

The ICP should practice by investigating situations in which several patients develop infections with the same organism identified on culture. In many of these investigations she will find that the infections were unrelated and that there was little epidemic potential. The ICP will have gained valuable practice in planning and conducting the investigation and probably will have increased her ability to recognize serious problems.

Dixon[4] reported that in the CHIP study, approximately 9% of the nosocomial infections appeared to be part of an epidemiological cluster. The CHIP study hospitals averaged six clusters of infection for every 10,000 patients discharged. These were community hospitals, and it could be assumed that the incidence of clustering infections could be higher in university hospitals and other tertiary centers.

Two underlying principles associated with epidemic investigations are worth mentioning specifically. First, the goal of conducting the investigation is to try to identify the source as promptly as possible and to control the spread of disease within the hospital. Second, the investigator should have a clear picture of the chain of transmission of infections. For an infection to occur there must be a susceptible host, a suitable pathogen, and a mode of transmission so that pathogenic microorganisms can reach the susceptible host. One can interrupt this chain of transmission by removing any link.

The ICP will probably become aware of the occurrence of a cluster or potential outbreak of infection by detecting it through surveillance or by being informed by someone in the hospital that something unusual is occurring. The source of the information could be nursing staff, microbiology personnel, or others. As soon as it is apparent that a problem may require epidemiological investigation, the ICP should sit down with a cup of coffee, and calmly consider the available information, and begin to plan a strategy for conducting the investigation. Lack of initial planning seriously hampers successful epidemic investigation.

Methods. Briefly, the steps in conducting an epidemic investigation follow:
1. Evaluating the information already available and developing the initial plan
   a. Verifying the diagnosis on all cases reported
   b. Confirming the presence of a cluster of infections

    c. Informing those who need to know about the situation
    d. Instituting the control measures that seem appropriate, based on the information available
    e. Developing an initial case definition
2. Searching for more cases
3. Characterizing cases by time, place, and person
4. Formulating tentative hypotheses or theories about the relationship between risk factors and the infections
5. Testing the hypothesis
6. Instituting and evaluating the permanent control measures
7. Writing the report

Evaluating the information available. The information initially available will be incomplete. All cases of the infections will not have been detected, and any decisions that will be made based on the incomplete information should be considered tentative.

Frequently in the hospital when people suspect that an infection problem may be occurring, they tend to view unlike patient situations as if they were alike, which leads to incorrect estimates of the size and severity of the problem. It is essential that the chart of each patient reported to be part of the outbreak be reviewed to verify the diagnosis. From this careful review and confirmation of each case will come the initial case definition and the confirmation of the existence of a cluster of cases.

The information to be obtained from the charts will, of necessity, be fairly extensive and will require the development of a convenient form for recording and summarizing the data (see p. 108). Specific information sought should be sufficient to place the patient geographically in the hospital, to determine the risk factors preceding the onset of the infection, and to determine the time of onset of each infection.

Occasionally, an error in laboratory diagnosis will produce a pseudoepidemic. With the laboratory person who performed the identifications, the ICP should review the methods used and note whether there were any changes in media, methods, or nomenclature that might influence the appearance of an epidemic. Also, she should determine whether the specimens were worked up sequentially, possibly reflecting laboratory error.

When the cases have been reviewed and the information recorded, the ICP may wish to consult others within the hospital, to involve others in the investigation, or to simply inform them that a problem may be occurring. If the ICP is inexperienced, the advice of others in confirming the presence of a cluster of infection and in planning the subsequent steps to be taken is essential. Initially, the ICP should compare the incidence of the infection with the incidence in a comparable period of time before onset of the suspected problem, a month or a year ago, for example. If a cluster of infections seems apparent, an investigation will probably be necessary.

Prevalence survey sheet

Month/year _____

Patient name	Number	Service	Date of onset	Infected site	Pathogen 1 antibiogram	Pathogen 2 antibiogram	Surgery	Comments

Several of these initial steps may be taken more or less simultaneously. The ICP may be informing others of the problem, as well as seeking advice as she gathers information. Developing the case definition is a process that will be occurring as some of the other actions are taking place, but it is such an important aspect of planning the investigation that the ICP and the physician responsible for the infection control program will need to work together.

The case definition is a written statement of the features that describe the case or infection problem that is occurring so it can be recognized and differentiated from noncases. The initial case definition will include broad descriptions of the facts known about the cases at the time and will be revised to become more specific as more additional information becomes clarified. The case definition answers the following:

- *Who* is developing the infection
- *What* the infection appears to be (site involved, pathogen, antibiogram, or clinical signs and symptoms)
- *Where* in the hospital the program is occurring
- *When* the infections began and for how long the situation has existed

It is important that the case definition initially be sensitive enough to identify all cases of the disease. It is tempting to try to narrow the definition early to make the investigation more manageable, but it is more important to define only the facts known to be true and thus keep the scope of inquiry broad. As the investigation proceeds, the case definition will be revised periodically. Investigations that appear to require complex methods and outbreaks that apparently are involving rapid spread of infection or serious morbidity may need to be evaluated by another skilled investigator. Most state or local health departments are able to offer such assistance, and it would not be unreasonable for an ICP without much experience to seek assistance from them or to consult a more experienced ICP.

People who will need to be informed about the presence of the outbreak will vary, depending on the situation. If there is any question of legal responsibility on the hospital's part, that is, if the hospital is liable for the situation, the administrator should be informed immediately, and the hospital attorney may also wish to be involved. In addition, the chairman and other members of the infection committee should certainly be informed, and the chiefs of services or departments in which the cases are occurring should also be informed. There is little to be gained from broadcasting information to others that an outbreak or epidemic may be occurring.

Occasionally, at this stage of an outbreak investigation, breaks in technique may be the obvious source for the infections. In such cases control measures almost suggest themselves. When the preliminary investigation suggests strongly that this is the case, then very likely the ICP will not have to investigate further except to institute the control measures that seem to be appropriate and to evaluate their success.

Situations are rarely this clear, and more commonly the investigation will need to be carried several steps farther. Deciding not to investigate a situation may have major consequences, and it is a decision that merits cautious consideration.

Searching for more cases. Diseases may produce a spectrum of severity of illness, ranging from asymptomatic infection or colonization to fulminant disease. Usually patients who are severely affected will be the ones identified first in a preliminary evaluation of available data; however, it is important to identify patients with less severe disease who are also part of the cluster. This is done to define the extent of the problem and to describe accurately the factors associated with it. All cases are never found on the first preliminary investigation. It may be necessary to classify cases as definite and probable or infected and colonized for accurate identification. The case definition should be constructed to accommodate this.

It is necessary to determine where to look for the additional cases and also how far back in time to search. If the case definition is based on culture results, a search of the laboratory log or records will most quickly identify additional cases. If the case definition is based on observable signs and symptoms of infection, patient charts and reports from patient care personnel will be the initial source for the case search. The case search should include present and former patients, including patients who have expired. The patients should be from the locations and population identified in the case definition.

The decision about how far back in time to search for cases is more difficult than the decision about where to search. Initially, the ICP should try to go back until the first case is identified, or until there is an abrupt rise in incidence, indicating a change in the endemic level. When this point is reached, the search should go back another month in the same population, or back at least two incubation periods, if the disease has a known incubation period. If there is a question that seasonality may influence incidence, a comparable season should be reviewed.

There are some practical limitations regarding the case search. If the records are voluminous or the documentation is unreliable, this may limit the amount of review that is possible without outside help. In situations in which review demonstrates that the problem is endemic over a long time, a decision to limit the search at an arbitrary point may be made. All pertinent data from all the cases together should be listed in a fashion that will display patterns and be easily summarized.

Characterizing cases by time, place, and person

TIME. An incidence histogram or epidemic curve will display the time of onset of each infection and can also be used to compare the epidemic period with a normal period. The vertical axis (ordinate) of the graph records number of cases, and the horizontal axis (abscissa) can record the date or hour of onset of each case. One square represents one case. The pattern of occurrence becomes clear when displayed in this way, and sometimes surprising information related to time emerges.

Experienced epidemiologists can determine the incubation period of a disease from a histogram and the nature of the disease, whether it is from a common source or transmitted by person-to-person contact. Fig. 7-2, A, with its sharp increase suggests that the victims were all exposed to a common source of infection at about the same time, whereas those in Fig. 7-2, B, probably

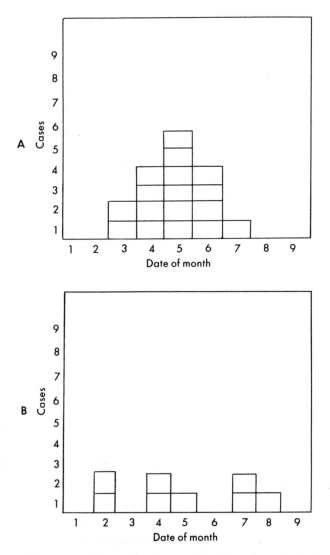

FIG. 7-2. A, Incidence histogram or epidemic curve suggesting a short incubation period, possibly a disease from common exposure. **B,** Incidence histogram or epidemic curve showing a few sporadic cases, suggesting an intermittent source or person-to-person spread.

acquired their infections from a sporadic source or by person-to-person spread.

Sometimes learning the reason for a gap in the cases on the horizontal axis is helpful, since the absence of cases may mean that the source of infection was absent the length of the incubation period. This is useful when risk factors are being analyzed.

PLACE. The geographical location of the patient at the presumed time of exposure, rather than the date of onset of the infection, is the important information to extract. In a large outbreak a diagram of the hospital may be necessary. More commonly this is unnecessary, and diagrams of small units such as the ICU or patient rooms on the nursing floor will be appropriate.

PERSON. This emphasis entails all the significant features of patients who acquired the infections (host factors), as well as all the features of the animate and inanimate environment that may become risk factors. This information can be displayed in a sortable, summarizable fashion, as shown in Table 7-1. It is essential to identify all the potential risk factors.

When all the information is recorded, the ICP can begin sorting the data by various risk factors to detect patterns. As the work proceeds, some information may need further investigation because of incomplete records or because more questions have been raised by the process of arranging and rearranging the data. The ICP should use whatever techniques suggest themselves to help clarify the patterns; many people use colored pencils, symbols, or summary sheets for this work because it makes the different important features stand out.

Attack rates may be calculated for the various factors at this point, with careful attention paid to obtaining the correct denominators for each calculation. There will always be several factors, such as persons, procedures, or supplies, that seem to figure prominently in the numerators but that become insignificant when placed with their proper denominator. For example, finding that the same operating room was used by nine out of ten patients who subsequently developed wound infection is interesting. The ratio for the risk factor, 9:10, can be computed as a rate:

$$\frac{9 \text{ cases exposed to risk factor}}{10 \text{ total cases}} \times 100 = 90\%$$

This looks very impressive. If, when searching for the correct denominator, the room was found to have been used for six cases a day for the entire time for a denominator of 360 procedures, 351 of whom did not get infected, the original rate becomes less impressive:

$$\frac{9 \text{ cases}}{360 \text{ at risk}} \times 100 = 2.5\%$$

It is always important to ensure that the denominators are valid, and it is absolutely essential to do so when the numbers being manipulated are small. The cases are included in the denominator, and all the individuals in the

TABLE 7-1. Seven patients with group A streptococcal infections*

Patients	Room	Site	Operating room 2	Operating room 3	MA-2 respirator 1	MA-2 respirator 2	Bronkosol	Saline (3%)	Surgeon A	Surgeon B	Anesthesiologist 1	Anesthesiologist 2	Assistant 1	Prep solution 1
Smith	418	WD	+	−	−	+	+	+	+	−	+	−	+	−
Jones	419	WD	−	+	−	+	+	+	+	−	+	+	+	−
Brown	420	LR	+	−	+	−	−	+	+	−	+	−	−	+
Black	418	WD	+	−	−	+	+	−	−	+	+	+	−	+
Ford	516	LR	+	−	−	+	+	+	+	−	+	−	−	+
Johnson	317	WD	−	+	−	+	−	+	+	−	+	+	+	−
Leckner	424	WD	+	−	−	+	+	−	+	−	+	−	−	+
Risk factors			$\frac{5}{7}$	$\frac{2}{7}$	$\frac{1}{7}$	$\frac{6}{7}$	$\frac{5}{7}$	$\frac{5}{7}$	$\frac{6}{7}$	$\frac{1}{7}$	$\frac{7}{7}$	$\frac{3}{7}$	$\frac{3}{7}$	$\frac{4}{7}$

*Key: WD, wound infection; +, risk factor present; −, risk factor absent; LR, lower respiratory.

denominator should meet the stated criteria and be at risk in the situation.

Close contact with a risk factor is more likely to be associated with an infection than with transient contact; the more peripheral a contact is, the less likely it is to be associated with infection. Air, furniture, sink traps, floor covering, walls, examination tables, and flower vases are examples of peripheral items. Although pathogenic microorganisms may be recovered from them, they are seldom responsible for infections and should rarely be the primary focus of an investigation. Selected microbiological sampling may be indicated and may add to the pool of information known; however, broad, undirected culturing never solves epidemiological puzzles and often actually hinders the investigation by providing confusing data.

Formulating hypotheses to explain infections. The hypothesis is the unproven theory or educated guess about infections and associated risk factors. The hypothesis or hypotheses should explain why some patients became infected and why others did not. It should be logical and consistent with the known epidemiology of the disease, and it should hold true for the cases investigated. The hypothesis should integrate the information regarding the infectious agent, the source of the organisms, and the mode of transmission.

Intervention to terminate the outbreak can be directed at interrupting the transmission or removing the source. If the hypotheses suggest that a risk factor may be associated with the infections, the risk factor should be eliminated as quickly as possible. Intervention should be prompt and vigorous, and the first test of the hypothesis is whether the infections cease. If the risk factor has been correctly identified and the intervention is successful, energetic surveillance for a recurrence of the problem is all that is necessary to test the hypothesis pragmatically.

Testing the hypothesis. There are several reasons for continuing the investigation to confirm an association between a suspected risk factor and subsequent infections. If the outbreak was unusual in the agent, source, or mode of transmission, publication of the results of the investigation should be considered. If the investigation points to a larger problem or if litigation or political pressure is a factor, the hypothesis should be tested. If the investigator would prefer to have the remaining loose ends tied up neatly, or if it is still difficult to determine that the problem is under control, the hypothesis should be tested. The hypothesis to be tested may be selected because it is the one most likely to be correct or because it is the one easiest to test.

There are several methods of testing most hypotheses, and selection of the proper method in a given situation may be influenced by cost, available assistance, and the benefits to be gained by using a specific method. Some methods are more precise and reproducible than others.

If the hypothesis is that a break in technique is responsible for the problem, the ICP may test the hypothesis by using one or more of these methods:

1. Questioning employees about how they perform the procedure. Employees who do not know how to perform correctly will be identified, but employees who do know the correct method and still fail to perform correctly will not be identified.
2. Observing employee performance directly.
3. Simulating the technique in question. If the procedure as it may be performed is potentially dangerous to patients, using a training device or other controlled condition may be useful.

If the hypothesis is that a human or other source in the environment is associated with the outbreak, careful culturing to isolate the implicated organism from the suspected source may be sufficient to test the hypothesis.

These methods are pragmatic and economical for use in hospitals much of the time; when performed carefully, they will be sufficiently reliable methods. If publication is being planned, if it is difficult to sort out several likely hypotheses, or if the hypothesis cannot be tested by the more direct methods, a case-control study should be considered. The purpose of the study is to determine whether the suspected risk factor occurs more frequently in the cases (those who have the infections) than in the controls (a sample of similar patients who do not have the infections).

Case-control studies. For the purposes of epidemic investigations a retrospective case-control study will be the most inexpensive and accurate way to test the hypothesis. In a retrospective case-control study chart review evaluates the differences in host or risk factors between the two groups. Infection has already occurred.

The control group may be selected on a randomized basis, or it may be matched with the cases for host factors, such as age, sex, and diagnosis, and for risk factors, except for the suspected causal factor.

The degree of care necessary for matching the cases and controls depends on how difficult it will be to get enough observations to ascertain the importance of the suspected factor. Generally, if it has been necessary to proceed this far with an investigation, it will be important to match the cases and controls carefully for all pertinent susceptibility factors and for factors such as time and location. The suspected cause of the infections is the variable being measured. In addition, a large enough control population to ensure several observations of each variable being measured is important. If there are many possible controls and few variables to match, the matching may not be necessary. The ICP can increase the number of controls to compensate and may select the controls on a random basis. This may be done by assigning consecutive numbers to the total group of possible controls and selecting the sample numbers from a table of random numbers, available in the appendix of most statistics textbooks. Other facets of randomizing are discussed in Chapter 8.

When the control charts have been selected and reviewed, data may be recorded on forms similar to those described earlier. The case group findings will be compared with those of the control group, using statistical formulas to determine whether significant differences are present. Several tests for significance may be suitable for this analysis, but the average ICP probably only needs to be familiar with the 2×2 contingency table from which to calculate a chi-square value and t tests for differences between means to ensure equivalency of case and control groups with respect to age, length of stay, and other factors. A chi-square or 2×2 contingency table allows one to compare two groups, one with infection and the other without, on the basis of their exposure to a single risk factor. The frequency of infection in the control group that is not exposed to the risk factor is established and then compared with the frequency of the event in the case group. If the groups are really alike except for their exposure to the risk factor, it may be reasonable to assume that there is an association between that factor and subsequent infections. Some difference between the expected value (control group) and the case group could be attributed to chance. The purpose of validating the data statistically is to show that the difference between the two groups is not likely to be caused by chance alone because the frequency of occurrence of the infections is greater than coincidence would allow. This sounds as if it should be so obvious that one could easily detect significant differences between the groups, but that is not so. Additionally, the ICP will often be dealing with small numbers that are even more difficult to interpret than large ones.

Constructing a 2×2 table is explained in some detail in Chapter 8, which also includes the method for calculating the chi-square value. Several other authors will be of substantial help at this point.[3,4,10,11,16]

For example, an investigation has begun to determine the source of seven group A streptococcal infections on the thoracic surgery service. Table 7-1 lists the patients and the risk factors. If the patient was exposed to the risk factor, a plus sign is entered in the appropriate box; if the patient was not exposed to the risk factor, a minus sign is entered. Several risk factors seem overrepresented on the vertical column: column 6, the MA-2 respirator 2; column 9, surgery A; column 11, anesthesiologist 1. Several questions should be answered by further investigation, assuming that the investigator has already verified the cases, searched for more, and characterized the cases by time, place, and person.

More of the cases were exposed to anesthesiologist 1 than any other risk factor, so the first questions focus on this. To determine whether any infection existed in the rest of this anesthesiologist's cases, all or a representative sample of these cases should be reviewed. The ICP can interview the anesthesiologist to learn whether he has a health history of pharyngitis, skin infections, or any perianal disorders. Since group A streptococcal colonization occurs most frequently at these sites, cultures should be taken. In this case the controls will be drawn from the total of other surgical cases and matched for all factors except exposure to the anesthesiologist.

The ICP can assemble the completed information on a 2 × 2 table, assuming that anesthesiologist 1 only worked with these patients and no others and no other streptococcal infections were found.

	Streptococcal cases	Controls
Risk factor present	7	0
Anesthesiologist 1	a	b
Risk factor absent	0	7
	c	d

As expected, the large numerical values are in cells a and d. In a situation less clear, such as the example in Chapter 8, it is impossible to tell with certainty whether the risk factor is significant unless further statistical tests are performed.

Writing a report. The ICP should describe the problem investigated, the methods used, the results, and the implications for the patient care practices that were involved and for those that are similar. This report should be distributed through the infection committee to everyone who was interested in the investigation or who assisted, as well as those who should have been interested or need to know for other reasons. As much attention as possible should be focused on the importance of the control aspects and the investigation. The program will benefit from the attention and increased support.

SUMMARY

Nosocomial infection control programs presently exist in most U.S. hospitals, either by choice of the facility or mandate of the Joint Commission on the Accreditation of Hospitals, or a combination of both. Most of these programs attempt to reduce the incidence of infection by (1) collecting and recording information about infections and the people who acquire them, (2) analyzing the information to identify probable causes of some of the infections, and (3) instituting control measures designed to prevent transmission of infections to susceptible patients. These methods are based on sound epidemiological principles and will produce an effective program when the ICP and the other members of the infection control team understand and apply them.

REFERENCES

1. Austin, D.F., and Werner, S.B.: Epidemiology for the health sciences, ed. 2, Springfield, Ill., 1978, Charles C Thomas, Publisher.
2. Axnick, K.J.: Surveillance of nosocomial infections. In Barrett-Connor, E., et al., editors: Epidemiology for the infection control nurse, St. Louis, 1978, The C.V. Mosby Co.
3. Barrett-Connor, E., et al., editors: Epidemiology for the infection control nurse, St. Louis, 1978, The C.V. Mosby Co.
4. Bennett, J.V., and Brachman, P.S., editors: Hospital infections, Boston, 1979, Little, Brown & Co.

5. Binger, J.L., and Jensen, L.M.: Lippincott's guide to nursing literature—a handbook for students, writers and researchers, Philadelphia, 1980, J.B. Lippincott Co.
6. Britt, M.R., Schleupner, C.J., and Matsumiya, S.: Severity of underlying illness as a predictor of nosocomial infection, J.A.M.A. **239**:1047-1051, 1978.
7. Britt, M.R., et al.: The noneffectiveness of daily meatal care in the prevention of catheter associated bacteriuria. In American Society for Microbiology: Abstracts from the Sixteenth Interscience Conference on Antimicrobial Agents and Chemotherapy, Chicago, 1971, The Society.
8. Britt, M.R., et al.: Infection control in small hospitals: prevalence surveys in 18 institutions, J.A.M.A. **236**:1700-1703, 1976.
9. Burns, S., and Dippe, S.: Postoperative wound infections detected during hospitalization and after discharge in a community hospital, Am. J. Infect. Control. **10**:60-65, 1982.
10. Castle, M.: Hospital infection control: principles and practice, New York, 1980, John Wiley & Sons, Inc.
11. Castle, M., and Mallison, G.: Effective investigations of nosocomial outbreaks, A.P.I.C. Journal **5**:13-16, June 1977.
12. Centers for Disease Control: Proceedings of the first international conference on nosocomial infections, Atlanta, August 3-6, 1970.
13. Centers for Disease Control: Outline for surveillance and control of nosocomial infections, Atlanta, rev. June 1972, Hospital Infections Program, Centers for Disease Control.
14. Centers for Disease Control: Prevalence survey for nosocomial infections, Atlanta, rev. March 1980, Hospital Infections Program, Centers for Disease Control.
15. Centers for Disease Control: National nosocomial infections study reports, Atlanta, Hospital Infections Program, (published annually), Centers for Disease Control.
16. Chavigny, K.H.: Descriptive biostatistics. In Barrett-Connor, E., et al., editors: Epidemiology for the infection control nurse, St. Louis, 1978, The C.V. Mosby Co.
17. Chelgren, G., and LaForce, M.: Limited periodic surveillance proves practical and effective, Hospitals **52**:151-154, 1978.
18. Cruse, P., and Foord, R.: The epidemiology of wound infection, Surg. Clin. North Am. **60**:27-39, 1980.
19. Friedman, G.D.: Primer of epidemiology, ed. 2, New York, 1980, McGraw-Hill, Inc.
20. Haley, R., et al.: Nosocomial infections in U.S. hospitals, 1975-1976, Am. J. Med. **70**:947-959, 1981.
21. Joint Commission on Accreditation of Hospitals: Accreditation manual for hospitals, Chicago, 1982, The Commission.
22. Latham, K., et al.: The prevalence survey as an infection surveillance method in an acute and long term care institution, Am. J. Infect. Control **9**:76-81, Aug. 1981.
23. Lennette, E.H., Spaulding, E.H., and Truant, J.P., editors: Manual of clinical microbiology, ed. 2, Washington, D.C., 1974, American Society for Microbiology.
24. McGuckin, M.B., and Abrutyn, E.: A surveillance method for early detection of nosocomial outbreaks, A.P.I.C. Journal **7**:18-21, March 1979.
25. Thompson, E., and Hayden, A.: Textbook and guide to the standard nomenclature of diseases and operations: guide to service classification, Berwyn, Ill., 1967, Physicians Record Co.
26. Trunet, P., et al.: The role of iatrogenic disease in admissions to the intensive care units, J.A.M.A. **244**:2617-2620, 1980.
27. Wenzel, R.P., et al.: Hospital acquired infections. I. Surveillance in a university hospital. Am. J. Epidemiol. **193**:251-260, 1976.

8 MARGUERITE M. JACKSON

Research

analytical study The process of making comparisons.
case-control study Identifies individuals who already have a particular disease and compares them with those individuals who do not have the disease; frequency of characteristics is also assessed.
cohort study Assesses whether people develop diseases more frequently when they display specific characteristics.
descriptive study Shows distribution of disease by describing events in terms of the person affected, the place the event occurred, and the time frame involved.
experimental epidemiological study Deliberate manipulation of a population by exposing part to a proposed risk or benefit factor and leaving another part unexposed.
SENIC Study on the Efficacy of Nosocomial Infection Control.

For infection control to be effective, practitioners (ICPs) must understand the epidemiology of nosocomial infections and identify techniques that can change the epidemiology of the nosocomial infection. There are many unanswered questions and unquestioned answers in infection control practice today.

The Study on the Efficacy of Nosocomial Infection Control (SENIC Project)[1] is a large-scale effort to answer some of these questions and reevaluate some accepted practices. Results from this study will be published for the next several years and will provide guidance for the future of infection control programs.

Additional questions will be answered through research at the clinical level. Clinical research is especially pertinent in such areas as the nature of antimicrobial resistance within and between various microorganism groups.

Traditionally, most infection control research has been conducted and published by physicians and medical microbiologists in large teaching institutions. This chapter is presented to suggest ways that the ICP can make valuable contributions to the field of nosocomial infection epidemiology through research in her setting.

Before beginning the "how to" section, it is appropriate to review briefly the current state of the art and some expectations for the next decade.

PERSPECTIVES FROM THE 1970 AND 1980 INTERNATIONAL CONFERENCES

At the First International Conference on Nosocomial Infections in August of 1970 Kass[35] described the three functional levels of infection control programs. At the first level are those measures *proven* effective; at the second level are practices considered prudent on the basis of strongly suggestive evidence; at the third level are measures of dubious value that are often expensive in time and materials. In 1970 most components of infection control programs fell into levels two and three.

At the Second International Conference on Nosocomial Infections a decade later Eickhoff[27] challenged participants to assess the technological progress made to date and, in the coming decade, to upgrade more practices into level one based on controlled studies.

At the 1980 Association for Practitioners of Infection Control (APIC) Seventh Annual Educational Conference, it was announced that new Centers for Disease Control (CDC) guidelines would include recommendations categorized by the following ranking scheme*:

> *Category I: Strongly recommended for adoption*†
>> Measures in Category I are strongly supported by well-designed and controlled clinical studies that show effectiveness in reducing the risk of nosocomial infections or are viewed as useful by the majority of experts in the field. Measures in this category are judged to be applicable to the majority of hospitals—regardless of size, patient population, or endemic nosocomial infection rate—and are considered practical to implement.
>
> *Category II: Moderately recommended for adoption*
>> Measures in Category II are supported by highly suggestive clinical studies or by definitive studies in institutions that might not be representative of other hospitals. Measures that have not been adequately studied, but have a strong theoretical rationale indicating that they might be very effective are included in this category. Category II measures are judged to be practical to implement. They are *not* to be considered a standard of practice for every hospital.
>
> *Category III: Weakly recommended for adoption*
>> Measures in Category III have been proposed by some investigators, authorities, or organizations, but, to date, lack either supporting data or a strong theoretical rationale. Thus, they might be considered as important issues that require further evaluation; they might be considered by some hospitals for implementation, especially if such hospitals have specific nosocomial infection problems or sufficient resources.

Shortly thereafter at the Second International Conference on Nosocomial Infections, Dixon[26] again emphasized these criteria and urged participants to

*From Centers for Disease Control: Guidelines for the prevention and control of nosocomial infections, Atlanta, 1981, 1982, and 1983, Guidelines Activity, Hospital Infections Branch, Bacterial Diseases Division, Center for Infectious Diseases, Centers for Disease Control.

†Recommendations that advise against the adoption of certain measures can be found in the guidelines. These negative recommendations are also ranked into one of the 3 categories depending on the strength of the scientific backing or opinions of the members of the working group. A negative recommendation in Category I means that scientific data or prevailing opinion strongly indicate that the measure not be adopted. A negative recommendation in Category III means that, given the available information, the measure under consideration should probably not be adopted; such a measure, however, requires further evaluation.

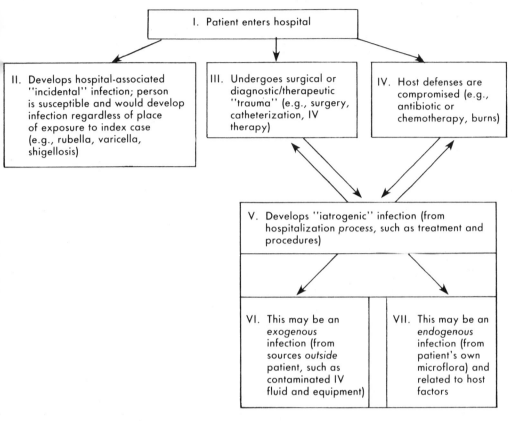

FIG. 8-1. Various sources for infections classified as nosocomial.

design controlled studies to answer questions about the efficacy of certain infection control practices. At the same conference Axnick[6] encouraged participants to look to the behavioral sciences for studies of communication patterns, management skills, motivation factors, and other techniques that contribute to behavior and behavioral change. Such areas need to be explored in the next decade to increase the effectiveness of infection control programs.

UNANSWERED QUESTIONS AND UNQUESTIONED ANSWERS

Fig. 8-1 illustrates one way to categorize nosocomial infections. The following outline lists a number of potential research questions arising from the categories in Fig. 8-1 and elsewhere. (Many of these problems were posed at the Second International Conference on Nosocomial Infections; others are suggested by Chavigny.[17]) Some of the questions have been answered and several are under investigation, but most still await controlled studies to solve them.

The list is not intended to be exhaustive but only to stimulate thought:

   I. Patient enters hospital: problems for investigation
      A. What are *patient* characteristics most frequently associated with nosocomial infections?
      B. What are *hospital* characteristics most frequently associated with nosocomial infections?
      C. What physical layout for a hospital ward or intensive care unit promotes infection control effectively? How will this be measured?
      D. Is there a clinically relevant association between length of stay and infection rate?
      E. Is there an important association between preoperative length of stay and infection rate?
      F. What patient characteristics are most frequently associated with preoperative length of stay?
      G. What is the mean increase in length of stay, stratified by prognosis, compared to the category of nosocomial infection? What is the cost of this prolonged hospitalization?

  II. Patient develops hospital-associated *incidental* infection: problems for investigation
      A. Will an employee immunization program reduce the risk of patients and employees contracting certain communicable diseases (e.g., rubella, influenza)?
      B. Will a preadmission screening program for pediatric admissions reduce the risk of patients and employees being exposed to certain childhood diseases (e.g., varicella)?

III. and V. Patient undergoes surgical or diagnostic/therapeutic *trauma* and develops *iatrogenic* infection: problems for investigation
      A. What is the rate of phlebitis associated with IV therapy in the hospital? What variables affect this rate? How can the rate be reduced?
      B. Is there an association between urinary catheterization and urinary tract infection rate? How direct is this association?
      C. What is the efficacy of daily urinary meatal care regimens for nosocomial urinary tract infections?
      D. Is there an association between the use of respiratory therapy devices and lower respiratory tract infections?
      E. What proportion of iatrogenic infections in this category can be prevented? How? How will this be measured?

 IV. and V. Patient's host defenses are compromised and he develops *iatrogenic* infection: problems for investigation
      A. What are the antimicrobial prescribing patterns by physi-

cians on staff for certain types of patients? Are patterns appropriate when compared with recommendations based on controlled studies?

B. What is the infection rate among patients on specific chemotherapy regimens? What factors affect infection in these patients? How will these factors be measured?

C. Are certain procedures or treatments associated with a higher infection rate in immunocompromised patients versus normal patients?

D. Can selected preventive measures reduce infection rates in immunocompromised patients, thus increasing survival from underlying diseases?

E. How can patients who are especially susceptible to nosocomial infections be identified?

F. What proportion of iatrogenic infections in this category can be prevented? How? How will this be measured?

VI. Patient develops *exogenous* infection: problems for investigation

A. Can the use of a "special" precautions system for patients with multidrug-resistant organisms reduce cross-contamination to other patients?

B. When an unusual microorganism is identified from several patients in the hospital, what is its source(s) and mode of transmission?

C. When an outbreak occurs in a particular unit in the hospital, what is/are its source(s)?

D. Can surveillance of selected discharges to long-term care facilities reduce the risk to other patients there of acquiring multidrug-resistant organisms? How will this be accomplished?

E. Can the use of private rooms for patients with superficial wound infections reduce the risk of cross-contamination to other patients? How will this be measured?

VII. Patient develops *endogenous* infection: problems for investigation

A. Will suppression of patient's normal bowel flora before bowel surgery modify patient's risk of infections?

B. Will a particular skin preparation regimen before surgery affect infection rate (e.g., antiseptic scrubs; clipping versus shaving)?

C. What are factors responsible for or related to colonization of the urethra with gram-negative organisms?

VIII. Additional problems for investigation
   A. What motivates patient care personnel to practice infection control techniques? How can this be measured?
   B. What management styles are effective for the ICP? How can this be measured?
   C. What methods are effective for teaching employees infection control information? How can this learning be measured and evaluated?
   D. In what other areas of hospital risk management can epidemiological methods be applied?
   E. What are the environmental and occupational risks of the hospital environment?

Examples of problems that have already been addressed by epidemiological studies include those pertaining to length of stay, urinary tract infections associated with urinary catheterization, and various outbreak investigations that pinpointed a common source. More difficult are questions that require evaluation of multiple patient and hospital variables or risk factors. Such studies require experimental, analytical, and statistical techniques (e.g., multivariate analysis) beyond the scope of this chapter and beyond the resources of many infection control programs.

Because infection control is a multidisciplinary effort, it involves the shared responsibility of many individuals. Rarely are research projects accomplished by a single individual, although small studies and outbreak investigations may be accomplished by the ICP with limited outside help. The ICP may recognize the problem, initiate the investigation, and see the project through to completion; however, cooperation and assistance from the infection control committee, the hospital epidemiologist (if there is one), the microbiology laboratory, the hospital's nursing and medical staff, a medical librarian, a statistician, and others may be required to complete the project. In large hospitals, where research is emphasized, the hospital epidemiologist, physicians, or research microbiologists may take primary responsibility for infection control research projects. The ICP often participates actively in the data collection phase and may have input into other aspects as well.

After this preliminary introduction to the expectations for research in infection control, discussion of some "how to" information needed by the ICP is appropriate.

USING THE EPIDEMIOLOGICAL APPROACH TO DESIGN THE STUDY

Table 8-1 presents a simplified classification of epidemiological approaches to research. Fig. 8-2 shows the interrelationships of the various epidemiological approaches when applied to observational studies.

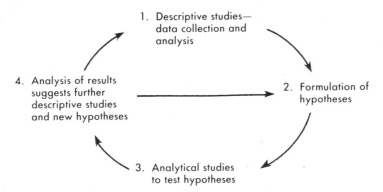

FIG. 8-2. Scheme for epidemiological study cycle as it pertains to observational studies. (Modified from Mausner, J.S., and Bahn, A.K.: Epidemiology: an introductory text, Philadelphia, 1974, W.B. Saunders Co.)

OBSERVATIONAL EPIDEMIOLOGY
Descriptive studies

All ICPs do descriptive studies in their daily work. Outbreak investigations are a type of descriptive study as are monthly surveillance reports. Both types of studies describe disease, events, or trends with regard to person, place, and time. Such studies provide useful information about infection control, can suggest causal associations, and will always be of value to answer epidemiological questions.

Descriptive studies describe factors found among patients with similar diseases or conditions. The frequency of occurrence of any one particular factor provides clues that a possible association may exist between the factor and the disease or condition.

The first step in designing a descriptive study is to define the particular disease or condition in clear terms. After writing the definition, the next step is to determine which factors will be examined. The purpose of this type of study is to look at a number of factors, one or more of which may be associated with a particular outcome (e.g., infection). (Chapter 7 describes an outbreak investigation and the report that should result after completion.)

Descriptive studies are a particularly useful first step for suggesting the analytical studies needed to verify or explain suspected associations. They also serve to determine what variables or characteristics need to be controlled, that is, held constant in the case-control comparison groups.

Descriptive studies can use several approaches. If data are to be collected from existing records, then the approach is *retrospective*. If data are to be collected in the future, then the approach is *prospective*. Many descriptive studies include retrospective and prospective components.

TABLE 8-1. A simplified classification of epidemiological approaches to research

Classification	Stem question	Knowledge base	Purpose of study	Time frame
I. Observational epidemiology				
A. Descriptive studies	Who? Where? When?	Person Place Time	To *describe* amount and distribution of disease, events, and trends To *formulate* hypotheses	Retrospective and/ or prospective
B. Analytical studies	What are the *relationships* among or between . . .?		To *explain* associations and relationships; to *test* hypotheses	
1. Prevalence, cross-sectional, or sample surveys		1, 2. Disease already present in cases	1, 2. To look for risk factors and strength of association with existing disease	1. Single point in time or a period of time
2. Case-control studies				2. Usually retrospective
3. Incidence or cohort studies		3. Disease not yet present; classify cohorts by risk factors	To look for development of disease and strength of association with classified risk factors	3. Prospective or historical prospective
II. Experimental epidemiology				
A. Intervention studies	Why? If–then?	Full knowledge of topic	To *manipulate* variables to *test* hypotheses To establish *causal associations*	Always prospective, although controls can be historical or from literature (nonconcurrent; nonrandom methods)

Analytical studies

Analytical studies are used to answer questions about association of factors with outcome. Analytical studies include descriptive information about the population under study (e.g., age, sex, underlying disease) but also include the use of more complex methods for data analysis. There are several types of analytical studies detailed in the following section.

Prevalence, cross-sectional, or sample surveys. These studies are used to determine the distribution of one or more factors in a cross section of a popula-

Data collection methods	Data analysis methods	Expected answers	Examples
Chart review Interviews Questionnaires Participant observation	Descriptive statistics (e.g., mean, standard deviation, coefficient of variation, percents); content analysis; graphs, tables, and charts	Description of situation; identification of variables meriting further study; validity and reliability data	Case reports; outbreak or epidemic investigations; monthly reports of surveillance data; nosocomial infection trends by category (e.g., site versus organism)
Chart review Structured observation Interviews Questionnaires	In addition to above—inferential statistics (chi-square, *t* tests); correlational analysis; relative risk/odds ratio; attributable risk; *note:* consult with a statistician *before* attempting most analytical studies	Explanation of relationships between and among variables; strength of associations; validity and reliability data; possible causal associations	1. Prevalence surveys for nosocomial infections 2. Case-control studies of the association of Foley catheters with urinary tract infections 3. Cohort studies of association of *Staphylococcus aureus* umbilical site colonization with subsequent neonatal S. aureus infection; the Framingham cohort studies
All available structured methods Investigator controls some variables	All available structured methods All available statistical procedures; *note:* consult with a statistician *before* attempting any experimental study	Support or reject hypotheses Causal associations established	Clinical trials of experimental drugs Community trials of vaccines

tion, of an entire population at a specific point in time, or during a specified period of time. Such studies are relatively quick and inexpensive and may help establish relationships. A prevalence survey for nosocomial infections present on a particular day is an example of this type of study (p. 108). Prevalence includes both existing and new cases of disease and is expressed by calculating a prevalence rate.

ICPs should be encouraged to explore the uses of prevalence surveys. The CDC[14] recently revised its guidelines for conducting prevalence surveys for nosocomial infections. These surveys require less time and effort than some other forms of surveillance and can be used as the basis for answering such questions as "How many patients on a given day are on isolation precautions, and what types of isolation are in use?" or "How many of these patients have nosocomial infections?"

In addition, sample surveys can provide extremely useful information to the ICP about such things as attitudes, opinions, and educational programs. Self-administered questionnaires and personal or telephone interviews with a fixed questionnaire format are the most frequently used tools for sample surveys. Mechanisms for conducting sample surveys are discussed in many social science and nursing research textbooks.[10,29,30,36,51]

Case-control studies. Case control studies identify individuals having a particular disease (i.e., the case) and compare them with a control group(s) of individuals who do not have the disease. The objective is to determine what risk factors ("host exposure factors") are associated with the disease and to assess the strength of the association.

Case-control studies are usually retrospective and in infection control are most often accomplished by chart review.

In retrospective studies the cases and their controls are selected and compared for the presence or absence of one or more risk factors. The investigation of cases of nosocomial pneumonia complicated by *Pseudomonas* organisms compared to a control group of patients with pneumonia who have remained free of *Pseudomonas* organisms, looking for antecedent risk factors (such as the use of a particular type of respiratory therapy device), is an example of a case-control study. The case-control method is particularly useful for identifying possible causal associations, as in this case when there may be an epidemic organism that can be traced easily.

Caution: The selection of appropriate control groups is not always easy. The major objective is to select a control group that is as *similar* as possible to the case group, except, of course, for the control group not having the disease. Age, sex, underlying chronic disease, and other factors enter into the selection of control groups. Cases and controls should also be *concurrent*, that is, studied over the same time period. Because of the enormous variability of human beings, it is apparent that there are many factors that may affect the relationship between the risk factor under study and the outcome (i.e., development of infection). To reduce the effect of confounding, some matching may be done. Matching means selecting controls so that they are similar to cases in specific restrictive characteristics (usually age, sex, and underlying disease) but are unmatched for the factor or factors to be assessed.

Another method for choosing a relatively small number of controls from a large population is the use of random selection. Random selection is a deliberate process for ensuring that each individual or item in a population has an equal chance of being selected. Random selection attempts to obtain a sample that is truly representative of the population as a whole. For example, if patients with nosocomial urinary tract infections during June form the case group, then an equal sized or twice equal sized random sample selected from among all other June patients could constitute the control group. If nosocomial infections among surgical patients were being studied, however, the controls should be randomly selected from other surgical patients and not from the entire hospital population. By retrospective chart review the ICP can determine the proportion of each population in which various risk factors were present (e.g., Foley catheters). Such a study can answer questions about Foley catheters and other variables associated with urinary tract infections.

It must be emphasized that if a variable is used for matching, it cannot be investigated for its etiological role in the development of disease. For example, if all cases had Foley catheters and all controls also had Foley catheters (but were not infected), Foley catheters cannot be studied as a risk factor. However, such a study can show the association between length of catheterization and infection and answer numerous other questions.

Incidence or cohort studies. A cohort is a group of persons who share a common experience within a defined time period. At the beginning of the study there are no cases of disease. Cohort study approaches may either be prospective or historical prospective. Risk factors are specified at the beginning of the investigation, and the cohort is observed over a time period to determine the rate at which disease develops in relation to exposure to the risk factors.

The length of time required for a cohort study varies directly with the frequency of the disease in the population being studied, the incubation period for the disease, and whether or not the disease has a long latent period. To accumulate enough cases of disease to make a statistically meaningful analysis, the ICP needs to know something about each of these factors. The long follow-up period for cohort studies is especially apparent in the investigation of chronic diseases (e.g., heart disease, carcinoma, black lung).

In the hospital setting where nosocomial infection is the outcome the follow-up period may not be so long; however, the frequency with which the event occurs in the population and the time it takes for the condition to develop will affect the design of the study. An example of the need for a fairly long follow-up period is that of postoperative complications (e.g., infection) following joint implant surgery.

A type of infection that has been studied successfully with the cohort approach is nosocomial urinary tract infection. Reasons for this include the fact that urinary tract infections are the most common nosocomial infections and that they are defined by standard quantitative microbiological data whether symptoms are present or not. On the other hand, to study an infection with low frequency (e.g., surgical wound infections following "clean" surgical procedures) can take a very long time. For example, one desires to compare patients of surgeon A (one cohort) with patients of surgeon B (another cohort, or a cohort without the risk factor of surgeon A). Some hypothetical numerical values follow:

> Community Memorial Hospital performs 300 surgeries per month. Of these, 60% are classified as "clean" procedures. Cruse and Foord[21] quote an attack rate of 1.8% for "clean" procedures. Therefore the expected numbers of infections would be as follows:

> 300 surgeries $\times$ 60% = 180 clean surgeries (expected number of wound infections = 1.8% of 180, or 3.24 per month)

> Number of surgeries per month for surgeon A = 30, of which 60% are clean = 18 surgical cases (expected number of wound infections = <1 per month)

> Number of surgeries per month for surgeon B = 30, of which 40% are clean = 12 surgical cases (expected number of wound infections = <1 per month)

To obtain any meaningful information with such a prospective cohort study would take a very long time. In addition, there are many variables that cannot be controlled by the ICP (e.g., surgical technique, type of patients each surgeon sees). Thus, even if surgeon A has more infected patients than surgeon B, it may turn out that surgeon A's patients are older and have more underlying disease. The ICP should be aware that such information may be requested by infection control committees when a particular surgeon has had a few infected patients in a short time period. There is usually little thought or knowledge of the time required to accumulate enough information for meaningful analysis. If the request is made for this information, a retrospective descriptive study or a retrospective case-control study would be a much better approach than a prospective cohort study.

Another method is the historical prospective approach. In this approach a cohort is identified at some point in the past, and the subsequent morbidity and/or mortality is analyzed forward in time from existing records. At the beginning of such a study cases have not been identified, but risk factors have been enumerated. An example of a historical prospective study would be to investigate in 1981 the cohort of patients of surgeon A undergoing surgery in 1980, compared with the cohort of patients of surgeon B. If the ICP had no knowledge of infections among surgeon A or surgeon B's patients in 1980, she would begin her study with no cases. After reviewing the records for the cohorts (i.e., all of surgeon A and surgeon B's patients) the ICP could classify them as infected or not infected, and each patient would be classified for exposure to the enumerated risk factors (e.g., age, sex, underlying illness, length of surgery, type of surgery). This differs from a case-control study because cases were not identified at the beginning of the study.

Fig. 8-3 compares retrospective and prospective studies with respect to time factors.

Fig. 8-4 is a 2×2 table comparing case-control (retrospective) and cohort (prospective) study designs.

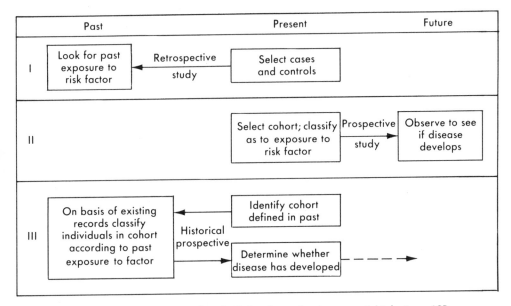

Interpretation: When using analytical methods for the study of nosocomial infections, ICPs can adapt methods developed for the study of chronic diseases. A principal difference is that chronic diseases develop over a long period of time, whereas most nosocomial infections develop over a much shorter period of time.

In a retrospective study (I) people diagnosed as having a disease (cases) are compared with persons who do not have the disease (controls). The purpose is to determine if the two groups differ in the number or proportion of individuals who have been exposed to specific risk factors. This type of study is retrospective because it compares cases and controls with regard to the presence of some element or risk factor in their past experience.

In a prospective study (II) the starting point is a group of people (a cohort) all considered to be free of a given disease but who vary in exposure to a specific risk factor. The cohort is observed over time to determine the rate at which disease develops in relation to exposure to the risk factor.

In a historical prospective study (III) a group or cohort is identified at some point in the past, and their subsequent morbidity and/or mortality is analyzed from existing records. At the beginning of such a study, cases have not been identified.

FIG. 8-3. Comparison of three different study designs. **I**, Retrospective (case-control). **II**, Prospective (cohort). **III**, Historical prospective (cohort). (Modified from Mausner, J.S., and Bahn, A.K.: Epidemiology: an introductory text, Philadelphia, 1974, W.B. Saunders Co.)

Case-control studies
(retrospective)

DISEASE

		Present (cases)	Absent (controls)
RISK FACTOR	Present (exposed to factor)	ⓐ	b
	Absent (not exposed to factor)	c	ⓓ

Cohort studies
(prospective)

Interpretation: The essential difference between the
two types of studies lies not in the time sequence but
in the way the groups for study are assembled.
   In retrospective studies cases (those with disease)
and controls (those without disease) are selected and
compared for presence or absence of a risk
factor. If there is an association between the risk factor
and the disease, the largest numerical
values are expected to be in cells *a* and *d*.
   In prospective studies, individuals who
are free of the disease under consideration are examined. They are
classified by exposure or lack of exposure to a risk
factor, and are observed over time for development of disease.

FIG. 8-4. Contingency (2 × 2) table showing case-control (retrospective) and cohort (prospective) study designs. (Modified from Mausner, J.S., and Bahn, A.K.: Epidemiology: an introductory text, Philadelphia, 1974, W.B. Saunders Co.)

EXPERIMENTAL EPIDEMIOLOGY

Experimental studies are designed to manipulate variables (risk factors) to test hypotheses. These studies have many designs and require considerable statistical consultation before implementation.

A type of experimental study that is sometimes conducted by ICPs is an *intervention study*. Intervention studies are those in which the ICP actively attempts to alter the cause of the infection and then evaluates the effects of this intervention on disease risk. The most common intervention study conducted by ICPs uses the "before and after" method: a problem is identified and studied retrospectively; a change is made to alter the presumed "cause"; and the effects of the change are evaluated prospectively. Such studies are subject to several types of errors or biases, the major one being that the ICP is using a historical control rather than a concurrent control. For such comparisons to be valid, it is important that major variables (e.g., personnel, types of patients, standard procedures) remain unchanged in both study periods. Although this approach may be the only one logistically possible in many facilities, caution is necessary about making generalizations from the results and attributing the change solely to the intervention.

Another type of experimental study is the randomized controlled trial. This method has been used many times to test vaccine efficacy. In hospital infection control the studies of the efficacy of immune globulin to prevent hepatitis B after an accidental needlestick were randomized controlled trials.[33,46] To ensure enough subjects both studies required input from several medical centers.

The double-blind technique is often used in experimental clinical trials for drugs. This phrase implies that (1) the treatment is identified by a code only, and the actual content of the material is unknown to those giving and receiving it, and (2) the assessment of outcome is also made without knowledge of the treatment given or whether any treatment has been given. Unfortunately, all studies do not lend themselves to a double-blind technique. An example is one in which the medication being tested has a peculiar taste that cannot be replicated in the placebo. Also, it is not always possible for the assessment of outcome to be made by persons other than those administering the treatment and under conditions in which they cannot identify the group to which the patient being assessed belongs. When double-blind assessment is not possible, reliance must be placed on the selection criteria of outcome that are as objective as possible.

If the experimenter knows the assignment of the subject, the study is called a single-blind approach.

Mechanisms such as those previously mentioned are designed to eliminate bias in assessment of outcomes from the expectations of the investigator and the participant. For additional information about epidemiological methods the reader is referred to basic textbooks in epidemiology.*

DEFINING THE PROBLEM

The first steps in any research project are to define the problem in specific terms and to be realistic about what can be accomplished in a particular setting. Is the ICP aware of any infection control problems in her facility that need to be investigated? Has she read a study recently in which results differ dramatically from what she would expect in her facility? Does the ICP have an adequate microbiology laboratory? If not, then answering questions based on culture results may require additional funds and medical support. Is the ICP's facility research oriented? If not, then the project may need "selling" under a different name.

*References 5, 31, 40-42.

Most problems for investigation come from the environment in which the ICP works. What situations or problems chronically recur without adequate solutions? Are there procedural questions that merit study (e.g., IV site care or the protocol for starting IV infusions in emergency situations)? Is the ICP satisfied with nursing and medical staff compliance with handwashing routines? If not, she may want to consider an observational study of current practices and then focus on behavior modification. Does her new employee orientation program need revision? How does the ICP measure learning in the orientation program? How does she measure effectiveness of other teaching programs she presents?

The ICP should permit her ideas to crystallize, write them down, discuss them with colleagues, and clearly establish the purpose for the study. She should list points she and others raise and then move on to the review of the existing published literature.

REVIEWING THE LITERATURE

An adequate review of the published literature is an important early step in every study. Literature review should tell the ICP if her question or problem has already been answered and may suggest methods of study and analysis. Alternately, review of the literature may indicate reasons why some questions have not been answered.

A good starting place for the ICP to learn more about her topic is any recent textbook on hospital infection control.* She will quickly get an overview of the selected subject by reading one or more chapters of these textbooks. Because it usually takes many months (and sometimes even years) for a book to be published, most books will not reflect the most current references on a topic.

To obtain more recent information, a search of the periodical literature is required. This search may be done in several ways:

1. By consulting the reference list in a recently published review article in a major periodical and then obtaining those references of interest.
2. By consulting the Cumulative Index Medicus,[22] the Cumulative Index to Nursing and Allied Health Literature,[23] Current Contents,[24] or other periodical literature.
3. By requesting the medical librarian to run a MEDLINE search. This is a computer-assisted literature review using as a data base more than 3500 journals in the health care field. For access and the cost of MEDLINE search, the ICP may consult her hospital library, a nearby health science library, or a resource library in her area. Resource libraries number about 800 and are usually affiliated with medical schools. The next level is the Regional Medical Library (RML). The 11 RMLs in the United States are

*References 4, 7, 8, 11, 12, 52.

designed and funded by the National Library of Medicine in Bethesda, Maryland. A current listing is available in the *Cumulative Index Medicus*.[22]

4. By consulting recent issues of the journals where infection control studies are published, such as the *American Journal of Infection Control*, *Infection Control*, *Annals of Internal Medicine*, *Journal of Infectious Diseases*, *Journal of the American Medical Association*, *New England Journal of Medicine*, *American Journal of Medicine*, *Journal of the American Public Health Association*, *American Journal of Epidemiology*, and others. Occasionally, an infection control article will be published in the *American Journal of Nursing*, *Nursing*, *R.N.*, *Nursing Research*, and other nursing journals. The journals in the behavioral sciences and education may also be helpful for some topics. Reviewing recent issues of journals will locate papers published in the past 3 months that have not yet appeared in the *Cumulative Index Medicus*, the *Cumulative Index to Nursing and Allied Health Literature*, or other indexes.

5. By asking researchers with expertise in the field of interest for access to their reprint collections of journal articles on the particular topic.

A fairly comprehensive guide to nursing literature has been published recently[9] that covers many aspects of the literature review. An article specific to literature review for infection control has also appeared recently.[34]

Before progressing very far with the literature review, it is helpful to establish a filing and retrieval system for references. This can serve both as a resource for the ICP and for the hospital. Several systems have been developed.[28,32,47] One that is particularly useful for infection control information is the marginal punch-sort card system because many articles contain information on several topics. The marginal punch-sort card system permits a single article to be sorted by any of several topic headings, depending on where the margins are punched. Emerson and Jackson[28] describe the system step by step. If the ICP's system includes bibliography cards be certain that *complete* citation information is on each card, including the original source for the reference. This is some insurance against errors in transcription, although a citation will occasionally be printed incorrectly in the primary reference list (e.g., from a reference list in a book or periodical).

After the ICP has accumulated several articles on her selected topic, she should spend some time digesting their contents. Has the original question been asked? Has it been answered? If so, was the problem solved by methods that the ICP can use in her facility? If not, is it practical to conduct a study in the facility, and does the facility have the personnel and financial resources to do so? In assessing practicality, does the ICP have the time and administrative support to proceed? Does she have the laboratory support for cultures if indicated? Does the event occur with enough frequency to provide sufficient numbers for meaningful analysis? If not, would a collaborative effort with one or more hospitals provide better data? The South Florida Consortium for Infection Control (Miami) is an example of a collaborative effort by several hospitals that has yielded some interesting data.

FORMULATING THE PROBLEM STATEMENT

Problem statements vary from simple to complex, depending on the nature and purpose of the study and the questions being asked.

A simple problem statement gives information about time, place, and person characteristics of the population studied. For example, "What are the characteristics of patients who develop nosocomial wound infections after cesarean section delivery by the obstetrical service?" Answers to this question should include information about age, parity, type of section (i.e., elective versus emergency), and length of stay. Such a question will not necessarily provide information about infection rates unless denominator data (all cesarean sections for a certain time period) are obtained.

To learn more about the total population who had cesarean sections during the time interval, and something about how those infected differ from those not infected, a more complete problem statement can be developed. For example, "What are the characteristics of all patients who had cesarean sections performed by the obstetrical service during a specific time interval?" Such a question will yield data about nosocomial infections and denominator data for use in generating a *rate* of wound infection after cesarean section.

By stating the questions as "Is there a difference in nosocomial postcesarean section wound infection rates between those having elective cesarean sections and those having emergency cesarean sections?" information will be obtained that can be analyzed and compared.

Problem statements that are written to test the supposed relationships or associations between two or more variables are called *hypothesis* statements. A hypothesis, simply stated, is an educated guess.

To study the relationships between two or more characteristics (variables) requires classifying the variables into categories. An *independent* variable (designated X statistically) is the presumed antecedent event. In the previous example cesarean section delivery is the independent variable. A dependent variable (designated Y statistically) is the presumed "effect" or outcome. In the previous example nosocomial wound infection is the dependent variable.

A third important variable is called a *confounding* variable. Confounding variables are those that "confuse the issue" by indirect association. Confounding variables are related both to disease and to the risk factor under consideration. To actually confound, a variable must fulfill both of the following criteria: (1) it must be related both to frequency of risk exposure and to frequency of disease recognition, and (2) it must occur with differing frequencies in groups being compared (cohorts or cases and controls). A knowledge of confounding variables will assist in ensuring comparability of groups being studied. The topic is discussed briefly by Friedman[31] and in more detail by MacMahon and Pugh.[41]

When a suspected relationship exists between one independent and one dependent variable, it can be designated as a simple hypothesis. When the relationship involves two (or more) of these variables, it is referred to as a complex or multivariate hypothesis. Such complex hypotheses require sophisticated statistical procedures for testing, and computer assistance is usually necessary.[40,41,49]

For most infection control studies a case definition must be established early in the project. A case definition is a statement containing the criteria by which a "case" will be defined. Adoption of case definitions used elsewhere makes an ICP's data comparable to those of others and is often the preferred method. Diagnostic criteria used in the case definition should be clear and reproducible. In nosocomial infection studies case definitions usually follow criteria established by the CDC. However, the ICP has the option of making a case definition anything she wishes.

For example, in investigating an outbreak of shigellosis in the ICP's hospital where a particular meal or day is implicated, the case definition could be "any individual with a positive stool culture for *Shigella flexneri* who ate lunch in the hospital cafeteria on June 1." Another example is "any patient from whom *Pseudomonas cepacia* is cultured from the blood 24 or more hours after admission to the hospital." By using specific case definitions, it is much easier to search for additional cases of diseases among the population under review.

SELECTING DATA COLLECTION METHODS

To be of much use, data acquired by an ICP must consist of observable, measurable items for analysis. Because most infection control studies have concentrated on measuring rates of infection and changes in rates of infection, reasonably clear definitions of various nosocomial infections have been established. Such definitions form the basis for the National Nosocomial Infections Study reports and for the SENIC Project and can be obtained from the CDC.[13]

Data collection methods useful to the ICP will be discussed in the following sections.

Chart review

Chart review involves (but is not limited to) seeking information about positive cultures, elevated temperature, radiographic reports, medication regimens, and other factors that determine whether or not an infection meets the case definition. The accuracy of this method depends on how accurate and complete charting is in the particular facility.

Various sections of the chart will yield pieces of information. If the ICP is in a teaching hospital, *physicians' progress notes* are probably most useful because charting of the same information is done by several different individuals. Usually the medical student's notes are followed by those of the intern, the resident, and finally the attending faculty physician. In community hospitals the completeness of physicians' progress notes varies tremendously.

Another place to seek information is in *nurses' notes*. These notes may be very helpful or else of little assistance, depending on the type and style of charting. Information usually found in the nurses' notes includes elevated temperature, wound drainage, patient complaints about pain, bowel and bladder problems, and requests for medication.

The *medication record* can provide information about antibiotic usage and the frequency of pain and antipyretic medications.

Microbiology laboratory data can provide information about a patient's cultures and sensitivities; however, correlation with clinical data is mandatory in determining whether the patient is infected or only colonized.

Other laboratory data include information about the patient's urinalysis, hematology, enzymes, and multiple other host factors that contribute to the patient's ability to withstand iatrogenic insults. Information about viral studies is also becoming important in nosocomial infection epidemiology.

Radiographic reports lend information about pulmonary infections and, if frequent enough, can show clear progression of a lower respiratory tract infection.

Surgical records provide data about surgical procedures and may provide information about breaks in technique (this is not always the case, however).

Chart review has a number of limitations, not the least of which is deciphering illegible handwritten notes! Because of the time lag in getting reports from the laboratories, the x-ray department, and other hospital areas into the patient's chart, more current information about a particular patient who is still hospitalized can be obtained by observation and consultation with those providing care.

If the ICP's study is a retrospective one, however, her data will be only as complete as her facility's charting, assuming this is the only method being used, and there may well be questions she cannot answer with such a study.

Participant observation

Participant observation is a technique of unstructured observation in which the ICP participates in the functioning of the group under investigation. A log (or field notes) is kept daily to record such things as observations, time of events, and behaviors. Such notes can provide the basis for both data collection and data analysis if they are complete; however, there is always some observer bias and often observer influence because of the subjectivity of the approach. For example, if the ICP has been having a problem with a particularly resistant organism in an intensive care unit, it may be worthwhile for the ICP to go to the unit and participate in patient care activities for 1 or more days. During this period of participant observation, it is possible to observe care techniques, handwashing frequency, and other procedures. However, because her identity is clearly that of the ICP, the stay would need to be long enough to minimize the staff's behavioral changes in response to the investigator's presence. Indeed, in such a case, the ICP's presence may serve as a control method.

Structured observations

Structured observation methods differ from unstructured techniques in that specific behaviors or events are selected for observation. Record keeping forms are prepared in advance; the observer uses a formal observational procedure for data collection.

In the structured approach a category system is useful so that a checklist may be used for the presence or absence (frequency of occurrence) of events. For example, if the ICP is interested in observing the frequency and method of suctioning secretions in patients in a particular unit, the checklist would include such things as gloves—one hand, gloves—both hands, new suction tubing each event and, number of times secretions were suctioned in an hour.

Structured observation methods of various types are especially useful for observations of behavior and are discussed at length in nursing research textbooks.[10,44,45,51]

Questioning subjects

Direct questioning of subjects may take the form of an unstructured interview or the use of formal structured tools, called questionnaires or interview schedules. Such questionnaires may be self-administered or interviewer administered in person or by telephone. An example of a large study in which several questionnaires were used is the SENIC Project.[1]

The usefulness of data obtained this way is related to a number of factors. In general, interviewer-administered questionnaires provide better data than self-administered questionnaires. Unstructured interviews and interviewer-administered questionnaires take more time and cost considerably more to administer than do self-administered questionnaires. Accordingly, the selection of a method for questioning subjects may be determined by factors such as cost and time, outweighing the ability to obtain optimal results from the largest number of respondents interviewed in person.

The development of questionnaire questions requires skill and practice. Brevity and lack of ambiguity are essential. There are various forms that questions can take if this method is selected. Such questions should be validated and pilot tested before use. Before deciding to use a questionnaire, the ICP should consult one or more of the textbooks that include chapters on the subject.*

Closed-ended (fixed alternative) questions offer the respondent several alternative responses from which to select one. These choices may be of the yes/no variety or offer several choices. Closed-ended questions are difficult to write but relatively easy to analyze. A type of widely used opinion scale, known as the *Likert scale*, offers several choices along a continuum from negative to positive poles:

> *Statement:* Handwashing is the most important means of preventing the transmission of infection.
>
> *Instructions to respondent:* Select the response that most closely matches your opinion:

Strongly agree   Agree   Indifferent   Disagree   Strongly disagree

Such scales may have numerical values assigned to each response category, and various statistical tests can be made on the data.

ICPs will find these scales useful in the development of questionnaires for evaluation of teaching programs, opinions about patient care practices as they pertain to infection control, patient and staff behavior, and other information.

Open-ended questions permit participants to respond to questions in their own words. Such questions are easier to write than closed-ended questions but present greater difficulty in analysis.

One difficulty encountered with mailed, self-administered questionnaires is the problem of nonrespondents. If fewer than half of the distributed questionnaires are returned, as is often the case, it is risky to generalize from the results because of nonrespondent bias. In fact, many investigators aim for an 80% to 90% response rate for this reason. The acceptable nonresponse rate depends somewhat on the sample surveyed and the representativeness of the responder group. To reduce the effects of nonrespondent bias, it behooves the ICP to obtain as large a sample as possible and then to follow up in some way to secure responses from as many nonrespondents as possible. This is because nonrespondents are often not representative of the population being surveyed. Obtaining maximal response may require a telephone call to the nonrespondents, but results will be more meaningful if this extra effort is made.

An example of a questionnaire used by ICPs is for postdischarge follow-up for infections not recognized until the patient has left the hospital. Most such surveys entail sending a questionnaire to the physician for completion at the patient's first follow-up visit. The effectiveness of such questionnaires varies directly with the level of cooperation by the respondent group.

*References 10, 30, 36, 45, 49, 51.

SELECTING THE GROUP TO BE STUDIED

The appropriate group or population to be studied depends on the type of study one desires to conduct.

"How large should my sample be?" is a common question asked by ICPs. This may be a difficult question because the answer sometimes depends on information that can be obtained only by conducting the study and obtaining results. For many planned investigations, it is not possible to estimate in advance the sample size that will be needed to ensure statistically significant results.

By definition, a sample is a portion selected from the existing entire population. Ideally, a sample should then be representative of the whole. The theoretical and statistical components of sampling are the topics of entire texts[18,39] and cannot be covered here. However, a few points need attention.

Fig. 8-5 represents the relationship between sample size and the likelihood of departure of the sample from being representative of the "true" picture. Clearly, the larger the sample, the less likely it will convey a false impression of the population.

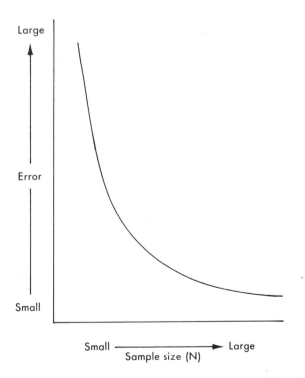

FIG. 8-5. Relationship between sample size and "sampling error" (possibility that sample is not truly representative of the population).

Samples may be classified into two types: *probability* samples and *non-probability* samples.

Probability sampling means that every element in the population has an equal chance of being selected for inclusion in the sample.

Nonprobability sampling includes haphazard sampling (such as a study of patients in the hospital at a particular time), quota sampling, and purposive sampling. Purposive sampling is frequently used in hospital infection control in which patients are deliberately included because they have an infection or are subjected to various risk factors.

Most infection control studies have been conducted using nonprobability samples not only because those were the most convenient kinds of samples to obtain but also because the ICPs often did not know the difference. Nonprobability sampling introduces the likelihood of bias that can affect the results and limits the ICP's options for statistical analysis of the data.

The best advice for the novice ICP is to use as large a sample as possible. Larger samples tend toward being more representative of the population, and they also maximize the sensitivity of the analysis for detecting weak associations and small differences between groups. The list on p. 143,* based on a formula published by the research division of the National Education Association, can be used for determining sample size from a given population when random sampling is done. As one can see, the smaller the population, the larger the proportion needed to ensure accurate results. To use this list for survey research, the ICP can assume that her hospital nursing population is 600, and she wants to take a random sample of the group for a questionnaire survey about infection control. She would need to randomly select 234 nurses and then attempt to get as large a return from that group as possible. The list should not be used to assess whether the number of respondents to a questionnaire distributed to the entire group was adequate because nonrespondent bias may occur.*

Brink and Wood[10] suggest that if the ICP has some choice in planning sample size but cannot use probability sampling, then the size of the sample will depend on the number and type of variables being measured. If one is looking for relationships between variables, a handy rule-of-thumb is to plan for at least five observations for each category of each variable. For example, if the investigation is going to categorize urinary tract infections by "duration of catheterization" divided into 24-hour units over a 10-day period, the ICP would want to include at least 50 subjects with urinary tract infections (five subjects times ten 24-hour periods). If the ICP also wanted to look at the variable of sex (males versus females), then she would need to double the number of subjects because

*From Krijcie, R.V., and Morgan, D.W.: Educ. Psychol. Measurement **30**:607-610, 1970.

Population size	Required sample size	Population size	Required sample size	Population size	Required sample size
10	10	220	140	1200	291
15	14	230	144	1300	297
20	19	240	148	1400	302
25	24	250	152	1500	306
30	28	260	155	1600	310
35	32	270	159	1700	313
40	36	280	162	1800	317
45	40	290	165	1900	320
50	44	300	169	2000	322
55	48	320	175	2200	327
60	52	340	181	2400	331
65	56	360	186	2600	335
70	59	380	191	2800	338
75	63	400	196	3000	341
80	66	420	201	3500	346
85	70	440	205	4000	351
90	73	460	210	4500	354
95	76	480	214	5000	357
100	80	500	217	6000	361
110	86	550	228	7000	364
120	92	600	234	8000	367
130	97	650	242	9000	368
140	103	700	248	10000	370
150	106	750	254	15000	375
160	113	800	260	20000	377
170	118	850	265	30000	379
180	123	900	269	40000	380
190	127	950	274	50000	381
200	133	1000	278	75000	382
210	136	1100	285	100000	384

the number of categories has doubled. In general, to double the precision of an analysis, it is necessary to quadruple the sample size. It is easy to see why studies using multiple variables require a much larger number of subjects. Although this is a useful approximate rule, it may not always be possible to use it for infection control studies.

Whenever possible, the random sampling method is preferred over other methods. Random sampling may be used for selecting control groups with which cases will be compared. The most frequently used random sampling method is the *simple* random sample. A table of random digits is used for this method (p. 144). Another approach is systematic sampling in which every third, fifth, and tenth person (and so on) from a list is selected. This is legiti-

A small table of random digits

Instructions for use: close eyes and place finger anywhere on the table. This is your starting point. To use table you must follow the numbers in order but may elect to do this horizontally, vertically, or diagonally. If your population numbers up to 999 and you are selecting 100 members of the population, you must select digits three at a time. For example, if your starting place is at the point of the circled number 98, your numbers would be 985, 951, 929, 666, 334, 171, and so on until you had selected 100 numbers. Tables of random digits are in most statistics texts and books of statistical tables.

83	56	27	04	20	75	83	95	68	63
22	73	49	77	07	29	48	82	92	83
64	97	51	88	99	40	76	54	84	39
22	91	47	28	24	75	21	26	68	30
94	90	22	33	96	53	27	38	26	38
51	18	18	57	03	34	56	85	99	14
15	13	(98)	59	51	92	96	66	33	41
71	74	03	46	04	26	94	39	44	55
64	48	42	85	04	39	43	59	45	27
42	78	42	74	88	71	71	69	63	73
84	75	11	33	94	73	29	37	04	76
23	52	74	22	14	88	30	53	17	87
12	72	67	21	61	74	14	20	48	68
74	14	40	68	43	99	12	73	66	18
91	20	69	70	46	23	57	27	17	83
56	85	79	94	34	22	55	08	68	86
59	00	78	10	89	98	18	79	52	02

mate *only* if there is no prearranged method of assignment to the list (e.g., it is inappropriate for alphabetical listings but may be acceptable for selecting from lists of assigned hospital identification numbers).

Finally, if the ICP's study involves human subjects, she may need to obtain "informed consent" before data collection. Most facilities have human subjects committees or institutional review boards for the purpose of reviewing requests for such studies because there are a number of ethical considerations to be taken into account when performing research. For example, an ICP using patient charts for a retrospective study needs to be aware that the patient's right to privacy must be protected. The institutional review board would want to know what plans had been made to ensure confidentiality (e.g., coding of patient names, using no specific identifier information in published material).

For prospective studies in which the patient or employee is required to make a choice about participation, provisions may be needed for informed consent of the participants. A major concern of the institutional review board is that participants are aware that a study is being done and that they have a choice about participation.

In the early stages of study design it is a good idea to check with the hospital's administrative office and/or legal council about the need for review of the study by the institutional review board and the need for informed consent of the participants.

DEVELOPING THE DATA COLLECTION INSTRUMENT

Design of the data collecting instrument depends heavily on methods available for data analysis. If the ICP has access to a computer for data analysis, she should consult with personnel in her data processing department before preparing the final version of the data collection form. Some entries may be directly coded on sheets for computer analysis, and the ICP needs to know how to do this at the beginning.[49]

Two methods in common use when computers are not available are the data card or page for each subject and the line listing sheet. A single information card or page for each subject has the advantage of allowing the ICP to sort the cards into different stacks according to different variables being analyzed. It is also easier to use if the ICP wishes to examine other variables at a later date. For example, after the initial analysis, another question arises that can be answered from data recorded on each card but not analyzed in the first sort. A useful system for handling larger numbers of cards (100 or more) is a marginal-punch sorting system available commercially (McBee, Indecks).[28] Some ICPs find this system a useful one for collecting nosocomial infection surveillance data, but it can be equally as useful for studies. A major advantage is that if the cards are properly coded initially, information retrieval is much faster than it would be by reading each card for every item. In essence, this system serves as a hand-sorting simple "computer."

Date form filled out _____ Worksheet for study of _____

Completed by _____

Name _____ Identification no. _____ Age _____ Date of birth _____ Sex _____

Date of admission _____ Service _____ Nursing unit preoperative _____ Nursing unit postoperative _____

Admission diagnosis _____

Infection at time of admission _____ Yes _____ No   If yes, type of infection _____

Onset (date/time) of nosocomial infection and type _____ No infection noted/date _____

Surgical procedure(s) _____

Date of procedure _____ Type of procedure _____

                                                                            From   To

Operative team

Surgeon _____ Assistant _____ Anesthesia staff _____ Anesthesia resident _____ Scrub nurse _____ Circulating nurse _____ Other

Operating room no. _____ Skin prep _____

                                  Solution   Lot no. (if known)

Devices

_____ Lot no. _____

_____ Lot no. _____

_____ Lot no. _____

Progress notes

Date _____

Date _____

Date _____

Antibiotic listing preoperative and postoperative

Date on	Date off	Antibiotic	Dose	Route

Notes (underlying illness, steroids, etc.):

DATE	SPECIMEN AND CULTURE NUMBER	SMEAR AND STAIN H Heavy F Few M Moderate R Rare O None								AMOUNT OF GROWTH	ORGANISM IDENTIFICATION	Penicillin	Oxacillin	Cefazolin	Streptomycin	Kanamycin	Tetracycline	Chloramphenicol	Erythromycin	Colymycin	Trimethoprim	Ampicillin	Carbenicillin/ug	Gentamycin/ug	Tobramycin	Amikacin		
		Gram + cocci	Gram − cocci	Gram + rods	Gram − rods	Yeast cells	Mycelial ele	PMNs	Lymphocytes																				

FIG. 8-6. Example of data collection form for study of surgical infections in which one risk factor is implantable devices.

Another method for data collection is the line listing. Line listing of information has been a traditional method for infection control data. It is most useful, however, as a compilation listing rather than for large quantities of original data. The usefulness of the line listing is also dependent on the size of the sample and the complexity of the questions being asked. It is difficult for an individual to examine a long list of data and locate *every* entry consistently; thus data may be easily overlooked. (For example, a line listing of 50 patients with nosocomial infections is not overly difficult to handle, but a list of 500 would be very burdensome and have high potential for overlooked entries.) Additional information about line listing is readily available.[7,13,14] This method is also discussed in Chapter 7.

Fig. 8-6 is an example of a data collection sheet that could be used for a retrospective study of surgical infections in which one risk factor is implantable devices.

COLLECTING DATA

Actual data collection depends on all of the previous steps and is individualized according to the type of study being done.

Experience will teach the ICP that if she does not ask questions, she will not get answers! This may lead the beginning investigator to try to answer every conceivable question and may result in enormously cumbersome data collection forms. Conversely, asking too few questions can lead the ICP to miss important pieces of information. The key lies in seeking a reasonable middle ground. While reviewing the literature, the ICP should be observant of the questions asked and the variables discussed. From a compilation of the items in these resources, she can prepare a list of needed information.

In general, as the number of items collected increases, the quality of the end result decreases. If a questionnaire survey is being used, the more questions asked, the greater the likelihood of a decreased response rate. When using statistical analyses, the more data there are to analyze, the more difficult becomes the task of analyzing them. A rule-of-thumb of the experienced investigator is "Don't collect information you don't intend to use." To determine what will and will not be used takes skill and practice, and there will be times when the ICP will collect too much data (and, unfortunately, times when she will collect too little). Her skill at answering the "how much" question will improve with time.

Caution: Data should not be overly reduced before analysis. For example, the ICP may ultimately classify ages by 5-year categories, but when collecting the data, she should present the *exact* age of the subject. It is important not to calculate rates until all data are collected and an accurate denominator is determined. Summation means loss of information. Summarizing should not occur until the end of the data collection period.

Relevant variables may not have been recorded in the chart (e.g., travel histories, occupation), and if such information is important to the investigation, methods must be developed to retrieve it elsewhere (e.g., by interview, questionnaire).

All data collection methods are subject to potential bias. Bias in prospective studies results from a number of factors. There is potential bias in the ascertainment of disease because factors about the disease are not apparent at the outset and are not included in the case definition. Prospective studies require larger numbers of subjects than do retrospective studies, and if an extensive time period is involved, there will undoubtedly be attrition of subjects. For example, when infections develop after discharge, there may be no reliable method of postdischarge follow-up for the patients affected.

Retrospective studies are relatively inexpensive and usually require fewer numbers of subjects. However, rarely are all data available in a retrospective study, especially if the principal data collection method is chart review. In most medical records departments, charts are not always available on the first request, and their retrieval may cause additional delays in data collection. Retrospective studies are less accurate in quantifying risk, and one must assume that bias exists.

When an epidemic or outbreak is being investigated, standard steps for data collection should be followed. Outbreak investigations are described on p. 105 and elsewhere.[7,8,31,52]

The "Hawthorne effect" can also affect data collection adversely. The Hawthorne effect refers to the effect on subjects' responses that results from their knowledge that a study is under way. In intervention studies care needs to be taken that the resultant changes in the dependent variable (Y) can be attributed to the independent variable (X) and not to the special attention given to the group experiencing the change.

ANALYZING AND DISPLAYING DATA

Analysis and display of collected data are paramount to the value of any study. Depending on the type of study design, data are analyzed by many methods (Table 8-1).

Tables, graphs, and charts are concise, effective ways to display data. In the initial phase of analysis it is helpful to rough out table and graph outlines and then fill them in with information about the groups being studied. Every study should include the compilations of basic demographical information about the who the subjects were, where the study was done, and when the events occurred. In other words, basic "person, place, and time" information should be recorded. In organizing analysis of data the ICP may start with characterizing the subjects by age, sex, and underlying illness. If other events occurred that might affect subjects' susceptibility to the infections being studied (e.g., surgery or exposure to respiratory therapy devices), the ICP should include this information. Next she should look at the time the events in question occurred (e.g., surgical procedures, hospital admissions). These data are often best analyzed by preparing a graph where time (hours, days, weeks) is the X or horizontal axis (abscissa) and cases are on the Y or vertical axis (ordinate). If the patients were moved from one place to another (e.g., ICU to ward to ICU again), these data can also be examined by making a graph.

After these data are sorted, some statistical analyses are called for. Swinscow[50] presents basic statistics in a simple and easily understood manner. An especially good treatment of tables, graphs, and charts is provided in the training materials of the CDC.[16] Data analysis and statistics are also discussed in several of the other references.* Because these topics are well covered elsewhere, this chapter will mention only a few statistical techniques that are particularly useful to the ICP.

Caution: Before beginning an analytical or an experimental study of any type, it is always wise to consult a statistician. This individual can help design the study so that data may be analyzed in a meaningful way. Failure to heed this advice has often resulted in wasted time and effort in accumulating data that were not amenable to statistical analysis.

A useful measure of the amount of infection in a population is obtained by calculating rates. There are three types of rates used with infection control data:

1. An *attack rate* is a type of incidence rate, but it pertains to a population at risk for a limited period of time only. Attack rates are often used with common source outbreaks and for nosocomial infection statistics.
2. An *incidence rate* is a direct indicator of risk of disease because it measures the rate at which individuals become ill. Accordingly, it is a reflection of the factors that affect *development* of disease.
3. A *prevalence rate* reflects and is affected by factors that influence *duration* and *development* of diseases. Point prevalence rates are usually higher than incidence rates because they include both existing and new cases.

Calculation of many other statistics may be useful to the ICP. Means, standard deviations, percentages, and other simple descriptive statistics can be calculated easily with pocket calculators presently costing under $25. Such calculations permit the ICP to take a preliminary "look-see" at the data. To determine whether or not two mean values are significantly different statistically (e.g., Are the ages of the cases and controls really different?) requires the technique called *t testing*. This procedure is not difficult and can be learned from any of the statistics books listed in the references. Also, there are calculators available that can be programmed to calculate chi-square values and *t*

*References 19, 36, 37, 40-42, 45, 49.

values and perform many other statistical procedures. If one is serious about learning statistics, it is worthwhile to enroll in a basic course in statistics and to invest in a good calculator.

One of the most useful analytical statistical procedures for the ICP is the construction of a 2 × 2 contingency table and the calculation of a chi-square (χ^2) value.

Fig. 8-7, A, illustrates a 2 × 2 contingency table in which disease presence or absence is compared with exposure to a single risk factor. Such a table should seem familiar because it resembles that used for simple case-control and cohort study designs (Fig. 8-3).

Fig. 8-7, B, is the same table in which hypothetical data (numbers) have been entered in the cells. A χ^2 value has been calculated to be 5.730. To determine if a statistically significant association exists between the disease (in this case, urinary tract infection) and the risk factor (presence or absence of Foley catheter), the χ^2 value is searched for in a χ^2 table.

χ^2 tables are lengthy, but for a 2 × 2 contingency table, only the first line is consulted. The first line of numbers in a χ^2 table follows:

	p value (probability)				
	.1	.05		.01	.001
1 degree of freedom	2.706	3.841	5.730	6.635	10.827

The value of 5.730 falls between the numbers 3.841 and 6.635. This means that statistically less than 5 times out of 100 will this pattern of numbers in the cells of the 2 × 2 contingency table occur by chance alone. In other words, the statistical probability is greater than 95% that there is really a significant linkage or connection between Foley catheters and urinary tract infections. Accordingly, probability (or the p value) is said to be less than .05 ($p < .05$). P values simply indicate the probability of an event occurring by chance alone. That is, if a p value is $<.05$ or $<.01$, there are less than 5 chances out of 100 or less than 1 chance out of 100 that the event occurred by chance alone. χ^2 testing is a relatively easy, quick, and extremely useful method for data analysis for which there are a small number of independent variables (risk factors) being compared with the dependent variable (disease).

Another use for a 2 × 2 contingency table is the calculation of a relative risk (RR) or an odds ratio. The formula for relative risk follows:

$$RR = \frac{a}{a + b} \div \frac{c}{c + d}$$

Theoretically, relative risk can only be used for prospective studies because it is a measure of the incidence rate among exposed persons, compared to the incidence rate among nonexposed persons, and all individuals at risk must be included in the total. Only in prospective studies can one be confident that the numbers represent the total population under investigation.

A

	Disease present	Disease absent	Row totals
Exposed to risk factor	a	b	a + b (R₁)
Not exposed to risk factor	c	d	c + d (R₂)
Column totals	a + c (C₁)	b + d (C₂)	Grand total (N) a + b + c + d

$$X^2 = \frac{(|ad - bc| - \frac{1}{2}N)^2 \, (N)}{(R_1)(R_2)(C_1)(C_2)}$$

B

	With urinary tract infection	Without urinary tract infection	
With Foley catheter	15	10	25
Without Foley catheter	6	20	26
	21	30	51

$$X^2 = 5.730 \quad p < .05$$

FIG. 8-7. **A,** A 2 × 2 contingency table for calculation of chi-square values. **B,** Hypothetical example with calculated chi-square value.

The calculation of relative risk is one of the measures of the *strength* of an association and is used most often in prospective cohort studies.

For *retrospective* studies an odds ratio can be used to calculate an *estimate* of relative risk. The formula for calculation of an odds ratio follows:

$$\frac{a}{b} \div \frac{c}{d} = \frac{ad}{bc}$$

This is an indirect estimate of relative risk because *all* members of the population at risk may not have been identified retrospectively. Such estimates of relative risk are used most frequently with retrospective case-control studies and are interpreted to mean the odds in favor of having disease with the risk factor present compared to the odds of having disease with the risk factor absent.

Mausner and Bahn[42] and other authors of textbooks on epidemiology listed in the references provide more information about the calculation and uses of relative risk and odds ratios. One or more of these texts should be consulted before using and interpreting these calculations.

DRAWING CONCLUSIONS

When drawing conclusions based on the various types of studies described in this chapter, there are two important aspects of data quality that need consideration.

First, validity or accuracy is a measure of how closely the observations correspond to the "real" situation. Are ICPs measuring what they think they are measuring? The emphasis in the question is on *what* is being measured. For example, an ICP has constructed a questionnaire to measure *attitudes* about infection control programs and has included questions of only factual information about infection control practices. The survey is not valid because while it is measuring the respondent's factual knowledge of infection control, it is *not* measuring her attitudes about infection control programs. In other words, it may measure some factor well but not measure the factor that the ICP intended. The subject of validity is complex and in this context is particularly important in behavioral research. The reader is referred to Kerlinger[36] for an outstanding discussion of the topic.

Second, *reliability* is a synonym for dependability, stability, consistency, and predictability. The concept of reliability may be approached in several ways. For example, if the ICP measures the same set of objects repeatedly with the same or a comparable measuring device, will she get essentially the same results? If a patient's blood pressure is measured with the same sphygmomanometer several times in quick succession, will the reading be essentially the same? This definition implies stability and dependability of the measuring device.

In epidemiology, validity and reliability are often discussed with criteria for the evaluation of a screening test to detect disease (e.g., skin testing for tuberculosis; eye testing for glaucoma).

In this context the two components of validity are *sensitivity* and *specificity*. Sensitivity is defined as the ability to correctly identify those who have disease. Specificity is defined as the ability to correctly identify those who do *not* have the disease. (See Chapter 7 for discussion of these terms for nosocomial infection control.)

Observations may be highly reliable but not valid. For example, bacterial cultures reliably measure the presence of organisms cultured but alone are not valid indicators of infection. Sampling variation or inadequate sampling can produce results that are not valid; that is, the results are not representative of the "real" situation.

Clinical observations are the primary basis for decisions about the presence or absence of infection. However, all ICPs know that if the primary criterion for the presence of infection is that documentation of nosocomial infection is included in the patient's discharge diagnosis, many infections normally counted as nosocomial would not be identified. Reasons for this are many, but the point is that the discharge diagnosis is neither a valid nor a reliable single indicator of the presence of nosocomial infection.

Conclusions are often based on statistical analyses of the results. It is tempting to make broad statements of association and even causality if the statistical associations are highly significant. However, it is risky for the ICP to assume that because she has supported her hypothesis statistically that she has identified the "cause" of the problem.

What are the special features of certain relationships that lead epidemiologists to describe them as causal? Epidemiology has a practical purpose in the discovery of relationships that offer possibilities of disease *prevention*. For this purpose, a causal association may be defined as an association between two categories of events (e.g., risk factor versus infection) in which a change in frequency or quality of one is observed to follow alteration of the other.

There are several criteria of judgment of causal associations. Such judgments are reached by weighing available evidence, and different investigators often come to conflicting conclusions. The five criteria for judging causal relationships are discussed in detail in the epidemiology texts referenced at the end of the chapter, so they will only be briefly outlined here:

1. *Consistency.* Has the association been found in other studies of other populations by different investigators?

2. *Strength.* How strong is the association between two categories of events? That is, the higher the ratio of incidence of disease following exposure to the risk factor compared to the incidence of disease without exposure to the risk factor, the stronger the association. Strength measures the extent to which the risk factor affects the outcome (disease). Relative risk is a measure of the strength of an association.

3. *Specificity.* What is the extent to which the occurrence of one factor can be used to *predict* the occurrence of another factor? Specificity describes the precision with which the occurrence of one variable (risk factor) will predict the occurrence of another (disease). Rarely is an association true 100% of the time; rarely does a single factor cause disease.

4. *Coherence.* Does the proposed causal factor make sense biologically?

5. *Temporally correct association.* Is the sequence of events related such that the risk factor preceded in time the development of disease? Is this

sequence of events consistent? Associations in which the related events occur simultaneously or with varying precedence cannot be considered causal.

ICPs need to understand the basic concepts of causality and exercise caution in using the term *causal association*. However, criteria for causality are much easier to meet for some infectious diseases than for chronic diseases or diseases for which the cause is unclear and probably a result of multiple factors. For example, in an investigation of an outbreak of gastroenteritis caused by a *Shigella* organism, the criteria for causal association could be applied as follows:

1. *Consistency.* A *Shigella* organism has been the etiological organism for many outbreaks of gastroenteritis, and the association is well documented.
2. *Strength.* Attack rates among those exposed tend to be fairly high; attack rates of gastroenteritis among the unexposed are usually very low.
3. *Specificity.* Exposure to *Shigella* organisms will not always lead to gastroenteritis but will do so with fairly high frequency. This is partly related to a dose-response relationship and the fact that it takes only a small number of *Shigella* bacteria to produce gastroenteritis.
4. *Coherence.* Ingestion of the organism has been shown to cause gastroenteritis, and this association is biologically sound.
5. *Temporally correct association.* Ingestion of the *Shigella* bacteria must precede gastroenteritis caused by the organism.

Thus, in investigating an outbreak of shigellosis, it is safe to say that there is a causal association between the organism and disease.

It is more difficult to assess causality for some infections for which there is no common organism and there are multiple possible causes (e.g., postoperative wound infections or pneumonia).

PREPARING A REPORT

At the conclusion of any study the ICP has the responsibility of writing up the results. Because most studies are instigated at the request of or in consultation with one or more individuals (e.g., the infection control committee, the hospital epidemiologist), these persons need to know the results. A well-written report will go far to increase the credibility of the ICP both to the infection control committee and to the hospital administration. The following outline can be used for writing most reports. With a little modification, such reports are sometimes suitable for publication. The outline also includes instructions for submitting manuscripts for publication:

    I. Organizing content (it may help to prepare an outline)
       A. Title
       B. Author(s) with credentials and address(es)

C. Acknowledgments (may be footnoted on title page or as separate section at end of chapter)
D. Introduction (including some or all of the following points)
  1. Why? Purpose of study
    a. Background information; pertinent references
    b. The problem or interests that instigated study
  2. What? What was proposed in study (problem statement and/or hypothesis)
  3. When? Time period of study
  4. Where? Geographical limitation (hospital, units in hospital)
  5. Who? Population studied and sample size
E. Methods (how study was conducted)
  1. Type of study (e.g., descriptive, analytical)
  2. Definition of a case (ICP's or "standard" definition; if "standard" definition, it should be referenced)
  3. Copy of data collection form and/or methods used for data collection
F. Results (what was learned)
  1. Demographic information about population
  2. Results in logical sequence
  3. Tables, figures, and statistical analyses (each table or figure should have complete legend that is self-explanatory)
G. Discussion
  1. Interpreting data presented in results section as they pertain to question or problem posed in introduction
  2. Including additional literature review to compare study with previous studies
  3. Do data provide answers to questions?
  4. Is evidence adequate? Was sample large enough to reveal statistically significant differences?
H. Summary or abstract
  1. Approximately 200 words
  2. Succinct points about purpose, study, design, results, and conclusions
I. References (citations should be consistent in style)
  1. Numerical system in which references are numbered in sequence as they appear in text (numbers appear as superscripts or in parentheses when referenced in text)
  2. Name and year system (Harvard system) in which author's last name and publication year appear in text; reference list in alphabetical order
  3. Numerical system with references in alphabetical order; cited by number in text

II. Preparing manuscript for publication
   A. Requesting "Instructions to Authors" from journals to be considered
   B. If desired, writing letters of inquiry to one or more journals to learn which one(s) may be interested in the topic
   C. Having manuscript critiqued by one or more colleagues before preparation of final copy
   D. Typing all pages *double-spaced* on good bond paper throughout with ample margins (4 cm on all sides is not too much); many journals do *not* want manuscripts on erasable paper
   E. Numbering all pages with page number and last name
   F. Preparing each table and each figure on separate pages
   G. Typing references *double-spaced* in selected style
   H. Proofreading final draft
   I. Submitting original and one or two copies (as requested by "Instructions to Authors") to only *one* journal at a time
   J. *Always* including a cover letter to editor; preferably addressed by name

There are many other references for preparing manuscripts for various purposes.*

Authorship

A word of caution about publishing reports is necessary. It is usually desirable at the beginning of a project, study, or investigation planned for possible publication to determine *who* will author the report and in what order the author's names will probably appear. It can be very distressing and disappointing to an individual who has invested considerable time and effort in the footwork, headwork, and hard work of a study to be merely acknowledged in a footnote. Unfortunately, ICPs are sometimes in this category. To avoid such disappointment, ICPs should insist that authorship reflect each individual's contribution. Getting such issues settled initially can save embarrassment and other problems when it is time to write up the results. As infection control continues to develop as a multidisciplinary team effort and ICPs become more sophisticated in research methodology, their names should appear with increasing frequency in the authorship of infection control publications.

USING RESEARCH RESULTS TO IMPLEMENT CHANGE

In many instances studies were done because the ICP wondered if a practice, procedure, or other element of hospital infection control could be improved. If conclusions show that improvement can be made, it is important to follow through with implementing the needed changes throughout the facility. For example, if the ICP were studying alternative surveillance methods and

*References 2, 3, 9, 20, 25, 38, 43, 48.

found that prevalence surveys would yield acceptable results with less time, is it necessary to have such a change approved by the infection control committee? If the answer is yes, then such approval should be solicited as soon as possible after the study is completed so that the impact of the ICP's findings is not diminished.

Does the implementation of the recommended change require in-service education of nursing and medical staff? How frequently does this need to occur? Such questions can best be answered by the ICP because she knows the situation in which she works and the factors that will effect change there.

SUMMARY

This chapter is intended to give the reader a taste of the research process as it pertains to infection control. ICPs have considerable potential to do meaningful studies about infection control topics. However, it requires practice and time to develop such skills. As more undergraduate programs in nursing include research methodology in the curriculum, ICPs of the future can expect to have some methodological background. For experienced ICPs who did not receive such background, there are courses in research methodology available in most institutions of higher learning. There are also short courses and workshops available through numerous continuing education providers. The learning guide by Pavlovich[44] can be used for some self-instruction.

Another way to learn the research process is to work with someone who is already engaged in research. The ICP should ask questions, thereby participating, and read as much as possible about the person's field. When the ICP reads for any literature review, attention should be paid not only to content but also to methods used, as well as the style of writing.

When the ICP designs a study, she should ask others to critique it before beginning. She should get to know other ICPs who are interested in research and participating in research projects. If the facility has a research nurse, the ICP can get to know this person and see how she can be of assistance. If the ICP is in a position to seek an advanced degree, she may have considerable opportunity to learn the research process as part of the graduate school program.

Finally, it is hoped that when the Third International Conference on Nosocomial Infections is held in 1990, there will be many more infection control practices upgraded to category I and considerably more information about the behavioral aspects of infection control. It is also hoped that the keynote speaker will acknowledge that a substantial proportion of the studies have had input and authorship by ICPs.

ACKNOWLEDGMENT

I am grateful to the following individuals who provided valuable assistance with various phases of the preparation of this chapter: Franklin M.M. White, M.D.; Elizabeth Barrett-Connor, M.D.; Crawford G. Jackson, Jr., Ph.D; Dianne Niemeier, R.N., Ph.D; Mary Anne Sweeney, R.N., Ph.D; and Douglas C. Dechairo, M.D. Cecelia Ross kindly typed several drafts of the manuscript. I also thank Nancy Muravez, R.N., M.S., for her encouragement and support in this and other professional endeavors.

REFERENCES

1. American Journal of Epidemiology: Special issue—the SENIC project, **111:**464-653, 1980.
2. American Medical Association: Manual for authors and editors: editorial style and manuscript preparation, Los Altos, Calif., 1981, Lange Medical Publications.
3. American Psychological Association: Publications manual, ed. 2, Washington, D.C., 1974, American Psychological Association.
4. Arking, L.M., and McArthur, B.J.: Infection control, Nurs. Clin. North Am. **15:**615-917, 1980.
5. Austin, D.F., and Werner, S.B.: Epidemiology for the health sciences, ed. 2, Springfield, Ill., 1978, Charles C Thomas, Publisher.
6. Axnick, K.J., et al.: Commentary: infection control: the next 10 years, Am. J. Med. **70:**979-986, 1981.
7. Barrett-Connor, E., et al., editors: Epidemiology for the infection control nurse, St. Louis, 1978, The C.V. Mosby Co.
8. Bennett, J.V., and Brachman, P.S., editors: Hospital infections, Boston, 1979, Little, Brown & Co.
9. Binger, J.L., and Jensen, L.M.: Lippincott's guides to nursing literature—a handbook for students, writers, and researchers, Philadelphia, 1980, J.B. Lippincott Co.
10. Brink, P.J., and Wood, M.J.: Basic steps in planning nursing research, Belmont, Calif., 1978, Duxbury Press.
11. Burke, J.F., and Hildick-Smith, G.Y.: The infection prone hospital patient, Boston, 1978, Little, Brown & Co.
12. Castle, M.: Hospital infection control: principles and practice, New York, 1980, John Wiley & Sons, Inc.
13. Centers for Disease Control: Outline for surveillance and control of nosocomial infections, Atlanta, rev. June 1972, Hospital Infections Branch, Bacterial Diseases Division, Center for Infectious Diseases, Centers for Disease Control.
14. Centers for Disease Control: Prevalence survey for nosocomial infections, Atlanta, rev. March 1980, Hospital Infections Branch, Bacterial Diseases Division, Center for Infectious Diseases, Centers for Disease Control.
15. Centers for Disease Control: Guidelines for the prevention and control of nosocomial infections, Atlanta, 1981, Guidelines Activity, Hospital Infections Branch, Bacterial Diseases Division, Center for Infectious Diseases, Centers for Disease Control.
16. Centers for Disease Control: Training materials: descriptive and analytic statistics, Atlanta, (no date), Instructional Services Division, Center for Professional Development and Training, Centers for Disease Control.
17. Chavigny, K.H.: Microbial infections in hospitals: a review of the literature and some suggestions for nursing research, Int. J. Nurs. Stud. **14:**37-46, 1977.
18. Cochran, W.G.: Sampling techniques, ed. 3, New York, 1977, John Wiley & Sons, Inc.
19. Colton, T.: Statistics in medicine, Boston, 1974, Little, Brown & Co.
20. Council of Biology Editors: Style manual, ed. 4, Arlington, 1978, American Institute of Biological Sciences.
21. Cruse, P.J.E., and Foord, R.: A five-year prospective study of 23,049 surgical wounds, Arch. Surg. **107:**206-210, 1973.
22. Cumulative Index Medicus: Washington, D.C. (published monthly), U.S. Government Printing Office.
23. Cumulative Index to Nursing and Allied Health Literature: Glendale, Calif. (published monthly), Cumulative Index to Nursing and Allied Health Literature Corp.
24. Current Contents–Clinical Practice and Life Science Series: Philadelphia (published monthly), ISI Press.
25. Day, R.A.: How to write and publish a scientific paper, Philadelphia, 1979, ISI Press.
26. Dixon, R.E.: Forging the missing link in infection control, Am. J. Med. **70:**976-979, 1981.

27. Eickhoff, T.C.: Nosocomial infections—a 1980 view: progress, priorities, and prognosis, Proceedings from the Second International Conference on Nosocomial Infections, Am. J. Med. **70**:381-388, 1981.

28. Emerson, S.G., and Jackson, M.M.: Organizing your references with the marginal punch-sort card system, Nurs. Management **13**:33-37, 1982.

29. Ferber, R., et al.: What is a survey? Washington D.C., 1980, American Statistical Association.

30. Fox, D.J.: Fundamentals of research in nursing, ed. 4, New York, 1982, Appleton-Century-Crofts.

31. Friedman, G.: Primer of epidemiology, ed. 2, New York, 1980, McGraw-Hill Book Co.

32. Fuller, E.A.: A system for filing medical literature based on a method developed by Dr. Maxwell H. Wintrobe, Ann. Int. Med. **66**:684-693, 1968.

33. Grady, G.F., et al.: Hepatitis B immune globulin for accidental exposures among medical personnel: final report of a multicenter controlled trial, J. Infect. Dis. **138**:625-638, 1978.

34. Jackson, M.M., and Blaise, S.A.: Developing your own resource library, Infect. Control Urol. Care **5**:6-9, 1980 (Travenol Laboratories, Deerfield, Ill.).

35. Kass, E.H.: Surveillance as a control system panel, Proceedings 1970 International Conference on Nosocomial Infections, Chicago, 1971, American Hospital Association.

36. Kerlinger, F.H.: Foundations of behavioral research, ed. 2, New York, 1973, Holt Rinehart & Winston.

37. Knapp, R.G.: Basic statistics for nurses, New York, 1978, John Wiley & Sons, Inc.

38. Kolin, P.C., and Kolin, J.L.: Professional writing for nurses in education, practice, and research, St. Louis, 1980, The C.V. Mosby Co.

39. Levy, P.S., and Lemeshow, S.: Sampling for health professionals, Belmont, Calif., 1980, Wadsworth, Inc.

40. Lilienfeld, A.M., and Lilienfeld, D.E.: Foundations of epidemiology, ed. 2, New York, 1980, Oxford University Press.

41. MacMahon, B., and Pugh, T.F.: Epidemiology—principles and methods, Boston, 1970, Little, Brown & Co.

42. Mausner, J.S., and Bahn, A.K.: Epidemiology—an introductory text, Philadelphia, 1974, W.B. Saunders Co.

43. O'Connor, A.B.: Writing for nursing publications, ed. 2, Thorofare, N.J., 1981, Charles B. Slack, Inc.

44. Pavlovich, N.: Nursing research—a learning guide, St. Louis, 1978, The C.V. Mosby Co.

45. Polit, D.F., and Hungler, B.P.: Nursing research: principles and methods, Philadelphia, 1978, J.B. Lippincott Co.

46. Seeff, L.B., et al.: Type B hepatitis after needle-stick exposure: prevention with hepatitis B immune globulin, Ann. Intern. Med. **88**:285-298, 1978.

47. Singer, K.: Where did I see that article? J.A.M.A. **241**:1492-1493, 1979.

48. Strunk, W., Jr., and White, E.B.: The elements of style, ed. 2, New York, 1972, MacMillan, Inc.

49. Sweeney, M.A., and Olivieri, P.: An introduction to nursing research: research, measurements, and computers in nursing, Philadelphia, 1981, J.B. Lippincott Co.

50. Swinscow, T.D.: Statistics at square one, ed. 5, London, 1979, British Medical Association.

51. Treece, E.W., and Treece, J.W., Jr.: Elements of research in nursing, ed. 3, St. Louis, 1982, The C.V. Mosby Co.

52. Wenzel, R.P.: CRC handbook of hospital acquired infections, Boca Raton, Fla., 1981, CRC Press.

9

Communication

communication Process of sharing information whereby one person sends a message to another with the conscious intent of receiving a response.

feedback Verbal and nonverbal responses to a sender; serves the function of acknowledging receipt of a message and checking the accuracy of the transmission.

feedforward Process by which the sender initiates a thought or idea that starts the communication and elicits feedback.

filters Two types of filters (barriers) distort communication: psychological filters (people) *distort* communication; environmental filters (things) *interrupt* communication.

jamming A form of communication that disrupts or obscures attempts to communicate.

language skills Skills used to construct and deliver intelligible messages.

perceptual skills Skills used to adapt messages to fit a specific listener.

small groups Groups of people who are psychologically and physically related and who communicate face-to-face.[1]

Communication calls for dynamic personal involvement and close sympathetic relationships. In itself, communication is a search for a common union. However, many do not understand the elements of communication, do not realize how to acquire the skills, or do not choose to initiate the dynamic personal involvement or close sympathetic relationship that effective communication requires.

The effectiveness of an infection control practitioner (ICP) depends not only on her personal knowledge and capabilities but also on how well she interacts with other people. The primary tool for interaction is communication. What most lose sight of is that communication is a frail and imprecise process. It is not a process that can be taken for granted.

An ICP spends a great deal of time, energy, thought, and money getting ready to practice infection control. How much of that time was devoted to skills in dealing with people? Unfortunately, in the ICP's approach to education, getting along with people is left for the most part either to chance or to a social nature all ICPs are thought to possess.

The effective communicator (the effective ICP) has two sets of skills: *language skills* and *perceptual skills*. Language skills are used to construct and deliver intelligible messages. Perceptual skills are used to adapt messages to fit a specific listener. Success in almost any endeavor depends on how good the ICP is at relating to, communicating with, and understanding others with whom she comes in contact. Although the ICP can come to some valuable conclusions through trial and error in communicating, it is not necessary for her to take risks with her success. Why should she stake her professional and personal life on a horse that wanders aimlessly down a track when some practical approaches to improving her ability to communicate will get her squarely on the road to success?

Once, all fine craftsmen signed their work. A craftsman's mark was a symbol—it stood for quality in workmanship and for a job well done. It was a mark of pride. Craftsmen took pleasure in what they did, and they signed their work to prove it. It is important for the ICP to remember that the words she speaks and writes bear her mark. They should be the mark of a craftsman.

THE DEFINITION

When trying to describe communication, one is reminded of the 1960s film *Cool Hand Luke* in which Paul Newman portrayed a rebellious inmate in a Southern chain gang prison. He continually tried to escape but was always caught and punished harshly. The warden looked over his sunglasses and said blandly, "What we've got here is a failure to communicate."

For the warden, communication had a very limited definition. It meant agreement with what he wanted. However, what the warden failed to understand was that communication is much more complicated than having others support his rules and regulations. By acting in a rebellious manner, Luke was communicating a definite message, but it was one that was impossible for the warden to comprehend.

Many see the communication process in a rather simplistic way, as did the warden. They believe that because they talk all the time, listen to the radio, or watch television they are "communicating" effectively. This view is deceptive and can very easily lead to situations in which silence is perceived as agreement, people and events are stereotyped, and people fail to realize that their views do influence the world around them.

My approach will be to look at interpersonal communication—verbal, nonverbal, and written—for small or large audiences or readerships. Interesting research is afoot today on communication that includes nonhuman components, but I will concentrate on how the ICP, a single yet powerful human, can interact effectively with people. The fundamental value of any interpersonal association is the enhancement and growth of the individual.

An ICP must communicate. She manages people, not machines. Machines have buttons that one pushes to make something happen; people do not. *Communication is what makes things happen with people.*

The single most important facet of the ICP role is communication. If the ICP makes a decision, that decision is meaningless until it has been communicated. She lends her experience to decision making by others, but how can she do that without communicating? She gives in-service education, which is a job of communicating. The ICP solves problems, but a solution not communicated is the same as no solution. She writes reports or memoranda that supply information to others. She motivates people, makes suggestions, offers ideas, and answers questions. All of these require effective and skillful communication.

However, with all the emphasis on and demand for communication, much of it is ineffective. The communication of even the best manager is only about 80% effective; the average is closer to 60%. Something will be misunderstood or misinterpreted or will produce the wrong reaction one out of every five times the ICP expresses an idea, explains a problem, or writes a report.

THE PROCESS

Perhaps the biggest reason for imperfect communication is the imperfection of the communication process itself. There is a vast difference between the ideal and the real communication process. In the communication process the message is whatever the ICP wants to communicate to someone. In the ideal situation the message she sends and the one that is received will be identical and produce complete understanding (Fig. 9-1). It rarely happens. The sender is the ICP; the receiver is whomever she is trying to communicate with. The medium is the way the message is sent, such as speaking to someone, writing a letter or report, putting a meeting notice on the bulletin board, issuing an infection control manual, and even waving a greeting or smiling at someone (Fig. 9-2).

All messages are sheathed in emotion.[6] Human experiences tell the ICP that she can trigger responses in receivers by derogatory words, slurs, racial overtones, or innuendos. The emotional state of the sender and the receiver can play havoc with communication. On the other hand, grasping the positive use of emotions in communication can work to the ICP's advantage.

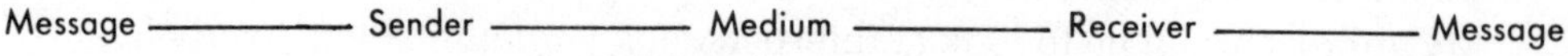

Message ——————— Sender ——————— Medium ——————— Receiver ——————— Message

FIG. 9-1. Ideal communication process.

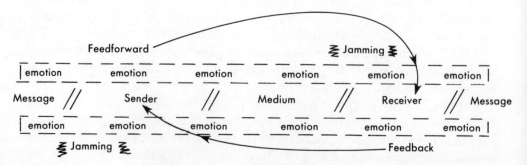

FIG. 9-2. Real communication process.

The response to a message is fed back to the sender verbally or nonverbally. *Feedback* serves the function of acknowledging receipt of a message and checking the accuracy of the transmission,[4] such as nodding approval, frowning to indicate puzzlement, rephrasing the communication, and even silently evaluating the group reaction before making another point. Sometimes it is explicit feedback, such as, "I think we should discuss in-service education."

In *feedforward* the sender initiates a thought or idea that starts the communication sequence and elicits feedback. Feedforward suggests the direction and content of further communication.[4] These preliminary messages alert others to what is to come or get a reading as to whether or not the sender should continue in a given direction. Although abbreviated, these preliminary messages are potentially valuable because they can set the stage for productive communication.

Jamming is a form of communication that disrupts or obscures attempts to communicate.[4] This includes inaccurate illustrations; humor that embarrasses, overamuses, or offends; or any reason that the receiver misinterprets a message or follows some tangent. Speakers and listeners can control jamming, but a large share falls on the listeners, for they do the actual jamming. The speaker is responsible for a clear, directed message; the listener, on the other hand, is responsible for not jamming the path.

Between each step of the communication process are barriers called filters. These imperfections distort communication. It is impossible to list all filters that the ICP may encounter. Any one attempt to communicate almost always involves several filters, all working at the same time. Although numerous, all filters are either *psychological filters* (people) or *environmental filters* (things).

Thing filters interrupt communication; people filters distort communication. Thing filters are the physical elements that either interrupt or confuse the flow of communication, such as noise that keeps the sender from being heard properly, a sender who mumbles, a receiver who is hard of hearing, or a typographical error in a report. Other distractions, such as a glaring light behind the speaker, a warm stuffy room, or a third party who arrives late, will break up the conversation to the point that the speaker never quites gets back on the track again.

Thing filters can cause severe damage to the flow of communication, but they are usually easy to identify. If it is too noisy, the sender can hear this and compensate for it by talking louder or moving the conversation to a quiet place. Interruptions and distractions can usually be seen by the sender, as well as the receiver, and can be corrected.

People filters relate to the minds of the sender and receiver. Does the sender select the right words to get the thought across? What kind of mood is the receiver in? What are the receiver's preconceived ideas about the subject? Does the sender act or sound bored or excited when she sends her message? What else does the receiver have on her mind? Does the receiver like, trust, or believe the sender? What is the receiver's attitude toward the medium of communication (she may never read the bulletin board because she thinks there is never anything there for her).

Because it is extremely difficult to know exactly what is going on in the receiver's mind, people filters are critical. They are filters that cause misunderstanding or misinterpretation. They produce results, such as, "But that's not what I thought you said," "I remember discussing it, but I didn't know you wanted me to do anything about it," or "I didn't realize you were serious about it."

What can be done about people filters? The ICP should constantly keep in mind that people filters exist. She must not assume that she got through and should ask questions (feedback) to find out if the message (feedforward) did get through. The following will help to minimize people filters:

1. The brain should be engaged before starting the mouth. The ICP must think through what needs to be said.

2. The eyes have it. The ICP should watch the receiver's eyes; they tell a lot about the mindset. The receiver is probably paying attention if she is looking at the ICP. If the receiver is looking away, she may be distracted or thinking about something else. The ICP should watch the receiver's eyes as she reads a report the ICP has submitted. If they move at a steady pace, the message is probably getting through. If they skip around, the reader is skimming and probably is not absorbing much. If they stop moving but stay on the paper, the chances are the reader is either confused by some point or something has peaked her interest. The ICP should ask! If the reader is confused, the problem should be cleared up. If the reader is interested, the ICP can grab the opportunity to lend understanding.

3. The unusual gets in the way. Knowing the receiver and how she normally acts will help. If something unusual is occurring, a people filter is at work. If a normally quiet, calm nurse is jumpy and loud, something is bothering her. That something may just distort communication. If a normally talkative nurse suddenly "clams up" during a discussion, it may be a sign of defensiveness, one of the most dangerous of the people filters. The ICP can apply the waiting rule to herself. If the ICP is under pressure or is moody, she should save anything important for another time when she will do a good job of communicating. Margerison[7] describes five interpersonal reactions—regressive, fixation, defensive, aggressive, supportive—and typical comments for each reaction that arises during an interpersonal discussion.

4. It is important to pay attention, listen closely, and read thoroughly.

The ICP should ask for clarification and not be ashamed to admit ignorance.

5. The best message should be put first. If the ICP has to make a point she knows the receiver may resist, she should deliver something the receiver likes first. That way the ICP will have the receiver's full attention when she gets to her point.

Because the ICP receives all messages through her own perceptual screen, communication seems difficult. She sees things in terms of herself. Her message seems more important than the pipeline of feeling that will allow it to flow to the receiver. Simply saying something does not make the receiver "get it" or "see what you are saying." The ICP sees with her "I," the totality of her personality—all things that have happened to make up her unique goals, purposes, and values.

Even the simplest words are often poor instruments. They are loaded for misunderstanding, misinterpretation, and misuse. Each word is strained through the hearer's values, goals, experiences, and emotions.

Communication begins where the other person is, not where the ICP is. The ICP must develop skills in building bridges over which a message can travel. The first bridge is feeling. Communication is sheathed in emotion. She must have patience to tune others in and to become a master of the art of building readiness for the individual and the group. No communication is perfect; at best, the sender and receiver may have the pleasure of sharing ideas.[7]

The ICP, as an effective communicator, should know her own likes and dislikes and have them under control. Is it possible that she is more interested in the message than in the receiver? Too often the message is prepared with such great care and precision that this well-structured message is delivered as if the listener(s) were secondary.

A single communication explodes in many directions.[1] It carries varying tones and intensities of meaning for its receivers. The ICP may take careful aim and hope to activate the intended receiver to give a favorable response. Once launched, a communication may reach the receiver or may miss the intended target. It is in the ICP's hands to direct her messages—complex and far-reaching missiles—across the barriers inherent in the process of communication.

SMALL GROUPS

Most of the daily activities of an ICP are related to or conducted in small groups: the ICP and one other person or staff meetings between the ICP and up to 12 or 15 others. To be an effective communicator, the ICP should examine the nature of small groups and think critically about the communication roles that she adopts as a member of all these groups.

No specific number of people makes up a small group. A five-person family, a two-person tennis team, a surgical team, or a hospital staff may all be considered a small group. If not defined by numbers, what is a small group? According to Allen,[1] members of a small group—2 or 102—are psychologically and physically related, and they communicate with each other face-to-face.

It is not enough that people be in the same place at the same time. They must be psychologically and physically related; they must have a feeling of identification with each other. Nine people in a hospital elevator are physically related in that enclosed space. If the elevator stalls between floors, they become aware of each other as persons. They become a group when they interact purposefully to solve their common problem, that is, to exit from the elevator at their intended destination.

How many small groups does the ICP belong to? By origin, there is the casual group, the self-motivated group, the ongoing group, the appointed group, and the constrained group. If groups are classified according to purpose or function, they fall into social groups, learning groups, problem-solving groups, or action groups. If small groups are considered in the context of large group communications, they are classified as panel discussions, symposiums, or workshops.

Small groups may have varying numbers of members. As a small group increases in numbers, it becomes increasingly difficult for the group to maintain psychological identification in which face-to-face communication exists.

As the number of people increases in the group, the number of possible links continues to rise by geometrical progression. As the number of people increases, the task of experiencing psychological identification and a sense of direct communication becomes more and more difficult. The links possible in a 12-member group and a 15-member group are numerous and complex. Since small group communication is an integral part of life, the function of a sender and receiver of messages in that setting is at the core of successful communication.

ANALYZING COMMUNICATION

One-to-one communication—two people, one link—is deceivingly simple. The ease in diagraming this mode of communication belies the complex forces at work (Fig. 9-3). ICPs find themselves daily in one-to-one communication. The ICP might survey the variety of communication groups she finds herself in during one day's hospital work and note the times she was a subordinate, a peer, or a supervisor. How often did she talk to herself?

If a picture is worth a thousand words, then a diagram is invaluable in pinpointing unbalanced communication (Fig. 9-4). Keeping score and charting the most frequent mode of communication can open the ICP's eyes and ears, and perhaps she will be able to see what she says and how she says it during interpersonal communication. Charting communication between a supervisor

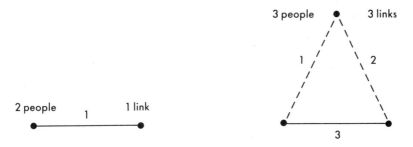

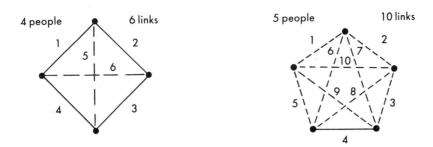

FIG. 9-3. Communication links in small groups.

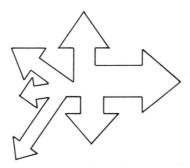

FIG. 9-4. Exploding nature of a single communication.

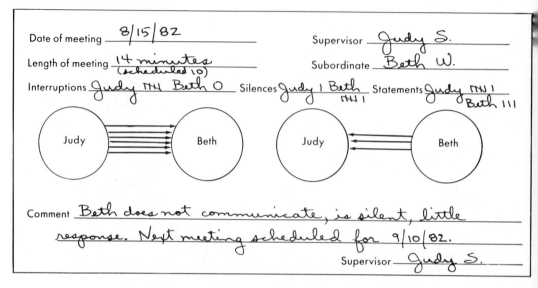

Date of meeting ___8/15/82___   Supervisor ___Judy S.___

Length of meeting ___14 minutes___   Subordinate ___Beth W.___
                  (scheduled 10)

Interruptions ___Judy THL Beth 0___ Silences Judy 1 Beth   Statements Judy THL I
                                                        THL 1   Beth III

Judy → Beth   Judy ← Beth

Comment ___Beth does not communicate, is silent, little___
___response. Next meeting scheduled for 9/10/82.___
                                          Supervisor ___Judy S.___

FIG. 9-5. Communication dominated by supervisor.

and subordinate on a file card will help the ICP check the quality and equality of communication.[6] Does she dominate the conversation, interrupt, or remain silent? How long are the silences? When she is silent, is she listening or is she filled with emotion and plotting her next defensive move, thus blocking out the other person's ideas? In Fig. 9-5 the low participation by the subordinate, the high number of interruptions, and the low number of silences suggest that the subordinate tried to participate but was cut off by the supervisor. The meeting was obviously dominated by the supervisor. Of importance is the supervisor's incorrect assessment that the subordinate does not communicate. The supervisor correctly sees that the subordinate is silent but fails to see that she has dominated this interpersonal communication. A scheduled 10-minute meeting dragged on to 14 minutes possibly because the supervisor thought that quantity of input from her would make up for the quality that she was lacking. Fortunately, another meeting was scheduled, and if the supervisor analyzes this communication using the diagram, a more productive meeting may result.

In Fig. 9-6 the diagram indicates that a balanced one-to-one communication was achieved. Another positive change, the allotted time, was used productively. The supervisor's comments reflect the value of quality and equality in this meeting.

Diagraming can be applied to any small group, in any role the ICP may be playing, and in her personal and professional life. As a leader of a discussion group or chairman of a meeting, the ICP can mentally keep score to pinpoint

Date of meeting ——————————   Supervisor ———————————

Length of meeting ——————————   Subordinate ———————————

Interruptions ————————— Silences ————————— Statements —————

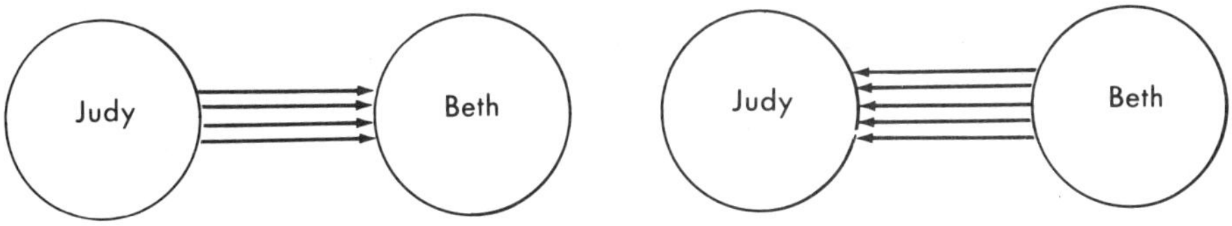

FIG. 9-6. Balanced one-to-one communication.

the dominant participant(s) and then shift the participation to those reluctant communicators, unearthing treasures that once were silent.

SIDEWAYS COMMUNICATION

One of the toughest communication challenges is the horizontal or sideways communication, that is, communication between managers on the same level who represent different areas or different functions within the hospital. It is also the form of communication that results in the most serious problems when it breaks down.

Sideways communication is one of the toughest because it has peculiar pitfalls that do not exist in up-and-down (up to supervisor, down to subordinates) communication and requires peculiar skills. It causes the biggest problems when it breaks down because it commonly involves things that affect the hospital as a whole. Breakdown of vertical communication within one department usually affects only that organizational unit (Fig. 9-7).

Certain characteristics of managers can frequently get in the way of communicating effectively with other managers. A manager's primary obligation is to do her own job. That preoccupation can result in insulating herself from the duties and responsibilities of others. Once she is insulated, the ability to consider the other managers' viewpoints or problems or assess things in terms of "the bigger picture" is seriously impaired. One of the reasons the manager got to be a manager is a sense of competition. Competition has two elements:

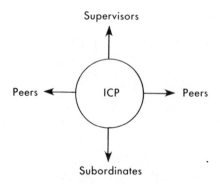

FIG. 9-7. Personal communication network.

offense and defense. Unfortunately, many managers carry over these same attributes to their dealings with other managers on the same team. It results too often in strained relations that interfere with cooperation. Friendly competition becomes conflict, defensiveness, and the constant suspicion of an ulterior motive.

An important element of vertical communication is missing in sideways communication: the boss-subordinate relationship that predetermines who has the most authority. Manager-to-manager communication involves unconscious sparring intended to establish authority, but it usually does not.

The challenge of sideways communication has no alternative. Without effective communication between managers, the whole management process breaks down.[7] With it can go the success of the entire organization. How does the ICP meet this challenge? Some suggestions follow:

1. The lines of communication with other managers should be kept open no matter what. The ICP should talk with the other manager, not behind her back. Even if talking does not solve the problem, silence guarantees that the problem will get worse.

2. Offering cooperation rather than finding fault, assigning blame, or accusing others of being careless or inefficient will help. The ICP should not make another manager oppose her just to save face.

3. The ICP must never hesitate to let her requirements, objectives, or problems be known. She should share challenges and solutions and speak up without demanding. She will be hurt in the eyes of her supervisor if another manager says, "Of course I could have helped, if only she'd let me."

4. Preparing schedules or timetables is important. The ICP cannot expect others to know her work intimately; she needs to tell them. Many projects involving more than one department or unit often fail because everybody waits for someone else to act.

5. The ICP should learn how to promote a plan. If she can show that her proposal will benefit the hospital as a whole, half the battle for gaining cooperation is won. If, instead, it seems only to favor her or her area of responsibility, total support is diminished.

6. Knowing how to disagree is an advantage. It is possible to disagree with another manager without making an enemy. The ICP should not lose her temper or attack the manager's intelligence, integrity, or competence. The ICP must not brush off the manager's ideas, good or bad; they are hers, and she has a right to express them. If the ICP has to disagree, she should do so in straightforward, unemotional, and impersonal words. She should disagree with the idea, not with the person who suggested it.

7. The ICP must be prepared to compromise. She should not automatically shoot down other managers' suggestions or assume that every objection or modification of her own plan is an attempt to trip her up. Fighting for her own ideas is good, but the other manager may have sound reasons for her ideas, too.

8. Worrying about who has authority will get the ICP nowhere. If the question bothers her that much, it is probably because she is not very secure in her own position. (She will have to resolve this within herself, not in conflict with others.) She should either accept authority jointly with another manager or recognize that a higher authority will have to be called in anyway. The first alternative is better by far. It is the quickest way to get results. More important, if the subject will have to be taken to a supervisor anyway, the ICP and the other manager are both better off by presenting a united front. Finally, having to call in a higher authority may resolve the problem, but it also puts the supervisor on notice that the ICP and manager are squabbling.

9. In every dealing with another manager, the ICP should honestly ask herself, "Is she saying something about me and my job, or is she really saying something that she has a perfect right to say because it also affects her job?" If it is the latter (and it usually is), the manager deserves the most cooperative response the ICP can give.

PERSONAL COMMUNICATION

Fig. 9-7 illustrates the players in the ICP's personal communications network that functions within the hospital and within her personal life. Talking with oneself is a valuable tool. The thought processes that go into assessing a situation in a meeting before making a point and how to verbalize it silently are valuable feedback in the overall communication pattern. Uris[11] points out that rehearsing a difficult message or running through a joke before a presentation are signs of a successful communicator. The notes the ICP writes on her memoranda pad or appointment calendar, such as "Meet with Dr. Weiss—budget," are written self-reminders. If the ICP brings herself to a fine performance point (talking herself into it), she will reinforce the value of her inner talks.

MEETINGS

Every person at a meeting is caught between a desire to participate and a fear that factors present in the situation will make it impossible to offer ideas.[8] The leader must do her best to eliminate those factors that block participation—people and thing filters—and give full attention to the basic needs of all participants[9]:

- To receive information
- To tell something of their unique interests
- To ask questions for clarification
- To be asked for advice from their experience and background
- To be creative and give of themselves

Effective participation in discussion involves more than just talking. Skill in reflective thinking processes and flexibility in interpersonal relations are basic to an effective participation pattern in discussion. Individuals may participate in ways that are goal centered, group centered, or ego centered.[4] If the leader is not respected and trusted as one who believes in hearing others out, people will not communicate clearly and honestly no matter what techniques are used. The following suggestions for improvement of participation apply equally to members and to those designated as leaders:

1. Listen critically and thoughtfully to others; use critical faculties when listening; accept new facts, information, and opinions; and demand backup for unsupported generalizations.
2. Be sure you know the goal of the discussion and the time limit at the start. If you do not know where you are going, you may never get there.
3. Speak your mind freely. Besides the responsibility of listening, you have the duty to share ideas.
4. Strike while the iron is hot. If you wait too long, your point may be lost.
5. Let the other participants talk, too. Be concise and precise; do not speak for more than a minute or two. Who is carrying the ball toward the goal is unimportant. Reaching the established goal of the meeting is vital.
6. Stay on top of the discussion. Ask for clarification because you cannot make wise decisions based on misunderstandings.
7. Freely share the ownership of ideas. Present an idea to the group and let it become their property.
8. Disagree in a friendly and positive way. Raw emotion always hinders sound thinking.
9. Stay on target. Show how your remarks are relevant to the discussion, and do not repeat what has already been said.

10. Try to maintain an open mind. Discussion is not debate. Try to be unprejudiced and objective.

11. Come to the discussion prepared to participate. Think through the issues, collect the facts, and list the questions you would like to have answered.

12. Try to make the experience a pleasant one. A smile or a bit of humor may do more for the discussion than your best argument.

13. Help others to participate. Help to draw out the timid because their knowledge and opinions are important. Call them by name and refer specific questions to them. Everyone is a resource.

14. Chart the progress of the discussion. From time to time, ask for a summary or give one yourself. Call attention to the group's goals and the progress made toward those goals, pointing out the ground to be covered and the time remaining.

15. Avoid interrupting the progress of the discussion. Do only those things that move the discussion toward the goal. Be a booster, not a blocker.

16. Keep the communication channels open. Be sure to listen to what is said. Direct remarks to the entire group in clear and temperate language, checking to see if you have been understood as you intended and asking for feedback.

SEATING

The leader must take advantage of every opportunity to promote working together, trading ideas, and understanding difficult and different points of view. A wise leader knows that conflicts can arise before the meeting begins.

If the members of one department, group, or school of thought are lined up on one side of the table and their opponents are on the other, what could be more natural than a battle? The sides have already been drawn up for a fight. This type of "versus" seating stresses conflict, disagreement, and distress. The ICP can counteract this by breaking up groups, separating them physically so that they begin to think separately. A wide, centrally placed table can be used. The ICP can surround them with good space, air, temperature, light, and supplies. A good meeting room gives the group a feeling of coming together for a purpose and puts the ICP in a favorable position of control.

The secret ingredient of the meeting situation is cooperation of the members and control by the ICP as leader.[10] The ICP should be in a central position at the head of the table or on the side. Long narrow tables should be avoided. They make it impossible for one member to see another and put the ICP in a bad control position (Figs. 9-8 and 9-9).

If there are more than 12 members, the ICP, as a leader, should sit in the center on the side so that she will face more of the group. A judge in a court-

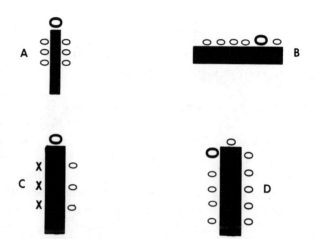

FIG. 9-8. Some seating plans work against leader to build tension and promote conflict and dissension, thus strangling communication. **A,** Table too narrow. **B,** Poor leader visibility. **C,** Conflict of groups. **D,** Poor leader position.

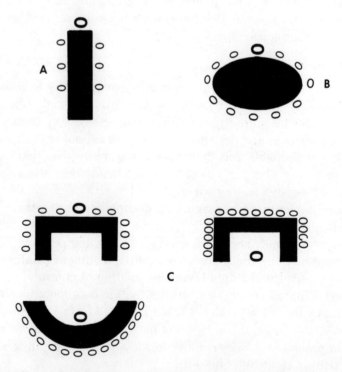

FIG. 9-9. Seating will work for leader and group when there is good visibility and good leadership position. **A,** Smaller meeting. **B,** Good visibility—oval or round table. **C,** Excellent visibility for larger meeting.

room is not at the front of the room on a raised platform for whimsical reasons. That is a power position. The meeting should be given every chance of success. The members will recognize the ICP's efforts and will contribute generously.

ASSERTIVE COMMUNICATION
Pushy people

Nowhere is skilled communication needed more clearly than in the face of pushy people. These living obstacles to the clear communication path are described by Bramson[2] as Sherman tanks—they push, charge, and attack on a psychological rather than on a physical level. Most evident is their strong commitment to a single cause: their view of the world is always right. If they perceive the ICP's resistance to their own plans, their short fuse is ablaze. Impatience turns to irritation, indignation, or caustic anger. They expect one thing: others will run from them. It is critical that the ICP not fulfill their hope that, through fear or rage, she will be put out of commission or her message will die. She must avoid an open confrontation, not man the verbal battle stations. She should "bite the bullet" and apply assertive communication:

1. The ICP must stand up for herself. If she lets herself be pushed around, she will fade into the scenery; pushy people will act as if the ICP is not a part of their world, and for a Sherman tank, she is not. It is all right for her to feel angry, awkward, or distraught, but she should say something assertive: "I'm not sure you heard what I was trying to say" or "Here's the point I was trying to make."
2. The ICP should give time and room to run down. Whatever the assault phase, she should remain firmly in place, look directly at the Sherman tank, and wait. When the attack begins to fade (and it will), she can jump into the situation.
3. The ICP should forget about being polite and just jump in. Cutting Sherman tanks off before they are through is a necessity. If she is cut off in turn, she can say firmly and loudly, "You interrupted me!"
4. The ICP should get their attention, carefully and firmly. Since they expect the ICP to run away or fly into a rage, she must get their attention and dispel the idea that she is going to respond according to their expectations. She should clearly and loudly address pushy people by their names, names that fit the ICP's level of relationship (e.g., Dr. Bartlet, Mr. Meade, Kim, Joe—not name calling). To get rapid attention and interrupt the interaction, the ICP can either stand up deliberately, drop a pencil, or upset a glass of water. This sounds drastic, but opening up the communication in the ICP's favor is the objective.
5. The pushy person should be asked to sit down. Sherman tanks cannot run over people and move over the fallen bodies when they are seated. Most people behave less aggressively when seated. The ICP can offer a

chair and say firmly, "If we're going to argue, we might as well be comfortable and sit down."

6. The ICP should speak from her point of view by selecting words and phrases that project self-assertiveness. Her words must express her viewpoint, yet she does not need to launch a direct attack on the other person's ideas: "In my opinion, it's a good idea" or "My experience was such that I disagree with you."

Bramson[2] cautions that the fear and confusion that are felt after being attacked by a pushy person are natural "fright and flight" feelings and are appropriate human reactions. The ICP should go with those feelings but clear up the distorted message.

The other sex

If the ICP feels cheated or defeated in conversations with men, it may be because she is not playing the communication game by the same rules. In conversations between the sexes, typically the woman reacts more and asks more questions. Her properly placed nod, "Mm hmm," or "Yes" encourages the speaker to plow on. Men are masters of what may be called the "delayed minimal response," an infuriating grunt that comes seconds too late. A woman may interpret this as a lack of interest, often bringing the conversation to a halt. A man is much more likely to interrupt and change the subject abruptly. Zimmerman and West[12] made some startling discoveries when studying taped conversations between men and women. Women may contribute in various ways to their own victimization in a conversation. In the study men repeatedly butted in when speaking with women, not to agree with what the women were saying but to take over and change the subject. In all too many cases the women relinquished the floor and fell silent.

Men who commandeer conversations are believed to be "flexing their muscles," since through interruptions, men control and dominate women trying to communicate. Perhaps the conditioning a woman receives, with its emphasis on being polite and cooperative, may be responsible for her willingness to let a man take the floor. Between the ages of 5 and 12 girls learn how to get along and master diplomatic indirect conversation. Boys who usually hang out in larger groups learn domineering conversation.

Lakoff[5] suggests that some women put themselves at a disadvantage in conversation with men by the words they choose, their intonation, and the structure of their sentences. Speaking "like a lady" ends up sounding insecure and nonassertive. Empty adjectives (e.g., "divine," "lovely," "cute"), tag questions hung at the end of a statement seeking confirmation from the other conversation partner ("It's nice here, isn't it?") or superpolite language ("Would you be so kind as to remove that wheelchair?") all make the woman appear weak, unsure, and insecure. Another hallmark is rising terminals; questioning intonations at the ends of sentences can be interpreted as being apologetic or lacking confidence. Since both sexes do this, it may be a way of indirectly expressing some potentially hostile questions. In either case rising terminals sound hesitant and weak.

If the ICP wants to sound more assertive, she should speak in a positive tone without a questioning ending. If she needs to question, she should make it a powerful, explicit question instead of a weak implicit question. Practice strategies for handling conversation power grabbers, such as "Please don't interrupt me" or "I'm not finished yet," should work. In the ICP's work environment she may have to be more deferential with this strategy: "Excuse me, I have just one more point to make."

In dealing with a delayed response the ICP may slip in a ridiculous statement or ask her male conversation partner what was just said. Zimmerman and West[12] believe that this may elicit a change in the male's conversational behavior.

Sensitivity to her own and others' communication tactics should improve the ICP's one-to-one communication skills. Like any muscle, assertive communication requires repeated use, and the ICP needs constant awareness of the power in the messages she sends.

POSITIVE COMMUNICATION

Initiating positive messages calls on the initiator's whole being to give a positive mindset and a graceful performance. Like the batter smashing a home run, the communicator brings all the positive energy into play when connecting with the receiver. A healthy mind and healthy body not only assist in sending messages that activate a positive response, but also back up the sender who may receive an unwanted response from the receiver. Unlike the film industry's series of "takes" until every performance by the artists and the technicians is just right, a communicator often does not have the luxury of dress rehearsals or a series of tries before a "final take."

Every communicator can be up, ready, and prepared with a total, positive mindset. There are dress rehearsals for written communications; the ICP can write and edit her writings or ask a colleague or friend to review them. Written messages can be spoken, recorded, and played back until the message that she wishes to carry her imprint is ready. She can rehearse a spoken presentation in her mind and use notes for guidelines. The ICP should make use of all the hardware to get her software (messages) honed for positive transmission. When she gives form and shape to her thoughts and communicates well, it is akin to the most graceful ballet performance or to the most inspiring of paintings: it is her performing art. A message from the ICP is all hers; it is the purest replica of her mind, body, and being. There is power in positive thinking and communicating.

HUMOR

Like a fine oil, humor lubricates human minds and makes the difficult easier. Successful humor in the ICP's communications springs from her personal experience. Telling a joke on herself says she is human like everybody else.

Humor has many uses in the work environment. In small group meetings tension mounts and tempers are short; members start snapping at each other. Humor can defuse tensions and lower the blood pressure; a good laugh is very relaxing and opens the way to clearer understanding. It is important not to make someone else the "victim" of humor. The ICP may get a laugh at the time, but the embarrassing memory lingers. Good fellowship is enhanced by "laughs at my own expense."

Surprise is a big measure of humor. Saying something unexpected often produces the greatest laughter. A recipient of a nursing award unexpectedly thanked not those who supported her efforts but those who had opposed her. It was the opposition who had triggered her to rethink, reevaluate, and redo until she had produced a slice of creative genius. A crisis report was lightened with "We know now that the light at the end of the tunnel is not a train coming the other way!" Quick wit and an ability to ad lib are fast becoming recognized as important elements in career success. However, the secret is in the sincerity of the humor. Put-on humor is as detectable as clown makeup.

Both women and men who have attained a level of success admit that humor has helped. Humor in the work environment comes with great difficulty to many, especially to women. Early cultural training of girls too often promotes suppression of social assertiveness. Unfortunately, from that same assertiveness springs the easy expression of adult humor. Traditionally, society encourages women to respond to, rather than generate, humor. A survey of male executives cited "lack of a sense of humor" high on the list of reasons women should not hold top executive positions. Even if not culturally encouraged, women and men can learn fellowship, congeniality, and their own style of sincere humor.

Many believe that humor is something people are born with or that delivering a well-placed humorous remark is a sixth sense. However, even professional humorists consciously develop their humor and practice it. The first step is to relax; tension does not cultivate a quick wit. Intense, harried, serious people are not fertile spawning grounds of smiles, titters, or belly laughs. The ICP can teach herself to recognize the humor in many work situations. Irritations at work can seem funny if she lets go of her anger. Tough as it may be at times, the ICP should learn to laugh, even if she uses records and tapes by comedians to feel the warming glow of laughter.

Telling jokes is a small slice of the personal humor the ICP can nourish.

Simple humor has its own comfortable place in self-expression. One type of humor the ICP can ease into is the "silly series," or a sequence ending in the unexpected. An ICP discussing the possibility of a staff opposing an in-service program might remark, "That's impossible—the staff is too loyal, too decent—too complacent." Another trick is altering or paraphrasing a cliche: "We have nothing to fear but failure itself." The technique of reversal (e.g., "the worst of all possible worlds") gives a comfortable, humorous touch. Wearing silly clothes is not always possible in the work area, but perhaps the ICP could incorporate some humorous clothing in in-service, especially if it supports a point that needs to be made.

The ICP should try out new skills in the infection control arena. She will probably reap a positive change in the quality of her communication and interpersonal relationships.

SPEAKING

Anna in *The King and I* had a solution to a very human problem: "Whenever I feel afraid, I hold my head erect and whistle a happy tune, and no one will suspect I'm afraid." However, the ICP cannot whistle instead of speaking, especially in the work setting.

Americans fear speaking in public more than they fear heights, bugs, or death. Speech-anxious ICPs may use a variety of techniques, including quiet whistling, to counteract their consuming fear of speaking. Speech anxiety causes adrenaline to pour into the body, halting the digestive system and making the heart beat faster. Meanwhile, the brain relays that failure is imminent. The ICP's sweaty palms and shaking knees give away her secret: speaking in public is a fate worse than death.

Appreciating the distinction between distress and stress, the ICP will never be able to rid herself of the butterflies in her stomach. A good speaker needs stress to perform and may hope for making the butterflies fly in formation. In other words, the ICP can control her fears and distress.

A tried and tested technique that will help the ICP present better talks is the "5-P Plan":

1. *Prepare.* The ICP should consider her objective, think, write, read, listen, organize, and practice. She should choose a topic that she knows something about (if she has the choice of topics). She should select a subject that will mean something to her audience and write ideas down. It is not necessary to worry about grammar, spelling, or organization; writing is important. These ideas will represent about 80% of the final speech. Reading varied materials with a selfish viewpoint will be beneficial: "What's in here that I can use to support one of my talks?" A well-prepared speech is nine-tenths delivered. Organizing and outlining

the speech ahead of time is vital. Practice makes the difference between a good speech and an excellent speech or between butterflies fluttering and flying in formation. The ICP should memorize a short opening (three or four typewritten lines) and the conclusion. This will get her through the first moments at the podium. A memorized conclusion will tell her when to stop and can be used if she forgets what comes next. Most of all, a memorized conclusion will allow the ICP to have good eye contact with the audience and support her sincerity, which comes from the heart rather than the notes.

2. *Pinpoint.* It is unnecessary to try to cover too much ground. If the ICP talks about everything, her listeners will remember nothing. She should cover only one point in a 5-minute speech and a maximum of three main points in a 30-minute speech. A simple outline is easy for her to remember and for the audience to understand.

3. *Personalize.* The ICP should establish common ground with her audience. She should develop interest by bringing the topic close to home and making it mean something to the listeners. She should aim at their wants, wishes, drives, and desires. She must make it personal for the listeners, not for herself.

4. *Picture.* Creating mental pictures for your listeners is beneficial. The ICP should make them use both their ears and their eyes. Demonstrations, displays, drawings, models, charts, chalkboard, colors, equipment, examples, quotations, questions, cartoons, clippings, posters, and paintings are all examples. Painting vivid mental pictures for the listeners so that they can "see what you mean" is helpful.

5. *Prescribe.* The ICP can close the presentation by answering the questions that listeners always have in mind: "So what?" "What does this mean to me?" "How's it going to help me?" or "What do you want me to do?" She must always think of her listeners as having those questions in mind and give them her prescription.

On the other side of the speaking coin are five common mistakes made by speech-anxious speakers:

1. They try to imitate the style of another speaker.
2. They fail to project a sense of confidence and use poor posture, inappropriate gestures, and little variety in pitch, voice, and tone.
3. They tend to speak down to the audience, using jargon or technical references that the listener cannot identify.
4. They do not prepare enough supporting information to back up their own statements; they use aids that jam the message or fail to practice integrating the aids smoothly into their presentation.
5. They tend to lack dynamic openings and closings.

It is important to keep in mind that 55% of the meaning of the presentation is conveyed through body language, 38% through tone of voice, and only 7% through actual words. What the ICP says can often matter less than how she says it.

Understanding nonverbal cues that are communicated is indispensable to understanding other people. The ICP must also read her audience for their response to her presentation. There is immense power in nonverbal cues. Not all pick up quickly on nods, folded arms, or leaning toward the speaker. The ICP should tune up her body language, voice, and words and speak up.

UNEXPECTED SPEECHES

If the ICP is called on to make an impromptu speech, she may experience a moment filled with fear. Such a reaction is emotional. Fear feeds on itself and makes the moment more intense. Relaxing, taking a few deep breaths, and meeting the situation squarely will help ease the tension.

Perhaps a specific question has been asked that requires a specific answer. If the ICP can answer it, she can start walking toward the place from which she will answer it. While walking, she can formulate what the answer will be. If she must only rise and speak from her seat, then she can ask for the question to be repeated. This will give the ICP the necessary time to gather her thoughts. If she has notes, she should glance at them and use them. She is not expected to jump up and blurt out the first fear-filled thought that enters her mind. A pause to collect thoughts will show that the ICP is skilled in presenting coherent information on short notice.[8]

A speech, no matter how short, has an opening, a body, and a closing. An off-the-cuff speech can embody rational thinking and organization, which are signs of a good leader.

If the ICP is totally ignorant of the subject, she should still follow the pattern, but the body of her very brief speech will be that she does not have sufficient knowledge of the subject and if permitted will gather the information and present it at the time most advantageous to the group.

In any question-and-answer session the ICP should think first and avoid pouncing on a question. She should pause long enough to form a rough outline in her mind, determine if her ideas make sense, and follow a logical plan.

INFORMAL PRESENTATIONS

Somewhere between the demanding presentations that give the ICP plenty of forewarning and the unexpected impromptu speeches lie the informal speeches the ICP may be called on to deliver as a part of her work. When she has time to prepare, a notecard outline offers a good security blanket that helps her remember her main points and keeps her from straying off the topic.

1. The cards can be mounted in a small ring notebook. The ICP will not have to worry about dropping them or flipping cards. The cards should be numbered.
2. To avoid confusion, no more than two main ideas should be placed on a card.
3. Notes should be printed in *large* letters, and abbreviations should be avoided unless the ICP can remember them.
4. Punctuation should be overemphasized. The ICP can use dashes to remind her of pauses.
5. Essential points can be underlined in another color.
6. Color stickers can remind the ICP to smile, use a visual aid, or stop a bad habit, such as hanging onto the lectern, shifting from foot to foot, or making no eye contact with the audience.

The best advice is to use all these as guideposts, not as crutches. Practice is still the greatest aid to a successful speaker.

VISUAL AIDS

A successful ICP lost the case containing all her visual aids on her way to an educational conference. When she arrived, she asked for a black marker and a flipchart and then made up all the visual aids as she spoke. The audience was fascinated, and the vehicle was an unexpected, but fruitful, way to convey the message. One trick that helped was that the ICP was able to outline in pencil on the flipchart all her exhibits before the presentation started. She was familiar with her material, and she was creative under pressure. Unfortunately, many could not duplicate this clever way of saving a presentation by inspiring the audience with the smooth "on-the-spot" creation of visual aids.

Perhaps the most obvious suggestion is for the ICP to always carry her exhibits with her. She may invest in a carrying case or art portfolio and never let her support materials out of sight. Luggage does not always arrive at the expected destination on time.

Often what is meant as a visual aid turns out to be a distraction for the audience or, even worse, a stumbling block for the speaker. The visual technique was meant to help but it becomes a jamming of the communication. Some ideas for the ICP to make her audience glad that she brought visual aids follow:

1. Having someone else check them before she uses them. She may be too familiar with the content to spot omissions or a simpler way to convey the message.
2. Making one point per page. She may have a graph or chart that illustrates several factors. She may have a separate and distinctive exhibit made up for each message she wants to get across.

3. Covering each exhibit when she is not talking about it. The audience will look at the exhibit instead of listen to her. If she is using a series of exhibits side by side, she can have a blank cover for each chart so that no one can see what is ahead of the visual aid she is working with. When she finishes using a chart, she should cover it up again before going on to the next. If her exhibits are on cardboard, she can place each on the floor out of sight both before and after she has put it on display. If using slides, the ICP can use black filler slides to darken the screen when information is not to be displayed.

4. Prompting herself with penciled cues. At an easel there is no greater surprise than turning a page and discovering an unexpected chart. The ICP can avoid surprises and lightly pencil in a cue to what is coming. She can also pencil information along the margins so she does not have to leave the easel to make a point: "These figures show a 30% variance from the chart for 1971."

5. Knowing the exhibits. Many speakers keep turning their heads like a lighthouse from the exhibits to their notes. The ICP can either have the exhibit memorized or have smaller models of them in her notes so that she can let go of the exhibit or notes while speaking. She should not talk to the exhibits rather than to the audience; the aids may have a jamming effect on the message.

6. Using exhibits to illustrate or to highlight. Exhibits are intended to be aids, not duplicates of all information. Repeating everything on a chart will make the audience wonder how the ICP estimates their intelligence. Repetition is a waste of their time and hers. She should expand on a chart, not repeat it.

Exhibits should be used to reinforce the speech, dramatize it, and make it stronger. Otherwise they will detract from both verbal and visual communication.

TELEPHONE COMMUNICATION

To some ICPs using the telephone to get information or to solve a problem is a terrifying tangle of wires and switchboards. With the further annoyance of being put on hold, it becomes more difficult to see that the telephone is a tool, not a trauma.

The phone call is a short speech. What is the most important thing the ICP wants to say or know? She should prepare questions before dialing so everything in her conversation leads to that conclusion. She should also be prepared to leave a message. She should take notes during the conversation so that she can ask any questions that enter her mind and so she can remember the information she asked for.

Treating the call as a face-to-face communication will help. The ICP must leave a good first and last impression by being courteous and pleasant. On the phone, people have a tendency to copy the tone of the other person. It helps to be friendly. The ICP can offer a cheerful greeting, identify herself, and try to use the other person's name. She should check to see if she has called at a good time, listen carefully, and not hold another conversation with someone else near the phone.

The ICP should avoid breaking her thoughts with a string of pauses that may confuse the listener. She should pause only once before uttering a sentence.

The ICP must speak directly into the telephone transmitter, pronouncing words clearly and carefully. She should use simple language and avoid technical terms and slang. Talking at a moderate rate and volume, but varying the tone of voice to add emphasis and vitality to what is said, will be beneficial.

If the ICP is taking a message for another, she should afford the same courtesy to the caller and leave a brief, but clear and concise, message.

Table 9-1 suggests that the telephone embodies advantages and disadvantages in communication.[11] When the telephone fails, the ICP may need to consider another method to complete a successful communication.

TABLE 9-1. Advantages and disadvantages of methods of communication

Method	Advantages	Disadvantages
Phone	Speed; give-and-take of questions	Words and figures might be misunderstood or garbled; usually no record of conversation; may be an interruption of ongoing work
In person	Visual; can show and explain for better understanding	May have to leave work area; lose time; an inconvenience to ICP or to other person
Informal note or memorandum	Brief; memorandum and copies can be filed for reference; permits considered statement; greater impact than spoken word	ICP does not get immediate reply; must allow for routine delivery time and receiver's interest in opening or reading mail
Formal report	Complete; permits time for organizing material; can be reported to others; can include other data; authoritative	May require much time to write; may suffer from receiver's delay in reading; may present problems of organizing and presenting material

WRITTEN COMMUNICATION

In addition to being unable to escape death and taxes, the ICP also cannot escape the need for communicating via the written word. The ICP probably writes a letter, memorandum, or report every week—maybe every day—as part of her work. Her writing touches her entire communication network of peers, supervisors, and subordinates.

An odd paralysis akin to speech anxiety often strangles the writer of communication. The most engaging conversationalist, the most knowledgeable ICP, and the most enthusiastic person can turn stilted and ponderous on paper. How many times in the last month has an internal memorandum from the ICP been misinterpreted and resulted in unnecessary questions? Has she spent days composing an immense report for a hospital committee who never bothered to read past the first paragraph?

Writing is far from being the best way to handle significant matters, but not all communication can be accomplished face-to-face. Much is left to skill in written communication.

Part of the problem stems from years of English classes in which teachers urged the expansion of thoughts. Many people in the business world believe bigger is better; long, complicated sentences and weighty words in a memorandum show that a person really knows a subject. This is wrong! Perhaps the ICP is insecure about her writing skills and does not trust her own use of the language enough to write naturally. Because of her exposure to badly written memoranda, she believes somehow that jargon, wordy expressions, the passive voice, and complex sentences will make her appear more educated and more polished. Perhaps the ICP is timid about putting certain information—especially bad news—too bluntly in writing. Direct, clear, concise writing that approximates the way reasonable people speak will never be embarrassing.

DiGaetani[3] suggests a useful way to revise written communications: the conversational test. As the ICP revises, she should ask herself if she would ever *say* to her reader what she is writing. She can imagine herself speaking to the person instead of writing. Although a valid method for revising written communication, the conversational test is not an encouragement to use slang. Written words still require a good balance of formality.

Where does good written communication begin? Step one in the writing process should always be the same for the ICP: determining what she wants to communicate by asking herself three basic questions:

- What is the real reason I am writing this?
- What is the main point I want to get across?
- How do I want the reader to react to what I am about to say?

Once she has mentally defined her purpose, she can put it down on paper as the first paragraph. She should state her case as quickly and precisely as possible. If her letter bears bad news, it may be appropriate to provide the necessary background for understanding the problem. However, she should get to the point as quickly as the background has been established. Will that point be clear at first reading? What would the ICP decide to do if, in a memorandum, she were given these instructions:

> Assist local and regional public health agencies in determining whether to provide infection control education subsidies to maintain in operation particular hospital infection control programs by establishing criteria for determining whether particular components of an infection control program are effective and suited for training subsidies.

That memorandum will suffer and die from benign neglect. A memorandum that falls short of making its point clear at first reading is in trouble because it is giving the reader trouble.[11]

The lead to a newspaper story contains everything: who, what, when, where, why, and how. The lead in the ICP's memorandum, letter, or report should too. It may be the only thing the reader takes time to read. Writing's six basic concerns are answered in the following memorandum:

> We expect problems this week while the electric company workers replace and check the building's electrical fixtures. The work will bring the building up to code.

If the ICP is giving instructions, she should be explicit. As a backup, someone else might test her instructions before they are written in a memorandum or letter. It is surprising how many significant details the instruction giver takes for granted or leaves half-explained in written communication.

Tone, tact, and courtesy in a straightforward manner with positive overlays arm the reader with the right expectations and fewer frustrations. Managers intent on correcting certain behavior can easily come across as patronizing to subordinates. Angry or cute memoranda may offend readers. Thus the ICP should provide her reader with a positive statement that acknowledges the receiver and then give the reasons why she must say no if that is the response to a request.

Most readers expect two out of three reports to be boring. Unfortunately, two out of three usually are. Page after page of material, dull and unappealing to the eye or the intellect, deters the reader. The general rule is that shorter is better. If background material is necessary for reader comprehension, it should be included, but overwriting must be avoided.

If it will take more than a page and a half (single-space typing) to get the message across, the ICP should make it easier to read and digest. She should double-space and break up paragraphs into small messages. The goal is to make the memorandum look appealing so the reader notices something besides its length.

When the ICP is faced with a multipage report that cannot be reduced, she

TABLE 9-2. Situations in which a memorandum may be the effective medium

To	Subject	Purpose
Head nurse	In-service class	To confirm dates, times, and topics
Head of purchasing department	New urinary drainage system	To recommend purchase for trial and evaluation
Hospital administrator	Standards of the Joint Commission on Accreditation of Hospitals	To apprise of compliance and variation with new infection control standards
Director of nurses	New isolation pamphlets	To compliment the nursing staff on efforts to orient patients to isolation procedures
Department heads	Infection control policies and procedures	To inform of need; to offer assistance in development
Medical and hospital boards	Quarterly report	To inform of current activities of the infection control program
Director of facilities	Office space	To outline needed space for expansion of services; to request review of situation
Chairperson, nursing procedure committee	IV catheter care	To inform of recommendation of infection control committee; to request change in procedure

should break the monotony with a few tricks that magazine editors use. Enormous blocks of typewritten copy are hard to tackle. Breaking up long paragraphs, even if logical development does not require it, is helpful.

Subheadings visually break up large copy blocks and work as guideposts to key issues the ICP is trying to communicate. If subheadings are written correctly, they can tell the story at a glance. Graphs, tables, and pictures can successfully augment written communication. These are especially helpful tools for readers who have a better aptitude for spatial relations than for written communication (Table 9-2).

Although writing is far from being an exact science, the following general guidelines will improve written communication:
1. Definite, specific language should be used.
2. Statements should be put in a positive form.

3. Unnecessary words should be deleted.
4. Active verbs can be used to convey more action in less space.
5. Revising and rewriting is essential; the material should be put aside and read anew.
6. Sentence style and length can be varied.

The ICP should make her written communication the mark of a craftsman.

SUMMARY

Effective communication is the foundation of successful role development for the ICP. Although the skills required for this process seem deceptively simple and are often taken for granted, a successful communicator must continually monitor interactions to ensure mutual understanding.

The successful ICP employs language and perceptual skills in both verbal and written communication. Language skills are used to construct and deliver intelligible messages, whereas perceptual skills are used to adapt messages to fit a specific listener or reader. These two sets of skills, coupled with a proactive approach to role development, enable the ICP to design and implement an infection control program that addresses institutional, patient, and personnel needs.

REFERENCES

1. Allen, R.R.: Speech in American society, Columbus, Ohio, 1978, Charles E. Merrill Publishing Co.
2. Bramson, R.M.: Coping with difficult people, New York, 1981, Doubleday & Co., Inc.
3. DiGaetani, J.L.: Conversation: the key to better business writing, Wall Street J. **52**:24, Feb. 8, 1982.
4. Harnack, R.V., Fest, T.B., and Jones, B.S.: Group discussion, theory and technique, ed. 2, Englewood Cliffs, N.J., 1977, Prentice-Hall, Inc.
5. Lakoff, R.: Language and woman's place, New York, 1975, Harper & Row, Publishers, Inc.
6. Levine, E.L.: Tools for correcting communication problems, Health Serv. Man. **14**:7, March 1981.
7. Margerison, C.J.: Managerial problem solving, New York, 1974, McGraw-Hill, Inc.
8. Phillips, J.D.: For those who must lead, Chicago, 1966, The Dartnell Corp.
9. Potter, D., and Andersen, M.: Discussion: a guide to effective practice, Belmont, Calif., 1963, Wadsworth, Inc.
10. Snell, F.: How to hold a better meeting, New York, 1958, Harper & Row, Publishers, Inc.
11. Uris, A.: Memos for managers, New York, 1975, Thomas Y. Crowell Co., Publishers.
12. Zimmerman, D., and West, C.: Taped conversations and personal interviews, University of California (Santa Barbara and Santa Cruz), 1981.

SUGGESTED READINGS

Clement, J.: And out of her mouth came toads, Cosmopolitan, pp. 152-154, Dec. 1981.
Copeland, L., and Copeland, F., editors: 10,000 jokes, toasts, and stories, New York, 1965, Doubleday & Co., Inc.
Doblin, J.: The map of media: understanding the contexts for communications, Indust. Design Mag. **28**:35-37, Jan.-Feb. 1981.
Maccoby, E.E., and Jacklin, C.N.: The psychology of sex differences, Stanford, Calif., 1974, Stanford University Press.

Rocke, R.: The grandiloquent dictionary, Englewood Cliffs, N.J., 1972, Prentice-Hall, Inc.

Schaef, A.W.: Women's reality: an emerging female system in the white male society, Minneapolis, 1981, Winston Press, Inc.

Weintraub, P.: The brain: his and hers, Discover **2**:14-20, April 1981.

Wicklein, J.: Electronic nightmare: the new communication and freedom, New York, 1981, The Viking Press.

Wittig, M.A., and Petersen, A.C.: Sex-related differences in cognitive functioning: developmental issues, New York, 1979, Academic Press, Inc.

10 LU ANN W. DARLING

Consultation

consultative relationships A voluntary relationship between a professionally trained person and a client system, in which the consultant is attempting to give help to the client in solving some current or potential problem.

educational model A philosophy of consulting in which the client is viewed as a learner; the philosophy emphasizes client education and the mutual use of knowledge and expertise and places high value on actions leading to client independence.

line management The full responsibility and authority for directing the activities of people in an organization.

medical model A philosophy of consulting in which the physician or other health care provider focuses on the defect or dysfunction within the person, using a problem-solving approach; focuses on the physical and biological aspects of specific diseases and conditions; the result is client dependence.

staff roles Positions providing specialized counseling, service, and advice to line management.

THE NATURE OF THE CONSULTANT-CLIENT RELATIONSHIP
Consultation as a staff relationship

Classical management theorists divide all roles in organizations into either *staff* or *line* positions. Line management has the full responsibility and authority for directing the activities of people in the organization; the staff role, on the other hand, is one of counsel, service, and advice.[28] Seen in this perspective, the infection control practitioner (ICP) role is a staff role. ICPs do not have full and final responsibility for the infection control program nor do they have authority to direct the activities of the employees in various hospital departments. Instead, ICPs have a special role to provide counsel, service, and advice in the area of infection control.

It is important to underscore this point, for the use of the word *control* in the title of the position and in the name of the program can be misleading. It can suggest to persons in the position that inherent in the role is the authority to direct and control. This is not true. They must become influential and effective without having the authority to direct and control. They must develop and use their specialized knowledge about the control of infections in such a way to assist hospital managers maintain an effective infection control program. Just how to do this is given scant attention in their training. Like other staff specialists, such as accountants, planners, personnel specialists, and computer analysts, ICPs learn a great deal about the content of their specialty but are likely to be completely naive about professional relationships and roles.[29]

Consultation is an important facet of the ICP's function; it is through the consultative process that the ICP interacts with hospital staff. This chapter outlines the nature of the consultant-client relationship, the range of possible consultant role behaviors, the processes involved in consultation, and considerations for marketing the consultant role and for maintaining effective relationships with client systems. In this chapter *consultant* refers to the ICP; *client* or *client system* refers to the manager or work group with whom the ICP interacts on a given project or problem.

Consultation as a helping relationship

The consultative relationship is a voluntary relationship between a professionally trained person and a client system, in which the consultant is attempting to give help to the client in solving some current or potential problems.[27] The consultative relationship is temporary, and the consultants are "outsiders" to the specific system in which they are consulting.

Stated more simply, the consultative process is a helping relationship. It is a personal relationship between the individual, the client trying to solve a problem, and the consultant trying to help. The consultant, the person in the helping role, always enters the relationship as a person with some specialized knowledge or skills. The consultant must use this in a way viewed as helpful by the client. "Help" is always defined by the receiver of the help. If the client does not feel helped, the consultant is not engaged in a helping relationship.[9,16,23,28]

The emphasis in these definitions is on the "relationship." Consultation involves an interdependent interaction between a help seeker or receiver and a help giver. Consultation is a dynamic process.

There are two major aspects to any consultative relationship: the work on solving the problem or completing the task and the work on the relationship between the consultant and client, that is, the process. The difficulty in establishing collaborative staff-line relationships was identified by McGregor[29] 20 years ago; it remains a key problem today: "The problem we face is that of creating a climate of mutual confidence around staff-line relationships which will encourage collaboration in the achievement of organizational objectives rather than guerilla warfare." Building collaboration appears to be a significant concern as the ICP relates with various client systems throughout the hospital. It is common for ICPs who rise from the ranks of staff nurse to experience role conflict; as they approach client systems without the skills to gain cooperation, they are seen by hospital managers as finding fault. Such a problem arises, I believe, because of an erroneous view of the ICP role, because of a lack of understanding of consultant-client relationships, and because of the lack of skill to resolve the interpersonal issues unique to the consultative relationship.

Relationship issues in consulting

There are twin issues that must be worked through in any consultative relationship. The influence issue is often prominent.[23] How much is each person concerned with influencing and controlling the other? The act of asking for help or accepting help can put clients in a dependent position and make them feel weaker and more vulnerable. There is also a common tendency for the helper or consultant to feel superior and to let feelings of power and control overshadow the client's best interests.

Influence must be balanced with empathy.[23] How much knowledge and understanding does the consultant have of the client, and how does the client perceive infection control problems and practices? The ability to see the problem from the point of view of the other party is absolutely essential. The consultant must be willing to influence the client, but this must be balanced with empathy for the views and feelings of the client. As these twin issues of influence and empathy or affiliation are worked through, the consultant and client can more readily set mutual task goals for the consultation activity.

CONSULTANT ROLE BEHAVIOR

The role of a consultant is not limited to one specific type of behavior. A number of consultant role behaviors have been identified, ranging from those that are primarily client centered to those that are primarily consultant centered.* The approach used should be based on the client's diagnosed need; it should be appropriate to the focal issue, that aspect of a situation presently causing the client's difficulty.

Criteria for choosing consulting role behavior

Three factors influence the consultant's choice of role behavior. One is the consultant's view about the *goal* of the consulting effort. Is the goal education of clients to increase their ability to handle problems now and in the future, or is the goal limited to assisting the client so that the client's present problem is solved? Second, who has the *knowledge and expertise* to work on the problem? Does the consultant assume the client has knowledge and expertise that can be brought to bear on the problem in conjunction with the consultant or that the consultant alone has the necessary expertise to work on the problem? The third factor is *client dependence or independence*. Does the consultant intend to help the client become independent, or does the consultant consider that client dependence is acceptable in these circumstances? Has the client already gained sufficient independence so that the consultant's efforts would not undercut the client's autonomy?

One can look at these three criteria and identify two distinctly different

*References 9, 12, 19, 30, 39, 40.

philosophies of consulting.[19,35,37] The traditional medical model views the client as a patient. This philosophy emphasizes assistance over education. The use of the physician's knowledge and expertise results in client dependence. Conversely, the educational model views the client as a learner. This philosophy emphasizes client education and the mutual use of knowledge and expertise and places high value on actions leading to client independence.

In the traditional medical model the emphasis is on the solution of the immediate problem of the client with little provision for handling recurrences. The client is passive in the diagnosis; there is no passing on of diagnostic skills. Problem solving is fast and expedient. However, the client may be reluctant to reveal information, so the information in the diagnosis may be distorted. The client may also be unwilling to believe the diagnosis or accept the prescription. Another cost is the dependence the method fosters.

The educational model, in contrast, assumes the client must learn to examine problems, share in the diagnosis, and become actively involved in the solution. The emphasis is on working with the client in the client's frame of reference to increase the client's problem-solving ability now and in the future. The educational model takes longer and is more costly, but it taps greater motivational forces for change while maintaining the client's autonomy. There are times and situations when the medical model is appropriate for the ICP, as in a major infection outbreak, but in the long run the educational model has far greater benefits.

In the educational model the consultant draws on existing resources in the group and through education may even help develop additional resources to deal with the problems of the client system. The use of expertise in any given situation is a pooling of consultant-client knowledge. There is a joint assessment of the problem and use of resources of both client and consultant as they are relevant and available. In this model consultants must have a realistic picture of their own skills, knowledges, and limitations and have a similar assessment of the client system. Based on the assessment, ICPs will use their skills differentially. In a client system well informed in the area of infection control, for example, consultants would primarily tap into the energies and resources within the system and link them to the hospital's objectives of infection control. In an uninformed client system they would apply their knowledge and skill extensively in education and in the solution of problems.

As long as consultants focus on the goal of client growth and autonomy, they are free to draw on all of their skills and experiences that are relevant in the situation.

Possible consultant roles

Keeping in mind the three criteria that influence the consultant's choice of role behavior, I will discuss the range of possible consultant roles of the ICP.

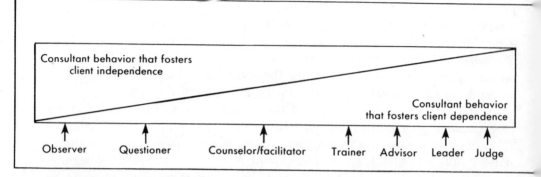

FIG. 10-1. Possible consultant roles of the infection control practitioner. (From Darling, L.A., Cox, C., and Axnick, K.: A.P.I.C. Journal **5:**11, March 1977.)

Schuttenberg[39] places these on a continuum according to the impact on client independence or dependence. Those at the left of the continuum foster independence. As one moves farther to the right, the behaviors tend to foster client dependence. Each role has its time and place. If the consultant's role behavior tends to be characteristically at one end or the other, there are consequences and implications for client growth and autonomy. One needs to assess the costs and benefits in choosing an appropriate role on the continuum.

On the continuum in Fig. 10-1 the consultative roles of *Observer* and *Questioner* tend to foster client independence. The *Advisor, Leader,* and *Judge* roles move in the direction of client dependence. *Counselor/facilitator* and *Trainer* roles are midway. Clearly, the more directive the consultant is toward the client, the more dependent the client becomes on the consultant. At times each of these seven roles is appropriate for the ICP to assume. The ICP needs to become familiar with these roles, see how they look in operation, and develop needed skills to function in each. Armed with this understanding, the ICP can make role-taking decisions that will advance the hospital's infection control program.

Observer. The observer may be present at meetings or in a work area without being an active participant. The purpose may be to gather data or to get the feel for what is happening. Later the consultant may give feedback of her observations to the supervisor of the area. The role should be distinguished from that of a spy, for a spy gathers information about a person or group to assist someone else to impose change. The observer feeds back information to the head of the area to help bring about needed change.

EXAMPLE:
In performing surveillance rounds the ICP observes poor techniques in the management of indwelling urinary catheters (disconnected drainage systems and drainage bags resting on the floor). Feedback is given to the head nurse to promote changes in nursing care.

Questioner. This role involves asking searching questions and raising fundamental issues that lie beneath the client's actions and decisions. Such questions may confront the other person with the consequences of an action or invite him to examine basic assumptions. Although the role of questioner may be somewhat threatening, it can be very helpful because it requires individuals or a group to examine their thinking.

> EXAMPLE:
> A physician refuses a request to isolate his patient. The nurse feels it is required and asks for assistance in obtaining the order. Through questioning, the ICP discusses with the nurse the criteria she is using as a rationale for isolation.

Counselor/facilitator. In this role the consultant spends much time talking with individuals or groups about their infection control goals and problems, giving information, and helping them to clarify their thinking, to make choices, and to plan courses of action.

> EXAMPLE: INDIVIDUAL
> The in-service education instructor is developing the curriculum for a course in critical care nursing. She is aware that the critically ill patient is at high risk for the development of a nosocomial infection. She has asked the ICP for suggestions to incorporate infection control theory into the course content.

> EXAMPLE: GROUP
> Recent repeated cultures from physical therapy equipment reveal high counts of *Pseudomonas* and gram-negative organisms. The ICP knows the present product for cleaning to be good. The physical therapy staff says the product is "no good." The manufacturer's representative states that the problem is improper use of the product. The ICP arranges a meeting with the manufacturer's representative and physical therapy staff to discuss the problem and find the solution.

Trainer. In the trainer role the consultant acts as a resource person and educator for a work group to help them achieve learning goals in the area of infection control. At times the consultant presents theory sessions and leads discussions. At other times the consultant may help group members explore their own feelings and interrelationships.

> EXAMPLE:
> The head nurse on a medical unit reports that some of the nursing staff are reluctant to care for patients with tuberculosis. There seems to be a lack of understanding of the disease process, and thus confusion arises in patient care. The ICP leads a unit conference by presenting information on tuberculosis and then serves as a resource person as the head nurse explores the feelings of the staff.

Advisor. In the role of an advisor the consultant identifies problems in the organization and recommends ways of solving these problems. An astute advisor can have a great deal of influence on the formation of policies and the making of decisions.

EXAMPLE:

The hospital administration has approved funds for the construction of a 10-bed surgical intensive care unit (ICU). The ICP is asked to serve on the planning committee to ensure the inclusion of infection control principles in the environment.

Leader. A consultant may exert leadership in a group and gradually gain the respect and trust of the group members to such a degree that the group looks to the ICP for direction and guidance.

EXAMPLE:

The chairperson of the infection control committee expects the ICP to develop an agenda for committee meetings and to introduce and lead discussions on appropriate topics.

Judge. In the role of judge the consultant reviews policies and practices of the organization and evaluates them. The role may also include the evaluation of individual staff members to determine their effectiveness and to identify areas where they need additional training and development.

EXAMPLE:

In preparation for accreditation survey the administrator and director of nurses ask the ICP to evaluate infection control measures in various departments and provide recommendations to correct deficiencies noted.

THE CONSULTATIVE PROCESS

Thus far the reader has seen that the consultative relationship is a helping relationship and that "help" is evaluated by the receiver of the help, or the client. It is clear that the ICP role is one of advice and counsel rather than direction and control. I have examined the variety of possible consultant role behaviors open to the ICP. Now I will turn to a summary description of the consultative process; I will put the pieces together and explore the dynamics of this human, interactive process (Fig. 10-2).

Model of the consultative process

The ingredients of the consultative process are the consultant (helper), the client (receiver), and the focal issue or problem. The interaction between the consultant and the client is intended to lead to increased functioning on the part of the client in four areas, following the educational model: increased understanding, skill, effectiveness, and autonomy.[33]

In infection control the desired outcomes are improved understanding, skill, and effectiveness on the part of the hospital client regarding the prevention and control of hospital infections. Furthermore, the client's ability to function independently of the ICP should show a marked increase. Since the ICPs cannot do the entire job, they will only be effective to the extent that hospital personnel become more knowledgeable, more skillful, and more vigilant regarding the control of infections. They must work toward a goal of

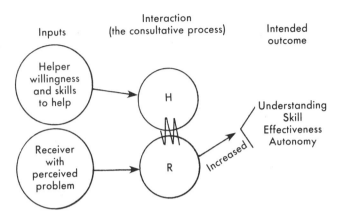

FIG. 10-2. Consultation process. (From Darling, L.A., Cox, C., and Axnick, K.: A.P.I.C. Journal **5**:11, March 1977.)

having many hospital leaders able to assess situations and make decisions independently.

Requirements for effective help

There are four requirements for help to be truly effective[33]:
1. There must be a real desire on the part of the consultant to provide help and a real desire on the part of the client to receive help. (Numerous barriers that often make it difficult for a consultant-client relationship to develop from the outset follow.)
2. The consultant must be able to establish an effective human relationship with the client and develop the confidence of the client. There must be mutual trust and acceptance. The issues of influence and empathy or affiliation discussed earlier must be resolved.
3. The consultant must have adequate conceptual, technical, and interpersonal skills to diagnose the situation.
4. Both parties must be able to engage in joint problem solving. There must be mutual exploration of alternatives, with the client free to make the final decision. Freedom of choice is essential if the client is to achieve increased autonomy and independence.

Barriers to effective help

In addition to diagnosing problems and goals of the client, consultants must be able to realistically assess their own motivations and limitations. This may be hard to do. Some of the difficulties the consultant faces in giving help follow:
- Lacks understanding of the helping role
- Lacks awareness of own limitations and resources
- Likes to give advice

- Is insensitive to resistance
- Responds to own needs and overrides the needs of others
- May overpraise
- May fail to confront
- Lacks awareness of self and own motivations
- Lacks interpersonal skill
- Likes to be a crusader

People often assume that it is easy to receive help, but quick examination shows that this is not true. Some of the barriers a client has in receiving help follow:

- Perceives problem to be unique
- Finds needing help hard to admit
- Distrusts the consultant; doubts consultant's competency and motivation
- Fears what will happen
- Fears what others will think
- Fears losing control; finds it important to be independent
- Only wants sympathy, not help
- Does not see that he must change
- Is defensive; stops listening
- Has a strong need to lean

Questions guiding the consultative process

Recognizing the importance of working on the relationship between the consultant and client, not just the task, leads the consultant to a broader set of questions to work through during the course of a consulting relationship[27]:

Question 1: What seems to be the client's difficulty? Where does it come from? What is maintaining it?
Consultants need a theory about what to see and how to understand it; they also need ideas about the symptoms or source of trouble.

Question 2: What are the motives in becoming involved in this helping relationship? What is the basis of the desire to promote change?
Consultants need to be clear about their justification for intervention. Is an individual manager calling for help, or is it a matter of hospital welfare? Who set the goals for change? Is action justified when the goals are formulated solely by the consultant?

Question 3: What present or potential motivations does the client have toward or against change?
A force-field analysis (Chapter 12) is an important part of the initial assessment.

Question 4: What are the consultant's resources for giving the kind of help that may be needed?

Question 5: What preliminary steps are needed to explore and establish a consulting relationship?
If the client is not well motivated toward change, how can awareness of the need for help be developed?

Question 6: How does the consultant guide and adapt to different phases of changing?

There are several phases to changing.[26] In the "unfreezing" phase the need for change and for establishing the consultation relationship is developed. The "moving" or "changing" phase involves several steps, namely, clarifying the client problem, examining alternate solutions and goals, and transforming intentions into actual change efforts. Finally, in the "freezing" or "refreezing" phase, the focus is turned to the generalization and stabilization of a new level of functioning or a new structure.

Question 7: How does the consultant help promote a continuity of the created change?

The most challenging task is to discover ways to train groups to use procedures of data collection and analysis on a continuing basis so they can, on their own, identify infection control problems and possibilities and solve their problems without the aid of a consultant.[14,26]

Starting up the consultative process: scouting and entry

Scouting. Most ICPs have hospital-wide responsibilities in the area of infection control. This can create an overwhelming feeling and pose a dilemma about where in the system to start. Where can intervention make a difference? What is the best point to enter, considering legitimate power and authority, readiness of the system, and its criticalness for the infection control program? In the scouting stage the ICP is exploring various potential client systems to determine where it is best to intervene.

ICPs will want to conduct some interviews and rounds to build their own understanding of the hospital system, establish contacts, and generate goodwill for the program. They need to establish a network of relationships[32] to obtain current information about actual or potentially infectious situations, as well as to assess the readiness of a system for change. They use these linking relationships to keep informed, to disseminate appropriate information, and to be spokespersons or educators for infection control.

There are three factors in determining where to intervene in the system: leverage, accessibility, and readiness.[26]

Leverage. Leverage is perhaps the most important factor. This requires the ICP to assess priorities and impact. Risk is the key: what are the areas of high risk in the hospital now, or potentially so? She also has to consider the return on the investment of her time and energies. Here the 80:20 rule can be useful.[24] In what 20% of the organization will an active consultation effort generate 80% of the improvement in the control of infections? The concept of "critical mass" is also helpful.[3] What is the minimal number of people needed to support a particular infection control program to guarantee its success and its diffusion in the system? Who are the opinion leaders in the organization whose support or active involvement would make a difference? What systems, if left untended, could get worse and create major problems?

Accessibility. Which of those areas identified as having high leverage for the infection control program are accessible to the ICP? Does she have contacts to enter the system? Is the system a manageable size? Does the client system have staff available to work on the program? Is this an appropriate time to approach the client system in terms of their priorities and ability to work on the program?

Readiness. Progress is much faster with client systems that are ready and eager to work. A department head who asks for help or a nursing unit where the head nurse is worried about the control of infections is likely to be receptive to the ICP's efforts. So would a client system where the ICP has established good-will and where the staff is very interested in more effective infection control. Conversely, it is extremely difficult to intervene effectively in a system where key staff members feel threatened, indifferent, or hostile to either the consultant or the infection control program.

Entry. Once the consultant determines the appropriate client system and makes an initial contact, the next step is making an appropriate entry into the system. In this stage the consultant and client discuss their expectations of each other, agreeing on the contributions to be made by both parties. The concern is through negotiation to gain sufficient influence to implement the agreed on program or action.

When sufficient interest has been generated and the client does want the services of the ICP, the progress leads to contract setting.

Contract setting. In the sense it is used here a contract is not a legal document; it is a psychological or interpersonal agreement, or an explicit exchange of expectations. This takes the form of dialogue between the consultant and client, supplemented with some written documentation, when desirable, that clarifies for the consultant and client three critical areas[42]:
- What each expects to get from the relationship
- How much time each will invest and at what cost
- The ground rules under which the parties will operate

The clarity of the agreed on expectations can be crucial to the consultant-client relationship. Unnecessary role confusion can inhibit the success of the infection control program itself.

Action research as a consulting methodology

For motivational reasons many consultants use a special method of problem-solving called *action research* in consulting with client systems. This can be a useful methodology for the ICP. Action research is a data-based, problem-solving model that uses the steps of the scientific method of inquiry and involves participants of the client system in the process. Three processes are involved: data collection, feedback of the data to clients, and joint action planning based on that data.[12]

Action research operates with several premises. Realistic fact-finding and

evaluation is essential to any learning. For persons to be interested in changing their behavior, they must first be dissatisfied. Only when those who have
to change feel that they have a problem is there likely to be any movement.
Most change efforts flounder because carefully executed plans are ignored
or sabotaged.[36] Therefore, wherever possible, those persons in the client
system who are to take action should be involved in fact-finding from the
beginning.

In action research the role of the consultant is to help the managers of client
systems plan their actions and design their fact-finding procedures in such a
way that they can learn from them and solve their own problems. Before action
there should be an objective, so planning is the first step of a cycle. Action
follows, but it is taken one step at a time. After each step it is usually desirable
to do some fact-finding to see whether the objective is realistic, whether it has
been reached, or whether it needs alteration. So the action research cycle is one
of planning, acting, fact-finding, evaluation, and then planning for the next
cycle.

People tend to support what they have helped create, so client system members and the consultant jointly define the problems they want to address, the
methods to be used for data collection, and the hunches they have about the
problem situations and, whenever possible, jointly evaluate the consequences
of the actions taken. There is a collaborative ingredient in action research that
sets it apart from other forms of problem solving.

Action research uses a motivational and evolutionary approach to change.[36]
It is particularly suited for situations in which the goal of consultation is client
education, growth, and autonomy, and hence it has much potential value for
ICPs. Action research would not be the method of choice when the goal of the
consultation is limited to solving an immediate problem or correcting an immediate situation and when time is urgent.

MARKETING THE CONSULTANT ROLE

Consultant effectiveness is measured by the extent to which others seek
advice and counsel and by the extent to which advice, when followed, leads to
improvement.[34] A beginning task of a new ICP is to obtain clients, that is, to
have hospital supervisors and managers recognize the value of the program
and seek her advice and counsel in controlling infections.

Any new role or newly created role requires educating those persons who
are likely to interface with the role. People have to be taught how to use the
consultant and what resources and services are available. For a person new to
the role, this requires personal role development and some comfort and familiarity with the role as well. The introduction of innovative roles is much easier
when ICPs have been involved in creating, defining, and articulating the role to
management. If the role is new, a certain amount of evolution is likely to be

necessary. Unless someone else has been preparing the way, potential clients will not be waiting to request the consultant's services.

Marketing refers to activities that cause others to seek out a specific product or service. The ICP role involves a service that must be marketed. Marketing is a proactive process of getting business and may be an alien experience for ICPs who have come from traditionally structured roles such as nursing.

Drucker[8] differentiates between marketing and selling. Marketing requires asking who the customer is and who they should be, determining what the value is to the customer, and producing services or products to meet those values and needs. Relating Drucker's questions to consultant-client relationships, the questions become who the client is, who they should be, and what the value is to the client. Drucker maintains that as these questions are thoughtfully and effectively answered and services developed to meet client needs, selling becomes relatively unimportant. The more effectively the ICP identifies and meets client needs, the more clients will seek out and use her services.

However, consultant-client relationships in a hospital infection control program are fairly complicated. ICPs have hospital-wide responsibilities, so their clients are potentially all managers and their organizational units involved in or affected by infection control throughout the hospital.

Although for practical purposes their active clients are likely to be limited to those areas of greatest risk, at certain times ICPs will be concerned with a much larger number of clients. Given the variability of clients and client systems, ICPs need an understanding of the differing orientations and needs of each client system and must have sufficient flexibility in their approach to clients to meet those needs. Good communication skills and an understanding of change processes will help them in the broad areas of marketing the consultant role and stimulating interest in change.

In discussing marketing two approaches will be highlighted: first, the informal marketing of a new role or a role that is unfamiliar to the client, and second, strategies to stimulate interest and involvement of client systems that have not yet recognized any need for change.

Informal marketing

Marketing is both formal and informal. Formal marketing includes formal presentations, papers, proposals, brochures, written descriptions of services, and the like. Informal marketing takes advantage of ongoing contacts and relationships. Information shared, service provided, and questions raised can all be the base for establishing further links throughout the hospital and broadening the infection control program.

Some informal methods of marketing the consultant role require planting ideas and patiently waiting for them to germinate. Other methods are more immediate and more concrete. All of these methods work toward making the role of the ICP visible in a positive, nonthreatening way in the health care

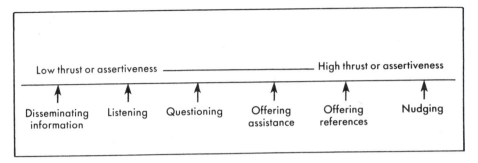

FIG. 10-3. Informal marketing strategies.

facility. In the following discussion it is important to note that in all methods the decision to use services or follow advice is in the hands of the client. A consultant cannot force help on a client. Also, methods differ in the degree of thrust and assertiveness used (Fig. 10-3).

Disseminating information. Disseminating information is used to inform others of the role and its value or to broaden another's perception of the role. In a concrete way the ICP makes known her availability, her readiness to help, and her position as a resource. This provides visibility for the role in a safe, non-threatening way, since there is no need for the client to express any interest or commitment at this time. Any setting in which the ICP is involved in a positive, constructive way may have possibilities for marketing by disseminating information. Discussing various aspects of the role in in-service classes is one marketing technique. Distributing written material, such as a newsletter on infection control or copies of pertinent articles, to selected key staff members informs potential users of services. ICPs can also make known their availability as speakers.

> EXAMPLES:
> "Perhaps it would be helpful if I told you some of the things I do and am able to do."
> "My title may be confusing; I'd really like to tell you something about my work and why the role was set up."
> "There is a good article in the current issue of _____ on this subject; would you like me to send you a copy?"

Active listening. Active listening is an invaluable tool for the ICP. It is one of the best ways to see the problems as the potential client sees them, and it demonstrates the ICP's capacity to understand problems from the client's point of view. Active listening is an essential foundation for any effective consultant-client relationship.

> EXAMPLES:
> "So you're concerned about. . . ."
> "If I understand correctly, you see the problem as. . . ."
> "Let me see if I am following you. . . ."

Questioning. Coupling active listening with raising questions is a useful way to suggest ideas.

EXAMPLES:

"So you're concerned about. . . . Had you considered . . . ?"

"So you're concerned about. . . . What did your examination of . . . turn up?"

"Would a study of that situation be useful at this time?"

Offering assistance. Providing support or direct help can be quite general or quite specific.

EXAMPLES:

"Should you decide to go in this direction and you want help, just give me a call."

"Would you like me to set up a class?"

"If you feel it would be helpful, I would be happy to. . . ."

Offering references. Sometimes the ICP may offer assistance, but the potential client will still be reluctant. The client may harbor some doubts about the ICP personally or the process involved. References from other clients or consultants can provide needed information and reassurance.

EXAMPLES:

"I would encourage you to talk to . . . about what's involved in. . . ."

"You might want to talk to . . . to see how useful he found it. . . ."

"Nudging" or urging. This technique assumes that previous contact with the client was positive and encouraging and that some trust and acceptance between the consultant and potential client has been established. Without this initial bond, "nudging" can be perceived as threatening and cause the client to back off or to respond reluctantly to the pressure, whether real or perceived. Without a positive relationship, such assertiveness can be risky. There is a fine line between urging and forcing. The difference may not be words but tone of voice. Forcing belongs to line management; it is usually not part of the role of the ICP.

EXAMPLES:

"The lab reports are very clear . . . and action certainly seems indicated; what do you plan to do?"

"It seems to me that no matter how much you go in this direction, you'll still have problems to face. What about. . . ."

"It doesn't sound as though it's going to get any better with the methods you are now using. How about trying. . . ."

Initiating planned change

In the beginning of marketing a new role, neophyte ICPs are likely to feel tenuous and have doubts about their competence and expertise. The informal marketing methods described earlier are low-key ways to get started. As ICPs gain experience and confidence, marketing is likely to be more dynamic and proactive and take the form of program development. At this point ICPs are initiating planned change. In addition to the processes mentioned earlier, they will have distinct strategies for stimulating the desire for improvement, for heightening sensitivity to problems, and for offering help in solving acknowledged problems.[26] They are likely to engage in these strategies more each succeeding year as they reactivate client relationships, as they extend the consulting cycle, and as they involve themselves and clients in more comprehensive infection control programs.

Stimulating a desire for improvement. A consultant can stimulate a desire for improvement by choosing specific topics for talks to hospital groups. This can allow the consultant to focus attention on successful changes that have been made in other hospitals or in other areas of the hospital. She can also prepare and distribute special case studies of significant change in other hospitals, take potential clients on tours or rounds to areas of the hospital where successful changes have been made, and encourage an open house or showcase of successful demonstrations.

Heightening sensitivity to problems. There are a number of ways in which a consultant can heighten and make more widespread an awareness of infection control programs and practices. One way is to highlight the discrepancy between professed values and actual practices in the unit's routine: "This is what you say, but look what you are doing." If this is done judiciously, a new ICP can be a persistent questioner, making thoughtful inquiries about aspects of hospital infection control that need improvement. This can help staff members see problems to which they had become accustomed in a new light. The consultant could develop a collaborating network of persons throughout the hospital who are concerned with infection control, that is, persons who are sensitive to the problem and could help stimulate sensitivity in others and help locate sources of trouble.

Offering help in solving an acknowledged problem. Often a consultant can encounter a problem situation in which people are very sensitive to the problem but have little energy to solve it; they are blocked or apathetic. Here the consultant can find some means of transforming the awareness into some practical, "do-able" action. She might bring people together, serving as a catalyst to get persons who do have ideas and energy together to work on the problem. This helps to combat "pluralistic ignorance," in which people individually are dissatisfied with a common concern, but each feels the others do not share the dissatisfaction. This is a way to point out the mutuality of their concern.

CHANGES IN CONSULTATIVE RELATIONSHIPS
The consultative cycle

Each consultative cycle has a point of entry, diagnosis, planning, action, evaluation, and termination.[23] Each consultative activity starts with entry and ends with termination or renegotiation. In between are problem-solving stages: diagnosis (fact-finding and problem identification), planning (setting of goals and deciding on specific action strategies), action (implementation of the plan), and evaluation (additional fact-finding to assess the action and to lead to further planning). At the conclusion of one cycle the consultative relationship either terminates or is renegotiated. Usually, renegotiation is done to cover another project or activity on an "as needed" basis, or the consulting activities may continue as is for some indefinite period of time. Given the limited resources of the ICP, she can afford to maintain ongoing activities requiring a high level of effort with only a few client systems, and these are likely to be those at high risk for infection. Other client "contacts" may be on an as needed basis or may be initiated by the ICP according to the surveillance findings.

To maintain effective contact with hospital departments, the ICP must decide how to use time most effectively and how to terminate, maintain, and pick up relationships that have had to become inactive after, for example, inspection by the Joint Commission on Accreditation of Hospitals.

Terminating consultative relationships

The limits of the consultation effort should be discussed at the beginning in terms of the amount and nature of activities and the nature of the termination. This can be open for renegotiation at any time, but both the consultant and client should be clear at the outset about the nature and amount of activities and the role to be performed by each. (Difficulties the consultant may have in the termination process are discussed under "Letting Go.")

Maintaining consultative relationships

If action research is used as a consultative methodology, the nature of continuing consultative relationships is made clear during each phase of the cycle; the end of one cycle leads either to the decision to terminate or to planning for the next cycle. Each cycle is discrete, and with each cycle new commitments are made. The ICP is likely to have such ongoing commitments with high-risk units of the hospital.

Reestablishing consultative relationships

Reactivating a consultative relationship after a period of inactivity can be perceived by the ICP as a frustrating new start or as an opportunity for developing a new level of infection control sophistication. Having to start over for whatever reason can be tiresome, but it can be an opportunity as well because with each "re-start" the consultant and client are at a different place. The ICP now has more experience and expertise. She can enter the system with more poise and confidence. She can have as a potential goal for the relationship a more sophisticated program in that particular area. When the staff in the client system is new, she can present herself and her role freshly and more articulately.

The re-start can also provide an opportunity for the client system to participate in the process at a deeper and more responsible level, drawing on previous experience. The consulting contract can be negotiated more speedily, since there is less time needed for explanations and education, and a certain amount of bonding has taken place.

On the other hand, the ICP may be reentering a client system in which the relationship between the two previously was difficult and ineffective or floundered in some way. Here the initial negotiation will be more difficult, since the ICP must deal with uncomfortable or negative feelings in herself or in the client. A high level of self-awareness and interpersonal skill is helpful here. If the previous fiasco was caused by ineptness or inappropriate consultant behavior, a simple acknowledgment of the problem may be enough to get the relationship on course again. For more difficult situations some of the techniques of role negotiation and conflict management can be useful.[10,17,41]

ISSUES IN CONSULTING

Thus far the discussion has been fairly straightforward, but there are issues in consultation that add complexity. Two such issues are dealt with in this section: the question of who the client is and the question of who the consultant is, an internal or external person. (Other often discussed issues such as trust and dependency are examined in the section "Consulting Tips for the ICP.")

Who is the client?

The question "Who is the client?" is more complicated than might appear at first glance. Is the client one person or an organizational unit? Is it a system or subsystem of the hospital, or is the client the entire hospital? Obviously, the ICP will make initial contacts with individuals at the managerial or leadership level. This could be at any level in the hospital but is likely to be managers of operating units, such as the head of dietetics, the ICU, or neonatal ICU.

French and Bell[12] recommend that in the initial contact the consultant view a single manager as the client, but that as trust and confidence develop, both the consultant and client begin to view the manager's organization as the client. This seems relevant to the ICP role, since the intent is to control hospital infections throughout the institution, starting with systems or subsystems most involved.

One task of the ICP is to identify key client systems in the hospital for high-priority attention. She will need to develop effective consultant-client relationships with managers in high-risk areas and establish ongoing relationships with them. She may have less frequent contact with managers in other areas, providing consulting services to them on a more cyclical basis.

Individual nonsupervisory employees are not clients, since they do not represent an organizational unit of the hospital. A nonsupervisory employee who calls the attention of the ICP to an undesirable or hazardous practice has no authority to enter into a consultant-client agreement, but such a call can alert the consultant to negotiate entry with the manager of the department or unit in question.

Who is the consultant?

Traditionally, consultants to organizations have been independent of and external to the institution. In recent years the use of internal consultants who are employees of the organization has been growing rapidly. The ICP role is such an internal role.

External consultants, coming from outside the organization, are freer to examine the organization from a broad, systems viewpoint. They also have easier access to the top people and can be more confrontational on problems. Employees of the organization who are assigned consultative roles have more difficulty explaining and articulating their role to their organizational clients. They are also more ready to accept the system as given and to accommodate themselves to the needs of the intact system. Organizational structure, climate, and norms have a great impact on the internal consultant. By accepting the given norms of the organizations, internal consultants tend to spend less time helping the organization move toward self-renewal, growth, and change.[19]

There are advantages and handicaps in being an internal consultant. The ICP is more likely to be caught up in and influenced by the system. She is less likely to have an objective view and is more likely to be influenced by the personal impact that recommendations might have on staff members. As an insider she may be unable to see glaring problems. On the other hand, a consultant who does not create a wide gap between herself and her client is more effective, since a client can identify with her more easily.[6] This gives an edge to the internal consultant. Also, program continuity is easier to maintain with an internal consultant because of her accessibility.

Schuttenberg[39] points out the difficulties internal consultants can have in developing the role in light of the line manager's expectations that they function as other members of the organization. It is common for the manager to expect the internal consultant to produce results and "do for" the manager. In a number of cases this is appropriate, but when the need is to educate managers to solve their own problems in infection control, this expectation generates a dependency on the consultant that can prove handicapping, since the number of ICPs is limited and the range of responsibility to provide service is hospital-wide.

There is a hazard at the other extreme as well. If consultants attempt to impose "help" authoritatively, whether directly or by accepting assignments of control from supervisors, they place themselves in the role of policemen.[29] The policeman posture can be fostered by ICPs, since they usually report to a high or influential level in the organization. For example, ICPs can be unsuccessful in getting middle managers to follow their advice. If they discuss the difficulty with the chairman of the infection control committee or other key organizational figures, the result may be an order from the organizational leader to the manager that accomplishes the purposes desired by the consultant. Under such conditions it would not be surprising for ICPs to be seen as spies or powerful police agents. Furthermore, by their own activities they may directly or intentionally convey a threatening message of "I am here solely to advise and counsel you, but you take my advice or else." The policeman role, McGregor[29] pointed out, is completely incompatible with the professional role.

In summary, the internal consultant has a number of advantages and handicaps that are different from those of the external consultant. The hazards of the internal role are clearly evident, but the internal consultant's identification, continuity, and familiarity with the organizational intricacies are considerable advantages. By being sensitive to these aspects of the role, the ICP is in a far better position to maximize the advantage of the internal role and chart a thoughtful and effective course of role development.

CONSULTING TIPS FOR THE ICP

This last section is devoted to a discussion of a number of short consulting tips for the ICP.

Attitude

The attitude of the consultant shows through in the stance taken with the client. In terms of transactional analysis the consultant needs to build "Adult-Adult" relationships.[5] ICPs who come through as "Critical Parents" will generate defensiveness and threat. An attitude of respect is essential. Attitudes of condescension, judgment, or blame create defensiveness in the client and cannot be tolerated.

Building cooperation

People support activities in which they participate and in which their needs and values are respected. Understanding the underlying needs, feelings, and concerns of the client to help the client meet those needs while working on the infection control program is one way to build cooperation.

Cooperativeness is a function of the identification of one person with another. Identification may range from positive identification to indifference or hostility. If the consultant and client have agreed on important issues in the past or agree on common ends, they are more likely to have a base of goodwill from which to approach disagreement collaboratively.[41]

Filley[10] provides several guidelines for increasing cooperation. Cooperation is increased when one person shares the likes and dislikes of another either by common language, frames of reference, reminders of mutual success, or de-emphasis of differences. Common association between the two persons may generate positive feelings between them in problem-solving situations, so simply increasing the interaction between the two persons can be useful. When one person is identified with or associated with something positively valued by the other, cooperation may be enhanced. This is particularly true if one person helps others enhance their reputations. Cooperation is facilitated when one person acknowledges help received from the other. Finally, if there is conflict or disagreement brewing, depersonalizing the situation can be helpful; that is, both persons address the issues or the sources of antagonism rather than the person. Filley[10] urges people to "fight the antagonism, not the antagonist."

Building trust

To become effective in the consultant role the ICP must be able to develop trusting relationships with clients. She must be seen as trustworthy and competent to be sought as an advisor or counselor. This is especially true because the consultative relationship is voluntary, and the client has free choice to accept or reject any help that is forthcoming. Trust is built with a pattern of open, honest communication and reliable performance.[12] If consultants create a climate in which they are distrusted and seen as spies for management, trust breaks down and the relationship is seriously threatened, if not severed completely.

Dealing with defensive behavior

Defensive behavior occurs when an individual perceives or anticipates threat. Six types of behaviors create defensive climates, in contrast to behaviors that build supportive relationships.[13] Speech or other behavior that appears judgmental increases defensiveness; descriptive speech does not. Speech used to persuade and control the client evokes resistance; an attitude of seeking a solution to a mutual problem does not. Hidden messages or agendas spark defensiveness; openness does not. Lack of concern for the other person's welfare generates defensiveness; empathy and valuing the other person does not. An attitude communicating superiority and unwillingness to enter into a shared problem-solving relationship builds defensiveness; an attitude conveying willingness to enter into participative planning with mutual trust and respect does not. Seeming to know all the answers and being certain of the answers puts others on guard; an attitude of tentativeness and a willingness to experiment does not.

Dealing with resistance

People resist change in direct relationship to the perceived amount of loss that the change represents. Some changes are "lightweight" and easy to handle, and some are "middleweight" and somewhat more difficult. However, "heavyweight" changes that represent distinct loss or create a disruption particularly in social relationships, are usually strongly resisted.[15,25,31] The ICP needs to understand the personal meaning a proposed change in the infection control program has for the client system and help the people involved manage the change so that trauma is minimized and emotional loss is worked through.

Researchers are also discovering that changes that are instituted without advance notice or preparation are particularly stressful to the people affected.[1,2] People need to become used to a proposed change. Providing advance notice and a regular flow of information will ease the stress. ICPs would do well to adopt a "doctrine of no surprises" whenever possible in their work.

Handling "expertise"

The ICP needs to be visible for her expert knowledge and skill but in appropriate ways. Educational endeavors are especially suited to this, as is advice and counsel, provided she does not use her expertise in a way that limits client growth and autonomy.

Influencing the system

ICPs can build stature for themselves and for the program by having a clear understanding of the role and of the change process, by developing positive personal power skills, and by understanding the pathways to power in the organization. The nature of the role provides a unique perspective in and of the organization. ICPs need to use that perspective with thoughtfulness, with a clear sense of their own value system, with interpersonal skill, and with restraint. (See also "Models and Strategies of Change," "Pathways to Power," and "Positive Personal Power Styles.")

Information flow

The ICP needs to maintain an effective network of relationships throughout the hospital to keep informed of present or potential infection control problems. Mintzberg[32] stresses the importance of maintaining a system of contacts throughout the organization to build goodwill, gain cooperation, and obtain information. Such liaison activities make it possible to build and maintain a predictable, reciprocating system of relationships.

The ICP needs to establish links throughout the hospital to have a regular flow of information from those areas of the hospital identified as critical. She may wish to develop informal systems of monitoring to augment formal audits and rounds. Linkage with selected members of the clinical laboratory staff, for example, would be valuable in developing an effective infection control information network.

Letting go: avoiding dependency

A consultant can easily feel torn between working to increase client resourcefulness and independence and at the same time wanting to remain involved with the client to feel needed and competent. Although logically this problem can be handled by a gradual reduction of the consultant's role or by less frequent contacts, the process of letting go can be difficult for the consultant. Letting go can be further complicated if the consultant measures her success primarily by the number of people who call or feel they have to call for advice.

Some clients can also be very satisfying to work with, and it can be tempting for the consultant to hold onto a relationship that otherwise would be terminated. One remedy is for the consultant to have a number of client relationships active at any one time and to have attractive new projects waiting to be started, so the "letting go" process is not so difficult.

Models and strategies of change

Given the extent to which the ICP is engaged in organizational change, she would do well to seek out useful models of the change process, both as to how individuals change and how organizations can be changed. A change that is minor or lightweight is relatively easy to accomplish. Change that is complex or involves more of the central core or essence of the person or organization is exceedingly difficult to achieve. (For a general introduction to the change process see Darling[7]; for information on loss and change see Marris[31] and Goodman[15]; for the unfreezing-changing-refreezing mechanisms of change see Schein[38]; and for managing complex organizational change see Beckhard and Harris[3] and Sayles.[36])

Pathways to power

Kanter's research[20,21] on pathways to power would suggest that the ICP look for program ways she can engage in activities that are relevant to the hospital, are out of the ordinary rather than routine, and are visible. Kanter would advise her to be aware of the value of alliances with specific individuals above her in the organization, either superiors or mentors, as well as maintain effective contact with peers and junior personnel who are "comers." (See also "Positive Personal Power Styles.")

Positive personal power styles

Traditionally, managers have drawn on position-based sources of power to achieve their goals. In a classic article French and Raven[11] identified five bases of social power: position, coercion, reward, expert, and referent. The first three power bases come from one's official position, that is, the power that comes from rank, authority, and the ability to reward and punish. By contrast, expert and referent power are person-based sources of power. Expert power refers to the technical and interpersonal knowledge and ability and skills possessed by the person, whereas referent power refers to attractiveness, identification, and simple liking.

ICPs, along with other persons in staff or consultant roles, must draw on person-based sources of power, since they do not carry the "clout" of line management positions. Since they are involved in an organizational program in which their influence must be felt, they must develop competence in personal power and influence. Harrison[4,17] has focused on organizational roles in which authority alone cannot produce results and personal skill and self-confidence is needed to work effectively in face-to-face situations with others. He has developed a program to help persons develop their positive personal power and increase their ability to influence others in a way that does not damage or weaken others and, conversely, that is intended to make others stronger. Harrison maintains that an effective influencer needs the flexibility and competence to use four personal power styles. The ICP would do well to build her competencies in these styles:

1. *Assertive persuasion.* Using the power of logic, facts, opinions, and ideas to persuade others
2. *Reward and punishment.* Using pressures and incentives to control the behavior of others
3. *Participation and trust.* Involving other persons in decision making or problem solving
4. *Common vision.* Identifying and articulating a common or shared vision of what the future of an organization, group, or individual could be; mobilizing the energy and resources of others through appeals to their hopes, values, and aspirations

SUMMARY

The ICP has a special role as a consultant relating to clients in the hospital. Consulting is a helping relationship in which influence is balanced with affiliation with the client system. Consultants have a range of role behaviors from which to choose, each behavior having implications for client independence or dependence.

Two consultant models are described. One is the traditional medical model, in which the consultant uses expertise to assist the client, and dependence of the client on the consultant is an accepted outcome. The other is the educational model, in which the consultant emphasizes the use of education, joint sharing of expertise and resources, and the development of the client's ability to solve problems independently. Although the traditional medical model is appropriate for certain situations, the educational model has more overall value for the ICP.

The consultative process is examined, including scouting and entry, action research methodology, various informal methods of marketing the consultative role, and strategies for initiating planned change. In addition to scouting and entry, the consulting cycle is seen as involving diagnosis, planning, action, evaluation, and termination or renegotiation. Areas are identified where the ICP will want to maintain relationships and others where consultation would appropriately be shifted to an "as needed" basis or re-started for specific short-term goals.

REFERENCES

1. Adams, J.D.: Understanding and managing stress: a book of readings, San Diego, 1980, University Associates.
2. Adams, J.D.: A workbook in changing life styles, San Diego, 1980, University Associates.
3. Beckhard, R., and Harris, R.T.: Organizational transitions: managing complex change, Reading, Mass., 1977, Addison-Wesley Publishing Co., Inc.
4. Berlew, D.E., and Harrison, R.: Positive power and influence program trainers manual, Boston, 1979, Situation Management Systems, Inc.
5. Berne, E.: Transactional analysis in psychotherapy, New York, 1961, Grove Press, Inc.
6. Blake, R.R., and Mouton, J.S.: Consultation, Reading, Mass., 1976, Addison-Wesley Publishing Co., Inc.
7. Darling, L.: Communication and change. In Barrett-Connor, E., et al., editors: Epidemiology for the infection control nurse, St. Louis, 1978, The C.V. Mosby Co.
8. Drucker, P.: Management: tasks, responsibilities, practices, New York, 1973, Harper & Row, Publishers, Inc.
9. Ferguson, C.: Concerning the nature of human systems and the consultant role. In Bennis, W., Benne, K., and Chin, R., editors: The planning of change, ed. 2, New York, 1969, Holt, Rinehart & Winston.
10. Filley, A.C.: Interpersonal conflict resolution, Glenview, Ill., 1975, Scott, Foresman & Co.
11. French, J.R.P., Jr., and Raven, B.: The bases of social power. In Cartwright, D., editor: Studies in social power, Ann Arbor, Mich., 1959, University of Michigan.
12. French, W.L., and Bell, C.H.: Organization development, ed. 2, New York, 1978, Prentice-Hall, Inc.
13. Gibb, J.: Defensive communication. In Kolb, D., Rubin, I.M., and McIntyre, J.: Organizational psychology: a book of readings, ed. 2, New York, 1974, Prentice-Hall, Inc.
14. Glidewell, J.C.: The entry problem in consultation. In Bennis, W., Benne, K., and Chin, R., editors: The planning of change, ed. 1, New York, 1961, Holt, Rinehart & Winston.
15. Goodman, E.: Turning points, New York, 1980, Fawcett Columbine Books.
16. Goodstein, L.D.: Consulting with human service systems, Reading, Mass., 1978, Addison-Wesley Publishing Co., Inc.
17. Harrison, R.: Role negotiation. In Burke, W.W., and Hornstein, H.A.: The social technology of organization development, Fairfax, Va., 1972, National Learning Resources Corp.
18. Harrison, R.: How to design and conduct self-directed learning experiences, Group Organization Stud. 3:149-167, 1978.
19. Huse, E.F.: Organization development, St. Paul, Minn., 1975, West Publishing Co.
20. Kanter, R.M.: Men and women of the corporation, New York, 1977, Harper & Row, Publishers, Inc.
21. Kanter, R.M.: Power failure in management circuits, Harv. Bus. Rev. 57:65-75, July-Aug., 1979.
22. Kolb, D.: Organizational psychology, Englewood Cliffs, N.J., 1974, Prentice-Hall, Inc.
23. Kolb, D., and Frohman, A.L.: An organization development approach to consulting, Sloan Mgt. Rev., 12:51-65, 1970.
24. Lakein, A.: How to get control of your time and your life, New York, 1973, Peter Wyden Publishing Co.

25. Lawrence, P.R.: How to deal with resistance to change. In Kolb, D., editor: Organizational psychology: a book of readings, Englewood Cliffs, N.J., 1974, Prentice-Hall, Inc.

26. Lippitt, R., Watson, J., and Westley, B.: The dynamics of planned change, New York, 1958, Harcourt, Brace & World.

27. Lippitt, R.: Dimensions of the consultant's job. In Bennis, W., Benne, K., and Chin, R., editors: The planning of change, ed. 1, New York, 1961, Holt, Rinehart & Winston.

28. McGregor, D.: The staff function in human relations, J. Soc. Issues **4**:5-40, 1948.

29. McGregor, D.: The human side of enterprise, New York, 1960, McGraw-Hill, Inc.

30. Marguilies, N., and Raia, A.: Organization development: values, process and technology, New York, 1972, McGraw-Hill, Inc.

31. Marris, P.: Loss and change, Garden City, N.Y., 1975, Anchor Books.

32. Mintzberg, H.: The nature of managerial work, Reading, Mass., 1973, Addison-Wesley Publishing Co.

33. Nylen, D.J., Mitchell, R., and Stout, A.: Handbook for staff development and human relations training, Washington, D.C. (undated), National Training Laboratories for Applied Behavioral Science, National Education Association, pp. 112-117.

34. Reddin, W.J.: Effective management by objectives, New York, 1971, McGraw-Hill, Inc.

35. Rubin, I., Plovnick, M., and Fry, R.: The role of consultation in initiating planned change: a case study in health care systems. In Burke, W.W., editor: Current issues and strategies in organization development, New York, 1977, Human Sciences Press, Inc.

36. Sayles, L.: Leadership, New York, 1979, McGraw-Hill, Inc.

37. Schein, E.: Process consultation, Reading, Mass., 1969, Addison-Wesley Publishing Co.

38. Schein, E.: Mechanisms of change. In Bennis, W., Benne, K., and Chin, R.: The planning of change, ed. 2, New York, 1969, Holt, Rinehart & Winston.

39. Schuttenberg, E.M.: Organization development in industry: an inquiry into the role of the internal consultant. OD Practitioner 1971 (mimeo)

40. Steele, F.I.: Consultants and detectives, J. Appl. Behav. Sci. **5**:187-202, 1969

41. Thomas, K.: Conflict and conflict management. In Dunnette, M.D., editor: Handbook of industrial and organizational psychology, 1976, Rand, McNally and Co.

42. Weisbord, M.: The organization development contract, O.D. Pract. **5**:1-4, Summer 1973.

11 KAREN J. AXNICK

Education

Learning is finding out what you already know.
Doing is demonstrating that you know it.
Teaching is reminding others that they know just as well as you.
You are all learners, doers, teachers. ·
Richard Bach*

---

andragogy The art and science of teaching adults.
behaviorist orientation A model of human behavior that views the individual as a passive organism whose behavior can be manipulated, molded, and controlled through appropriate control of external environmental stimuli.
operant conditioning Behavior is controlled by its consequences; stimuli follow rather than precede the behavior and influence the probability of the behavior being repeated.
paradigm A framework of thought by which aspects of reality are explained and understood.
paradigm shift Occurs when knowledge is generated that does not fit into an old framework.
phenomenological orientation A model of human behavior that views the individual as a source of action who is free to choose different modes of behavior; freedom stems from human consciousness and self-awareness.
universal process A model that views learning as a lifelong endeavor; seeks to address the whole person, viewing the teacher and students as learners in a joint process of discovery.

Education or training is a primary component of the infection control program. Although the act of teaching is often regarded as a special, formal activity in which the infection control practitioner (ICP) engages only a relatively small portion of time, it is in fact impossible not to teach. Each interaction is an exchange that facilitates teaching and learning by both participants.

The scope of this chapter is the exploration of the learning and teaching process common to the patient, staff, and ICP. This discussion will include an overview of adult learner characteristics, a review of the learning process, and the application of these topics to the development of goals, teaching strategies, and evaluation methods for educational programs.

*Excerpted from the book ILLUSIONS by Richard Bach. Copyright © 1977 by Creature Enterprises, Inc. Reprinted by permission of DELACORTE PRESS/ELEANOR FRIEDE.

NATURE OF LEARNING

Teyler[16] defines learning as "a relatively permanent change in behavior as the result of experience." How this change is effected has been the subject of intense debate. In the past two decades the understanding of how learning occurs has been influenced by psychological insight and neurophysiological research and manifested in changing educational theories and practice.

Psychological contributions

Two contrasting models of human behavior have been drawn by both philosophers and psychologists. The *behaviorist* orientation views the individual as a passive organism whose behavior can be manipulated, molded, and controlled through appropriate control of external environmental stimuli. Universal laws govern human behavior, making it amenable to study through scientific methodology. The *phenomenological* orientation holds that the individual, as the source of action, is free to choose different modes of behavior; the freedom stems from human consciousness and self-awareness. Observable behavior, therefore, is only a reflection of an internal private experience of being.[13] The application of these models to teaching and learning yields interesting concepts.

Behaviorist orientations. Skinner,[13] a renowned researcher in behaviorist psychology and an outspoken critic of the U.S. educational system, notes that teaching is simply the arrangement of reinforcing factors under which students learn. The cornerstone of Skinner's premise is *operant conditioning.* The perspective of classical behaviorism, which states that behavior is the result of a stimulus-response reflex, is too narrow to explain much of human behavior. Skinner builds on this model but notes that behavior is operant; that is, it changes or modifies the environment. Therefore Skinner postulates that in operant conditioning behavior is controlled by its consequences. Stimuli or reinforcers *follow* rather than precede the behavior and influence the probability of the behavior being repeated.

In the educational setting the effects of reinforcement are so pervasive that they are seldom part of a person's awareness. Verbal and nonverbal reinforcement takes the form of praise or criticism and smiles or frowns. All of these responses influence whether or not the student will risk answering a question or performing a behavior. The absence of reinforcement or feedback quickly extinguishes the likelihood of continued performance.

The ICP needs to give careful consideration to the concept of operant conditioning in planning educational activities. Reinforcement by the ICP for behavior demonstrated in class is quickly forgotten if the employee's supervisor does not continue to reinforce the behavior in the clinical setting. For example, an ICP may encourage the staff to perform IV catheter care daily. However, the head nurse believes that inspecting the site and changing the dressing that often only increases the risk of infiltration. With these conflicting expectations, the staff member is more likely to follow the dictates of the head nurse, since that reinforcement is given more frequently and is perceived as having greater consequences.

Phenomenological orientation. Whereas behaviorism focuses on only the objective, observable behavior of human beings, the phenomenological orientation encompasses the inner world or private experience of the individual, manifested in behavior.[13] This viewpoint is the basis of the humanistic-existential movement in psychology. Carl Rogers, founder of patient-centered therapy, is a key figure in this movement.

Rogers' view of learning[13] is based on the assumption of the individual's ability to adapt and propensity to grow in a direction that enhances his existence; the absence of positive growth occurs when an individual's unique world view is incongruous with reality.

Fully functional human beings, and thus those who are most able to grow and learn, live fully with the entire spectrum of feelings and reactions. At each moment in each situation these individuals are fully aware and trust their total being. They are then creative, constructive, and trustworthy and need affiliation and communication; their behavior is not predictable but dependable.

In a rogerian mode the goal of education does not differ from the behaviorist model, but the process is strikingly different. An educated person is one who has "learned how to learn."[13] Learning is viewed as a natural and required *internal* process directed by the *learner* who is engaged with the environment as it is perceived.[8]

Schein[15] illustrates the importance of incorporating humanistic approaches into professional education in what he calls "training for uncertainty." He notes that situations frequently arise in which attitudinal and emotional components are called into play with the knowledge base to determine professional practice. The humanistic attributes for successful ICPs include the following:

- Self-confidence when a clear answer to a problem is not evident
- Responsibility for decisions that rest on incomplete or partial information
- Decisiveness in a high-risk climate
- Ability to inspire confidence in situations of uncertainty

These attributes evolve from learning situations that value the inherent ability of an individual to use both externally gained knowledge and the internal awareness of choice. The ICP creates a climate conducive to this process by providing principles of practice and encouraging the staff to generalize this knowledge to a variety of clinical situations. For example, the decision-making process for isolation is relatively uncomplicated for a patient with a diagnosis of hepatitis B confirmed by radioimmunoassay. However, a patient coming to the hospital with overt jaundice and elevated liver enzymes is more difficult to assess. The decision-making process in the latter case requires the staff nurse to perform a physical assessment and obtain a medical history through specific questions used to solicit an epidemiological assessment based on a broad understanding of the pathophysiology of liver disease. Working with incomplete information, the nurse then evaluates the likelihood of an infectious etiology and the risk of crossinfection based on an understanding of modes of transmission. The difference between observing guidelines in the isolation procedure and performing the nursing assessment lies in sophisticated cognitive functions leading to a clinical judgment.

Neurophysiological research

While psychologists were forging new models of human behavior, concomitant advances in biological science contributed to the changing perspective of the learning process. Neurophysiologists distinguish between two major modes of human consciousness expressed in *split-brain* or lateralization theories.

Split-brain refers to the right and left hemispheres of the cerebral cortex. The characteristics of these two modes of consciousness follow:

Left hemisphere	Right hemisphere
Intellectual	Sensuous, intuitive
Time, history	Timelessness, eternity
Active	Receptive
Analytical	Gestalt
Explicit	Tacit
Linear	Nonlinear
Sequential	Simultaneous
Focal	Diffuse
Masculine	Feminine
Time	Space
Verbal	Spatial
Causal	Acausal
Propositional	Appositional

Although motor and sensory systems are represented bilaterally in the human brain, language systems appear to be an unexplained exception to normal symmetry of neural functions (Fig. 11-1).[6] The left hemisphere, which corresponds to the right side of the body, excels in verbal processing. It possesses the abilities for analysis, linear arrangement, and temporal ordering necessary for speaking, reading, calculating, and writing. Behaviorist psychology places heavy emphasis on the left hemisphere aspects of learning, since these are most readily reflected in observable, measurable behavior.

Conversely, the right hemisphere corresponds to the left side of the body. Superior in managing visual and spatial tasks, this hemisphere deals in tactile, kinesthetic, and auditory modalities. It is important to note that the right hemisphere is verbal, as is the left hemisphere, but it seeks its mode for expres-

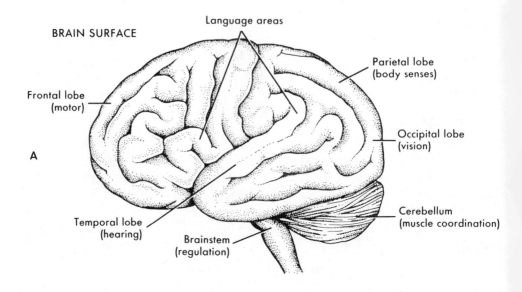

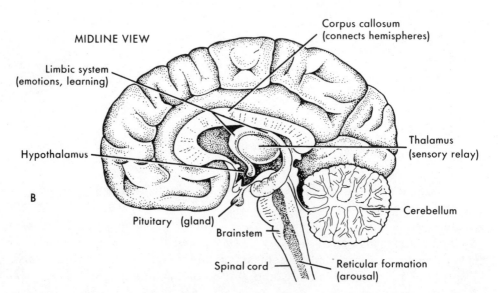

FIG. 11-1. A, Surface of left hemisphere of the human brain with major areas and their functions labeled. **B,** Midline view of right hemisphere with major areas and structures and their functions labeled.

sion in symbols, images, and metaphors rather than words and thought patterns.[3]

The two hemispheres, connected by a band of nerve fibers called the *corpus callosum*, represent coexisting modes of awareness that form a holistic view of reality (Fig. 11-2). These two types of cognition have been termed *appositional* (right side of the brain) and *propositional* (left side of the brain). Contrary to popular thought, the difference does not lie in intellect versus affect, or thinking versus emotions, for each hemisphere has its own affective apparatus in the limbic lobes (Fig. 11-1). Rather, the contrast is more process specific than content specific.[3]

Each lobe is capable of functioning independently in a different manner, but neither can substitute for the other. This unilateral function is readily apparent in the variation of sequelae observed in stroke patients; deficits in

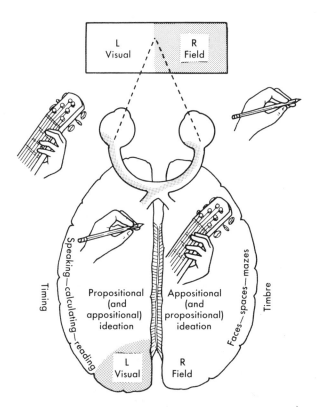

FIG. 11-2. Schematic outline of the brain as seen from above to suggest complementary dominance of cerebral hemisphere for various tasks, summarizing evidence from cases of lateralized lesions and from testing of patients with cerebral commissurotomy. (Redrawn from Bogen, J.E.: Some educational implications of hemispheric specialization. In THE HUMAN BRAIN. Edited by M.C. Wittrock © 1977 by Prentice-Hall, Inc., Englewood Cliffs, N.J. 07632; based on Sperry, R.W., Vogel, P.J., and Bogen, J.E.: 1970.)

communication or thought process are specific to the hemisphere and lobes of damaged brain tissue.

Creativity and learning require both modes of awareness. The intuitive right hemisphere arrives at insight or the gestalt experience only after the left hemisphere has been appropriately primed with information and the normal linear process has been temporarily suspended. The verbal, ordering ability of the left hemisphere is then required to organize, interpret, and communicate the discovery to integrate it into the existing body of knowledge.

Although inherent individual style may influence the learning process, past experience creates the appearance of a dominant left hemisphere. In actuality this exaggerated style is probably more a reflection of societal values than a neurological phenomenon. Western culture, as expressed in the traditional classroom, evokes the linear, rational mode of consciousness. The "Three R's," associated with the left hemisphere of the brain, have received great emphasis to the detriment of art and music.

To the ICP, application of the split-brain model requires awareness of its influence on the individual's learning process. Information through experience is assessed in three representational systems[1,2]:

- *Audio.* Verbal mode of reading, writing, or listening to words
- *Visual.* Imagery mode of patterns, pictures, or colors
- *Kinesthetic.* Sensory mode of feeling tones, body sensations, and gross or fine muscular movement

Although individuals use all three systems in learning, there is usually a dominant mode. Often this can be assessed by the vocabulary used.[2] The following statements all express a sense of understanding but are highly reflective of different representational systems:

"I hear what you say." (audio)
"I see what you mean." (visual)
"I am really in touch with your ideas." (kinesthetic)

Since adult groups are heterogeneous in their learning styles and past experiences, the ICP should attempt to include all three representational systems in learning activities. If the goal of the educational session is to learn to teach patients aseptic technique for home hyperalimentation procedures, the ICP can organize the content to include a discussion of aseptic principles using handouts (audio) and graphics of the procedure (visual). The kinesthetic mode can be addressed by role playing a patient teaching situation in which the technique is demonstrated.

Shifting educational paradigms

A paradigm is a framework of thought by which aspects of reality are explained and understood. A paradigm shift occurs when new knowledge is generated that does not fit into the old framework. Eventually these data accumulate beyond the tolerance point of the old paradigm, and the apparent contradictions are reconciled in a new, powerful, and more comprehensive theory.[5]

The revolutionary concepts of human behavioral change and the learning process stretched the limits of the educational paradigm. The resultant shift can be perceived as occurring in two phases. The first phase addressed a sociological phenomenon that began in the late 1950s and early 1960s; namely, adults began to return to the classroom to obtain high school diplomas or advanced education. Educators discovered that methodology successfully used with children seemed inadequate when applied to adults. This new approach was called *andragogy*.

Phase 1: andragogy. Andragogy, the art and science of teaching adults, has evolved from contemporary psychotherapeutic modalities in humanistic and existential psychology.[8] The premise of andragogy is that adults as learners differ from children. This distinction, as Knowles[8] suggests, is probaby more illusory than real, arising from a stereotypical picture of children as passive, immature, dependent personalities.

Knowles[8,9,17] has outlined four critical assumptions concerning adults as learners that distinguish between pedagogical and andragogical philosophies (Table 11-1).

Self-concept. Infants initially view the world as an extension of themselves; there is no separation or boundary between their consciousness or bodies and the external environment. As they mature, the differentiation is experienced as total dependency. Gradually this self-concept changes as they gain motor and speech skills. In the pedagogical model the dependency of children is reinforced and perpetuated by an orientation to conformity and authority. Knowles[9] expresses concern that this approach ignores the fact that school-aged children are equipped to engage in self-directed learning and require an environment that guides this process responsibly and efficiently.

Adults, in a psychological context, view themselves as self-disciplined, autonomous, and unique. Learning situations that thwart this expression of

TABLE 11-1. Assumptions about learners

Assumption	Pedagogy	Andragogy
Self-concept	Dependent on authority	Self-directing
Experience	Limited but open to change	Richer but often rigid
Readiness to learn	Biological development; socialization (by threat of punishment)	Developmental requirements of social roles
Orientation to learning	Postponed application of concepts (subject centered)	Immediacy of application (problem centered)

self-direction create incongruity between the circumstance and the self-concept. This results in either rebellious or accommodating behavior, depending on the perceived risk inherent in the response.

To illustrate this assumption, in one hospital an ICP and in-service coordinator made a series of videotapes addressing isolation procedures, IV catheter care, urinary catheter management, and dressing techniques. The videotapes were stocked on a cart with the recorder and television set and were made available to the nursing units on a contractual basis. Staff members could select the tapes based on their own learning needs and clinical situations. The tapes could be viewed individually or in small groups.

Experience. In contrast with children, adults have more life experiences, which result in richer resources for learning. For children, experiences are something that happen to them; they are passive recipients of events. Adults, however, perceive experiences as expressions of who they are. As sources of their experiences, situations that reject or undervalue personal experience are interpreted as a rejection of the individual.[8,9] By virtue of their experiences, adults may be more rigid, judgmental, and closed to new experiences because their self-concept is at stake. Teaching techniques must incorporate four principles to account for the adult experience base:

1. Adult educational technology focuses on experiential rather than information-transmittal techniques.
2. Experiences specifically designed to "unfreeze" perceptions and expectations may be necessary to initiate the self-directing adult.
3. Educational content must be broad enough to accommodate the heterogeneous needs of a group of adults.
4. Techniques must draw on the experiences of individual members of the group.

EXAMPLE:
The ICP has been requested to provide an in-service lecture on the management of indwelling catheters. In preparation for the class she conducts an informal survey of the staff to assess the specific problems of this nursing unit. During the session the ICP provides background information about the etiology and pathogenesis of infections related to catheter use and leads a discussion whereby staff members identify methods of nursing care that would be effective in preventing infections.

Readiness to learn. Readiness to learn, or the "teachable moment," is closely aligned with time orientation for adults.

Educators organize childhood education based on developmental phases that depend on biological maturation of the brain and body, coupled with the socialization process achieved through prior academic and life experiences. Developmental phases are not as clearly defined for adults. However, readiness to learn is again linked to the problem-specific needs of the adult, arising from a discrepancy between role performance and role expectations at home, at work, or in social situations. Timing learning experiences to coincide with the learner's developmental tasks is critical.

EXAMPLE:
After a staphylococcal outbreak in the newborn nursery the ICP finds staff interest and receptivity to new knowledge and skills in infection control. The shared experience and knowledge resulted in individual behavioral changes for both physicians and nurses in adhering to nursery policies.

Orientation to learning. Differing time perspectives of adults and children influence their orientation to learning.

Most childhood education is delivered with the idea that a broad, general education is necessary to train the mind. Immediate application of what has been learned is not a hallmark of primary or even most secondary education programs. This orientation to future application of knowledge results in a subject-oriented curriculum that often seems meaningless to the student. In Knowles' opinion[8] this is a gross misjudgment by those responsible for early education.

Adults have different time perspectives. Motivated by the recognition that they are unable to solve a problem with their current level of knowledge and skills, adults seek educational opportunities with *immediate* application. Adults also view time as a valuable, limited commodity and carefully select educational endeavors before investing time and energy.

This time perspective has major implications for curriculum design. Traditionally, in subject-centered learning, course material is organized sequentially in broad blocks from theory to application to practice. However, mature adults with a problem-specific orientation require more flexibility in course design. Problem sets, incorporating the theory–application–practice sequence, can be organized to foster more immediate benefits in self-esteem and competency.

EXAMPLE:
Few new ICPs have the luxury of taking courses in epidemiology, microbiology, and management theory before implementing this new role. Consequently, educational opportunities should be designed to address specific needs. One problem set could include basic microbiology from theory to clinical application in the laboratory and patient unit; a second problem set would address basic principles of surveillance and their application to the hospital. These two problem sets could then be linked in a practice session of chart review that draws on the clinical knowledge and skills of the ICP and requires immediate use of the new knowledge in microbiology and surveillance.

Phase 2: universal process. The second phase of the paradigm shift is beginning to occur at all levels of education. As Knowles[8] prophesized, the distinctions between pedagogy and andragogy are blurring as a more universal view of human learning emerges. This new view seeks to synthesize the artificial demarcations of the psychological, educational, and biological models and hence produces the shift in the educational paradigm.

The old paradigm stressed the transmittal theory of education; namely, the purpose of education was to transmit the totality of knowledge from one generation to the next.[5] In this context the teacher was the reservoir of knowledge and was responsible for conveying information in a controlled, orderly manner. This subject orientation of the pedagogical system leads to conformity in the search for the "right" answer.

The emerging paradigm, in contrast, views learning as a lifelong endeavor. It seeks to address the whole person, viewing the teacher and students as learners in a joint process of discovery. The new paradigm incorporates the paradoxical qualities of the human brain reflected in behavioristic and humanistic psychology (Table 11-2).

This new enlarged paradigm focuses on the nature of the learning process. At the heart of this change is an appreciation of the dichotomous nature of knowing expressed in the split-brain theory.[18] How does one "know" something? Is it through the rational process of the left brain sequentially organizing random information into a body of knowledge? Or is it through an intuitive

TABLE 11-2. Education and paradigm shift

	Emphasis	
Characteristic	Old paradigm: content ("right" body of knowledge; theoretical; abstract)	New paradigm: context (learning to learn; knowledge integrated with experience)
Viewpoint	Product (destination)	Process (journey)
Intent	Preparation for role	Lifelong process
Structure	Hierarchical and authoritative	Egalitarian
Rewards	Conformity	Autonomy (realized potential)
Progress	Compartmentalized movement	Flexible, integrated movement
Priority	"Correct" performance	Self-esteem of "student"
Methods	Analytical and reductionist	Intuitive (with analytical) and holistic
Environment (classroom)	Structured; rigid setting	Light colors; airy; flexible
Technology	Reliance on "tools" (audiovisual aids)	Balance technology and human interaction
Teacher	Reservoir of knowledge; one-way communication	Facilitator and learner; reciprocal communication

Modified from Ferguson, M.: The aquarian conspiracy, Los Angeles, 1980, J.P. Tarcher, Inc.

sense or experience of truth through insight of the right hemisphere? Both views are valid and hence the new paradigm.

Wittrock[18] suggests that a new concept of education is in order, one that successfully integrates the forces creating the paradigm shift. Learning must be "reconceived" as a generative, cognitive process; that is, learning is an active process whereby the individual must construct meaning for new information or experience using propositional (verbal) and appositional (imaginal) processing. To induce and elaborate these meanings or representations involves a process of transferring previous experience to new events and problems. Hence this premise addresses the assumptions of andragogy: the integral functions of both hemispheres and the experiential component of humanistic psychology. Furthermore, Wittrock reconciles the split between behaviorist and humanistic psychology:

> In this view, teaching is more than the reinforcement of correct responses in the presence of discriminative stimuli. In large part teaching is the process of organizing and relating new information to the learner's previous experience, stimulating him to construct his own representations for what he is encountering. Students learn by active construction of meaning, by what reactions the teacher causes them to generate.*

PROGRAM DEVELOPMENT

The purpose of learning is to improve or maintain competency in dealing wih life's situations. Within this context of learning a triad of needs must be considered.

Patient education is the promotion of both health maintenance and disease prevention and control. The emphasis and scope of patient education or information programs vary with the philosophy, resources, and patient population of the health care facility.

The extent of the ICP's involvement in this institutional effort should be addressed in phase 1 (identification) of the role development process. At a minimum the ICP should address the need for basic explanation of isolation techniques and communicable disease control measures. In more sophisticated programs the ICP has taken an active role in teaching patients and families about specific infectious diseases, as well as maintenance of the home environment, equipment, and supplies for infection prevention and control.

Continuing education and training of hospital *staff* is the backbone of every infection control program. Implemented either formally in a classroom or informally in the work setting, this aspect of the ICP's role is vital for the promotion of staff understanding and performance of infection control policies and procedures.

*From Wittrock, M.S.: The generative processes of memory. In Wittrock, M.S., editor: The human brain, Englewood Cliffs, N.J., 1977, Prentice-Hall, Inc.

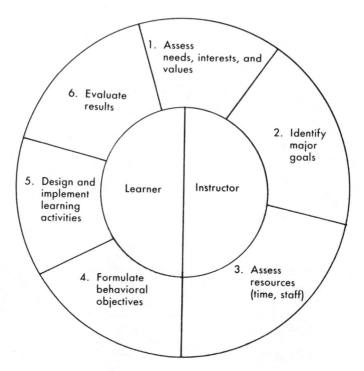

FIG. 11-3. Program developmental model.

Finally and equally as important is the commitment of the ICP to *self*-development. The nature of the infection control field is characterized by evolution and change. This nature, coupled with the lack of a defined curriculum for preparation for the role, demands that the ICP seek out resources to develop and maintain expertise in a wide variety of academic and skill areas.

In each of these situations a standard approach to planning, implementing, and evaluating the learning experience is used (Fig. 11-3).

Assessing needs, interests, and values

A primary tenet of the andragogical process is the relevancy of program content to life and work situations. The instructor's commitment to this process carries a responsibility: to base learning activities on objective performance criteria as defined by the line manager and on subjective feedback from the learners themselves.

Learning needs, defined by role expectations, interests, and values, are assessed at three levels: individual, organizational, and societal.

Individual. Adult learners, by virtue of their experiences and past educational activities, are a heterogeneous group. These two factors, coupled with a

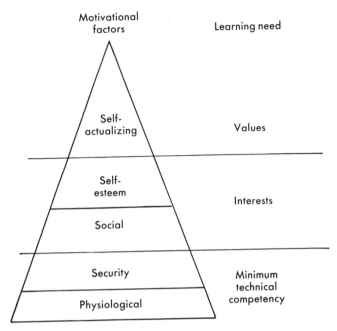

FIG. 11-4. A comparison of Maslow's hierarchy of needs and learning needs.

spectrum of skills, licensure requirements, current role responsibilities, and career goals, provide a challenge for the instructor. Defining the target population, the instructor further needs to assess the intellectual and physical maturity of the group.

Readiness to learn is often influenced by the perception of the individual's ability to perform well in a role. The lack of congruity between performance and expectations becomes a powerful motivational factor. Maslow[12] has described a hierarchy of needs (Fig. 11-4). The premise of his motivational theory is that behavior seeks to address a need; once the need is met, a new need emerges in ascending order in the hierarchy as a motivator. When this motivational theory is applied to learning theory, the lowest level needs, physiological and security, relate to basic technical competency; social and self-esteem needs correspond to behavior motivated by interest. Modifying values is undertaken by the self-actualizing individual. No one is ever permanently arrested at one level or is the transition from one level to the next linear and smooth. Consequently, the instructor must constantly assess the dynamics of behavioral change in the learner.

Organizational. Every health care facility has a responsibility to establish the scope and competency of practice at all levels within the organization. The "bottom line" in patient care is the *outcome* of an educational process: safe, quality care. It is critical for every educator to realize that the power and authority to determine the boundaries of practice and to evaluate performance rests with the line manager. Educators, possessing staff authority, may influence these expectations through the development of policies, procedures, job standards, and institutional goals and objectives, but managers have the final approval.

Societal. Community (local or national) health care regulations, professional standards of practice, and consumer expectations define role responsibilities and hence influence learning needs.

The means by which the educator assesses learning needs vary with the institution and the staff:

1. *Direct observation of practice.* Observation can be achieved on regular surveillance rounds. Frequently, problems, such as undated IV tubings, improper positioning of Foley catheter bags, or inappropriate isolation techniques, are readily apparent.

   Formal, planned observation times can also be arranged. In response to an increase in endometritis related to cesarean section, an ICP spent 5 days working with the staff in the delivery room. Recommendations for changes were first presented in a written report, followed by a series of in-service classes. Another ICP spent 2 days observing in a cardiovascular intensive care unit when a new cardiac output monitor was introduced. A procedure was jointly developed with the staff, and subsequent in-service classes included both the technological and infection control aspects of using this new equipment.

2. *Communication and feedback systems.* Informal education is a continuous process in the interaction between the ICP and the hospital staff. Questions regarding infection control practices are asked frequently during routine visits to the nursing units or departments. Spending time with staff members at breaks or lunch time and sitting in on reports can bring concerns to the surface.

   More formal assessment methods include reviewing care plans, distributing skill inventories and questionnaires, and meeting with individuals or groups to "brainstorm" topics.

3. *Reports, records, and literature.* Incident reports, audits, research studies, committee minutes, and professional literature will also yield problem areas that may be amenable to correction by educational means.

4. *External requirements.* Local, state, and national regulations may highlight educational needs. The Joint Commission on Accreditation of Hospitals outlines specific educational requirements for infection control in both orientation and continuing education for staff. In addition, some professional groups have specific continuing education requirements for relicensure.

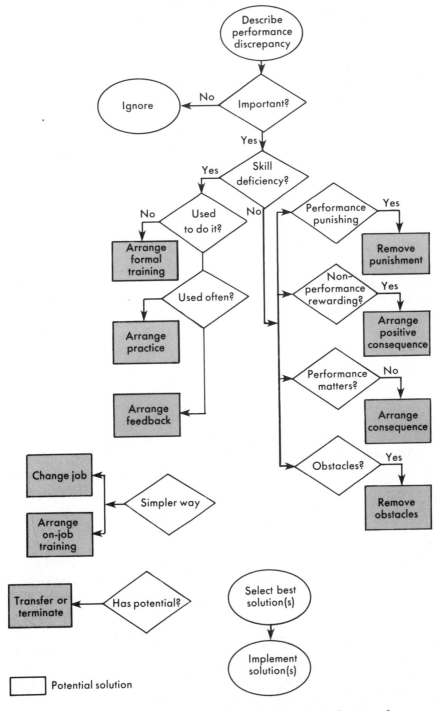

FIG. 11-5. Decision-making process. (From Mager, R.F., and Pipe, P.: Analyzing performance problems, Belmont, Calif., copyright © 1970, Pitman Learning, Inc.)

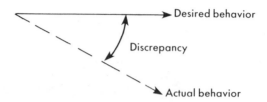

FIG. 11-6. Performance problem.

The goal of all these methods is to accurately assess learning needs to meet individual, organizational, and societal expectations. Before proceeding to the next step of program development, the ICP must become aware of the limitations of education as a tool for behavioral change. The answer to performance problems is often *not* an in-service class.

Mager and Pipe[11] have developed a model for analyzing performance problems (Fig. 11-5). A performance problem is a discrepancy between the *actual* performance of an employee and the *desired* or expected performance of the role (Fig. 11-6).

All people have performance problems in their daily lives: the sales representative who is 15 minutes late for an appointment, the head nurse who fails to rewrite a procedure within the agreed on time frame, the administrator who promises part-time secretarial support and does not provide for it in the final budget, and the physician who fails to order the appropriate isolation precautions.

Discrepancies that relate to infection control may become apparent when the ICP is performing the needs assessment: observing inappropriate technique, documenting an increase in the nosocomial infection rate, or questioning management of an infectious disease. Unfortunately, most ICPs respond with a knee-jerk reflex to problems by suggesting an in-service program. This approach presupposes that the problem is a skill or information deficit, which may not be true.

Skill deficiencies are amenable to resolution through educational activities. Non–skill deficits indicate a management problem (Chapter 12). Skill deficits may be modified by either increasing the employee's skill level or eliminating the behavior as a role expectation. If it is determined that the behavior is important and expected, then several questions must be asked:

1. Did the employee perform the behavior in the past? If no, then formal training is the answer. If yes, then the next question is asked.
2. Is the skill used often? If no, then practice should be arranged. If yes, then the ICP should observe and provide feedback.

Two additional aspects must be considered:

1. Is there a simpler way?

2. Does the employee have the potential to benefit from change? If the answer to this is no, then the employee should be transferred or his employment terminated.

EXAMPLE:
Performed behavior in past. A gastroenterologist, a new member of the medical staff, is ordering "enteric precautions" for his patients who are chronic HB_sAg carriers. This is creating confusion for the nursing, laboratory, and dietary staffs and havoc for the admitting department over room assignments. In assessing the problem with the nurses and then discussing the situation with the physician the ICP determines that he is following the protocol of another institution and was unaware of her hospital's policy. She arranges to have coffee with him. The problem is resolved. Had the situation continued, the problem then would shift into a management realm because it is no longer a skill deficit.

Skill not used often. The ICP observes an increase in the number of postoperative asymptomatic urinary tract infections following cesarean section. Tracing the problem, she discovers that one nurse seems to have been involved in 50% of the cases, although the organisms are different. She consults with the head nurse and then approaches the nurse. It seems that in the hospital where the nurse worked previously, physicians always inserted Foley catheters. Now she is expected to, and it has been 5 years since she performed a catheterization. The ICP agrees to observe her technique and arrange a practice session with a mannequin in the education department. The problem with urinary tract infections resolves.

Identifying major goals

Often the list of needs and interests far outweighs the limits of resources available for educational activities. Therefore some system for categorizing needs by high, medium, or low priority is essential. The system should address individual, organizational, and societal aspects of needs.

Following is a suggested format for assigning priority to assess the impact on nosocomial infections[4]:

I. Needs associated with actual infections
   A. Who has developed infections related to the need, and who is potentially at risk of infection in the future (e.g., patients in the nursery, patients in the ICU, personnel in the laboratory, personnel in the laundry, nurses in specific units, visitors, families of staff)?
   B. How frequently have infections related to the need arisen in the past? How frequently are they likely to arise in the future?
   C. How widespread has infection related to the need been? How widespread is it likely to be?
   D. How serious have the consequences of infection been? How serious are they likely to be (e.g., death, serious morbidity, discomfort, birth defects)?

    E. What are the probable consequences of failing to meet this need during the coming year (e.g., are infections likely to increase in number of seriousness)?

II. Needs associated with potential for infections

    A. Who is potentially at risk of infections related to the need (e.g., patients in the nursery, patients in the ICU, personnel in the laboratory, personnel in the laundry, nurses in specific units, visitors, families of staff)?

    B. Have infections related to the need been documented in the literature, or have such infections been brought to the ICP's attention by other ICPs? If so, how frequently have such infections arisen? How frequently would they be likely to arise in the hospital?

    C. If infections related to the need have been documented or brought to the ICP's attention, how widespread have those infections been? How widespread are they likely to be in the hospital?

    D. If infections related to the need have been documented or brought to the ICP's attention, how serious have the consequences of those infections been? How serious are they likely to be among patients affected in the hospital (e.g., death, serious morbidity, discomfort, birth defects)?

    E. What are the probable consequences of failing to meet this need during the coming year (e.g., are infections likely to increase in number or seriousness)?

III. Needs associated with staff development relating to infection control

    A. Who is interested in this need?

    B. How widespread is the application (e.g., one individual, a nursing unit, one or more departments, hospital-wide)?

    C. What are the benefits to be gained from meeting this need?

IV. Needs associated with external requirements

    A. What agency is recommending or requiring this need?

    B. Is there any evidence that infections may occur if this need is not addressed?

    C. What are the consequences of not meeting this need?

Needs assigned to categories I and II are usually assigned highest priority. The staff development needs in category III may not have a significant impact on infection but may improve the ICP's relationships with hospital personnel by providing recognition of their individual growth needs. This indirectly affects patient care through the staff's evaluation of the importance of infection control practices. Needs in category IV are generally related to legal, licensure, economic, or administrative issues and are thus considered low priority in their impact on infections. Feasibility through assessment of resources is not considered until the infection control priority is assigned.

Assessing resources

The availability of resources influences the program content, the formulation of behavioral objectives, and, most important, the type of learning activities. The assessment includes physical, human, and financial resources.

Physical resources include a meeting room, laboratory facilities, and audiovisual aids. *Human* resources address the issue of interest and availability of the learners, as well as the availability of competent instructors. Handout materials, supplies, and equipment may be restricted by *financial* limitations. Almost any need can be met with unlimited resources, but in the current economic market facing health care institutions the ICP is required to creatively meet needs within increasing constraints.

Formulating behavioral objectives

Writing objectives is often viewed as an unpleasant task, required for form but not clearly influencing the learning process. Arguments can be made for both views. Behaviorists (Skinner) view objectives as vital when they describe *terminal* behaviors. Humanists view objectives set by a teacher as *antithetical* to the self-directed adult learning process.

Objectives are helpful for three primary reasons:

1. They become the foundation for the *evaluation* process of learning.
2. When jointly agreed on, objectives provide a bond between the instructor and learners to share experiences to reach mutual goals. Learners can, in fact, become *more* responsible for their own learning by providing and getting feedback when they are not achieving objectives. This enables learners to actively seek out additional resources.
3. Well-defined objectives guide the selection of appropriate learning activities for the target population and for content to be learned.

Mager[10] defines an objective as "a description of performance which the learner exhibits to assure competency." The focus is on the *learner*, not the instructor, and the description is of the *result*, not the process of instruction. Three important components of a meaningful objective follow:

1. *Performance.* The objective states an expectation of what a learner is able to do.
2. *Conditions.* The objective includes a description of the condition(s), if appropriate, under which the performance is expected to occur.
3. *Criteria.* There is a clear description of the level of acceptable performance; these criteria may address speed, accuracy, or quality factors.

Clarity in writing objectives is a critical skill. Mager[10] notes that a meaningfully stated objective is one that succeeds in communicating the expected performance; the wording must be precise, not vague or ambiguous. Objectives must be formulated, agreed on, and fully understood by the line manager, the learner, and the educator.

The first pitfall of ambiguity is the selection of the action verb. Verbs that are open to broad interpretation force the learner to "psych out" the instructor's expectations. The resultant anxiety may divert the learner's energy away from the actual learning process in attempting to cope with the interpersonal conflict. Some objectives concerning choice of action verbs follow:

Broad interpretation	Precise interpretation
To know	To identify
To understand	To list
To be familiar with	To contrast
To enjoy	To interpret
To feel	To analyze
To appreciate	To classify
To realize	To describe
To believe	To state
To value	To apply
To be aware of	To demonstrate

Another problematic area is the use of a highly technical vocabulary or "flowery" phrases that obscure the intended communication. Intellectualism may impress peers or superiors, but it does little to establish a bond between the instructor and learner.

A final caution in formulating objectives is to avoid listing multiple behavioral expectations in a single objective. Multiple objectives, each expressing a single expectation, are better than awkward or misleading statements. If two or more objectives are related, the main objective can be supported by subobjectives, often called enabling, subordinate, or supportive objectives.[13]

EXAMPLE:

Main objective: To perform isolation techniques in accordance with the infection control manual
1. To select the correct category of isolation for the disease entity
2. To obtain an isolation cart
3. To wear appropriate isolation apparel
4. To correctly perform double-bag technique

Formulating behavioral objectives emphasizes the difficulty in knowing that learning is taking place. The behaviorist orientation in psychology addresses the objective, observable behavior as the only valid criterion for learning. In health care, since competency of practice is the first concern, objectives must be stated in overt, measurable terms. Covert behavior, which involves cognitive or affective functions, is highly valued in a humanistic learning environment; however, objectives concerning covert behavior are statements of inference rather than performance. Mager[9] suggests that the solution to this dilemma is to analyze behaviors that would indicate a change. Care must be taken to formulate these indicators by involving the line manager, learner, and ICP, since each person brings different educational backgrounds, life experiences, and values to the job.

EXAMPLE:
To develop an awareness of infection control in admitting new patients to the unit (covert behavior: awareness)
Indicator behaviors:
1. The admitting note will include a physical assessment, including signs and symptoms of infection.
2. The care plan will reflect nursing orders for appropriate infection prevention and control measures.
3. An order for isolation is obtained for appropriate precautions when needed.

In the late 1940s psychologists and educators collaborated in defining levels of behavior according to complexity and in developing standardized terminology. Three areas, or *domains*, reflected in the action verb of the objective were identified and then ordered in a taxonomic form of hierarchy[14]:

1. *Cognitive.* Addresses intellectual abilities to recall information, apply knowledge, or solve problems
2. *Affective.* Includes the expression of feelings, attitudes, values, and interests
3. *Psychomotor.* Deals with motor skills and neuromuscular coordination

TABLE 11-3. Examples of objectives: integration of component and domain models

Domain	Objective	Components
Cognitive	Following a 1-hour discussion, the new employee will be able to list the five categories of isolation with 100% accuracy	*Condition:* Following a 1-hour discussion, the new employee *Terminal behavior:* will be able to list *Criteria:* the five categories of isolation with 100% accuracy
Affective	After reading the isolation pamphlet the patient demonstrates interest by asking relevant questions about his visitors and his activities.	*Condition:* After reading the isolation pamphlet the patient *Terminal behavior:* will demonstrate interest *Criteria:* by asking relevant questions about his visitors and his activities
Psychomotor	After observing the videotape on urinary catheterization the learner will perform a catheterization without breaking sterile technique.	*Condition:* After observing the videotape on urinary catheterization the learner *Terminal behavior:* will perform a catheterization *Criteria:* without breaking sterile technique

Most learning objectives for health care professionals focus on cognitive and psychomotor domains. The affective domain, which relates to Mager's concept of covert behavior, is poorly understood, not easily influenced, and hard to measure. Nonetheless, the affective domain is a vital component of the humanistic orientation in education. In addition, the adult learner's resistance to change is grounded in the self-concept and experiential base of the affective domain. A synthesis of the component model and classification by domain is found in Table 11-3.

Designing and implementing learning activities

Clear and comprehensive objectives are the foundation for the selection of learning activities to promote the desired behavioral change. Instruction that does not foster change is ineffective and powerless; if change occurs but is judged to be undesirable or has untoward effects, then the instruction is of poor quality.[10]

Once the objectives have been agreed on, the particular learning activity or teaching strategy must be compatible with the following conditions:

1. *Nature of desired behavioral change.* Cognitive, affective, and psychomotor domains influence different learning activities.
2. *Availability of resources.* Factors such as size and arrangement of meeting space, audiovisual equipment, learner availability, and learner/instructor ratio affect the selection of teaching methods.
3. *Philosophy of the institution, instructor, and learner.* In some instances the pedagogical premise is valid; the goal of the session is to transmit a definitive body of information quickly and effectively in an appealing package. Cardiopulmonary resuscitation or culturing techniques may be taught in this manner. Conversely, the andragogical assumptions of problem finding and solving to achieve maximal learner involvement may be more relevant for encouraging patient teaching by staff.

A great deal of latitude can be exercised in designing learning activities. The plastic quality of the human mind enables people paradoxically to be endlessly self-transcendent (humanistic, right hemisphere orientation) and to be equally capable of conditioning self-limited behavior (behaviorist, left hemisphere orientation).[5] It is appropriate to capitalize on both these qualities by mixing and matching activities to create a climate conducive to the learner and the content.

The learning climate. All environments hold potential for human learning, yet specific factors in the physical, interpersonal, and organizational environment seem to exert either a facilitative or disruptive influence on the learning climate. The optimal environment offers security enough to explore and excitement enough to move forward.[5] The instructor, in large part, is responsible for creating a learning climate.

Physical environment. Comfort is the key to setting a learning climate through the physical environment. Although often overlooked in contrast to content and form, the physical aspects can often create or destroy the "mood" of the learner before the first word is spoken.

Obvious physical aspects include the seating arrangements, heat and ventilation, acoustics, visual limitations, lighting, directions and parking, writing materials, refreshments, registration materials, and name tags. All these factors, when present or done well, seem irrelevant to the success of a program. However, if one or more of these basic "creature comforts" are overlooked, the entire tone of the experience changes. The ICP might imagine, or perhaps recall, arriving late for a conference because she circled the block looking for a parking space and could not locate the room once inside the building. She discovers that she did not receive her registration materials. Finally, entering the room, she discovers row upon row of hard seats in a room too dark to take notes. The room is alternatively too hot or too cold, and smoking is not restricted to one area. The speaker is struggling with an antique public address system that crackles mercilessly, and her slides are too small and cluttered to be meaningful. To top off the day, the ICP knew lunch was not included in the registration fee, but no one mentioned that the nearest eating facilities were eight blocks away with 30 minutes allotted for the break. This may be an exaggeration, but how much learning could take place in this environment?

Interpersonal milieu. The paradigm shift in education is most evident in the relationships between the instructor and learners and among the learners themselves. The "teacher" becomes a facilitator for the learner's behavioral change. This interpersonal climate does not depend on what a person does as much as who a person is. Teachers who manage the learning process with integrity, creativity, enthusiasm, genuine caring, respect, spontaneity, competency, and humor contribute to the emotional or psychological well-being of the learner. The fundamental truth for these instructors is that employees are the hospital's most valuable resources. The ICP as a teacher cannot "fake" this philosophy; it flows out of a sense of high self-esteem and well-being. Ironically, the best way she can effectively meet the learner's needs is to first address her own physical, emotional, intellectual, and spiritual needs (Chapter 6).

Warm-up exercises can be helpful in establishing rapport within the group.

CONCEPTUAL BLOCKBUSTING. When the purpose of the group is to mutually identify and explore problems by sharing new knowledge and pooling group expertise, a new approach to problem solving often is needed. Barriers to creative problem solving frequently arise from reliance on habitual or familiar methods and traditional concepts. To transcend these barriers and break through these concepts, it may be necessary to assess learners in their shift from left hemisphere analysis (logical, linear thought) to right hemisphere functions. In creative problem solving there are no unsolvable problems, only perceptual barriers to solutions.

One method of accomplishing this assessment is to lead the participants in a brief relaxation exercise (Chapter 6) and then ask them to silently answer the following questions while keeping the problem in mind:

- What color is it?
- Does it have a shape?
- What would it taste like?
- How could it be solved with humor?
- How would your father solve it?
- If you were 6 years old, how would you solve it?

Sharing the answers in dyads or small groups further expands the context of the problem, and "new" solutions become available and establish group rapport.

CONCEPTS INTO IMAGES. Two additional ways to create a more personal environment for adults involve art work—another function of the right hemisphere of the brain:

1. The instructor can provide paper and colored felt-tip pens, divide the group into teams of three to five people, and ask them to draw a concept (i.e., to visually represent a thought or idea). For example, the instructor might ask a group of ICPs to "draw" what an infection control program looks like.
2. An assignment to get participants involved before class begins is to ask them to bring a picture from a magazine that represents a concept relevant to the class topic. At the meeting each participant can be asked to explain the picture to the group. The instructor might request a group of staff nurses to bring pictures of what isolation techniques are like on their units.

POLL EXPECTATIONS. A method that encourages the group to share and facilitate communication and respect for the adult learner's needs is to verbally poll the group, one member at a time, for their expectations of the class. What specific questions or issues do they want covered? These answers can be listed on a blackboard or flipchart. The instructor then has the responsibility to address each area, unless it is noted that the issue may be beyond the scope of the class or the group's expertise. The list also serves as a good summarizing tool at the end of the session to ensure that the individual understands the content.

Organizational factors. Before I address specific techniques to ensure a smooth, consistent flow of learning activities, it is necessary to point out that the organizational milieu influences both instructor and learner perceptions of the importance of continuing education. How does the ICP's philosophy of practice meld with the hospital's philosophy of educating its employees?

As previously discussed in Chapter 6, many hospitals possess type A personalities, operating under the assumption of "caring for too many by too few." In this environment mixed messages will be given: "Yes, education is important for competent, fulfilled employees, but we haven't enough time, staff, classrooms, or dollars to provide it."

Management philosophy also influences the educational methods endorsed by administrators. McGregor[8] postulated that there are two types of management styles, theory X and theory Y, which are based on viewpoints of human beings and the nature of work. Knowles[8] suggests that skinnerian or behaviorist theories of learning match theory X management philosophy, whereas rogerian or humanistic theories are required in a theory Y milieu. The importance of matching educational content and teaching methods with the management philosophy of the institution or within a department should not be underestimated. The behavioral objectives must be compatible with the role expectations (see p. 242 for a comparative analysis of management philosophy and educational theories).

For the ICP with responsibilities for educational activities, answers to the following questions will provide some insight into the management philosophy of her institution:

1. Are line managers expected to be involved in staff development activities?
2. Is work time provided for education and training?
3. Is there a tuition reimbursement program, and, if so, how is it administered?
4. Are people promoted from within, or are positions consistently filled with "more qualified" people outside the organization?
5. How does the organization tolerate suggestions for improvement in management and work methods from the "grass roots" employees?
6. Are classes provided only because of external regulatory requirement?

Within this larger organizational context, the instructor also has an obligation for organizational issues for each educational and training program, many of which relate to the physical environment mentioned earlier. Whenever possible, enlisting the assistance of other members of the staff as a planning group increases commitment to the success of a program. Areas for consideration include registration, advertisements, physical location and setup, speakers, and audiovisual equipment. Planning for these activities ensures a smooth, professional approach to program development.

Learning activities. Learning activities can be focused on a single individual or on a group process. All methods are appropriate if consideration is given to the size and nature of the target population and the goal of the activity. Table 11-4 summarizes the orientation and dominant domain of a variety of learning activities.

A comparison of the assumptions about human nature and behavior underlying theory X and theory Y management philosophy

---

Theory X assumptions about human nature (McGregor)

The average human being inherently dislikes work and will avoid it if he can.

Because of this characteristically human dislike of work, most people must be coerced, controlled, threatened in the interest of organizational objectives.

The average human being prefers to be directed, wishes to avoid responsibility, has relatively little ambition, wants security above all.

Theory Y assumptions about human nature

The expenditure of physical and mental effort is as natural as play or rest.

External control and the threat of punishment are not the only means for bringing about effort toward organizational objectives. Man will exercise self-direction and self-control in the service of objectives to which he is committed.

Commitment to objectives is a function of the rewards associated with their achievement.

The average human being learns, under proper conditions, not only to accept but to seek responsibility.

A high capacity for imagination, ingenuity, and creativity in solving organizational problems is widely, not narrowly distributed in the population.

Under the conditions of modern industrial life, the intellectual potential of the average human being is only partially utilized.

Assumptions implicit in current education (Rogers)

The student cannot be trusted to pursue his own learning.

Presentation equals learning.

The aim of education is to accumulate brick upon brick of factual knowledge.

The truth is known.

Creative citizens develop from passive learners.

Evaluation is education and education is evaluation.

Assumptions relevant to significant experiential learning

Human beings have a natural potentiality for learning.

Significant learning takes place when the subject matter is perceived by the student as relevant to his own purposes.

Much significant learning is acquired through doing.

Learning is facilitated by student's responsible participation in the learning process.

Self-initiated learning involving the whole person—feelings as well as intellect—is the most pervasive and lasting.

Creativity in learning is best facilitated when self-criticism and self-evaluation are primary, and evaluation by others is of secondary importance.

The most socially useful thing to learning in the modern world is the process of learning, a continuing openness to experience, an incorporation into onself of the process of change.

From Knowles, M.: The adult learner: a neglected species, Houston, 1973, Gulf Publishing Co.

TABLE 11-4. Orientation and dominant domain of learning activities

Learning activity	Orientation	Dominant domain
Individual		
Self-instruction	Mixed	Cognitive
ICP rounds	Andragogical	Cognitive and affective
Group		
Lecture	Pedagogical	Cognitive
Symposium	Mixed	Cognitive
Panel	Mixed	Cognitive
Seminar	Andragogical	Cognitive
Workshop	Mixed	Cognitive
Institute	Pedagogical	Cognitive
Journal club	Andragogical	Cognitive
Case study	Andragogical	Cognitive
Demonstration and return demonstration	Andragogical	Psychomotor
Role playing	Andragogical	Affective

Individual

1. *Self-instruction.* Programmed instruction is the primary contribution Skinner has made to educational reform. The principles of reinforcement are built into the design of the instructional materials. Advantages of these materials are that the (a) staff or patients can work at their own pace, (b) the learning activity does not depend on the presence of an instructor, (c) content can be standardized and stratified by levels of responsibility and educational background, and (d) content that must be repeated or disseminated to a diverse group can be delivered efficiently. Drawbacks to the use of these materials is that there will be a low level of learner opportunity to discuss applications to past experience, commercially prepared materials lack specificity to the individual hospital, and preparation for materials is time consuming. Programmed instruction generally ignores the four assumptions of andragogy, but if used as one part of a learning activity, this obstacle can be overcome.
   - Written materials can be developed for use by staff or patients. A sample of a programmed instruction for orienting new employees to the infection control program is shown on p. 244.
   - Slide-tape presentations or videotape cassettes are another way to provide new information. These can be left on the unit where staff members can view them individually during breaks.
   - Computer-assisted instruction is enjoying broad application to health education. Programmed instruction to teach antibiotic selection or

Infection control orientation booklet—RN

Introduction

Because infections acquired in the hospital or brought into the hospital from the community are potential hazards for all persons having contact with the hospital, effective measures must be developed to prevent, identify, and control such infections.

The function of the infection control program is to help you in identifying and controlling infections and potential infectious hazards in the hospital environment.

The philosophy of the program, outlined in the introduction of the *Infection Control and Isolation Manual*, specifically states that it is, "vital for all personnel to read, become familiar with, and implement the recommended infection control practices."

This orientation booklet is a guide to help you review the major infection control policies and procedures and provides questions throughout for you to answer. When you have completed these questions, the answers should be *returned to the infection control coordinator* to document completion of the infection control orientation.

Infection Control Coordinator

Purpose

This booklet will present clinical situations that typically arise in the hospital environment and will pose questions that you will be required to answer. Sections in the *Infection Control and Isolation Manual* will be identified as a reference for you to use in answering these questions.

CASE STUDY

Mr. S., a 65-year-old patient, has just been transferred to your ward from a local hospital. Mr. S. suffered a massive cerebrovascular accident that left him comatose, necessitating a tracheostomy. He is on a respirator. On admission he has a 103° temperature and severe congestion, necessitating frequent tracheal suctioning. His admitting diagnosis is "staphylococcal pneumonia (second-degree); tracheostomy following CVA."

1. What isolation is necessary for Mr. S. (see "Infectious Disease Isolation Required" in manual)?
2. What routes of transmission of disease can occur from a patient with staphylococcal pneumonia?
3. What is the appropriate protective clothing for this isolation?
4. Where do you obtain isolation carts (see "Isolation Protocol" in manual)?
5. Tracheostomy care is a standing hospital nursing order. How often should it be performed (see "High-risk Procedure" in manual)?
6. List five precautions that are necessary for all patients who have a tracheostomy.
7. Tracheostomy care (e.g., suctioning, cleaning) is a sterile procedure. Only sterile catheters and gloves should be used.   True _____   False _____
8. You are suctioning secretions from Mr. S. The catheter becomes plugged with mucus. You should:
9. A week after admission Mr. S. expires. What do you do with:
   a. Disposable suction drainage bottle:
   b. Respirator:
   c. Linen:
   d. His body:
   e. Isolation cart:
10. Who is responsible for the terminal cleaning of an isolation room?

Written by M. Yarbrough and D. Potts, Veterans Administration Hospital, Palo Alto, Calif.

    diagnosis of infectious diseases has been used in medical student education.

2. *Infection control rounds.* Special times can be arranged for individual nurses to "round" with the ICP for a few hours. This affords the nurse familiarity with the responsibility of the ICP and encourages discussion of specific patient care practices. It is also an effective way for ICPs to share their experience with other ICPs new to the field.

Group. Many of the terms used to describe group activities are used interchangeably, often causing confusion. One general rule about group process is that the larger the number of participants, the more passive the participation and the more difficult it is to assess the experience and understanding of the individual.

1. *Lecture.* The lecture features a speaker who transmits knowledge in an organized format to a group of learners. Essentially communication is limited to a one-way mode.

2. *Symposium.* Two or more speakers give short, formal statements on one or more related topics. Audience participation in the discussion is encouraged.

3. *Panel.* Individuals with special knowledge give prepared remarks on some aspect of a general topic in front of an audience. Two-way communication through audience questions and comments usually follows.

4. *Seminar.* A small, informal group discussion is led by an individual who has some expertise in the subject. Learners come prepared to discuss the topic; there is no audience.

5. *Workshop.* One or more groups engage in an active learning process. Background information may be provided in the form of lectures, videotapes, or movies. Following this orientation to the topic, the participants are assigned to small groups to develop solutions for specific problems.

6. *Institute.* This format is a formal series of presentations with little audience participation. In contrast to the single focus of a workshop, the institute may address a variety of major areas.

7. *Journal clubs.* A group meets on a regular basis to review and discuss journal articles. The format may include individual reviewer presentations or discussion of an article reviewed by all members.

8. *Case study.* A discussion is conducted to review a particular case or situation, requiring judgment in the decision-making process. Table 11-5 illustrates application of isolation principles to a patient placement exercise (Fig. 11-7).

9. *Demonstration and return demonstration.* A skill or technique is demonstrated by a leader with expertise; participants then repeat the technique to demonstrate understanding and psychomotor competency.

TABLE 11-5. Bed placement exercise: patient profiles

Patient	Admission diagnosis	History
A	Probable viral hepatitis	22-year-old man with 5-day history of fatigue, malaise, fever, and joint pain; came to emergency room complaining of extreme nausea and jaundice; recent travel in Mexico
B	5% to 10% second- and third-degree burns	33-year-old woman came to emergency room with third-degree burns on right hand and second-degree burns on right thigh after cooking accident involving boiling water; grafting will be required on dorsal surface of right hand
C	Acute myelogenous leukemia with fever and bilateral pulmonary infiltrates	44-year-old woman with 2-day history of temperature readings higher than 102° F and increasing shortness of breath after last course of chemotherapy; *laboratory*: chest x-ray film indicated bilateral lower lobe infiltrates; white blood cell count—1500.
D	Wound infection after cesarean section	29-year-old woman 7 days postpartum; 2 days after discharge, abdominal wound from cesarean section drained copious amounts of purulent material; wound indurated and drained; temperature was 101° F; *laboratory*: white blood cell count—17,900; wound culture—*Staphylococcus aureus*
E	Hypertension	57-year-old man with complaints of dizziness and intermittent loss of consciousness; blood pressure taken on admission was 210/135; admitted for complete hypertension workup

TABLE 11-5. Bed placement exercise: patient profiles—cont'd

Patient	Admission diagnosis	History
F	Tuberculosis versus neoplasm	66-year-old man from Southeast Asia came to the hospital complaining of sweating at night and hemoptysis for 3 weeks; *laboratory:* chest x-ray film showed a 10 × 15 cm "coin" lesion in right upper lobe with prominent hilar nodes
G	Status after cerebrovascular accident with aspiration pneumonia	84-year-old man transferred from extended care facility with elevated temperature (second-degree) and aspiration pneumonitis; *laboratory:* chest x-ray film indicated right middle and lower lobe pneumonitis; sputum culture was unable to be obtained because patient could not cough
H	Heroin overdose	18-year-old woman brought into emergency room unconscious; friend reported heroin use; patient slowly regaining consciousness and extremely combative; *laboratory;* HBsAg pending
I	Pyelonephritis	35-year-old man with history of recurrent urinary tract infections; 2-day history of elevated temperature and flank pain; *laboratory:* urinalysis, white blood cell count—50 to 75 hpf
J	Fracture of left femur	27-year-old man in recent fall while mountain climbing; closed reduction of left femur

Nursing unit description: 12-bed medical/surgical unit. Four private rooms with bath; two 2-bed rooms with one bath each; one 4-bed ward with one bath.

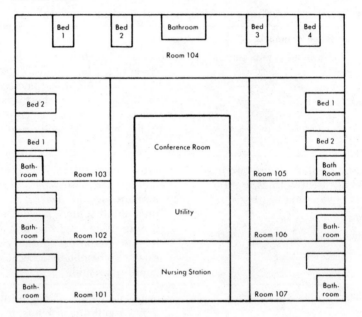

Nursing unit floor plan

Instructions: Read patient profile descriptions, and study floor plan. Decide on bed placement and isolation if necessary. Enter patient placements below. If isolation is required, specify type. Write brief justification for your decision under Comments.

Room 101 _____
Room 102 _____
Room 103 bed 1 _____
        bed 2 _____
Room 104 bed 1 _____
        bed 2 _____
        bed 3 _____
        bed 4 _____
Room 105 bed 1 _____
        bed 2 _____
Room 106 _____
Room 107 _____

FIG. 11-7. Bed placement exercise worksheet. (Developed by Trisha Barrett and Karen J. Axnick.)

10. *Role playing*. Through simulation of real-life characters or situations, the learner tries out new or different behaviors in front of an audience. This valuable experiential activity can deteriorate in quality if structure is not established concerning limits of behavior and audience feedback styles.

Evaluating results

The final step in program development is the evaluation process. Knowles[8] expresses the view that evaluation is the area of greatest controversy and weakest technology in adult education and training. Too often evaluation is used to demonstrate the *failure* of the learner to achieve the expected or desired behavioral change. Skinner[13] has been particularly critical of the role and means of testing in the educational system. The evaluation process should be designed to *improve* both teaching and learning by unveiling areas of misunderstanding. Feedback provided should reinforce positive behavior and redirect behavior that falls short of expectations.

Four phases of effective program assessment follow[8]:

1. *Reaction evaluation*. Data regarding participant response, including most or least liked aspects, positive or negative feelings, and suggestions for change
2. *Learning evaluation*. Data about concepts, facts, and techniques through pretesting and posttesting, demonstrations, role playing, and problem-solving exercises
3. *Behavior evaluation*. Data providing feedback on actual behavioral change after the training, including time and motion studies, observation scales, self-rating scales, diaries or field notes, questionnaires, and interviews
4. *Results evaluation*. Data from the organization about impact on turnover, costs, efficiency, and quality control

Most ICPs will solicit reaction and learning evaluations, but behavior and results evaluations are almost nonexistent in infection control literature and practice. The result is that although ICPs believe education is a primary component of an effective infection control program, there are no substantive data to demonstrate its efficacy. Two prime reasons for this situation are (1) the difficulty in controlling variables to demonstrate cause and effect relationships and (2) the fact that too few ICPs have the expertise, time, or resources to design a study with control groups. Despite these limitations, it is imperative that new educational modalities be carefully evaluated to establish their usefulness before extensive investments of resources are made.

Evaluation methods are designed with the learning objectives and activities in mind. The domain of the learning objective influences the evaluation tool. It makes little sense to give only a multiple-choice or written test on urinary

TABLE 11-6. Evaluation methods

Type	Description
Anecdotal records	Description of situation, behavior of learner, and evaluator's interpretation
Self-evaluation	Assessment by learner of situation and behaviors related to expected outcomes
Checklists	Listing of expected outcomes; answers usually limited to "yes" or "no" or "not applicable"
Rating scales	Range of varying degrees of achievement

Tests
  True-false
  Multiple-choice
  Matching
  Essay
	Written responses to questions or situations that demonstrate cognitive achievement

Questionnaires	Written responses to questions that solicit reactions to process and content of educational programs
Interviews	Discussion between learner and evaluator to assess achievement of expected outcomes
Return demonstration	Performance of psychomotor skills after demonstration by instructor

TABLE 11-7. Relationship between domain objectives, learning activities, and evaluation methods

Domain objective	Product	Learning activities	Evaluation methods
Cognitive	Knowledge and understanding	Lectures, reading, programmed instruction, crossword puzzles, and rounds with ICP	Written tests, problem-solving exercises and written care plans
Affective	Process and attitude	Role playing and rounds with ICP	Role playing, problem-solving exercises, field notes, interviews, and questionnaires
Psychomotor	Activity	Demonstration and rounds with ICP	Return demonstration, observation, and skill checklists

catheterization when a psychomotor skill is required for the desired behavior. However, this is a major pitfall in both school and hospital educational endeavors.

Evaluation may be either norm referenced or criterion referenced. Norm-referenced tools have been administered to a large number of individuals. The individual test is then measured against a statistical average. The Scholastic Aptitude Test (SAT) used to screen college admissions and licensing examinations for professionals are examples of norm-referenced evaluations. More likely to be used in hospitals is the criterion-referenced evaluation. This method measures progress toward achieving the behavioral objective. The learner is the source, and the evaluation is individualized. Criterion-referenced evaluation can employ andragogical, humanistic and split-brain concepts for design. Whatever method is used, three critical characteristics must be maintained.[7] The first is validity, or the capacity of the method to measure what it purports to measure. Next, the method must possess reliability. This means that there is consistency in its ability over time to measure change. Practicality is the final characteristic. The method should be both easy to use and interpret and economical in cost and time requirements.

Although the design of actual evaluation methods is beyond the scope of this chapter, Table 11-6 presents an overview of the variety available to the ICP. Table 11-7 summarizes the relationship between the domain of the objective, the learning activity, and the evaluation method.

A final dimension of the evaluation process is the fundamental concept of andragogical education as lifelong education: reassessment of learning needs, interests, and values. If the learning process has expanded the individual's experiential base, then the learner must reexamine old behaviors in light of new levels of competency. This aspect gives the program development model a dynamic quality.

CONCLUSION

A primary component of the ICP's role is education. To assure the desired outcome of behavioral change, the ICP must draw on principles of learning derived from psychology and neurophysiology. The goal of any educational endeavor is to help individuals or groups not only to achieve competency in role behaviors but also to strive toward new levels of excellence.

REFERENCES

1. Albrecht, K.: Brain power—learn to improve your thinking skills, Englewood Cliffs, N.J., 1980, Prentice-Hall, Inc.
2. Bandler, R., and Grinder, J.: Frogs into princes—neurolinguistic programming, Moab, Utah, 1979, Real People Press.
3. Bogen, J.E.: Some educational implications of hemisphere specializations. In Wittrock, M.C., editor: The human brain, Englewood Cliffs, N.J., 1977, Prentice-Hall, Inc.

 4. Centers for Disease Control: Management skills for infection control nurses, Atlanta, Jan. 1982, Centers for Disease Control.
 5. Ferguson, M.: The aquarian conspiracy—personal and social transformation in the 1980's, Los Angeles, 1980, J.P. Tarcher, Inc.
 6. Jerison, H.J.: Evolution of the brain, In Wittrock, M.C., editor: The human brain, Englewood Cliffs, N.J., 1977, Prentice-Hall, Inc.
 7. King, E.C.: Classroom evaluation strategies, St. Louis, 1979, The C.V. Mosby Co.
 8. Knowles, M.S.: The adult learner: a neglected species, Houston, 1973, Gulf Publishing Co.
 9. Knowles, M.S.: Gearing adult education for the seventies. In Popiel, E.S., editor: Nursing and the process of continuing education, ed. 2, St. Louis, 1977, The C.V. Mosby Co.
10. Mager, R.F.: Preparing instructional objectives, ed. 2, Belmont, Calif., 1975, Fearon Publishers, Inc.
11. Mager, R.F., and Pipe, P.: Analyzing performance problems or "you really oughta wanna," Belmont, Calif., 1970, Fearon Publishers, Inc.
12. Maslow, A.H.: A theory of human motivation, Psychol. Rev. **50:**370-396, 1943.
13. Milhollan, F., and Forisha, B.E.: From Skinner to Rogers: contrasting approaches to education, Lincoln, Neb.., 1972, Professional Educators Publications, Inc.
14. Redman, B.K.: The process of patient teaching in nursing, ed. 4, St. Louis, 1980, The C.V. Mosby Co.
15. Schein, E.H.: Professional education—some new directions, New York, 1972, McGraw-Hill, Inc.
16. Teyler, T.J.: An introduction to the neurosciences. In Wittrock, M.C., editor: The human brain, Englewood Cliffs, N.J., 1977, Prentice-Hall, Inc.
17. Tobin, H.M., Yoder Wise, P.S., and Hull, P.K.: The process of staff development, components for change, ed. 2, St. Louis, 1979, The C.V. Mosby Co.
18. Wittrock, M.C.: The generative process of memory. In Wittrock, M.C., editor: The human brain, Englewood Cliffs, N.J., 1977, Prentice-Hall Inc.

SUGGESTED READINGS

Foley, R.P., and Smilansky, J.: Teaching techniques, a handbook for health professionals, New York, 1980, McGraw-Hill, Inc.
Kemp, J.E.: Instructional design, ed. 2, Belmont, Calif., 1977, Fearon Publishers, Inc.
King, E.C.: Classroom evaluation strategies, St. Louis, 1978, The C.V. Mosby Co.

Management

autocratic leadership A leadership model that provides decisions that are usually unilateral (e.g., in schools or the armed forces).

conflict A clash or struggle that occurs whenever the harmony and balance among thoughts, feelings, and behaviors are threatened.

decision-making process A process by which one chooses among available alternatives for the purpose of reaching a conclusion and achieving a desired outcome.

delegation Assigning specific expectations to hospital personnel and practitioners.

democratic leadership A leadership model in which decisions are multilateral and subject to group authority and pressure.

directing Putting the plan into action within a defined organizational structure.

laissez-faire leadership A model in which there is almost an absence of leadership.

management The process of getting things done through other people.

planning The process of assessing the future and making provisions for it.

T he infection control practitioner (ICP) has the primary responsibility of managing the infection control program. Management is defined by Coventry and Burstiner[5] as "getting things done through other people, instead of doing the job himself." If one examines the role expectations of the ICP, one can see that the primary thrust of that role is to achieve the infection control program's goals through influencing the work of hospital personnel. This is accomplished by influencing physicians and employees to incorporate infection control practices in their daily activities.

This chapter will outline some of the basic principles of management and leadership that may be helpful for the ICP to use in formulating and maintaining a successful infection control program. These principles will be organized within four areas of management function: *planning, organizing, directing, and controlling.* This framework has been chosen because it is flexible and inclusive enough to permit presentation of the management and leadership principles relevant to the role of the ICP as a manager.

PLANNING

Planning is the process of assessing the future and making provisions for it. A well-developed plan serves as a road map. The road map provides a guide for the ICP and all those responsible for performing within the parameters outlined by the infection control program to reach a mutual end point (goal). This type of coordinated effort focuses everyone's talents and energies on specific infection control practices, reducing energy spent in moving toward different end points.

Management

Organizing	Directing	Controlling
	Planning	

FIG. 12-1. Planning is the base for the management function of organizing, directing, and controlling.

To accomplish a coordinated effort, planning should be the primary activity from which all other activities of the infection control program evolve.

As can be seen in Fig. 12-1, planning supports the activities of organizing, directing, and controlling, the other three areas that comprise the management functions discussed in this chapter. Planning is mental work that should be done before action is taken. Functionally, planning consists of the following[1,10,18,28]:

- Selecting and relating facts about the present
- Formulating assumptions regarding the future based on these facts
- Visualizing and formulating proposed activities necessary to achieve the desired results

Major areas within the infection control program that require planning as the primary activity from which all action should evolve will be discussed.

Maintenance programs. There are several areas within the infection control program that require maintenance functions; that is, once they have been developed, they continue on a routine, systematic basis. These activities include orientation, surveillance, and unit rounds. The ICP needs to have a clear purpose for these activities and a well-developed program for ensuring that maintenance programs are kept current and relevant and do not become routinized to the point of losing their effectiveness.

Expansion. Change is the rule, not the exception, for the ICP. As new technology, procedures, and regulatory agency demands develop, the ICP will be constantly challenged to incorporate these changes into the infection control program's objectives. Using an ongoing planning process provides a framework for efficient expansion of the infection control program when indicated.

Leadership. Through planning, the ICP becomes aware of what she wants to have happen and can give clear information to and set expectations for others to achieve this identified goal. This clearness of purpose projects strong leadership; the ICP knows what she wants to accomplish. This is especially important to the ICP, since her position within the organization requires results to be achieved through others. The ideal plan makes the ICP prepared, not rigid.

Clarity. Planning provides a clear guide to all personnel to the purposes of the infection control program and its associated activities. This clarity tends to stimulate a cooperative, integrated, enthusiastic approach to accomplishing goals.

Sequencing. Effective sequencing of effort can be accomplished through planning. Just as a house is best built by beginning with a good foundation, proceeding to the walls, and ending with a roof, most activities have a logical sequence for accomplishing an efficient, orderly outcome. Sequencing is the purposeful ordering of activities to accomplish a desired result. An example of sequencing is the typical nursing procedure for inserting a Foley catheter. The procedure first lists the equipment necessary to perform the procedure; then the procedure instructs the practitioner to wash her hands, open the package, assemble the sterile barrier, put on gloves, and so on. Sequencing reduces the execution of work in a haphazard manner and increases the understanding of which activities build on the next activity.

Use of resources. The planning process will help the ICP identify the appropriateness or necessity of involving resources outside of her control to accomplish a designated task. In the planning activity the ICP may recognize the opportunity to involve another member of the health care team, such as the director of nursing, in the planning process. When this type of involvement in planning precedes any management action initiated by the ICP, there is increased commitment to support the plan by those involved.

Planning, then, is equally as important as doing. Because this function is so important, each step in the planning process will be identified, and the specific skills needed will be detailed.

Steps in the planning process

There are four steps in the planning process[1]:
- Collecting and interpreting the facts of a situation
- Determining a line of action
- Making provisions to carry through with the plan
- Establishing checks and balances to monitor performance

Although the steps will be discussed separately, in actuality they are interrelated and interdependent in the activities necessary for each step.

Collecting and interpreting facts of a situation. Information needed for planning comes from three primary sources:
1. Those external to the hospital, such as Joint Commission on Accreditation of Hospitals (JCAH), state and federal regulatory agencies, and local and national standards
2. Those internal to the hospital, such as policies, procedures, hospital personnel, surveillance rounds, and written memoranda
3. The ICP through her own creative thinking, which challenges her to use

her personal experiences, vitality, innovation, energy, the information she has gained through education, and her ability to synthesize thoughts into workable concepts that reveal the interrelatedness of generalizations, impressions, and facts

Creative thinking. Because the ICP is such a valuable source of information, I will expand on the process of creative thinking.[23] Creative thinking can be defined as the ability to view the usual in unusual ways. By understanding the process, the ICP can develop the ability to be more creative.

HOW TO PRESENT AN IDEA. The most critical step in developing an idea and presenting it is to believe in the idea. Lupascu[23] explores two models of thinking: negative thinking and positive thinking (Fig. 12-2).

Positive thinking promotes clear communication, which in turn promotes understanding among people. New ideas, no matter how good, often create resistance. This resistance is usually expressed in statements everyone has heard:

1. We have never done it before.
2. Nobody else has ever done it.
3. It is not my job.
4. You are right, but. . . .
5. We are not ready for it.
6. It needs committee study.

When the ICP presents an idea, she should be prepared to listen to what others have to say. Sometimes, feedback and additional ideas from other people

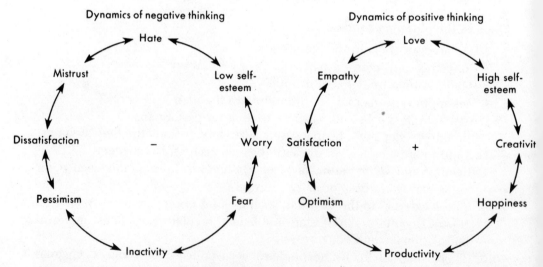

FIG. 12-2. Dynamics of negative and positive thinking. (From Lupascu, D.: Nurs. Manage. **12:**25-27, Sept. 1981.)

she has shared ideas with result in creating an altogether new and better solution than the one she first offered.

Once the ICP feels she has incorporated the best information into the idea, she will want to solicit support from her supervisor, the infection control committee, and colleagues. She will most likely need to present her idea both verbally and in writing. When she does, the presentation should cover the following points:

- Get attention
- Explain
- Listen
- Compare
- Consolidate
- Request

To get attention, the ICP should set up a date and time to discuss her idea. She can briefly give a background to the problem she is proposing to orient the audience.

The ICP may briefly list the benefits she feels will be of interest to the audience to gain agreement.

Because it is difficult, if not impossible, to have people agree if they do not understand the whole idea, the ICP must explain the idea carefully. She should be open to listening to disagreement, since this may lead to a positive adjustment of her original thoughts.

Because feedback is *positive* in that the ICP can determine how the audience has received her idea, she should not become defensive during the discussion phase. Instead, she should be open to compare benefits and liabilities for all ideas expressed. She should focus on points of agreement and restate the idea, incorporating the best points of all ideas that are mutually satisfactory.

The ICP should end the process by making specific requests that she feels are necessary to test her ideas further. One approach might be to present the idea to a larger group to determine their reaction.

Limitations in planning. There are limitations that should be recognized as information is collected for planning. First, the information the ICP is gathering will be used to apply to the future; therefore the accuracy of information and facts projected to the future will only be known when the future becomes the present. Second, the assumptions made about the future are limited by the accuracy of the information and facts from which the assumptions were made. Third, it is not practical to gather all the information. Accuracy will be affected by information not collected.

After the information has been collected, it needs to be interpreted for the purpose of forecasting its impact on infection control departmental operations.

Forecasting[6,18] is thinking ahead to assess the future, making provisions for the infection control program, and establishing where the present course of the infection control program will lead. Forecasting is accomplished through identifying trends that provide general direction for areas needing planning. Forecasting activities direct program operations by identifying advances in technical skill and knowledge. Two functions of the ICP that provide trends for the infection control program are surveillance and ongoing literature review.

Determining a line of action. Determining a line of action implies that a decision needs to be made. When faced with the need to make decisions, it is helpful to have a systematic process that will provide a reliable framework for decision making.

It is important to realize that the decision-making process is useful in planning, but it is only a tool within the whole planning process. It is also worth mentioning that decision making is influenced by the ICP's own values, beliefs, and biases.

Decision-making process. Decision making is a process by which one chooses among available alternatives for the purpose of reaching a conclusion and/or achieving a desired outcome (Fig. 12-3). The process has four steps[11,26,28]:

- Identifying problems
- Generating options
- Making a decison
- Evaluating results

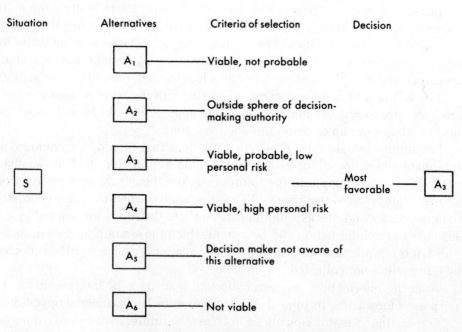

FIG. 12-3. Decision-making process model.

IDENTIFYING PROBLEMS. Problem identification is the most critical step in decision making. The way the problem is defined will dictate what solutions are considered. The solution chosen will only be effective when applied to the right problem.

Mager[25] has developed a model that illustrates how the solution evolves from how the problem is identified. His model deals with analyzing performance problems. The first step is to decide if the problem is caused by a skill deficit or something other than a skill deficit. This critical step really focuses on the kind of problem to be solved:

1. *Skill deficit* indicates an educational problem.
2. *Non–skill deficit* indicates a management problem. The challenge is to create conditions under which employees are expected to do what they already know how to do.

The solution to either the skill or non–skill deficit problem will be quite different.

Solving a skill deficit problem involves some type of education or training as a solution. Solving a non–skill deficit involves changing the conditions under which employees are expected to do what they already know how to do.

Mager further explores specific causes and reasons for non–skill deficit problems and places them in four categories:

1. It is punishing to perform the skill or task as desired.
2. It is rewarding to perform the skill or task other than desired.
3. It does not matter if the skill or task is performed.
4. There are obstacles to performing the skill or task.

Examples of these kinds of performance obstacles illustrate how identifying the correct problem is imperative to developing a solution.

The following guidelines will help in assuring correct problem identification.[32] All relevant facts should be gathered before diagnosing any problem. When gathering data, the ICP should ask herself how the chosen facts are related to the identified problem. This may reveal a personal bias that has limited her access to all the information. (The ICP should not rely on only one source of information.) The problem may be one of interpretation, the ICP's or someone else's. By using as many sources as practical, the ICP will be better able to separate facts from interpretation. She can make a systematic investigation of the scope of each presented problem. The goal is to identify the real issue, not become sidetracked by the symptoms of the problem. For example, the ICP might receive a phone call stating that all surgical patients are getting postoperative wound infections with coagulase-positive staphylococcal organisms. While gathering information, the ICP is told by the nursing staff that the housekeepers are the problem. The nursing staff have observed the janitors going from room to room without changing the water in the bucket, and they only use a new mop head once a month. Their cleaning is also inadequate, and the floors are an example of how the hospital environment really is unclean. If the ICP accepts the problem statement from the nursing staff in this example, she may be solving the wrong problem to effect a change in the postoperative surgical wound infection rate. It may be true that the housekeeping services are inadequate, but the etiological agent is most likely spread by person-to-person contact, not by the floors. Poor housekeeping may be a symptom of this problem but most likely not the real problem.

Problem identification is limited by the ICP's knowledge, skill, past experience, current situation, and perceptions. Limitations, however, do not mean that problem identification should be avoided. In solving the wrong problem the ICP at least has information of what the problem is *not,* and her attention needs to be directed back to the information gathered to identify the true problem.

GENERATING OPTIONS. Generating a large number of possible solutions will increase the chance that the potentially best solution will be present. The key to this statement is that the solutions are *possible.* Listing impossible solutions just to generate a larger number of options is not useful. Two methods to generate options include lateral thinking and brainstorming.

Lateral thinking is a method of looking at the problem in a different way, that is, moving from established ways to looking at things to find new ways. For example, the problem identified is that staff members do not wash their hands. Perhaps in the past the ICP's method to approach this problem was to give an in-service lecture to the staff about the benefits of handwashing in the prevention of cross-contamination. Lateral thinking would require generating additional options besides in-service education. An example of one option might be to add handwashing practices as a separate item to the employees' job description. Employees would then be evaluated annually on their handwashing practices. This type of solution would directly elevate the importance of handwashing in employees' eyes.

Another method for generating creative options is brainstorming. Brainstorming consists of exhausting all ideas the ICP can think of to solve a problem. The rule of brainstorming is that no idea is too ridiculous, and no judgments are made on the ideas during the brainstorming sessions. Brainstorming is best accomplished with other people so that one idea can be used to stimulate another. At the end of the brainstorming session it is appropriate to evaluate the quality of the ideas and select those that seem to have merit.

MAKING A DECISION. Making a decision is the critical point where thought leads to action. After all the options have been identified criteria for choosing one of the options as the preferred decision should be applied to each option. There are four criteria by which each identified option should be measured (Fig. 12-3). First, is it desirable? Is the option one that the ICP can support and that she feels best addresses the problem identified? Second, is it probable? Is the choice likely to be supported within the available resources in the health care institution (money, people, space, time)? Third, what is the risk? The selected option should have minimal personal risk or be a personal risk the ICP is willing to take. Fourth, is it compatible? The selected option should fit within the organizational goals and objectives. The option that meets the highest number of criteria is the most desirable option to solving the identified problem.

EVALUATING RESULTS. Objective criteria need to be developed that will indicate when the problem has been solved. This information will be useful in making provisions to carry through with the plan. The first step is to translate the identified plan into concrete tasks. These tasks are written in the form of objectives.[2,24,31] Objectives result from planning, and a plan requires objectives to provide a systematic evaluation of progress toward attaining the desired goal.

Each objective should contain a subject, object, and action verb; it should answer the question "Who will do what?"[24]

Subject	Action verb	Object
who	will do	what

A *specific* objective contains more criteria for measuring outcome than an objective does. In addition to a subject, action verb, and object, the specific objective also describes under what condition and to what extent the task will be accomplished.

Subject	Action verb	Object	Under what condition	To what extent
who	will do	what	when, where	how well

Objectives can relate to cognitive, affective, or psychomotor behaviors. Examples of objectives that reflect each area follow:

Cognitive (intellectual achievement) *Example:* To recognize organisms that are endemic to the hospital environment

Affective (relating to feelings, attitudes, and values) *Example:* To develop a code of general behavior consistent with prevention of disease transmission

Psychomotor (relates to motor skill development) *Example:* To change an abdominal dressing using aseptic technique

Identifying which of the behaviors the objective will influence provides immediate direction to the planning needed. For example, an objective directed to psychomotor skills will require a plan that includes demonstration and validation of the skill (see Chapter 11 for further discussion).

Making provisions to carry through with the plan

Strategy development.[18,34] The intent of strategy development is that the desired outcome is correctly incorporated into the work of the affected department. Once a plan has been formulated outlining *what* the ICP wants to do, a strategy needs to be developed that defines *how* she is going to do it. Some of the more common strategies include the following:

1. Obtaining approvals from the appropriate people, particularly the ICP's immediate supervisor and the infection control committee.
2. Assigning responsibilities. Personnel affected by the plan should have a clear understanding of their assigned responsibility.
3. Determining appropriate timing of the plan. The ICP should establish a timetable and keep the efforts on schedule. It is necessary to assign specific time periods to each work activity. Such a time frame provides vitality and practical meaning to the plan. As the steps are laid out, the time line allows for adjustments that may be needed. Such flexibility allows for unpredictable variables.
4. Developing a critical path. Once a time line has been developed, a critical path can be developed that will graph the series of related events and activities from beginning to end, indicating activities and when they should be accomplished (Fig. 12-4).

This type of critical path will help focus the attention on potential problems, help predict attainment, help focus on evaluation of progress, and indicate feasible adjustment.

Financial plan. Another important part of the planning process includes

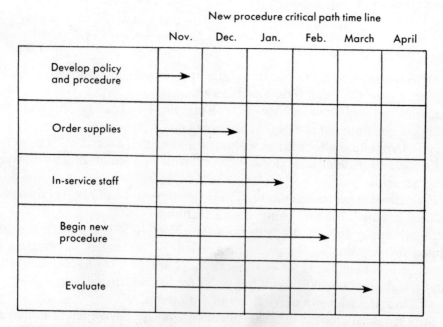

FIG. 12-4. Critical path time line example. Point of arrow indicates accomplished.

financial planning. A budget is a financial plan for the incoming or outgoing of money, personnel, purchased items, or other expense entities. The importance of planning for financial resources to support the total plan cannot be overemphasized. Just as ICPs experience restraints in their personal management of finances, they have the same type of financial restraints in professional resources.

In working with a budget it is necessary to understand some basic budgetary terms[1,3,28]:

cost center Specific area designated within the budget that has expenses and revenues recorded and monitored. The infection control program should have a designated cost center to record such items as expenses of salaries and supplies.

expense items Items within a cost center that must be purchased. Therefore they are an expense to the account. Usually these items are under a set amount of money (around $300) and are necessary for daily operations. These types of expenses are accounted for separately from capital expenditures and represent less money per item than capital expenditures. Examples of expense items are chart forms, paper items, stationery, and general supplies.

capital expenditure Equipment, such as microscopes and computers, costing over a set amount (over $300 in this example) that may be operable for a set number of years (approximately 5 years).

The ICP must determine financial considerations of the plan and outline needs for equipment, human resources, space, and in-service time. Once she has determined that the plan has financial implications, she can fill out the appropriate budget documents.

Besides having the plan affect the ICP's own budget, the plan may have indirect expense implications. Examples of these include in-service time and additional procedure time. Again, early involvement of the people whose budgets will be affected by indirect expenses is a critical strategy to employ. This will reduce any surprises caused by the ICP's plan and will promote support. Cost/benefit ratios should be calculated for proposed program change, and proposed expenses should be justified. The option to the cost passed on to the consumer should also be explored.

Establishing checks and balances. The critical path should be systematically reviewed to monitor progress. Ongoing surveillance data can also be used to monitor effectiveness of instituted changes. Policies and procedures should be updated to incorporate any new expectations.[28] It is also useful to review the organizational structure to determine if any changes in reporting or communicating need to be made. This will facilitate achieving unity of effort among the various components of an organization.

ORGANIZING

The purpose of organizing is to establish an intentional structure of roles by which people can identify how their role fits with others, what their tasks and objectives are, and what the scope of responsibility and accountability is.[13] The principles of organization include the following:

- Establishing clear lines of authority; assuring each individual has only one boss and defining authority and responsibility for each individual in writing
- Delegating to the lowest level of competency

Organizational structure

The formal organizational structure defines the areas of responsibility, the person to whom one is responsible, and channels of communication. Its primary purpose is directed at coordinating. It functionally accomplishes this by providing a road map that details to whom each person reports (Fig. 12-5).

Organizational relationships can take three basic forms[13,18]:

Line authority. Line authority is characterized by superior-subordinate relationships. A superior delegates authority to a subordinate and so on, forming a "line" from the top to the bottom level of the organizational structure. The authority relationship is a direct line between superior and subordinate. A person with line authority has charge of and is responsible for the work of the unit.

Staff authority. Staff authority is characterized by manager-to-manager relationships. Staff authority relationships are used to support line authority relationships. This is accomplished by performing tasks, functions required to supply information, and services to line components (see Chapter 10 for additional information).

Functional authority. This type of authority is delegated by management to a specialist. A specialist is defined as a person who has a single area of specialized information and knowledge in which she is authorized to act. Logan[18] states, "Functional authority is as binding as line authority, but does not carry the right to discipline in order to enforce compliance."

Establishing a clear line of authority. Authority is defined as the power or right to act, command, or direct action by others. Implicit in this definition is the responsibility for decision making.

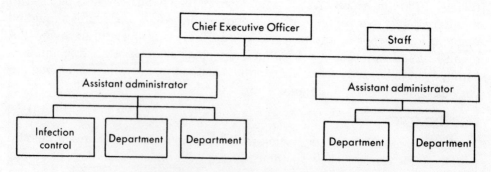

FIG. 12-5. Organizational chart reflects relationship within the structure.

Arndt and Huckabay[1] state, "The position vested with authority is the universal building block of all organizations. Incumbents of positions may come or go, but authority of position remains."

Authority is most specifically defined in the job description. A well-written job description will clearly state the following (see also box below):

- The position title
- Whom the position reports to
- Level of authority
- Level of responsibility
- Level of accountability
- Qualifications for the job

Department of Infection Control

Infection Control Coordinator: Job Description

The infection control coordinator (ICC) is a registered professional nurse who is assigned the responsibility of coordinating the multiple facets of the infection control program with 24-hour responsibility in his or her assigned area. This position involves professional responsibilities in the following areas: case finding, surveillance, reporting, analysis and interpretation, inspection, control measures, education, consultation, evaluation, and recommendations.

The major objectives of the ICC include the following:

1. To assure quality of patient care by:
   a. Reducing infection risks to patients and personnel through surveillance
   b. Teaching pertinent to infection control and isolation at all employee levels, including the medical staff
   c. Ascertaining the need for monitoring programs in any given area and instituting and maintaining such programs in an effort to identify and ultimately eliminate infection hazards in the environment
2. To support programs basic to the purposes of medical education and research as the hospital and medical school may implement that involve infection control activities.
3. To extend his or her services and knowledge beyond the walls of the institution, reaching into community health and education, and serve as a consultant in the area of infection control for other health care facilities.

Summary   Purpose

Plans, develops, coordinates and evaluates infection control activities. Develops and provides educational programs for all hospital personnel. Performs surveillance of patient units and laboratory data. Identifies and reports nosocomial infections and patients in isolation. Participates in medical research and research related to the improvement in infection control for patient care and personnel health.

Modified from Stanford University Hospital.   *Continued.*

Department of Infection Control—cont'd

Infection Control Coordinator: Job Description

Supervisory controls and guidelines

1. Responsible to the supervisor, department of infection control.
2. Appointed, oriented, directed, and evaluated by the supervisor, department of infection control, in conjunction with the hospital epidemiologist.
3. Responsible to the supervisor, department of infection control, for the quality of infection control and the overall administration of pertinent affairs of the patient units, personnel, and medical staff.

Intrahospital responsibilities

Surveillance

Surveillance is the dynamic process of systematic review of multiple data sources to document and evaluate the incidence of infection.

1. Examines laboratory (infectious disease) reports and consults with nursing staff to incorporate these data into the care of the patient.
2. Makes rounds to the nursing units for the purpose of case finding and supervision of environmental factors including isolation practices.
3. Establishes and maintains a record of all isolated patients and those patients and personnel who have nosocomial infections.
4. Reports daily and monthly on patients in isolation to selected departments to ensure safe practices in the management of patients with infections.
5. Prepares monthly and quarterly reports and summaries of special investigations on the occurrence of nosocomial and community-acquired infections.
6. Ensures reporting of reportable disease to the county health departments.
7. Assists the hospital epidemiologist whenever necessary in carrying out surveys of possible carriers among employees or patients and in tracing possible sources of infection within the hospital.
8. Institutes and maintains records and data pertinent to all assigned environmental and patient surveillance monitoring systems.
9. Consults housekeeping regarding the necessary terminal cleaning for specific isolation cases.

Education

1. Develops and evaluates programs (including objectives, content, lesson plans, and teaching materials) that pertain to responsibilities in infection control for the nursing staff (RNs, LVNs, nursing assistants, unit clerks).
2. Participates in weekly orientation for all new hospital employees.
3. Provides formal and informal educational sessions on infection control on the nursing units to clerical, nursing, and medical staffs.
4. Offers appropriate assistance with staff development on patient care units when requested to do so by the clinical nurse coordinator or head nurse.
5. Provides formal and informal training sessions relating to infection control for all hospital departments concerning patient care, personnel health, and environmental factors.

Consultation

1. Participates with the supervisor, the hospital epidemiologist, and the infection control officers in developing and implementing the appropriate management of problems that may be of an infectious or communicable nature.
2. Keeps the supervisor, the epidemiologist, and the infection control officer appraised of special problems in his or her assigned area.
3. Maintains close communication with all supervisors, clinical coordinators, head nurses, unit managers, and staff members ensuring that he or she is the primary focal point to which information will be directed in regard to patient or personnel infections and environmental factors.
4. Within the assigned area, acts as a liaison between the infection control department and all other departments in matters related to infection control.
5. Maintains a working rapport with the county health officer.
6. In consultation with the hospital epidemiologist, notifies all physicians who have inpatients with known exposures to a communicable disease during hospitalization.
7. Assists in the review of sterilization and disinfection methods (agents and procedures) used throughout the medical center.
8. Assists other departments in the development of policies and procedures for the care of patients, equipment, and the environment to provide optimal conditions for infection control.
9. Cooperates with other hospital departments engaged in research activities that require the facilities or assistance of the infectious disease laboratory or division.
10. As assigned, represents the infection control committee and department on hospital committees.
11. Participates in the activities of the health and safety committee, such as environmental surveys.
12. Assists other departments in incorporating infection control principles into plans for construction and renovation of the hospital environment.
13. Collaborates with appropriate representatives of other disciplines and agencies to provide coordinated services to patients for the improvement of overall patient care.
14. Assists in the evaluation and implementation of new products and equipment as relating to infection control.

Intradepartmental responsibilities

1. Assists in the development and implementation of the philosophy, goals, and objectives of the infection control program.
2. Attends all meetings of the infection control committee.
3. Attends Infectious Disease Journal Club and other relevant educational conferences.

Continued.

Department of Infecton Control—cont'd

Infection Control Coordinator: Job Description

Intradepartmental responsibilities

4. Participates in community educational programs and serves as a consultant to other infection control practitioners.
5. Assists in the development and revision of the infection control manual.
6. Relieves other infection control nurses in their absence and temporarily assumes their responsibilities and authorities.
7. Relieves the supervisor of the department as assigned.

Qualifications

Professional preparation and experience

1. Current licensure to practice professional nursing.
2. Advanced educational preparation with a baccalaureate degree desirable.
3. Progressive nursing experience with demonstrated leadership and teaching abilities.

Personal and professional

1. Shows evidence of good health and grooming.
2. Displays appropriate manner and conduct.
3. Has ability to work effectively with others.
4. Possesses integrity, imagination, initiative, and evidence of self-development.
5. Demonstrates ability in applying principles of administration in an organization.
6. Recognizes the responsibility of infection control to participate in appropriate community activities.
7. Demonstrates interest and ability in promoting the growth and development of others and self.
8. Demonstrates skill in using problem-solving methods.
9. Demonstrates ability in decision making based on fact and sound judgment.
10. Supports his or her professional organizations.
11. Displays willingness to engage in individual study.

Informal organization. The informal organizational structure evolves naturally whenever people work together.[13] These informal groups are not officially prescribed by the formal organization but can be very powerful. These groups are usually bound together by common interests. Information passed through the informal group is usually referred to as "grapevine" information. It seems wise to use these social groups to accomplish work goals, but this must be done with discretion. Information from the grapevine has a tendency to be distorted and inaccurate.

Delegation.[7,8] Delegation of authority is essential to the existence of an organization. The organizational units require the delegation of authority to the managers charged with their respective management. To delegate means to grant or confer, specifically, to confer authority from one executive or organizational unit to another. This topic will be developed more comprehensively in the next section.

DIRECTING

Directing is the process of putting the plan into action within the defined organizational structure.[7] In a discussion of the function of directing the following activities will be explored because they have specific application to the ICP role:

- Leadership theories
- Delegation
- Time management
- Planned change
- Motivational theory
- Conflict

Leadership theories[28,30,32]

Three basic types of leadership are normally found in industry:

- Autocratic
- Democratic
- Laissez-faire

The type of leadership that is given to a group depends on where the authority is located:

Authority in the leader—autocratic

Authority in the group—democratic

Authority in the individual—laissez-faire

Autocratic leadership provides decisions that are usually unilateral, such as those found in schools or in the armed forces. The autocratic leader tries to achieve major goals by means that often require personal sacrifice from those involved and, therefore, are not popular with the personnel.

In the *democratic* form of leadership decisions are multilateral and subject to group authority and pressure. With the democratic leadership technique, leaders derive and maintain a position of authority from the group and retain it as long as they satisfy the group members' needs and conform to their interests.

Laissez-faire leadership occurs when there is almost an absence of leadership. This is an intolerable situation for managing and operating a business or hospital. A lack of true leadership creates anxiety in people. People accept and actually prefer some degree of leadership in their daily activities. However, not everyone enjoys being a leader and doing a leader's job.

TABLE 12-1. Comparison of three leadership styles

Leadership style	Advantages	Disadvantages
Autocratic	Goals remain clear; concentration of effort; less confusion; faster, more direct action; permits maximal flexibility; with capable leader there are fewer mistakes	Group may resist decisions; serious errors from incapable leader; group knowledge not obtained; leaders not developed; could fall apart when leader is absent; ignores human needs; leader becomes isolated; tendency to go beyond capabilities
Democratic	Leadership fits need of the group; better quality decisions; better informed leadership; more and better ideas; participation develops acceptance, support, and cooperation; decisions are subject to criticism; helps develop leaders; good use of all talents	Can be slow in determining course of action; may be difficult to implement a decision that group does not support requires skill in leadership; decision could be influenced by some who lack adequate knowledge; group could feel that it and/or the leader is in charge
Laissez-faire	Natural leader will emerge; brings out group interests; leadership can change as situation changes	Wrong leader may emerge; confusion precedes selection; leadership rivalries may develop; may not stand pressure; may not be sustained; too disorganized

Each leadership type has certain advantages and disadvantages (Table 12-1), but sound business leadership is a hybrid between autocratic and democratic models. ICPs should seek to obtain the advantages of each.

Leadership styles are related to the types of leadership discussed earlier. They include the autocrat, democrat, and hybrid.

Each of these types can be effective or ineffective depending on how the leader employs the characteristics and under what circumstances the leader operates.

Autocrats can continue to place implicit trust in themselves and be concerned with both the immediate and long-run tasks. They become more effective when a skill is developed to motivate others to do what is wanted without creating big resentments. They strive to create an environment that minimizes aggression and maximizes obedience to commands.

Democrats can become developers. They can view the job as primarily concerned with developing the talents of others and providing a work atmosphere conducive to maximizing individual satisfaction and motivation.

Hybrids remain interested in both people and production, but they become most effective by setting high standards of performance and becoming decisive while recognizing individual differences and expectations and the need to treat subordinates as individuals.

It can be useful to recognize one's own leadership style and develop the ability to identify key leadership attributes in others.

If the ICP has the knowledge of her leadership characteristics, she can develop the ability to recognize her leadership strengths and weaknesses as she interacts in her role. This insight can help her seek help in addressing specific weaknesses she wishes to improve. For example, the ICP may discover that in stressful situations she becomes democratic, wanting a consensus from the group before she initiates action. When the situation involves exposure of large amounts of people to a highly infectious disease unless immediate action is taken, a democratic style will not only be ineffective but also inappropriate. In this situation the ICP needs to be autocratic and give exact directions.

Being aware of the leadership style of others can also provide the ICP with the insight to help plan responses to the situation in a way that effects outcomes she wishes to achieve.

Delegation[3]

It is impossible for the ICP to accomplish the goals of the infection control program alone. The act of delegation has a multiplying effect. The ICP essentially assigns the specific expectations for infection control to hospital personnel and health care practitioners.

The most functional method of delegation is through written, specific delegation of authority. Examples of this type of delegation can be found in most infection control manuals, such as the ability to culture or isolate without a physician's order or simply the responsibility to perform good handwashing in the work environment.

Other ways of delegation include verbal delegation, delegation by assumption, delegation by actions, and delegation by silence.

Verbal delegation tends to be less clear than written delegation and may expand to delegation by assumption. For example, the ICP may state to one nursing assistant that she would like to be called if a specific patient she is observing develops a fever. The ICP requests this because the nursing assistant is responsible for taking all vital signs on the particular nursing unit. The nursing assistant may in fact follow through with the request but may assume that the ICP has given (or delegated) an ongoing task that may or may not be acceptable. The ICP may receive feedback that the nursing assistant is responsi-

ble for monitoring all temperatures for her. The original delegation was specific, but because it was done verbally, the understanding of the delegation was
more global. In this example there may be no problem with the nursing assistant accepting the responsibility and accountability for the delegation, but the
nursing assistant's supervisor may have a problem, particularly if the subordinate relays the understanding of ongoing responsibility to monitor and report
all patients with elevated temperatures. As usual, communication is critical in
the delegation process, and every effort should be made to be clear about the
delegated functions. Perhaps one way to reduce this type of misunderstanding
when using verbal delegation is to review the specific request and assignment
with the employee's supervisor.

Delegation by assumption involves others making assumptions about
what they think the ICP has delegated. The usual outcome is that what the
ICP wanted done is not being done. For example, the ICP has delegated
the responsibility of routine IV catheter care to the staff nurse. If the ICP
does not have specific, written guidelines for how catheter care should be
performed, she may find that everyone does it differently. Each staff nurse
makes assumptions about what routine catheter care entails and performs
accordingly.

Delegation by actions is done by observing certain behaviors within the
practice of hospital personnel and health care practitioners, and through actions the ICP supports that what they are doing is, in fact, what she wants them
to do. This brings to mind a critical point that should be emphasized. The ICP
sets the tone for her expectations by each interaction she has with personnel.
When she observes behaviors that are inconsistent with her expectations, she
needs to bring them to the attention of those involved. The ICP's actions
(what she does) carry strong messages about what she approves or does not
approve.

Delegation by silence is very similar to delegation by actions. The only
difference is that the action is silence. Silence is usually perceived as approval.
If the ICP observes behaviors by others and is silent, the message is approval.

There are times when it is appropriate not to delegate. For example, in an
outbreak situation routine functions that the ICP does not usually get involved
with may become her priority, and she would not choose to delegate these.

Delegation can also have problems. There are traps for delegation that all
ICPs fall into occasionally. They use these traps to rationalize why they cannot
or do not delegate:

- They can do the job better.
- There is no one to delegate to.
- Not delegating keeps them in control.
- It is faster to do it themselves.
- There is a lack of confidence that others can or will perform.

- They choose to do the things they feel comfortable with, as opposed to less desirable role functions.
- They feel that others will accept them if they meet expectations.
- They are afraid they will be disliked.

Another trap for delegation is reverse delegation; that is, the ICP allows others to delegate their functions to her. There are many reasons this may happen:

- It is an unpleasant task; they do not want to do it, so they reverse it back to the ICP.
- They were not given authority.
- They avoid risk taking.
- They are afraid of being criticized.
- They lack confidence.
- Hospital personnel perceive that the ICP needs to be needed.
- Performance is punishing.
- It is an attention-getting ploy; they want some of the ICP's time.
- They know the ICP cannot say "No."

Time management[27,29]

Another critical area is the need for personal direction—the management of personal time. The place to begin with time management is to determine how time is spent (Fig. 12-6). The ICP's time will probably fall into the following categories:

1. *Routine work.* Making rounds; reviewing culture results; should be limited to 10% of time
2. *Special assignments.* Finding an answer to a boss's question; should be limited to 10% to 15% of time
3. *Regular role functions.* Most important tasks; serving on committees; approximately 70% of time

Following are seven ideas that may help an ICP save some time:

- Make up your mind quickly with most problems
- Be specific about dates
- Control the telephone
- Write down reminders
- Limit conversations
- Delegate work to others
- Reduce time spent on paperwork

Normally the ICP will have a number of special projects, activities, and jobs in process. It is necessary to control this work so that first things get done first and all jobs are completed satisfactorily on time.

Note taking is important. Many problems and situations are faced each day that require follow-up or action on the part of the supervisor.

	Daily time analysis		Date _____	
	Activity	Productive	Nonproductive	Reasons
7:00 AM				
7:30 AM				
8:00 AM				
8:30 AM				
9:00 AM				
9:30 AM				
10:00 AM				
10:30 AM				
11:00 AM				
11:30 AM				
12:00 M				
1:00 PM				
1:30 PM				
2:00 PM				
2:30 PM				
3:00 PM				
3:30 PM				
4:00 PM				
4:30 PM				
5:00 PM				
		Total	Total	

FIG. 12-6. Recording form for completing daily time schedules.

There are two basic ways to save time: do less or work faster. To do less, the ICP needs the art of delegation. To work faster, she should filter out interruptions, set priorities, and develop a paper flow system.

A. Common time management problems
   1. Telephone
   2. Meetings
   3. Visitors
   4. Delegation
   5. Procrastination
   6. Crisis intervention
   7. Special requests
   8. Delays
   9. Reading
   10. Documentation
B. Techniques of time management
   1. Daily tasks
      a. Set priorities.
      b. Identify those that can be delegated.
      c. Communicate to plan projects and complete in a timely fashion. Do not leave to the last minute.
      d. Do creative work; 5% to 10% of time; develop new procedures.
      e. Do paperwork; 5% of time; establish paper flow for three kinds of paper.
         (1) Active—immediate
         (2) Pending—after initiated action
         (3) Read and distribute or toss

Using these categories, the ICP should make a time budget for each week. It should be done in half-hour or hour increments. In addition, a list of tasks to be done during the day should be prepared first thing in the morning.

Committee work. Committee work is a key activity of the ICP, affording her direct access to influencing decision making within the health care facility. To understand this idea, it may be useful to review the basic definition and function of a committee. A committee is two or more people appointed for the purpose of acting or advising their superior about a subject that is not clearly within the competence of any one of them. Committees have delegated power and authority that may include one or all of the following:

• Power to make recommendations
• Power to create policy
• Power to initiate action on a set of well-defined tasks

Participation on committees, then, affords the ICP a variety of opportunities to investigate, recommend, participate in policy making, and act.

When the ICP is deciding which infection control concern she might defer to committee action, she should remember that committees work through consensus. It *does not* belong in a committee meeting when the following circumstances exist:

1. One person can do the job better. If so, the ICP should see that that person has the information and authority necessary to make things happen. For example, the ICP wants to have the laboratory begin to record all coagulase-positive staphylococcal isolates in one place. The ICP can establish this recording system with the laboratory personnel; it does not require committee action.
2. The matter is not important enough to require the time, attention, and energy of several people. Selecting a room to set up the yearly influenza vaccination program in is not a committee decision.
3. The ICP is not willing to accept a consensus recommendation. For example, a JCAH requirement cannot be changed by a consensus vote of the infection control committee.
4. The ICP needs immediate action. When the state department of licensure appears at the hospital to review how needles are disposed of, the ICP cannot defer handling this until there is a committee meeting.

The advantages of committee work follows:
- Pools experience
- Spreads responsibility
- Diffuses power

Committee effectiveness. Because of the amount of time the ICP spends in committee work, it is prudent to make sure that time is spent productively and economically. There are several methods that can increase the effectiveness of running (or participating in) a committee meeting:

1. Have a prepared agenda and send it out at least 1 week before the meeting date. This will give committee members time to review items that are going to be discussed and prepare their input when appropriate. It also provides a plan for the chairperson to use in keeping the discussions relevant to the issues under consideration.
2. Set strict time limits on meetings and keep them. Committee members are more likely to attend meetings that take a predictable amount of time. This also discourages members from presenting important items of discussion in the last 5 minutes of the meeting time, expecting other committee members to stay and act on the request.
3. Make clear the decisions that must be made by the time the meeting ends. Any decisions the ICP needs should be verbalized clearly during the discussion, with a clear answer from committee members before she allows the discussion to continue.
4. Develop strategies for meetings. Good ground work *before the meeting*

helps the ICP obtain support for her proposals. Actual committee time should be used for formal decision making. This type of political activity is included in the time the ICP should allot to committee activity.

When committee work seems to be stagnating or moving in directions the ICP does not necessarily agree with, there are strategies she can consider to improve committee meetings.

1. Planning is the key: consider any of the following activities to enhance the participation, learning, and/or commitment at your meetings:
   a. Small group discussions
   b. Role playing
   c. Simulations
   d. Field trips
   e. Brainstorming
   f. Total group discussion
   g. Video or audio taping
   h. Articles
   i. Written instructions
   j. Background papers
   k. Pamphlets and books
   l. Poetry
   m. Readings
   n. Quotes
2. Review the membership
   a. Are the key people there who need to make decisions?
   b. Who are the latecomers or frequently absent members of the group? Are they really needed?
   c. Are you getting enough input from people outside your committee?
   d. Who could you invite to your meetings to improve effectiveness?
   e. Which members of the group are high in influence? Low in influence?
   f. Who are the high participators? Low participators?
3. Know the purpose of your meetings
   a. How can you accomplish your objectives more effectively and efficiently?
   b. What functions could be dealt with more effectively by subgroups, task forces, or individuals?
4. Determine the atmosphere or climate of your meeting
   a. Can you improve seating, lighting, ventilation, noise, interruptions, or equipment?
   b. How can you promote cooperation and involvement?
   c. Are you aware of nonverbal communication?
   d. Is the leader recognized as the leader?

5. Assign follow-up responsibilities
   a. Do you consider participation and cooperation in meetings when doing performance evaluations of staff?
   b. Do you enforce deadlines?
   c. Are minutes meaningful and distributed?
   d. Do you and meeting participants evaluate the meeting regularly?

Planned change

Planned change has several interacting components[35]:
- The environment in which change is to occur
- The variation from the existing to the desired practice (the proposed change)
- The human element that needs to be modified (the change target)
- The change agent (ICP)
- The means for promoting and maintaining the revision (policies and procedures)

Lewin[21] describes the existing state as a dynamic equilibrium of driving forces and restraining forces of two types:
- Those that stem from the individual interacting with the environment
- Those that stem from the organizational structure of the environment

The latter can be divided into forces *within* the hospital environment and forces *outside* the hospital environment. Dynamic equilibrium, a balance between driving forces and restraining forces, is illustrated in Fig. 12-7. To change the present state, the dynamic equilibrium between the driving and restraining forces must be moved (Fig. 12-7).

Lewin also suggests that once the forces for change are identified, there are three phases of making the change:
- Unfreezing (if necessary) the present level
- Moving to the new level
- Freezing group life on the new level

In accomplishing the first, or unfreezing, phase the ICP needs to ascertain if the staff members involved in the change process are aware of the problem. Change should arise from a "felt need" of those involved. However, if their awareness is not evident, the ICP must be able to exercise referent power—the natural or learned ability to attract people to her ideas. The unfreezing process is complete when the individuals involved accept and understand the necessity for change and, indeed, view it as an alteration in their best interest.

The second phase, or moving to a new level, begins with mutual clarification of the problem and entails data gathering and interpretation.

The last phase, freezing group life on a new level, is measured by acceptance of the change and actual practice.

All three steps, unfreezing, moving to a new level, and refreezing, require a

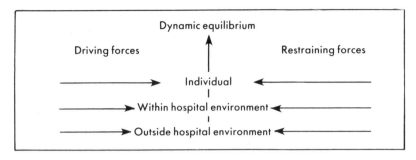

FIG. 12-7. Driving and restraining forces create a dynamic equilibrium. (From Yarbrough, M.G.: Effectiveness of the infection control practitioner as change agent: evaluation by participant observation, A.P.I.C. Journal **5:**48, June 1977.)

TABLE 12-2. Planning and implementing change

Objective	Activity	Evaluation
Change agent will: Identify problem with change target.	Change agent and change target will put problem in writing (unfreezing phase).	Statement(s) of the problem will be mutually agreeable and acceptable.
Identify level of needs of change target.	Change agent will keep written records in the form of Field Notes on how change target perceives problem.	Change agent will validate perceptions with change target.
Problem solve with the change target	Change agent and change target will prepare force field analysis on problem (moving to new level).	The force field analysis will be mutually agreeable and acceptable.
Select and implement with the change target appropriate force(s) in the force field analysis that have a possibility of being changed.	Written plan of action will be prepared to change driving and/or restraining forces (refreezing at new level).	Selection of change will be mutually agreeable and acceptable.
If change planning is not working within selected time period, choose another alternative.	Written evaluation criteria for acceptance or rejection of change will be prepared before the proposed change is implemented. Time limits will be established.	Written evaluation criteria will be mutually agreeable and acceptable.

From Yarbrough, M.G.: Effectiveness of the infection control practitioner as change agent: evaluation by participant observation, A.P.I.C. Journal **5:**48, June 1977.

concerted effort·by those involved in making the change. Promoting active involvement of the staff (change target) during this process has a twofold advantage: it increases the commitment of personnel and promotes the internalization of the proposed change.

It is also helpful to have a systematic process for implementing change. I have identified a five-step process for planned change (Table 12-2).

Step 1. The first step is to identify the problem with the change target (those whom the change will affect). To eliminate misunderstanding, this should be done in writing so that the statement is clear and mutually agreeable and acceptable to those involved. This is usually the most difficult step. As discussed under "Planning," this becomes the most critical step because all future steps will be directed at solving this identified problem. If the wrong problem is identified, the wrong solution will be developed.

The ICP must treat the cause, not the effect, if she is to reach the right solution to a problem.

Step 2. The level of needs of the change target should be identified. This can be accomplished through keeping and reviewing field notes on how the problem is manifested within the change target population. All perceptions identified should be validated with the change target.

Step 3. A force field analysis should be done with the change target.

Step 4. A change from the force field analysis should be selected. A written plan should be prepared (see "Planning" for details). It is critical to develop specific criteria for evaluation.

Step 5. Evaluating the change is entailed in this step.

The advantages of having such a planned change framework follow:

1. The ICP will always have an identified direction to follow. If the change is not working, perhaps the wrong problem was identified, or a different restraining or driving force can be selected and a plan developed.
2. The success of implementing the change is very rewarding.

A disadvantage in this type of planned change is that it takes time and commitment. As can be seen in Fig. 12-8, the change target should be involved all along the planning process to increase the cooperation, participation, and commitment of the change target to implementing the change.

A personal example of using this planned change strategy to resolve a typical infection control problem can best demonstrate its application. A unit in the hospital had an outbreak of urinary tract infections caused by highly resistant Serratia marcescens:

1. Discussion with the staff on the unit established the parameters of the problem. Together we prepared a written statement of the problem and put it in the unit communication book. The problem was identified as hand-to-patient transmission of the organism, especially in patients having indwelling urinary catheters.

2. I kept written records, in the form of field notes, of all conversations I had with the staff concerning this problem. This was an extremely difficult task but proved to be a valuable tool when disagreement and confusion occurred.
3. We developed a force field analysis (Table 12-3) of the driving and restraining forces on the unit that pertained to the *Serratia marcescens* outbreak. This was also placed in the communication book.
4. The practice of poor handwashing was selected by the staff as the restraining force they could successfully convert to a driving force. We developed a written plan of action and decided to evaluate the plan after 2 months.
5. Written evaluation forms were developed to determine if compliance to the handwashing requirements had improved. Evaluation criteria included (a) less than two new infections within the 2-month period and (b) 80% compliance of staff to the new handwashing policy (measured by a questionnaire and by the volume of soap used on the unit).

Keleman[16] proposes that the changes people experience in life are like "mini-deaths." He explains this by using the concept of formulative loops (Fig. 12-9).

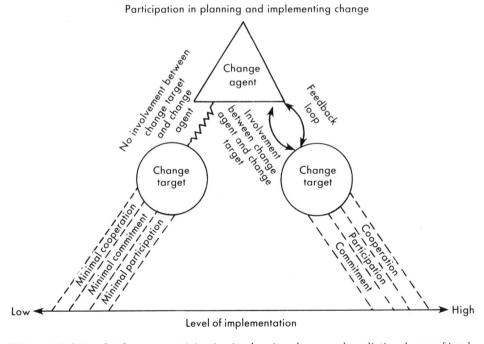

Participation in planning and implementing change

FIG. 12-8. Relationship between participating in planning change and predicting degree of implementation. (From Yarbrough, M.G.: Effectiveness of the infection control practitioner as change agent: evaluation by participant observation, A.P.I.C. Journal **5:**49, June 1977.)

TABLE 12-3. Force field analysis—*Serratia marcescens* outbreak

Focus	Driving forces	Restraining forces
Individual	Employees are motivated to stop outbreak.	Microorganisms cannot be seen—difficult to fight something you cannot see.
Within hospital environment	Patients have indwelling catheters to facilitate urinary drainage.	These catheters provide pathway for bacterial entry.
	Employees assist in many of the activities of daily living and interact frequently with patients.	Poor handwashing practices are observed between patients.
	Patients can remain in the hospital for extended periods.	Increased risk of infection is associated with increased hospital stay.
Outside hospital environment	Patients may move to other VA Hospitals for additional assistance.	Microorganisms may spread outbreak outside of hospital.

From Yarbrough, M.G.: Effectiveness of the infection control practitioner as change agent: evaluation by participant observation, A.P.I.C. Journal **5**:49, June 1977.

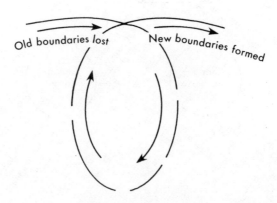

FIG. 12-9. Formative loop. (From Keleman, S.: Living your dying, New York, 1975, Random House, Inc. and The Bookworks.)

When entering a change situation, people enter the descending side of the formulative loop. During this phase, old thoughts, ideas, feelings, and action patterns are given up. During this phase, people experience a loss, much like a death. Because the change is a perceived loss, people deal with it emotionally just as with any loss.

Kubler-Ross[20] outlines the grieving process in five stages: denial, anger, bargaining, depression, and acceptance. When people experience change, they go through an emotional process similar to the grieving process. Once this has been completed, they can continue through the formulative loop to the ascending side and can take on new thoughts, intuition, and feelings. These are transformed into action patterns, and new connections are made. Movement into the ascending side is an energetic process.

Motivational theory

The ICP must influence others within the health care setting to incorporate appropriate infection control practices into their daily activities for the infection control program to be successful. Understanding and using concepts from motivational theory may lend insight to accomplishing influence on others.

Maslow[12,17] has described the needs of people, using a hierarchical arrangement, ranging from the basic physical needs such as food, water, clothing, and shelter to the highest level need of self-actualization. Maslow's motivational theory proposes that once any need has been met, it no longer exists as a motivator, and a new need, in ascending order on the pyramid, becomes a motivator. Based on the need that is motivating behavior, communication is "influenced through the selective quality of perceptions."[4]

For example, a new orienting nurse in the hospital may overhear the ICP discussing wound care of a patient, feels that the ICP is discussing her care, and feels threatened because the ICP is "reporting" her inabilities.

Hertzberg's theory of motivation[4] complements the work of Maslow by identifying job-related functions that are motivating factors (cannot motivate but can become source of dissatisfaction and lower performance) (Table 12-4 and Fig. 12-10).

Conflict

Conflict is defined as a clash or struggle that occurs whenever the harmony and balance among thoughts, feelings, and behaviors are threatened.[22] There are many sources of conflict (Table 12-5). Examples of conflict sources experienced within the health care institution follow:

- Lack of goal clarity
- Significant value differences
- Lack of well-defined tasks
- Lack of role clarity
- Lack of clearly stated policies and procedures

TABLE 12-4. Use of motivational factors

Factors	Examples of use
Achievement—to successfully accomplish something	Provide work assignments consistent with persons' capabilities; challenging but with minimal risk of failure
Recognition—to acknowledge; aware of sense of worth	Commend for good performance: "You did a fine job of that," "That was really great," "Good job," "Well done," "I appreciate your help; it really meant a lot," and "You are really good at that"
Work itself—to have intrinsic interest in and satisfaction with job content	Improve job content to include more planning, self-direction, and control; coach employees
Responsibility—to be answerable, accountable, and trusting	Delegate responsibility and the authority that goes with it; then allow the employee *time* to exercise both; get feedback; be helpful and supportive, but let employee be accountable for results
Advancement—to make progress; to rise in rank, amount, and value; move forward	Allow employees to advance fairly to limit of their potential when opportunities to do so arise; encourage qualified employees to try new job opportunities; give feedback to employees' supervisor for yearly evaluation
Growth—to develop and become more capable	Provide in-service programs, workshops, and related continuing education programs; encourage further formal education; help employees find learning opportunities based on their needs

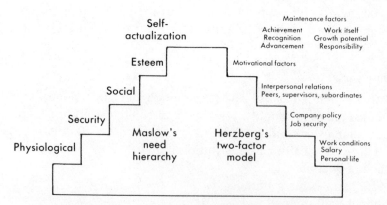

FIG. 12-10. Comparison of the Maslow and Hertzberg models. (From Donnelly, J.H., Jr., Gibson, J.L., and Ivancevich, J.M.: Fundamentals of management: functions, behavior, models, copyright © Dallas, 1971, Business Publications, Inc.)

TABLE 12-5. Possible underlying causes of conflict

Focus of the problem	Background factors	Formal system (possible causes)	Informal system
Individual	Poor match of individual with job; selection or promotion problem	Task too easy or too difficult; poor job definition; different expectations between subordinate and superior	Job fails to fulfill range of needs; little chance for learning; failure because of unclear expectations
Two persons	Personality clash; conflict in basic values	Poor role definition; poor communication; poorly defined expectations	Misunderstanding; unresolved feelings
Groups	Poor group composition; insufficient resources	Tasks poorly defined; role relationships unclear or inappropriate	Poor working process
Intergroup	Status and power conflicts of two professions; physical distance	Conflict on task perspective	Conflicting group styles
Leadership	Poor selection and promotion decisions; poor training	Overload of responsibilities; inappropriate reporting procedures	Individual not liked and/or respected; conflict with other sources of power

Conflict can be intrapersonal, interpersonal, intergroup, or interorganizational.

Marriner[28] describes three basic stages of conflict:

- Latent conflict
- Perceived conflict
- Manifest conflict

Latent conflict arises from anticipation. When considering all the consequences of a change, people often identify areas of potential conflict and develop strategies to reduce its occurrence. For example, when changing from an open urinary drainage system to a closed urinary drainage system, the ICP may anticipate conflict with the urologist and/or nursing staff. Although the conflict has not yet occurred, it is anticipated and planned for.

Perceived conflict indicates a cognitive awareness of a stressful situation. It may or may not be accurate, but it does exist for the person experiencing it. For example, the ICP may have heard through the "grapevine" that the purchasing department changed vendors for the purchase of handwashing solutions within the hospital, and this has not been approved by the infection control committee. This would be a perceived conflict to the ICP. It may or may not be real, but it will get her immediate attention to verify if a conflict actually exists.

Manifest conflict is conflict that exists through overt behavior that can be constructive or destructive.

In assessing a manifest conflict situation Kramer and Schmalenberg[19] identify the following findings present in a destructive course of conflict:
- The issue is broadly defined with tangentially related items included.
- The situation must have a winner and a loser.
- There is use of threats and coercion.
- There is mutual distrust and misperception.
- There is general frustration and dissatisfaction.

The result of destructive conflict is harmful and leads to stagnation.

They also define characteristics of conflict that is managed in a constructive fashion:
- The issue is focused and specific.
- There is action rather than reaction.
- There is demonstrated effort to reconcile.
- Differences are remedied by seeking new solutions.
- There is honest, open dialogue with a sincere attempt to understand each other's viewpoint.
- There are feelings of gain and satisfaction.

Constructive conflict can lead to feelings of well-being and growth.

There are three basic strategies for conflict resolution: win-win, lose-lose, and lose-win.[15] (These same strategies are used in negotiations. See Chapter 3.)

In a win-win strategy the focus is on goals. There is effort to obtain consensus and develop integrative approaches to problem solving. The focus is on the problem, not on each other. The ICP should strive to create a collaborative outcome that looks for ways to satisfy both parties' interests, such as looking for new alternatives and mutually solving problems.

In the lose-lose strategy neither side wins or achieves its goals. In this situation the parties seek outcomes that either compromise for partial satisfaction of both parties' concerns, such as exchanging concessions and bargaining, or seek to avoid the issues by sidestepping the issue through ignoring, passing the buck, and delaying. The issues become personalized, with the focus being on each other, not on the problem.

The lose-win strategy establishes a winner and a loser. One party strives to satisfy its concern at the expense of the other's through forcing, arguing, and pulling rank or through accommodation, when one party sacrifices its concern to satisfy the other party's concern through conceding and taking pity.

All individuals have a repertoire of modes for handling conflict that are selected as directed by the circumstances of the conflict situation in which they find themselves. However, most people are more adept at some modes and use them more frequently than others, just as a right-handed person favors the right hand over the left. The ICP should examine her conflict management style through examination of field notes with a goal to develop a style that can produce win-win situations. The most important behavior to incorporate to assure a win-win situation is to seek to preserve each person's self-esteem by mutually confronting the issues, not confronting each other personally.

Two strong reactions that occur during conflict situations that are a challenge to manage are anger and sabotage.

Anger is defined as a feeling of extreme displeasure, indignation, or exasperation toward someone or something; synonymous words include hostility, rage, wrath, and ire. Duldt[9] identifies two ways of dealing with anger. She defined a "destructive mode (one that is destructive to an interpersonal relationship) and a maintenance mode (one that tends to be constructive or maintain an interpersonal relationship)."

In the destructive mode communication is unclear, which makes it difficult, if not impossible, for others to help. Tension remains, and anger increases; tension is prolonged, and there is a potential for hostility, aggression, or violence. When energy is siphoned off for anger, there is little left for the individual to use in constructively managing the problem.

In the maintenance mode communication is clear, which can alert others to help. Tension is reduced, and the anger is dissipated.

When managing anger (one's own or others'), it is important to tell another person about the anger and carefully identify the source. This expression gets the anger out in the open so it can be dealt with.

Sabotage is defined as a "willful effort by indirect means to hinder, prevent, undo, or discredit (as a plan or activity); deliberate subversion (any act or process tending to hamper or hurt—wreck, destroy, damage)."[33] The ICP no doubt has felt the effects of sabotage in either her personal or professional life. An example might be her efforts to eliminate the dressing cart on the surgical floor. Everyone agrees that having a cart moved from room to room is a potential source of cross-contamination. The ICP establishes a new policy and procedure, removes the carts, and provides in-service education to the group only to find a cardboard box with dressing materials in it that is being taken from room to room.

Thorpe[33] outlines the following steps to counteract sabotage:

1. Identify the problem.
2. Let those involved know that you are aware of their tactics. Because your role is a staff position, you will need to do this with the immediate supervisor of those involved. This is the confrontation stage.
3. Spell out expectations of the group firmly and stick to them. Identify consequences of behavior.

4. Meet with all disciplines involved with the event, elicit their feelings, and clarify any misconceptions.
5. Record all meetings, and send copies to all the participants.
6. Make rounds frequently. Be consistent with the approach and persevere.

CONTROLLING

The real test of the effectiveness of the ICP as a manager comes from the results achieved through the infection control program: low infection rates, high consistent compliance of personnel to defined policies and procedures, compliance with requirements of accrediting bodies, and mutual satisfaction between the ICP and the hospital with the quality and quantity of the program. Nothing has been accomplished unless efforts bring about results. Controlling activities assumes that the work of planning, organizing, and directing has been completed and is an essential systematic process to measure if the performance has taken place according to the plan.

There are essentially three steps in the controlling activity[1,27]:
- Measuring performance
- Comparing it to a predetermined standard
- Implementing corrective action when necessary

Measuring the performance of the program deals with a single concept: finding out what is being accomplished. This is critical to validate the program, as well as to use as a guide for future direction of the program. The carrying out of this work can be achieved in many ways. I will discuss some of the more common ones:
- Personal observations
- Statistical data analysis
- Oral reports
- Written reports
- Audits

Personal observations

This step involves the ICP going to the area of patient care activities and indirect patient care activities to take notice of what is being done. Observations are made of the methods being used, the quality of work, the attitude of employees, and the general functions of people in the areas observed. There are many who feel that there is no adequate substitute for firsthand direction observation. Traditional activities of the ICP that fall into this category include surveillance rounds and on-the-spot in-service programs in individual departments. The ICP should consider some type of systematic, routine inspection program with the intent of making personal observations on the quality of performance of the infection control program throughout the health care institution.

Statistical data analysis

Collecting, analyzing, and reporting information on types, numbers, and general trends of infections in the health care institution are useful guideposts to reflect performance. This can be accomplished through monthly, bimonthly, or quarterly reports to the infection control committee and to the hospital administration. Although there are varying opinions about the frequency of generating such reports, there is little doubt that some type of systematic monitoring and reporting is useful. (For specific information about the generation of such data, the reader is referred to Chapter 7.)

Oral reports

Oral reports can be effective in personal meetings, group meetings, or committee settings. They maintain certain elements of the personal observation method in that information is transmitted orally and personal contact is included. The facial expression, tone of voice, and general evaluation of the performance by the reporter can be observed, and questions can be asked at the most opportune time to clear any misunderstandings or to gain additional information. Conditions needing remedial action can also be worked out at the time of the discussion.

Written reports

Written reports supply a permanent record of the activities of the infection control program. Simple, yet complete, summary statements about performance are effective. Other types of written documents that provide control to the infection control program include infection control manuals and policies and procedure handbooks. All of these documents provide a permanent reference for hospital personnel and clinicians to maintain the standards set by the infection control committee for infection control practices within the health care institution.

Audits

Establishing a systematic audit of how the ICP is accomplishing activities planned both through developing critical time lines and through developing objectives is a must for internal control. This can be accomplished easily by marking a calender in advance on each of the target dates. As the ICP sees these activities marked, it will be an automatic reminder to review the proposed plan and monitor progress. The ICP can pick key points where it seems reasonable to audit her progress in the action plan. At each of these points she will want to ask the following questions:

1. Am I progressing according to plan?
2. Am I achieving the objectives by doing these tasks?
3. Do the objectives still make sense? If not, what changes are necessary?

4. Am I achieving my objectives in a way that is beneficial to all involved?
5. What new variances can I now foresee for which I must design additional action steps? Add them.
6. What additional resources do I need, and how can I obtain them?
7. Is the time line still appropriate?
8. Is everybody still with me? Is there a shared sense of purpose? Of progress?
9. What is the mental state or attitude of those involved?
10. How is our group progress? How are we doing on managing our interactions?

Create improvements. In light of answers to the above what improvements can we make that will escalate our capability to work together and reach our objectives?

Check auditing process. Are we auditing well enough and often enough to catch and respond to variances before they take us too far off track? What improvements can we make?

Review goal. Review your larger goal at these audit points and at any time you feel discouraged, bogged down, or burned out.

Quality assurance

The primary aim of the JCAH has shifted emphasis from audits as a means to accomplish self-review within the health care setting to a total, integrated quality assurance program.

The goal of this change is to establish the need for strengthening the coordination and integration of all quality assurance activities within the health care setting. The specific JCAH criteria for quality assurance include the following:

1. Integrating or coordinating all quality assurance activities into a comprehensive program must occur. This particular requirement is meant to minimize duplication, enhance communications, and reduce costs.
2. The plan must be written.
3. There should be a problem-focused approach. This is a move from the previous practice of having diagnosis-specific audits to establishing a hospital-wide, problem-focused review.
4. There must be an annual reassessment.
5. There must be measurable improvement. This is a key item. This requirement represents a move from methods (audits) to results. The greatest challenge for ICPs may be to develop tools and methodologies that can document that the activities within the infection control program achieve measurable improvements.

As the ICP revises the infection control program to incorporate the standards of the quality assurance program, there are six basic steps that need to be addressed.

First, the infection control program must have identifiable standards for the control of infections and appropriate practice. Most infection control committees have outlined these standards in infection control manuals that are distributed throughout the health care facility.

Second, there must be ongoing review of how operations are complying with the standards. This can be accomplished through surveillance activities, special studies, audits, and daily rounds.

Third, the committee needs to analyze the findings from the review activities and measure them against the standards. The ICP can be invaluable in setting up this process and analyzing data before the committee meets. Meeting time can then be spent on developing a consensus of opinion about the findings and resolving problems.

Fourth, there must be an established corrective action plan. This is when the ICP's ability to plan will be a great asset to the committee.

Fifth, the action must be instituted. Many of the managerial skills outlined in this chapter will be needed to actualize this step.

Sixth, the results of the action plan must be monitored, reports must be prepared, and documentation should be developed, demonstrating how the action of the committee has resulted in measurable improvement in the health care setting.

CONCLUSION

ICPs have the challenge of influencing health care personnel to incorporate the principles of infection control into their daily practice. Management principles of planning, organizing, directing, and controlling can be helpful in accomplishing this challenge.

Developing skill and expertise in these areas will enable ICPs to plan for overall program effectiveness, set goals and expected outcomes, organize their personal and professional time, direct activities to accomplish the goals and outcomes, and evaluate the effectiveness of the program.

REFERENCES

1. Arndt, C., and Huckabay, L.M.D.: Nursing administration, St. Louis, 1980, The C.V. Mosby Co.
2. Bell, M.L.: Management by objectives, J. Nurs. Adm. **10**:19-26, May 1980.
3. Berger, M.S., et al.: Management for nurses, ed. 2, St. Louis, 1980, The C.V. Mosby Co.
4. Claus, K.E., and Bailey, J.T.: Power and influence in health care, St. Louis, 1977, The C.V. Mosby Co.
5. Coventry, W.F., and Burstiner, I.: Management: a basic handbook, Englewood Cliffs, N.J., 1977, Prentice-Hall, Inc.
6. Donovan, H.M.: Nursing service administration: managing the enterprise, St. Louis, 1975, The C.V. Mosby Co.
7. Douglass, L.M.: The effective nurse leader and manager, St. Louis, 1980, The C.V. Mosby Co.
8. Douglass, L.M., and Berris, E.O.: Nursing management and leadership in action, ed. 3, St. Louis, 1979, The C.V. Mosby Co.
9. Duldt, B.W.: Anger: an alienating communication hazard for nurses, Nurs. Outlook **29**:640-644, 1981.

10. Ewing, D.W.: The practice of planning, New York, 1968, Harper & Row, Publishers, Inc.
11. Ford, J.A.G., Trygstad-Durland, L., and Nelms, B.C.: Applied decision making for nurses, St. Louis, 1979, The C.V. Mosby Co.
12. Ganong, W., and Ganong, J.: Motivation, Maslow and me, Superv. Nurse **4**:25-32, July 1973.
13. Hamm, S.R.: The influence of formal and informal organization within a modern hospital, Superv. Nurse **11**:38-42, Dec. 1980.
14. Janis, I.L., and Mann, L.: Decision making, New York, 1977, The Free Press.
15. Karrass, C.L., and Glasser, W.: Both-win management, New York, 1980, Harper & Row, Publishers, Inc.
16. Keleman, S.: Living your dying, Berkeley, Calif., 1975, Random House: Bookworks.
17. Kistler, J.F., and Kistler, R.: Motivation and morale in the hospital, Superv. Nurse **11**:26-29, Feb. 1980.
18. Koontz, H., and O'Donnell, C.: Management: a book of readings, New York, 1976, McGraw-Hill, Inc.
19. Kramer, M., and Schmalenberg, C.E.: Conflict: the cutting edge of growth, J. Nurs. Adm. **6**:19-25, Oct. 1976.
20. Kubler-Ross, E.: On death and dying, New York, 1969, Macmillan, Inc.
21. Lewin, K.: Field theory in social science, New York, 1951, Harper & Row.
22. Lewis, J.H.: Conflict management, J. Nurs. Adm. **6**:18-22, Dec. 1976.
23. Lupascu, D.: Changing TGIF to TGIM, Nurs. Manage. **12**:25-27, Sept. 1981.
24. Mager, R.F.: Preparing instructional objectives, ed. 2, Belmont, Calif. 1975, Fearon Pitman Publishers, Inc.
25. Mager, R.F., and Pipe, P.: Analyzing performance problems or 'you really oughta wanna', Belmont, Calif., 1970, Fearon Pitman Publishers, Inc.
26. Marriner, A.: The decision making process, Superv. Nurse **8**:58+, Feb. 1977.
27. Marriner, A.: Time management, J. Nurs. Adm. **9**:16-18, Oct. 1979.
28. Marriner, A.: A guide to nursing management, St. Louis, 1980, The C.V. Mosby Co.
29. McCay, J.T.: The management of time, Englewood Cliffs, N.J., 1959, Prentice-Hall, Inc.
30. Moloney, M.M.: Leadership in nursing: theory, strategies, action, St. Louis, 1979, The C.V. Mosby Co.
31. Palmer, J.: Management by objectives, J. Nurs. Adm. pp. 55-60, Sept.-Oct. 1973.
32. Stevens, B.J.: The nurse as executive, ed. 2, Wakefield, Mass., 1980, Nursing Resources, Inc.
33. Thorpe, R.: Sabotage in nursing, Superv. Nurse **12**:24-25, May 1981.
34. Tregoe, B.B., and Zimmerman, J.W.: Top management strategy: what it is and how to make it work, New York, 1980, Simon & Schuster, Inc.
35. Yarbrough, M.G.: Effectiveness of the infection control practitioner as change agent: evaluation by participant observation, A.P.I.C. Journal **5**:46-49, June 1977.

PART THREE

Knowledge base

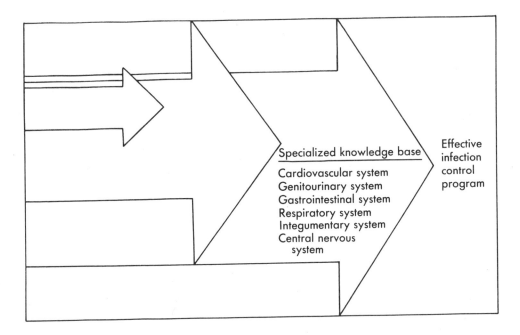

Specialized knowledge base

Cardiovascular system
Genitourinary system
Gastrointestinal system
Respiratory system
Integumentary system
Central nervous
   system

Effective
infection
control
program

Part Three represents the clinical content of the book and will review the current knowledge base of infection control practices related to the following six body systems:
- Cardiovascular
- Genitourinary
- Gastrointestinal
- Respiratory
- Integumentary
- Central nervous system

Each of these systems will be discussed in relation to current research data and general knowledge as it pertains to recommended infection control practices. Each system will be reviewed in the following areas:
- Important anatomical and physiological considerations
- Major infectious diseases
- Etiology of disease

- Signs and symptoms
- Predisposing practices and factors of infections
- Surveillance techniques
- Corrective actions
- Problem solving
- Employee health implications

The knowledge base presented in part three is the final component necessary for the infection control practitioner to effectively enact the role.

13

TRISHA BARRETT

Cardiovascular system

The heart and bloodstream are the pulse and river of life. This remarkable system brings life to the area it traverses, but it can also be the carrier of deadly pollutants. Nature has devised marvelous defense mechanisms to protect the cardiovascular system from invasion. However, the ravages of disease and the invasive practices of modern medicine often succeed in breaching these defenses in hospitalized patients. This chapter will examine salient features of the cardiovascular system, describe the major infections, and discuss important surveillance and prevention techniques.

ANATOMICAL AND PHYSIOLOGICAL CONSIDERATIONS

The infection control practitioner (ICP) must appreciate two basic features of the structure and function of the cardiovascular system (Fig. 13-1) to understand cardiovascular infections and develop appropriate infection control measures. The first is that circulating blood is a common denominator for all body systems. The cardiovascular system not only transports basic nutrients, oxygen, and metabolic by-products but also nonspecific and specific internal defense mechanisms. Examples of *nonspecific* factors include neutrophils, macrophages, lysosomes, and complement. Examples of *specific* circulating defense factors are antibodies, antitoxins, and opsonins. The commonality of circulating blood may be detrimental, as well as beneficial: circulating blood can act as a vehicle for infectious organisms to travel from one body site to another, even if the heart or blood vessels themselves are not primarily infected. This dissemination can occur from a specific infected focus, such as an intraabdominal abscess, or from a body site that is not infected but is normally populated with potentially pathogenic organisms, such as the oropharynx, colon, or perineum.

The second basic feature of the cardiovascular system is that circulating blood and nondiseased heart and vascular tissue are normally sterile. It should be recognized that a competent host may experience transient episodes of bacteremia that do not lead to serious clinical infections. Therefore the presence of any organism—bacteria, mycobacteria, fungi, viruses, or protozoa—in the blood, vascular, or heart tissue may have great importance to the ICP and the clinician.

A major function of the cardiovascular system is to act as the vehicle for the transport of vital substances during the inflammatory response. Inflammation comprises the reaction of hematological, microcirculatory, and connective tis-

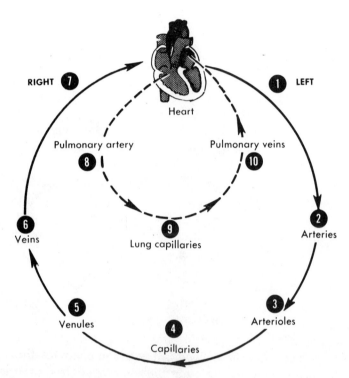

FIG. 13-1. Relationship of systemic and pulmonary circulation. As indicated by the number, blood circulates from the left side (ventricle) of the heart to arteries, to arterioles, to capillaries, to venules, to veins, to the right side of the heart (atrium to ventricle), to the lungs, and back to the left side of the heart, thereby completing a circuit. (From Anthony, C.P., and Thibodeau, G.A.: Textbook of anatomy and physiology, ed. 10, St. Louis, 1981, The C.V. Mosby Co.)

sue injury. Any injury to cells, whether caused by invading microorganisms or allergic reaction, will initiate the same enzymatic systems producing inflammation. These enzymatic systems are complex and many times overlap in their activities. For purposes of clarity each of the systems will be discussed separately, but they are not necessarily discrete in either space or time.

Complement system. The initial injury of the cell disturbs or physically damages the cellular membrane, allowing some of the cellular contents to leak into the extracellular space.[49] This initial contact of cellular protein causes the protein to become modified (lysosomal enzymes released from the cell react on the protein), which activates the complement system. The term *complement* refers to a complex group of enzymes in normal blood serum that, working together with antibodies or other factors, plays an important role as a mediator of immune reactions.[78] The complement system is activated in a set sequence, each step necessary to a particular activity of the inflammatory process (see Fig. 13-2 for a schematic depiction of this system). There is an alternate pathway (properdin pathway) that is capable of activating C_3, thereby sparing C_1, C_4, and

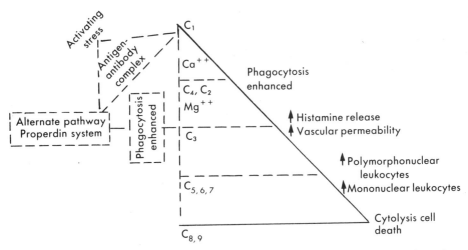

FIG. 13-2. Complement system. (From Blake, P.J., and Perez, R.C.: Applied immunological concepts, New York, 1978, Appleton-Century-Crofts.)

C_2. The alternate pathway that functions as a host defense before antibody formation may be important in neutralization of some viruses and some gram-negative bacteria.[12] The crucial aspect of the complement system is that phago-cytosis requires C_1, C_4, C_2, and C_3 to be activated before it can occur.

Plasmin system. Plasmin is an enzyme that is present in normal plasma as an inactive precursor. It can be activated by tissue damage. Once activated, it is capable of activating the complement system at the C_3 level. Plasmin is also the enzyme responsible for clot disintegration.[49,53]

Clotting system. The initial injury produces modified proteins that activate histamine. Once histamine has caused the vascular membranes to become more permeable, fibrinogen and platelets move into the extracellular space. Fibrin-ogen forms fibrin, which creates a reticulum of fibrin threads, causing the local extracellular and lymphatic fluids to clot. This clotting effect is an attempt to wall off the area of tissue damage, delaying the spread of bacteria or toxic products.[45,49]

Kinin-forming system. The kinin-forming system contributes to the general increased vascular permeability that exists in the inflammatory response. The primary activation of the kinin system is either factor XII of the clotting sys-tem[49] or the plasmin system.[56]

Histamine. Although the action of histamine is not in the form of a system, its contribution to the overall process of inflammation is major. Histamine acts by increasing local blood flow and increasing the permeability of the capil-laries in the area of the injured tissue. The increased permeability allows "large quantities of fluid and protein . . . to leak into the tissues."[56]

To summarize the cellular and microcirculatory responses to tissue damage, there are three primary mechanisms operating: (1) large amounts of histamine are released by various systems to initially open the vascular tissues and allow leakage of vascular substances into the interstitial spaces and to maintain the vascular tissues in a highly permeable condition, (2) a fibrin net forms around the injured tissue in an attempt to limit or delay the spread of bacteria or toxins, and (3) chemical messengers are released into the vascular system and tissues to summon specialized cells for phagocytosis.

Phagocytosis

Phagocytes receive the message to migrate to the injured cell through chemotaxis. Chemotaxis is the unidirectional migration of white cells toward an attractant. The attractant is released when cells become injured. The phago-cytic response operates on a gradient difference, moving from an area of lesser concentration to an area of greater concentration, following electrically charged particles. Once the phagocytic cells arrive at the site of cell injury, they line up on the sides of the vascular wall. This process is called *margination*. Because of the increased vascular permeability of the vascular wall, the phago-cyte is able to elongate a cytoplasmic stream through the enlarged pores of the vessel wall and migrate into the tissues. This process is called *diapedesis*.

Phagocytes ingest particles in a two-step process: first, the phagocyte must attach to the particle; second, the phagocyte surrounds the particle with cyto-plasmic streams and ingests the particle. Once the particle has been engulfed, the phagocytic vacuoles release granule enzymes that have either a bacterio-static or bactericidal effect.

Fever

Fever is defined as a body temperature above the usual range of normal. It can be caused by brain abnormalities or by toxic substances that affect the temperature-regulating center. Pyrogens secreted by bacteria during disease conditions and pyrogens released from degenerating tissues can affect the hy-pothalamic thermostat, causing it to rise. Once this thermostat is reset to a higher level, all the mechanisms for raising the body's temperature are actuated—chills, vasoconstriction and shivering—and the body temperature rises to match the new level. When the pyrogen effect no longer affects the hypotha-lamic thermostat, the hypothalamus is reset to normal. The body responds by lowering the temperature to match the reset of the thermostat with sweating or vasodilation. These signs and symptoms indicate that the fever will be falling. This reset-point is known as the "crisis" point.

Shift to the left

Leukocytosis-promoting factor (LPF) is also liberated by the injured tissue, stimulating the bone marrow to increase the production of neutrophils and platelets. The initial response of the bone marrow to the LPF is in direct response to the amount of LPF released. A large injury could deplete the neutrophils stored in the bone marrow. If the LPF continues to stimulate the bone marrow, immature neutrophils will be released in the blood. Large numbers of immature polymorphonuclear leukocytes in the blood result from a prolonged stimulation from LPF, and this process is termed a *shift to the left*.

MAJOR INFECTIONS OF THE CARDIOVASCULAR SYSTEM
Infective endocarditis

Infective endocarditis is caused by colonization and subsequent invasion of the endocardium by an infectious agent. The term *infective endocarditis* has replaced the term *bacterial endocarditis*, since pathogens other than bacteria have been shown to be etiological agents. *Acute infective endocarditis* (formerly called acute bacterial endocarditis) is the term used when the clinical course has been less than 6 weeks. Duration of 3 months or longer is termed *chronic* or *subacute infective endocarditis* (formerly called subacute bacterial endocarditis, or SBE).[60] Major distinguishing features of these two disease entities follow:

Acute endocarditis	Chronic endocarditis
Usually caused by pyrogenic, virulent bacteria	Usually associated with avirulent bacteria, fungi, and *Rickettsia* organisms
Previously normal heart structures often involved	Typically develops in tissue damaged by preexisting cardiovascular lesion, including prostheses
Usually sequelae of repeated microbial seeding from an obvious source	Source of microbial seeding is more occult
Embolization and suppurative complications more common	Embolization less common
Prognosis poor	Cure is probable

The classic lesion of both acute and chronic endocarditis is vegetation. The vegetative lesion is composed mostly of a necrotic, amorphous mass that abuts the endocardium or endothelium to which it is attached (Fig. 13-3). Over the necrotic core lies a thin layer containing colonies of the infecting microorganisms. Protecting the offending microorganisms is an outer layer of fibrinous, platelet-containing material that essentially protects the infecting organisms from humoral antibodies and circulating leukocytes.

A critical aspect of the vegetation is that emboli are generated as bits of the vegetation break off and are carried into the bloodstream. Catastrophic, cerebral, pulmonary, cardiac, or vascular infarction can occur, as well as less damaging, but nevertheless destructive, microembolization in other body organs.

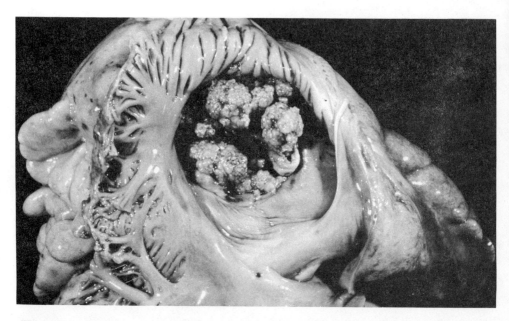

FIG. 13-3. Endocarditis. Dilated right atrium opened to expose valvular orifice. Note large cauliflower-like excrescences (vegetation) on leaflets of tricuspid valve. Causative organism was *Candida albicans*. Patient was a drug addict and hence a person prone to involvement of tricuspid valve. (From Smith, A.L.: Microbiology and pathology, ed. 12, St. Louis, 1981, The C.V. Mosby Co.)

There are two major reasons that the ICP should be familiar with acute and chronic infective endocarditis. First, infective endocarditis can originate from a nosocomial source. Prosthetic valve endocarditis develops in 1% to 2% of patients after prosthetic valve placement.[124] Infective endocarditis has also been documented after closed heart surgery.[41] Other invasive procedures have been associated with nosocomial infective endocarditis, such as hemodialysis,[36] intrauterine device insertion,[30,42] cardiac catheterization,[7] venous catheterization,[8] total parenteral nutrition,[54] and intraarterial monitoring.[55] Obviously not all infective endocarditis is hospital acquired. Structural, congenital, and luetic heart diseases, arteriovenous fistula, acute rheumatic fever, IV drug abuse, and even animal bites can predispose a patient to infective endocarditis. In an extensive review of infective endocarditis from the University of Washington Hospitals (1963 to 1972), Pelletier and Petersdorf[93] found 35 (28%) of 125 cases to be nosocomial in origin.

Aside from establishing a community versus nosocomial etiology, the second important consideration for the ICP is that patients with a history of infective endocarditis, or one of the predisposing factors mentioned earlier, should be monitored as compromised hosts. Once a valve surface is altered, it may become suitable for bacterial attachment and colonization. Any manipulation or contamination of the bloodstream that results in bacteremia or fungemia could result in infective endocarditis. Special care should be given to avoid such situations in these patients. There is also a role for the ICP in developing discharge teaching plans that include prevention and prophylactic treatment considerations. Every effort should be made to prevent the serious complication of infective endocarditis during and after hospitalization.

To complete the discussion of infective endocarditis a review of etiological agents is in order. Although many different bacteria and fungi have been implicated in causing endocarditis, streptococci and staphylococci account for 80% to 90% of the cases for which an identification is made.[106] Enterococci may be responsible for 5% to 18% of cases,[108] and the incidence appears to be increasing, perhaps related to increased drug abuse and medical genitourinary manipulations. Gram-negative bacilli account for 1.5% to 13% of cases.[106] One study[16] that reviewed 44 cases of gram-negative endocarditis revealed the following breakdown: *Escherichia coli,* 17; *Serratia marcescens,* 13; *Klebsiella* and *Enterobacter* species, 9; *Proteus* species, 2; *Providencia* species, 2; and *Citrobacter* species, 1. These organisms are commonly identified as nosocomial pathogens, and mortality rates in gram-negative endocarditis have been reported to be as high as 83%.[93] Fungi account for 2% to 4% of all cases.[106] Fungal endocarditis is usually associated with IV drug abuse, reconstructive cardiovascular surgery, or prolonged IV and/or antibiotic treatment. Many infectious disease experts predict that fungi will gain importance as nosocomial pathogens in the future. Therefore an increase in nosocomial fungal endocarditis would not be unexpected.

Septicemia—bacteremia and fungemia

Any discussion of septicemia should begin with a clear definition of terms. Physicians and nurses often use the terms *sepsis, septicemia, bacteremia,* and *septic shock* interchangeably. For the purpose of clarity I will define certain terms:

septicemia The presence of pathogenic microorganisms, or their toxins, within circulating blood.[85]
bacteremia The presence of bacteria in circulating blood.
fungemia The presence of fungi in circulating blood.
viremia The presence of virus in circulating blood.
septic shock A syndrome of circulatory insufficiency with hypoperfusion of body tissues resulting from an inadequate cardiac output caused by the systemic effects of pathogenic microorganisms, or their toxins, within the blood.[85]
sepsis The clinical picture that is consistent with the presence of microorganisms or their toxic by-products in circulating blood, as determined by a clinician.

Septicemia, like endocarditis, is a serious and sometimes fatal infection of the cardiovascular system. Although septicemia can be caused by virus (viremia), the remainder of this section will be devoted to a discussion of bacteremia and fungemia, the more common nosocomial manifestations of septicemia.

Bacteremias are generally classified as either "primary" or "secondary." Primary bacteremia occurs as a direct contamination of the bloodstream without another underlying, clinically evident site of infection. Secondary bacteremia is clinically, temporally, and microbiologically related to an apparent infection at another body site.[115] The incidence of primary and secondary bacteremia in hospital patients varies, depending on the author and type of hospital studied. Early reports were primarily from university hospitals and referral centers. McGowan reported a community and nosocomial bacteremia rate of 13 per 1000 admissions in 1977 from Grady Memorial Hospital[81] and 28 per 1000 admissions in 1972 from Boston City Hospital.[80] In contrast, Scheckler[105] reported a considerably lower rate of 3.4 per 1000 admissions over a 4-year period from a community teaching hospital in 1978. This variability is undoubtedly related to the severity of underlying disease in different patient populations. Scheckler demonstrated that there was a striking increase in the incidence of septicemia as the severity of underlying illness increased. Another factor that will lead to differences in the incidence of nosocomial bacteremia from hospital to hospital is the number of invasive manipulations that are carried out. Regardless of the type of hospital, all investigators report significant case fatality rates for gram-negative bacteremia from 25% to 58%.[115]

Bacterial pathogens will vary, depending on whether the bacteremia is community or hospital acquired. For instance, an analysis of 583 cases of bacteremia reported from Boston City Hospital in 1972 showed that 69% of community-acquired bacteremias were gram-positive, with Streptococcus pneumoniae, Streptococcus viridans, and Staphylococcus aureus the most frequent isolates in that order. Of the remaining 31% community-acquired gramnegative bacteremias, over half were caused by E. coli. In the same series hospital-acquired bacteremias revealed a markedly different bacteriological pattern. Of the nosocomial bacteremias, 52% were gram-negative, with Klebsiella and Enterobacter species, E. coli, Proteus species, and Pseudomonas aeruginosa the most common isolates in that order. Gram-positive hospitalacquired bacteremia was most frequently caused by S. aureus, followed by enterococcal species and S. viridans.[80] In general, nosocomial bacteremia will most frequently be caused by gram-negative organisms or S. aureus. Community-acquired bacteremia is most likely to be caused by a gram-positive coccus or E. coli.

Both gram-negative and gram-positive bacteremia can lead to septic shock. Gram-positive bacteremia is responsible for only about 25% of all episodes of septic shock. Far more common, septic shock is preceded by an episode of gram-negative bacteremia. The pathogenesis and treatment of gram-negative septic shock are described in great detail in other sources.[94] I mention it here only to highlight its clinical significance.

Fungemia has been less frequently reported than bacteremia, but it is becoming increasingly important. Community-acquired fungemia is most commonly associated with IV drug abuse. Nosocomial fungemia is usually caused by *Candida albicans*, *Aspergillus* species, or *Torulopsis* species and is associated with reconstructive cardiovascular surgery, prolonged IV therapy, total parenteral nutrition, and prolonged antibiotic therapy. Patients with fungemia are generally extremely compromised, and treatment with antifungal agents is fraught with difficulties. For these reasons the prognosis is poor, and the case fatality rate is high.[106]

Suppurative thrombophlebitis

Suppurative thrombophlebitis (ST) is an infection, usually bacterial, of the vein wall and is often associated with clot (thrombus) formation and bacteremia. The two major forms of ST that will be discussed here are *superficial suppurative thrombophlebitis*, associated with the superficial and subcutaneous veins, and *pelvic thrombophlebitis*, associated with the venous system of the female pelvic organs. Two other forms of ST, *cavernous sinus thrombophlebitis* and *pylephlebitis* (infection of the portal vein), have become relatively rare with the advent of antimicrobial therapy and will not be discussed in this chapter.

The pathophysiology of superficial ST is not completely understood. When ST is associated with IV invasion by a steel needle or plastic cannula, the route of invasion by the offending microorganisms is (1) by direct inoculation of contaminants from IV fluid into the vein, (2) migration from the dermal wound of insertion along the exterior wall of the needle or catheter, or (3) hematogenous microbial seeding of the IV device from a remote site of infection. It is generally believed that the clot that forms as a natural response to invasion of the vein acts as a nidus for the offending microorganisms in somewhat the same way that vegetation tissue houses pathogens in infective endocarditis. Those authors[21] that report a higher phlebitis rate with plastic cannulas than with steel needles suggest that the difference is related to this mechanism for fibrin sheath formation. Reports of superficial ST have highlighted specific risk factors such as burn injury,[98] cutdown insertion site,[116] lower extremity insertion site,[35,76] cannula insertion at the same site for longer than 48 hours,[32] underlying neoplastic disease, and steroid therapy.[106] In ST there are certain pathogenic changes that take place within the vein. The vein will become enlarged, thickened, and more tortuous as a result of internal pus formation, hemorrhage, and clot formation. When viewed microscopically, the vein wall reveals endothelial damage, fibrinoid necrosis, and thickening of the lumen. As liquefaction and fragmentation of the thrombi occur, there may be spreading of septic emboli, causing metastatic abscesses, pulmonary emboli, or endocarditis.[106] Removal of the infected intravascular device, surgical drainage of accumulated pus, and appropriate antibiotic therapy are necessary to cure superficial ST. If these interventions are not successful, it is sometimes necessary to surgically remove the entire infected vein.[88] One author of a recent review article on superficial ST pointed out that up until 1968 the most frequently reported causative agent for this infection was S. aureus, accounting for 65% to 78% of reported cases. However, review of the literature since 1970 reveals that Klebsiella and Enterobacter species are reported three times more frequently than S. aureus[106] (see box below). Whether these reports truly reflect a change in the microbiological aspects of superficial ST or are simply artifacts of over-reporting of unusual pathogens is not clear.

The other form of ST that warrants attention is pelvic thrombophlebitis. Pelvic thrombophlebitis is a cardiovascular infection that is generally limited to women of childbearing age. The intravascular changes are the same as those described in the discussion of superficial ST. Predisposing factors for the development of pelvic thrombophlebitis are childbirth, abortion, gynecological surgery, or precedent pelvic abscess. Any of the major veins that drain the pelvis may be affected in pelvic thrombophlebitis, but most commonly the veins draining the uterus and the inferior vena cava are involved. The common pathogens for pelvic septic thrombophlebitis are Bacteroides species, anaerobic streptococci, and gram-negative bacilli.[90] These organisms are normal flora in the vagina and perineum that gain access to a thrombus through the bloodstream or lymphatic channels at the time of childbirth or gynecological

Etiological agents of nosocomial superficial suppurative thrombophlebitis in 31 cases reported since 1970[8,116]

Organism	Number of cases
Klebsiella and Enterobacter species	12
Staphylococcus aureus	5
Providencia species	5
Proteus species	5
Serratia species	3
Escherichia coli	3
Candida albicans	3
Pseudomonas aeruginosa	2

Note: 14 cases were found at autopsy; five patients had two bacterial isolates from single vein; one patient had three cultures from three separate veins.

manipulation.[106] The ICP who monitors obstetrical and gynecological populations should be alert to this infection as a possibility in the febrile patient.

Intravascular graft infections

The science of surgical manipulation of the vascular system dates back to
1903 with the first experimental arterial transplants using animal tissue to
replace diseased, occluded vessels. These advances have been accompanied by
infectious complications. Infection can occur at the site of the implanted vessel
(autograft, plastic prosthesis, or animal implant) or at the donor site in the case
of autograft transfer. Reported rates of infection range from 0.2% to 7%, with
intraabdominal implants less frequently infected than implants placed more
distally.[39,106] Mechanisms for infection are generally believed to be (1) intraoperative contamination, (2) extension of infection from an adjacent tissue site,
or (3) hematogenous seeding of the implant during a bacteremic episode. The
microbiological factors of these infections vary with the anatomical location of
the vascular graft. S. aureus and Staphylococcus epidermidis are the most
common etiological agents when the graft is in the groin or popliteal site.
Aerobic gram-negative bacilli, principally E. coli, are the usual culprits if the
graft is in an abdominal site. Grafts at all sites are most likely to become
infected within the first month of implantation.

Vascular access sites for hemodialysis may be created by a prosthetic implant (usually Gortex), an animal heterograft implant (bovine), or creation of an
arteriovenous fistula. One large review[57] of 516 procedures in 444 patients
revealed a total infection complication rate of 2.1%. In this series peripheral
arteriovenous fistulas carried a lower infection rate (1.5%) than bovine heterograft fistulae (6.5%). The presumed mechanisms for infections at these sites
are either intraoperative contamination or, more commonly, contamination
during continual entry for hemodialysis and/or phlebotomy. The microbiological aspects of hemodialysis access site infections is probably similar to that
encountered in other distal vascular graft infections, as discussed earlier.
Onorato et al.[92] reported two cases of mixed fungal and S. aureus infection in
dialysis fistulas.

ENDOGENOUS AND EXOGENOUS SOURCES OF
CARDIOVASCULAR INFECTIONS
Endogenous sources

In the past health care professionals tended to consider hospital-acquired
infections as only those associated with an exogenous animate or environmental source. Since the Centers for Disease Control (CDC) published the Revised Outline for Surveillance and Control of Nosocomial Infections in 1972,
most ICPs and infectious disease experts consider infections occurring after

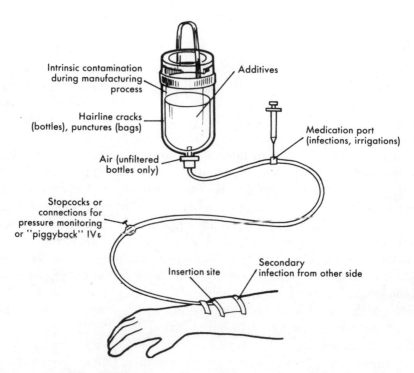

FIG. 13-4. Potential portals of entry for IV-associated infections. (Modified from Castle, M.: Hospital infection control: principles and practice, New York, 1980, John Wiley & Sons, Inc.)

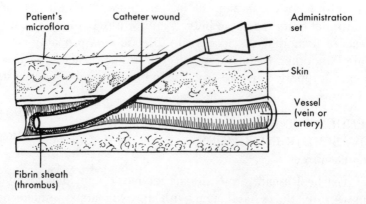

FIG. 13-5. Predisposing factors in percutaneous insertion of cannulas for IV therapy. (From Maki, D.G.: In Phillips, I., Meers, P.O., and D'Arcy, P.F., editors: Microbiological hazards of intravenous therapy, Lancaster, Eng., 1977, MTP Press, Ltd., p. 106.)

hospitalization from endogenous sources, as well as from exogenous sources, to be nosocomial (Fig. 13-4). There are two primary endogenous sources for cardiovascular infections. The most common endogenous source is the microbial milieu of the patient's skin through which may pass an indwelling or intermittent invasive device. In a percutaneous insertion of a needle or plastic cannula the wound through the skin is small, but bacteria that have not been removed at the time of insertion or bacteria that proliferate after insertion and migrate from the skin along the sheath of the wound can cause superficial suppurative thrombophlebitis and/or bacteremia (Fig. 13-5). The surgical wound created during a cutdown is much larger and more likely to develop a small surgical wound infection that will disseminate large numbers of microorganisms into the affected vessel. These organisms are the "normal flora" of the patient. Risk factors such as exposure to intensive care units, underlying disease, administration of total parenteral nutrition, and especially prolonged administration of antibiotics are known to change the composition of resident skin flora in hospital patients. Most cardiovascular infections originating from the skin are caused by S. aureus or S. epidermidis. Several authors have reported fungal complications when prolonged antibiotic use or total parenteral nutrition were involved[86] or when there was underlying neoplastic disease present.[59,73] If there is extensive injury to the skin, as in burn wounds, then aerobic gram-negative bacilli can be the endogenous organisms.[95]

Endogenous organisms can cause cardiovascular infections by another less obvious process. As mentioned earlier, the blood moves in a continuous flow through all body organs. A condition at any body site that results in microorganisms entering the bloodstream will constitute an endogenous source of septicemia. The septicemic episode may run the clinical spectrum from an asymptomatic, transient episode to a serious cardiovascular infection such as endocarditis or gram-negative septic shock, depending largely on the magnitude of the infective inoculum and the competency of the host to handle the assault. An active infection at another body site is always a potential source of bacteremia. Several investigators have pointed out the relationship between urinary tract infections and subsequent gram-negative bacteremia.[80,81,85,115] Abscess formation in any body organ will intermittently disperse microorganisms into the bloodstream. Vigorous manipulation of mucosal surfaces or lesions that are normally colonized with large numbers of microorganisms can result in endogenous contamination of the otherwise sterile bloodstream. Following are some procedures other than IV fluid administration that cause endogenous bloodstream contamination:

- Arterial puncture
- Nasotracheal suctioning
- Genitourinary manipulation
- Sigmoidoscopy

- Liver biopsy
- Use of oral WaterPik
- Dental manipulation
- Barium enema
- Fiberoptic bronchoscopy
- Upper gastrointestinal tract endoscopy
- Angiography
- Endotracheal intubation

Tumors that erode through skin, mucous membrane organs, or abdominal and pelvic viscera may also account for endogenous organisms invading normally sterile body tissues.

Exogenous sources

IV administration of fluids was first used as a medical treatment by Thomas Latta in 1832 during a cholera epidemic in a desperate attempt to replace fluids in his disease-ravaged patients. Along with the life-saving benefits of IV fluids came the inevitable complications.

The primary exogenous source for nosocomial cardiovascular infections is contamination of an IV or intraarterial fluid administration system. Such contamination can occur at the site of manufacture. Between 1965 and 1975 manufacturers recalled 608 large-volume parenteral products (involving 43 million already distributed containers) because of product contamination. The first report of contaminated IV fluid was made by Michaels and Ruebner[84] in 1953 but was largely ignored until 1971 when the CDC[17,18] reported a nationwide epidemic of bacteremia caused by IV fluid containers. In 25 U.S. hospitals 378 patients experienced bacteremia with Enterobacter cloacae or Enterobacter agglomerans, which was subsequently traced to contaminated Elastomer liners in the threaded caps that covered the bottle before use.[77] Investigation of this outbreak led to a change in bottle covers. This investigation also noted that visual inspection for fluid turbidity would not have identified contaminated bottles. In 1973, in England, Lapage, Johnson, and Holmes,[64] reported two similar outbreaks of bacteremia associated with IV infusion in which manufacturing processes were implicated as the sources for contamination. In one outbreak involving contaminated normal serum albumin the source of contamination was not identified, but the investigator[114] felt that contamination had occurred sporadically during filling of individual vials. The contamination was so slight that it was not detected at the time of manufacture or administration. Aside from contamination at the site of production, parenteral fluid can become contaminated during shipping and storage. The bottles or bags get hairline cracks or tiny punctures that may not result in obvious leakage but do allow for passage of organisms into the fluid. Common soil or water organisms like pseudomonal species, Klebsiella and Enterobacter species, and fungi can enter the fluid in small numbers only to grow and multiply to large inoculum sizes before the fluid is administered. Even in concentrations exceeding 10^6 organisms per milliliter the contamination may not be visually detectable.[71] Daisy, Abutyn, and MacGregor[38] surveyed 113 infectious disease specialists in 1979 to see how many had had experience with inadvertent administration of IV fluid contaminated with fungus. They found that 18 had seen a total of 24 cases. Fluid containers were often found to be defective, and the fungi were presumed to have entered the fluid after the defect had occurred.

Intrahospital manipulations of the parenteral fluid before or after beginning administration constitute a number of significant exogenous sources of contamination. *Enterobacter aerogenes* bacteremia[23] and *Candida parapsilosis* fungemia[95] have both been reported to be epidemiologically linked to the IV additive process in the hospital pharmacy. Multiple-dose vials for medication can be a source for contamination in a centralized pharmacy admixture program or on the nursing unit. Any point of connection or entry in the administration apparatus is a possible portal of entry for exogenous organisms. An outbreak of *Flavobacterium* bacteremias highlighted the opportunity for the organism to gain entry during blood gas determinations in patients with indwelling arterial catheters.[113] The organism was cultured from catheter hubs, stopcocks, and ice used to cool syringes. Unprotected stopcock ports undoubtedly become colonized with endogenous and exogenous organisms after prolonged exposure. Several authors[1,21,22,44,122] have identified nonsterile pressure transducers as potential reservoirs for exogenous contaminants.

A few other unusual exogenous sources of cardiovascular infections have been identified. In 1974 several types of intravascular devices including angiocatheters, subclavian catheters, and cutdown catheters were recalled because of microbial contamination.[26] Although unusual, the possibility of contamination of an IV product prepared and sterilized by a manufacturer must not be forgotten. Even commercially produced antiseptic agents have been epidemiologically implicated in nosocomial infections. Another obscure source of exogenous cardiovascular infection may be the use of unsterile products or devices. One example was a report of bacteremia associated with the use of Elastoplast occlusive dressing.[6] This product was used to create an occlusive dressing over central IV lines. The product is not marketed or advertised as a sterile product and has been linked to *Rhizopus* species infections in another report.[50] Even radiopaque contrast media have been identified as possible sources of cardiovascular infection.[109] It seems as though the possibilities of exogenous contamination of the cardiovascular system are unlimited with the increasing use of IV fluid administration, vascular access for diagnostic purposes, and intravascular hemodynamic monitoring. Table 13-1 depicts the common sources of exogenous IV fluid contamination and appropriate nursing interventions.

TABLE 13-1. Sources of exogenous IV fluid contamination

Source of contamination	Nursing approach
Manufacture, shipping, and storage	Inspect fluid for cloudiness or color change; notify infection control department
Hairline cracks in bottle or holes in bag	Inspect container for signs of leakage, cracks, holes, or other defects; remove from use immediately; return to storeroom; notify infection control department
Adding medications to bottle	Aseptic technique (in pharmacy when possible)
Stopcocks, manometers, and transducers	Aseptic handling; protect ports; change frequently; sterilization
Piggyback, IV, and push medications	Aseptic handling
Changes of bottles and tubing	Aseptic handling
Irrigations or declotting	Aseptic handling
Collecting blood	Aseptic handling; monitor laboratory or respiratory therapy technique
Unfiltered air if filter damaged (bottles only)	Prime correctly; discard if filter is wet or damaged

COMMON SIGNS AND SYMPTOMS OF CARDIOVASCULAR INFECTIONS
Fever

The healthy body maintains a temperature in its tissues and fluids within a relatively narrow range despite diverse environmental temperatures. Although allowances must be made for individual variation, most people will have a body temperature between 96.5° F (35.8° C) and 99° F (37.2° C). An elevation above 99° F with a concomitant elevation in pulse rate (about 10 beats per minute per degree Fahrenheit) is generally accepted as "fever."[61] Fever, as defined here, is one of the cardinal manifestations of infectious disease until proven to be noninfectious in origin. It is attractive as a diagnostic and surveillance tool because it can be easily and reliably measured.

Although fever has been recognized for centuries as a sign of infection, the exact mechanism for fever in the infectious process was not clearly understood. Since the mid-1940s, researchers have learned that infectious fevers are caused by exogenous pyrogens that upwardly displace the body's normal hypothalamic set-point. Microorganisms and their cellular components may be the source of the exogenous pyrogens. For example, it is well established that gram-negative bacteria contain a complex lipopolysaccharide in their cell walls that when introduced into the bloodstream evokes a mediator, or endogenous pyrogen, that is produced by some host cell.[10] Granulocytes appear to be the primary source of endogenous pyrogens, although monocytes and tissue macrophages have been shown experimentally to elaborate endogenous pyrogens. The higher hypothalamic set-point induces the body to raise its temperature, thereby diminishing loss of body heat by reducing cutaneous circulation and sweating. The body may also induce heat production through increased muscle rigors, creating the not uncommon symptom of hard, shaking "chills." Bernheim, Block, and Atkins[10] make the intriguing point that there may be a specific purpose for a fever in the resolution of an infection. They point out that higher temperatures increase uptake of thymidine in lymphocytes and increase the phagocytic activity of leukocytes. There is also experimental evidence to show increased leukocyte migration and localization of infection at higher than normal temperatures.

Infectious fever has been described as having several patterns in relation to time. Specific infectious diseases have been linked to specific fever patterns, such as sustained fever with typhus or tularemia, intermittent fever with tuberculosis or abscesses, or relapsing fever with malaria or brucellosis. These are generalities, and an individual fever pattern will be of limited diagnostic value. Most authors do agree that the vigor of the febrile response does diminish with age. Fever may vary in magnitude during the day. It is not uncommon to observe infected patients with temperature elevations at the maximum in the afternoon. This is probably an amplification of the normal body temperature cycle, which is highest in the afternoon and lowest in the morning.

Although the finding of fever is an important sign in identifying infected patients, the lack of fever does not exclude the possibility of serious infection. As already mentioned, extremes in age may decrease the body's ability to mount an appropriate fever response in the infant or the elderly patient. A suspicion of septicemia in such patients must be based on subtle behavioral or sensorial changes. Because the mechanism of fever depends largely on circulating, competent granulocytes, granulocytopenic patients may not run significantly high fevers even during massive infection. When the granulocytopenic patient does spike a fever, the endogenous pyrogens are probably supplied by macrophages. Other than extremes in age and underlying granulocytopenia, just the presence of overwhelming infection may result in an impaired fever response. In one large review[62] of gram-negative bacteremia in 612 patients 83 (13%) were found to have rectal temperatures of <97.6° F. Although shock and fatal outcome were no more frequent in the hypothermic group, it was noted that prior corticosteroid therapy appeared to blunt the febrile response.

Erythema and pus formation in superficial suppurative thrombophlebitis

Erythema, or redness, is another of the classical signs of infection. It is the cutaneous manifestation of increased circulation in the inflammatory response. From an evolutionary standpoint, erythema probably exists so that the host can visualize and therefore protect an area of injury. Erythema, redness, or cellulitis is a significant diagnostic finding in superficial suppurative thrombophlebitis. Phlebitis, or inflammation of a blood vessel, can be caused by mechanical injury, toxic local reaction to substances being infused, or microbial invasion of the vessel wall and/or surrounding tissues. When present, cellulitis or erythema is a sign of local reaction to invasion or infection. Evaluation of redness without evidence of purulence or pus formation is sometimes difficult. Rhame, Maki, and Bennett[100] give the following parameters for deciding if catheter-associated cellulitis is infectious or chemical: "When the inflammation is clearly separable from the vein, especially if it is distal to the insertion site, infection is usually present. Inflammation that is restricted to the course of the vein, however, may be caused by mechanical or chemical irritation from the cannula or the IV solution and its additives." A negative finding of erythema when IV site infection is suspected should not rule out the possibility. Various authors report different experiences with regard to local signs of erythema and proven IV device infection. Watanakunakorn and Baird[121] reported one series of 21 cases of intravascular device infection in which all but one patient had evidence of cellulitis. Stein and Pruitt[116] and O'Neill et al.[91] reported that swelling, tenderness, and erythema were rare in their series.

A finding of pus draining from the site of intravascular access devices is always considered a sign of infection. Pus is the liquid product of inflammation, composed of albuminous substances and leukocytes or their remains. Very often the purulent material will not be obvious until the phlebitic vein is "milked" from a site proximal to the insertion site. Even though this process may be painful to the patient, the diagnostic value of the material obtained for culture warrants vigorous attempts to remove the pus from the vein.

Positive blood cultures

Clinically significant cardiovascular infections will usually result in positive blood cultures if specimens are collected properly. In cases of endocarditis the bacteremia is nearly constant. A blood culture taken anytime will usually reveal the infecting organism. Other disease states, however, may not produce a state of constant contamination of the blood. When the bacteremia or fungemia is intermittent, it may be difficult to recover the offending organisms. The yield in these situations is greatest if blood cultures are obtained just before an expected rise in body temperature. Since this time is usually difficult to predict, the next best period is immediately after a temperature spike and/or chill.

Two or three specimens should be drawn from separate venipuncture sites. Multiple blood samples from separate sites will confirm the diagnosis when the same organism is obtained in separate samples. Separate venipunctures from several sites will also help rule out whether the organism recovered is a contaminant in one puncture or the responsible pathogen.[118] Distinguishing pathogens from contaminants in positive blood cultures is often very difficult. For instance, when one out of three blood cultures obtained is positive for S. epidermidis in a patient with a prosthetic heart valve, it may not be clear that this is a contaminant. The method of collection, clinical condition of the patient, type of organisms identified, and epidemiological information must all be considered. Regardless of the organism, all positive blood cultures should be viewed as bacteremia or fungemia until proven otherwise. (See "Surveillance" for a more complete discussion of blood culture contaminants, or "Pseudobacteremia.")

COMMON HOSPITAL PRACTICES RELATED TO CARDIOVASCULAR INFECTIONS AND PERTINENT PREVENTIVE OR CORRECTIVE ACTION

In this section specific cardiovascular manipulations will be discussed in detail. Each topic will be reviewed as to common practices, indications, complications, and pertinent preventive or corrective actions.

Insertion of peripheral IV devices (steel needle or plastic catheter)

Peripheral venous access is the modality of choice for the delivery of drugs, fluid, and blood products when the patient's condition requires parenteral administration of these substances. (In some cases the patient's condition is so complicated that central cardiovascular access is necessary for delivery of fluid, drugs, and blood products or for purposes of hemodynamic monitoring. Central cardiovascular access will be discussed later in this section.) Peripheral venous access devices should be inserted and maintained indwelling only as long as there is a specific therapeutic indication. IV administration of fluid or medication should be discontinued as soon as is therapeutically possible. The policy of "routine" insertion of IV devices in certain high-risk patients (e.g., emergency room, coronary care unit) should be carefully scrutinized in each institution. Devices inserted under such routine protocols should be assessed several times a day and removed as soon as the patient is stabilized.

Skin flora from the patient or from the health professional inserting the IV device can serve as the causative agent for IV site infection. These organisms gain access to the tip of the device and the bloodstream both at the time of insertion and subsequently by migrating along the interface between the catheter and tissue. A variety of antimicrobial agents have been studied for their antibacterial effects both as handwash disinfectants and site preparation agents.[76] Careful handwashing by health care personnel before inserting an IV device is a crucial preventive measure and cannot be stressed too frequently. Since IV insertion of a needle or catheter is a minor surgical procedure, it does not seem unreasonable that the health care worker be required to use an iodophor or chlorhexidine gluconate antiseptic handwash agent. These products have broad-spectrum activity against gram-negative and gram-positive organisms.[27] The CDC,[24] Maki et al.,[76] and Goldman et al.[53] all suggest the use of sterile gloves during insertion. Although this practice offers optimal aseptic protection in theory, widespread acceptance of and compliance with using gloves by those doing the insertions is doubtful. The use of sterile drapes for routine peripheral IV device insertion would also seem to be impractical. If scrupulous handwashing and aseptic "no touch" technique are taught and religiously employed, a similar degree of safety is probably achieved.

Adequate reduction of microorganisms on the patient's skin before insertion of the needle or catheter is of equal if not greater importance than reduction of organisms on the hands of the health care worker. The two generally accepted skin preparations are (1) 1% to 2% tincture of iodine, followed by removal with 70% isopropyl alcohol after the iodine has dried for at least 30 seconds,[24,53,76] or (2) a vigorous scrub for at least 1 minute with an iodophor solution that should not be washed off.[52,76] In rare instances when the patient is sensitive to iodine preparations, the IV insertion site should be vigorously scrubbed wih 70% isopropyl alcohol for at least 1 minute. In no situation should aqueous benzalkonium chloride or other quaternary ammonia compounds be used. These substances have been repeatedly implicated in epidemics when they have become contaminated by gram-negative rods.

Some other common insertion practices have not been completely studied for their infection prevention or control implications. Although it has never been studied, it is considered good practice to securely anchor the needle or catheter to prevent friction and trauma to the cannulated vein and to assure security and patency. Such taping should be done in a fashion that allows for easy observation of the insertion site and surrounding tissues. Shaving has never been studied specifically related to IV site infection, but Cruse and Foord[37] demonstrated an increased infection risk associated with razor shaving of surgical wound sites. One well-controlled study[107] showed a significant reduction of this risk when a depilatory was used instead of a razor. By extrapolating these data to IV sites, it would seem reasonable to use a depilatory if hair removal is required. Hair removal is more of a patient comfort issue than an infection control concern, since the presence of hair is relatively unimportant to the bacterial flora of the skin.[97] The various types of dressing applied after insertion, such as a Bandaid, gauze pad, or clear occlusive self-adhesive plastic, have not been adequately studied in well-controlled trials to make a definitive recommendation. Suffice it to say that the dressing should be sterile when applied, promote security and cleanliness of the insertion site, and be placed such that frequent observations of the insertion site and surrounding tissues can be easily made.

The skill and knowledge of the person responsible for insertion of the IV device is probably one of the most important factors related to the development of IV site infection. This has not been as carefully studied as some of the specific aspects of insertion technique, but there are a few intriguing studies in print that look at competency of the "inserter" as related to development of phlebitis. One study that looked at phlebitis alone, not specifically infection, showed rates of phlebitis highest when house staff started IVs and lowest when the IV was started by well-trained members of an IV team. The author[33] suggests that skill and knowledge of the inserter were the determining factors. A much better controlled study[13] that looked specifically at IV site infection and eliminated the variable of irritating drugs had similar findings. These authors showed that medical personnel improved their understanding of infection risk factors slightly after an education program but that they frequently ignored proper standards. The only significant reduction in infection occurred in a group of patients for which the ICP was a passive observer of the insertion procedure. Aside from education and competency, the more difficult question of procedure-by-procedure compliance must be addressed. The use of IV teams must be evaluated in each institution on the basis of available personnel, style of nursing care offered, cost effectiveness, and endemic IV-associated infection experience.

Choice of peripheral access device

One issue that has not been completely resolved by well-controlled clinical studies is whether steel scalp-vein ("butterfly") needles carry a lower infection risk than plastic catheters. Three factors that depend on the characteristics of the insertion device are phlebitis, or local reaction to the foreign body; thrombus formation; and trauma of insertion. Collins et al.[32] reported a 39% phlebitis rate in a prospective study of 213 plastic catheter insertions. Not all of these were infections, but the incidence of phlebitis increased with duration of the device in the same site. Since plastic catheters usually remain in place longer than steel needles, they probably carry a higher rate of phlebitis for that reason alone. Maki et al.[76] postulated that the clot that forms on the surface of a plastic catheter contains microorganisms from the dermal wound or circulating blood and accounts for higher rates of phlebitis. No such thrombus formation has been reported with steel needles. The last factor, trauma of insertion, is a function of the configuration and size of the device. A pliable plastic catheter necessitates the use of an interior needle to make the venipuncture. Therefore the tip is generally more blunt and has a larger diameter than a steel needle, and the added manipulation of removing the inner needle probably creates greater local trauma at the time of insertion.

Steel needles, however, are not without reported infection complications. Band and Maki[5] reported 36.1% local inflammation, 5.4% local infection, and 2.1% bacteremia when steel needles were used in 148 episodes in patients with granulocytopenia. These authors pointed out that previous combined prospective studies involving 778 needle insertions had shown a needle-related septicemia rate of only 0.16%, but these studies had not included immunosuppressed patients. There have also been anecdotal reports of suppurative phlebitis from scalp-vein needles.[73,96] In all these reports infections increased the longer the needle was left in the same site.

The heparin-lock device is an adaptation of either a steel scalp-vein needle or a plastic catheter. This is achieved by the insertion of an adapter with a multiple-puncture diaphragm into the needle or catheter. The device allows for intermittent chemotherapy infusions when the patient's condition does not require continuous fluid replacement. After each medication infusion, the heparin-lock device is irrigated with a heparinized solution to prevent clotting before the next medication dose, and the tubing is disconnected. This allows the patient to move around unencumbered by tubings, bottles, and poles. A prospective evaluation of complications with 221 heparin-lock needle insertions in 78 patients revealed a 12% phlebitis rate with no systemic infections.[47] A smaller study[34] showed an overall 10.8% phlebitis rate for 120 insertions in 97 patients. In another series,[46] which looked at site care for heparin-lock needles, the same investigators found a 36% phlebitis rate. Factors that were statistically linked to the increased rate in the last study were positive culture of a normal saline flush of the device at time of removal, number of different drugs infused, number of manipulations, and positive culture of the insertion site. All three of these reports were from the same investigators, and most of the patients were not immunosuppressed. There is one anecdotal report[2] of two patients with leukemia in whom cellulitis and septicemia developed subsequent to the use of heparin-lock needles. The observation in all the groups that phlebitis increased with time at the same site leads to a recommendation that heparin-lock sites be rotated every 48 to 72 hours as is recommended for all peripheral devices.

The heparin-lock device carries another risk: complacency. Heparin-lock devices are often put in on a routine basis to assure vascular access. Once the patient is stabilized, the heparin-lock device is overlooked and often remains in place for longer than is necessary. The other situation that is often observed is that as the patient improves and is switched to heparin-lock intermittent infusions from continuous infusion the scrutiny of the site and adherence to established policies slacken.

The choice of an IV access device should be based on the known infection risks and the condition of the patient. Steel needles should be the first choice for either continuous or intermittent infusions. Scrupulous handwashing and aseptic technique should be employed at insertion regardless of the device chosen. Heparin-lock devices and intermittent infusions must be handled with the same standard of asepsis that is applied to continuous infusion devices. All peripheral IV sites should be rotated every 48 to 72 hours, including heparin-lock devices. "Routine" or "standing order" placement of IV devices should be avoided or confined to very specialized situations. Any device that is inserted during a cardiopulmonary arrest or other less than favorable conditions should be so identified and removed as soon as is clinically feasible.

Care of peripheral venous site and administration tubing

Clinical studies have yet to provide a definitive answer to questions regarding the optimal agent and procedure for daily care of the peripheral IV site. Agents mentioned earlier during the discussion of insertion should be used for a regimen of daily site cleansing after careful inspection of the site for signs of inflammation. Studies of applications of antimicrobial (antibiotic or iodophor) ointments after insertion and during daily site care have not shown a conclusive beneficial effect.[87,89,125] The efficacy of these applications probably depends greatly on the most likely pathogen that will cause infection. Since this is difficult, if not impossible, to predict, the choice of antimicrobial ointments is usually based on user preference. Labet and Roderick[63] point out that aside from bactericidal activity, the ointment may act as a physical barrier to migration of skin organisms along the needle or catheter into the vein. The dressing used should provide protection from gross contamination from the environment. However, the use of a completely occlusive dressing is controversial, and the risks of external airborne or moisture contamination must be weighed against the proliferation of the patient's skin microorganisms in the warm, moist atmosphere under an occlusive dressing. Whatever is used should allow for easy inspection of the site and stability of the needle to prevent undue friction or dislodgment. The date of insertion should be on the dressing for easy reference to the date for site change.

From 1973 until recently, the standard CDC recommendation was that administration tubing should be changed every 24 hours. This recommendation was based on observations following nationwide outbreaks of bacteremia from IV solutions contaminated at the site of manufacture.[77] When this advice was reevaluated during nonepidemic situations by two independent groups[4,15] in 1979, both found that there was no increased risk for infection when administration tubing was changed every 48 hours instead of every 24 hours. These authors caution that this change in policy should take place only in institutions with low rates of infusion-related infections. Exceptions to the 48-hour interval for tubing changes are (1) fat emulsion (Intralipid) tubing and (2) blood product tubing.

Unprotected stopcock parts are often overlooked as a break in the sterile IV system. Little scientific literature exists to document the stopcock as the cause of infections related to infusions. However, common sense and the principles of asepsis dictate that unused stopcock parts need to have a sterile covering when not in use. If the sterile covering that comes with the stopcock is lost, as often happens, there are several suitable alternatives, such as a sterile heparin plug or the rubber stopper from a sterile 3 ml syringe barrel. If stopcock parts become contaminated with blood or other body secretions, they should be vigorously cleansed with sterile swabs or gauze pads, since dried blood is an excellent growth medium for microorganisms. Stopcock setups should be considered part of the tubing and changed at the same interval as the tubing. Preconnected, prepackaged systems are helpful in preventing use of nonsterile stopcocks, adapters, and extension tubing in elaborate setups. Any infusion tubing setup that is out of the ordinary should be carefully scrutinized for discrepancies in the concept of a sterile closed system. It might be helpful to include special instructions on the IV documentation sheet or nursing care plan in such situations.

Until recently there were conflicting reports in the literature regarding the effectiveness of an in-line filter in preventing IV site infections. In theory, placement of a 0.22 μm filter as close to the patient as possible should filter out bacteria that may have been introduced into the system. Maddox, John, and Brown[69] recently reported a prospective double-blind study involving 174 male patients undergoing elective surgery. They found no significant differences in the incidence of phlebitis after infusion or positive catheter cultures. From a practical standpoint in-line filters are fraught with difficulties. They cannot be used in medication infusions that are in suspension because they will filter out the medication. Viscous solutions and volumetric pumping frequently cause cracks and leakage of the filter. Whatever theoretical advantage the filter might offer is negated when the system requires frequent entry and manipulation because of its presence. The filter offers no protection from migration of skin organisms at the insertion site into the bloodstream.

Insertion and care of arterial catheters and pressure monitoring transducers

Arterial catheters are frequently used in the adult and neonatal intensive care unit populations. The reason that their use has become so popular is that they offer continuous access to the arterial blood system for purposes of arterial pressure monitoring and phlebotomy of arterial blood for blood gas determinations. Without arterial catheters, continuous arterial pressure readings would not be possible, and blood gas results would be available only by repeated arterial punctures.

First reports of infectious complications with arterial catheters were seen in the early 1970s in the pediatric literature. In critically ill neonates the umbilical artery is used. Colonization rates reported from three centers ranged from 6% to 60%.[122] In these neonatal populations contamination presumably occurred at insertion or shortly after from colonization of the umbilical stump. Interestingly, risk of infection did not appear to increase with duration of catheterization. In adults, however, the experience is different. The site most commonly used in adults is the radial or ulnar artery. Band and Maki[3] prospectively studied 130 arterial catheter episodes in 95 adult patients. They found a statistically significant increased risk with catheter placements exceeding 4 days. Other significant risk factors included insertion by surgical cutdown rather than by the percutaneous route and presence of local inflammation. An interesting feature of the microbiology of infections in this report was that C. albicans was the most frequently isolated organism (34%) in the 23 infected catheters. This is best explained by the fact that 80% of the study population was receiving systemic antibiotics.

Insertion of an arterial catheter should be done with sterile gloves and drapes after antimicrobial handwashing and skin preparation, as discussed earlier for peripheral IV insertion. An attempt should be made to pass the catheter percutaneously into the radial or ulnar artery. Cutdown should be done only when percutaneous cannulation fails. The femoral, brachial, or dorsalis pedis sites should be reserved as a last resort because they offer increased infection risks. Daily site care is the same as already outlined for peripheral IV lines. Daily assessment of the site for pain, inflammation, and purulent drainage are crucial for early detection and intervention of site infection.

An important cause of arterial infections is exogenous contamination of the system after insertion. Taking blood samples for blood gas determination occurs frequently and sometimes under emergency situations. One outbreak involving 14 patients highlighted risks involved with constant breaks in sterile technique during phlebotomy from the arterial line. A Flavobacterium species that had contaminated an ice source used for cooling syringes before blood gas draws was cultured from in-use arterial catheters, stopcocks, and syringes, suggesting extensive contamination of the system.[113] The stopcock used for blood withdrawal requires aseptic handling at all times. After removal of a blood sample the stopcock should be completely flushed. Any dried or adherent blood should be immediately removed aseptically. When not in use, all stopcock ports should be covered with a sterile heparin plug, stopcock cover, or fresh sterile syringe.

Another well-documented exogenous source of contamination in arterial artery infection is the pressure transducer. There have been many reports discussing the epidemiology and prevention of infections related to transducers. The early outbreaks were traced to improper cleaning of the transducer head and failure to sterilize the reusable transducer dome.[21,22,44,123] Even after recommendations were made to sterilize transducers and use disposable transducer dome protectors, problems were reported. Infections associated with disposable domes[14] and after recommended cleaning with glutaraldehyde[1] have been documented. In some of these reports the mechanism for contamination has not always been fully understood. A combination of ethylene oxide sterilization of the transducer and single use of a disposable transducer dome protecter appears to offer the best protection from epidemic bacteremia. When setting up the transducer system, it is necessary to wet the surface between the transducer head and the dome membrane diaphragm. Only sterile saline or bacteriostatic sterile water should be used for this interface. It is ideal to use a fresh single-dose vial for this purpose. Solutions containing glucose should never be used. All components of the system, including tubing, intraflow devices, stopcocks, and transducer domes, should be changed every 48 hours unless cracks, leakage, or damage to some component occurs earlier. Any disposable item cannot be reprocessed in any way and reused.

The complexity and expense of arterial monitoring equipment, combined with the complicated care of patients requiring arterial catheters, make it difficult for the ICP to impress ICU personnel with the importance of adhering to these recommendations. There are seemingly good excuses to avoid changing sites, sterilizing transducers, and so on until life-threatening infections or epidemics occur. Then, unfortunately, it is too late for the patients involved. Adherence to these guidelines requires a financial commitment to (1) provide enough transducers so that they can be sterilized between patients, (2) provide enough staff so that shortcuts in technique are not necessary, and (3) allow for adequate training and orientation so that all personnel handling the system are proficient in its use. The ICP should be knowledgeable in the use of arterial equipment and take time to observe how the equipment is handled in use from setup to sterilization. Smith[112] has published an excellent article outlining nursing practice in invasive pressure monitoring with several schematic diagrams explaining all components of the system.

Insertion and care of central lines

The term central line refers to lines that are placed so that the tip is resting in the superior vena cava, the right atrium of the heart, or in a distal branch of the pulmonary artery. Like arterial catheters, these lines are used mainly in the critically ill patient. There are two major indications for the placement of a central line. The first is delivery of drugs or parenteral nutrition when the patient's condition does not allow for oral delivery of these substances and/or when peripheral venous access has failed or is not adequate. Examples of this use of central lines are delivery of total parenteral fluid or Intralipid fluid or placement of a Hickman catheter for delivery of cancer chemotherapy. The second indication for use of central lines is to gather hemodynamic and cardiac measurement data, such as central venous pressure (CVP), pulmonary artery (PA) or wedge pressure, and thermodilution cardiac output (CO).

Whatever the indication for use, central line insertion should take place under optimal aseptic conditions. Since these lines will often be in place for long periods of time and the patients requiring their use are always compromised and often immunosuppressed, every effort should be made to minimize contamination at the time of insertion. Whenever possible, insertion should take place in the operating room under standard surgical conditions. If this is not possible, a sterile field can be created at the bedside with the appropriate use of sterile drapes, sheets, and towels. Since the catheters used are long and may flop during the insertion process, a large sterile field should be created to prevent touch contamination of the catheter. Personnel inserting central lines should wear sterile gloves, gowns, and masks. If the patient is awake and likely to talk or cough during the procedure, the patient should also wear a mask. The site is prepared as already mentioned in peripheral insertion. Many protocols call for "defatting" the skin with acetone. The efficacy of this practice was recently questioned by Maki and McCormick,[72] who found little benefit when clinical data were analyzed. Whenever possible, a percutaneous insertion should be attempted before resorting to a cutdown. Many authors suggest the use of an occlusive dressing, but the risk of exogenous contamination should be measured against the risk of increased proliferation of fungal skin flora under an occlusive dressing.

Infection risks associated with the administration of total parenteral nutrition (TPN) have been extensively discussed in the literature with reported septicemia rates from 2% to 33%.* A survey by the CDC of hospitals participating in the National Nosocomial Infection Study revealed a septicemia rate of 7% in 2078 patients. Of the septicemias, 54% were fungal.[19] Reasons for these high rates may be related to the ideal growth properties of the high-glucose, high-protein solution, combined with underlying deficiencies of patients to whom TPN is administered. Every effort should be made to minimize contamination of the solution. This includes mixing solutions in the pharmacy under a laminar flow hood and avoiding admixtures on the nursing units. One recent paper[48] showed that Intralipid, a common component of parenteral nutrition, can predispose the patient to bacterial sepsis because it impairs human neutrophil chemotaxis in vitro. Maki[70] recently demonstrated that 12 species of hospital isolates all rapidly proliferated in Intralipid to a mean 24-hour concentration of 8.3×10^5 organisms per milliliter. He concluded that lipid emulsions support luxuriant growth of a wide variety of hospital organisms. Since the fluid is opaque, visual inspection would not detect contamination at 10^6 orga-

*References 19, 43, 52, 86, 103, 104.

nisms per milliliter. He recommends that lipid bottles and tubing should not hang for any longer than 12 hours. Most published reports of infection associated with TPN are from the early and mid-1970s. More current TPN infection data are needed to evaluate how effective recommended prevention techniques have been and to see if the microbiological factors of the infections have changed.

Specific infection experience with central lines used for hemodynamic monitoring (CVP, PA, and CO) has not been frequently reported. One recent report[83] looked prospectively at culture results on tips of pulmonary artery catheters removed from 153 critically ill patients. Of those cases, 19% of the catheters were culture positive. There were no cases of sepsis definitely attributable to the catheter. Catheters were not cultured quantitatively, and 11 of 29 cases had positive blood cultures and positive tip cultures. All bacteremias were attributed to another focus of infection. These authors found that contamination of the catheter tip was associated with infection at another site and with placement of a catheter for more than 4 days. Lines used for PA, CVP, CO, or any other hemodynamic monitoring should be maintained and manipulated with the most scrupulous attention given to aseptic technique. Installation, flushing, measuring, calibration, and heparinizing practices should be scrutinized for possible breaks in techniques. If new hemodynamic practices are considered for use, the ICP should be involved in procedure writing and product evaluation before implementation. A step-by-step "dry run" should be done, even if it means wasting expensive materials. Otherwise, infection risks associated with a new procedure may not be addressed until an infection or epidemic occurs.

Administration of blood and blood components

Early reports of transfusion-associated sepsis in the 1940s and 1950s identified gram-negative bacilli and common skin organisms. Skin contaminants in low concentrations do not apparently cause clinical sepsis.[122] However, transfusion-associated sepsis can be caused by gram-negative bacilli that are able to survive at 4° C (39° F). With modern use of disposable closed infusion systems and careful collection techniques the risk of bacteremia after transfusion is minimal. Once the blood is not refrigerated, however, it carries an extremely high risk of supporting the growth of bacterial contaminants. For this reason it is imperative that the blood transfusion be started no longer than 30 minutes after the blood has left blood bank refrigeration. Blood not used promptly should be returned to the blood bank and not be kept in nursing unit refrigerators. The temperature of these refrigerators is not as carefully monitored as those in the blood bank.

Other than bacteria, organisms that can be transmitted through contaminated blood products are viruses (cytomegalovirus, hepatitis B, non-A, non-B hepatitis) and parasites (malaria, toxoplasmosis, babesiosis). Except for hepatitis B, these diseases cannot be screened for on a routine basis before blood is given.

A declining availability of whole blood, combined with increased knowledge of the benefits of blood component therapy, has led to a greater use of a variety of blood products. Hospitals, blood banks, and medical centers that collect, separate, store, and use these products should evaluate all steps in the process from collection to storage and distribution for potential sources of contamination. An outbreak of *Pseudomonas cepacia* related to the use of cryoprecipitate was recently reported.[101] These units became contaminated when they were thawed in a 37° C water bath. Small droplets from the contaminated water bath fell onto the outlet port where the infusion tubing was connected, thereby introducing organisms into the unit at the time it was spiked for delivery to the patient. Other components, such as fresh frozen plasma, that require thawing or warming before administration could become contaminated in this fashion. Substituting a dry warming environment rather than a liquid water bath would eliminate this potential for contamination. This is just one example of how these various components may be contaminated before use. Since these products cannot be subjected to sterilization processes, it is crucial that they be collected, prepared, stored, and administered employing the highest degree of asepsis. Difficulties involved when contaminated components or blood products are the cause of an outbreak were highlighted in a report of *P. cepacia* sepsis related to commercially produced human serum albumin.[114] One problem in identifying blood products as the cause is that there may be a low frequency of contamination, and unless large quantities of the components are used, it would be unlikely that the blood product would be readily identified in a common source epidemic. The other confounding factor may be that patients who receive component therapy will usually be exposed to risk factors more commonly linked to nosocomial sepsis (e.g., urinary catheters, assisted ventilation, IV catheters), obscuring the blood product as the source.

Other medical manipulations

This last section will briefly discuss several miscellaneous medical manipulations that have been associated with cardiovascular infection. As previously mentioned, at least two outbreaks of septicemia have been reportedly related to contamination during addition of medications to an IV infusion.[23,95] Even though one of the outbreaks occurred after admixture under the pharmacy laminar flow hood, it is recommended that as much manipulation of IV fluids be done in the hospital pharmacy as possible. The contamination in both cases was presumed to be related to multiple-dose vials that became contaminated during repeated entry. When medication additions are made on the nursing

units, small single-use containers of medication or irrigation fluid are preferable to multiple-dose vials. If multiple-dose vials are used, vigorous decontamination of the top diaphragm should be done using a sterile alcohol swab.
One unpublished study[50] showed that some nosocomial pathogens can survive
in multiple-dose vials at 4° C. Chemical preservatives did not reliably prevent
microbial proliferation. Multiple-dose vials should be dated, promptly refrigerated after use, and discarded after 24 to 48 hours.

Cardiovascular infection has also been associated with administration of
cancer chemotherapy through a hepatic artery infusion. In most cases infections have been confined to the site of catheter insertion[29] and, in one report,
septicemia with septic emboli.[74] A puzzling report of three cases of clostridial
sepsis attributed to hepatic artery chemotherapy infusion failed to show a clear
mode of transmission but was presumably endogenous in nature.[119]

Diagnostic procedures requiring cardiovascular access carried out in the
radiology, radioisotope, and cardiac catheter laboratories also offer risks for
infection. Many radiological procedures involve intravascular instillation of
radiopaque contrast media. These substances are usually prepared, stored, and
administered in the testing department by personnel who may have varied
levels of competency in aseptic technique. Two reports have epidemiologically
linked contaminated radiopharmaceuticals to common source outbreaks.[82,109]
In both cases the investigators pointed out that problems could have been
avoided by strict adherence to aseptic standards routinely recommended for
the handling of parenteral substances. Three investigators have reported infectious complications following cardiac catheterization. Two reported epidemic
pyrogenic reactions to endoxin,[6,99] and one reported a single case of endocarditis caused by a *Micrococcus* species.[102] In both reports of endotoxemia part of
the reprocessing procedure for the catheters employed the use of distilled
water contaminated with gram-negative organisms. Although final sterilization
had killed the organisms, the surviving endotoxin was responsible for the
pyrogenic reactions. In general, however, cardiac catheterization has not been
associated with high infection rates. The procedure should be done under
operating room conditions, including surgical preparation of the skin, draping
of the site, and gown, mask, and glove apparel for personnel involved in the
procedure.

SURVEILLANCE
Blood culture report review

The most reliable tool for surveillance of cardiovascular infections is a daily
review of positive blood cultures from the microbiology laboratory. With a
growing movement away from day-to-day ward surveillance by the ICP, the
daily review of blood cultures is still generally practiced. It can be argued that
bacteremia constitutes one of the most significant types of nosocomial infection

and therefore warrants careful observation. It is helpful if the laboratory makes a separate log or daily listing so that the ICP can quickly and easily find these results without having to review all reports. Information entered on the log should include the patient's name, room and bed number, medical record number, physician's name, date specimen drawn, date positive, Gram stain results, and final organism identification. It is also helpful to add a space so that it can be noted that the result was phoned to the physician and/or nursing unit. Keeping a log in this fashion not only facilitates prompt and timely review of the patients but also easily lends itself to summarization and analysis. The bacteremia experience should be summarized and analyzed at least yearly as to nosocomial or community origin, organism, nursing unit, and medical service.

Once the ICP has identified a patient with a positive blood culture, she should then review the case to ascertain the probable source of the infection. A decision about whether or not the isolate is a contaminant or clinically significant should be made, as well as a distinction made between nosocomial and community acquired. For guidelines the reader is referred to p. 326. These guidelines were adapted from medical records review instructions used in the Study for Efficacy of Nosocomial Infection Control Project (SENIC).[58]

Pseudobacteremia

The term *pseudobacteremia* (p. 326) refers to an isolate in the blood that is introduced during specimen collection or laboratory processing. Occurrences of pseudobacteremia are troublesome to the ICP and may result in unnecessary antimicrobial therapy to patients. Between 1956 and 1975 the CDC investigated 181 nosocomial epidemics of all types. Twenty (11%) were epidemics of pseudobacteremia. Causes for pseudobacteremia include the following[25]:

- Nonsterile blood collection tubes
- Skin and tube contamination during venipuncture
- Contaminated antiseptics used on skin and bottle tops
- Contaminated blood culture tube holders
- Contaminated commercial media
- Contaminated automated blood culture analyzer
- Contaminated bottle stoppers

Cultures in intravascular access infections

It has been repeatedly stated that IV devices suspected as the source of cellulitis, sepsis, or remote site infection should be removed promptly. Microbiological studies of components of the administration system and the insertion site can be invaluable in deciding appropriate therapy and in studying the epidemiological nature of the infection. When IV site infection is suspected, two peripheral blood cultures from independent venipunctures should be obtained. Before removing the device, the area should be cleaned with alcohol or

---

Bacteremia

Signs

Bacteremia (sepsis, septic shock, septicemia)
1. Hypotension or systolic pressure ≥90 mm Hg
2. Oliguria or anuria
3. Fever ≥99.6° F (37.5° C)

Pertinent definitions

1. Positive blood culture:
   Isolation of any organism from one blood culture
2. Pseudobacteremia:
   Isolation of an organism from blood that either:
   a. Physician diagnoses as contaminant or
   b. Epidemiological investigation proves to be probable contaminant during collection or processing

Criteria for infection

Bacteremia
1. Bacteremia is counted the following way:
   a. Positive blood culture and either:
      (1) No previous bacteremia this admission or
      (2) If previous bacteremia, both cultured and latest positive with Δ in pathogen
2. *Intravascular site infection (IVSI)*
   An IVSI will be counted if purulent drainage from the insertion site of an intravascular device even if no cultures are obtained. (Inflammation at such sites, without purulent material or strong clinical evidence of cellulitis, is not regarded as an infection unless a positive culture is obtained from the catheter or from aspirates of tissue fluid.)

Rules to determine nosocomial versus community-acquired infection

A bacteremia is nosocomial if it meets *either* of two criteria:
1. The date of onset is after day 3 of hospitalization
2. The infection is the second bacteremia this admission
3. Infections that do not meet either 1 or 2 are community acquired.

Modified from Haley, R.W., et al.: Am. J. Epidemiol. 3:638-639, 1980.

povidone iodine. Sterile gloves should be worn to prevent touch contamination of the device tip. Sterile suture removal equipment is useful and convenient for this process. The device should be carefully removed. A few drops of fluid should be allowed to drip onto a clean glass slide (for Gram stain), but touching the slide with the tip should be avoided. If the tip is of flexible material, it should be clipped with sterile scissors below the area of insertion interface and dropped into a sterile dry container with a screw-on cap. The tip should be cultured by the semiquantitative method described by Maki, Weise, and

Sarafin[75] or the quantitative method described by Cleri, Corrado, and Seligman.[28] If the device is a steel "butterfly" needle, the device should be cut above the winged area and placed in a sterile dry container with a screw-on cap. The laboratory should be instructed to culture the lower needle area, but the winged area should be considered contaminated. A sterile cap should be placed on the infusion tubing, and the entire system should be sent to the microbiology laboratory for culture. Any purulent material from the insertion site should be taken and swabbed for culture and Gram stain. Best results are achieved if one swab is made and immediately streaked onto a clean glass slide for Gram stain at the bedside before the material is dry. If this is done, a second swab of the site can be made to send for culture, since the first swab will be contaminated after contact with the slide.

Special studies

The surveillance activities discussed thus far will only detect those infections in which blood cultures or IV site cultures are obtained. Many cardiovascular infections may never come to the attention of the ICP without some additional scrutiny. The ICP may find it helpful to review all febrile patients if time and personnel allow for such review. To get a true attack rate for IV site infection and septicemia related to IV use, it is necessary to periodically review all patients receiving IV therapy. The best results are obtained in such studies when a special investigation team actually visually inspects all sites for signs of infection, as well as monitors medical record documentation of site condition, site care, and site rotation. These studies yield the best results when personnel directly responsible for IV administration are directly involved. It can be a valuable learning experience. Since IV infections are rare occurrences for patients of any one ICP or a single nursing unit, a collaborative effort with many units will result in more impressive findings for those involved. Findings of such studies should be presented in educational programs without the ICP being unduly critical or judgmental. A summary of nursing control measures in vascular access infections follows and might be a useful addition to such an education program:

A. Handwashing
B. Careful insertion technique
   1. Avoid cutdowns
   2. Avoid femoral or saphenous veins
   3. Use steel needle when possible
   4. Use skin preparation and aseptic technique
C. Patient assessment
   1. Inspect insertion site for 24 hours
   2. Watch for clinical signs of sepsis
D. Rotate insertion site every 48 to 72 hours

    E. Maintain sterile system
        1. Use aseptic technique when entering system
        2. Protect stopcocks
        3. Examine fluid
        4. Maintain sterility of transducers
    F. Remove device if infection occurs
    G. Culture
        1. Take Gram stain and culture of pus
        2. Culture catheter, tubing, and so on

SUMMARY

This chapter explores infection control aspects of the cardiovascular system. Although nosocomial infections of the bloodstream are less frequent than nosocomial urinary tract infections, pneumonias, and surgical wound infections, they are associated with significant morbidity and mortality when they do occur. The cardiovascular system is usually sterile in the normal host and is therefore ill equipped to handle the contamination that may occur in hospitalized patients who are invariably subjected to invasive procedures in the course of their care. I have attempted to cover pertinent anatomical and physiological considerations, common infections, sources of intrinsic and extrinsic contamination, surveillance techniques, and preventive measures specific to the cardiovascular system.

REFERENCES

1. Aduan, R.P., Iannini, P.B., and Salaki, J.: Nosocomial bacteremia associated with contaminated blood pressure transducers, Am. J. Infect. Control **8**:33-40, May 1980.
2. Agger, W., and Maki, D.: Septicemia from heparin-lock needles, Ann. Intern. Med. **86**:657, 1977.
3. Band, J.D., and Maki, D.G.: Infection caused by arterial catheters used for hemodynamic monitoring, Am. J. Med. **67**:735-741, 1979.
4. Band, J.D., and Maki, D.G.: Safety of changing intravenous delivery systems at longer than 24 hour intervals, Ann. Intern. Med. **91**:173-178, 1979.
5. Band, J.D., and Maki, D.G.: Steel needles used for intravenous therapy: morbidity in patients with hematologic malignancy, Arch. Intern. Med. **140**:31-34, Jan. 1980.
6. Bauer, E., and Densen, P.: Infections from contaminated Elastoplast, N. Engl. J. Med. **300**:370, 1979.
7. Becker, A.E., et al.: Bland thrombosis and infection in relation to intracardiac catheter, Circulation **46**:300, 1972.
8. Bentley, D.W., and Lepper, M.H.: Septicemia related to indwelling venous catheter, J.A.M.A. **206**:1749, 1968.
9. Berger, S.A., et al.: Bacteremia after the use of an oral irrigation device, Ann. Intern. Med. **80**:510-511, 1974.
10. Bernheim, H.A., Block, L.H., and Atkins, E.: Fever: pathogenesis, pathophysiology, and purpose, Ann. Intern. Med. **91**:261-270, 1979.
11. Berry, F.A., Blankenbaker, W.L., and Ball, C.G.: A comparison of bacteremia occurring with nasotracheal and orotracheal intubation, Anesth. Analg. **52**:873, 1973.
12. Blake, P.J., and Perez, R.C.: Applied immunological concepts, New York, 1978, Appleton-Century-Crofts.

13. Brown, B.J., Mackowiak, P.A., and Smith, J.W.: Care of veins during intravenous therapy: incidence of phlebitis as related to knowledge and performance, Am. J. Infect. Control **8**:107-112, 1980.

14. Buxton, A.E., Anderson, R.L., and Klimek, J.: Failure of disposable domes to prevent septicemia acquired from contaminated pressure transducers, Chest **74**:508-513, 1978.

15. Buxton, A.E., et al.: Contamination of intravenous infusion fluid: effects of changing administration sets, Ann. Intern. Med. **90**:764-768, 1979.

16. Carruthers, M.: Endocarditis due to enteric bacilli other than salmonella: case reports and literature review, Am. J. Med. Sci. **273**:203, 1977.

17. Centers for Disease Control: Follow-up on septicemias associated with contaminated Abbott intravenous solutions—U.S.A., Morbid. Mortal. Weekly Rep. **20**:91, 1971.

18. Centers for Disease Control: Nosocomial bacteremias associated with intravenous fluid therapy—U.S.A., Morbid. Mortal. Weekly Rep. vol. 20, suppl. 9, 1971.

19. Centers for Disease Control: Guidelines for infection control in hyperalimentation therapy, reprint, 1973.

20. Centers for Disease Control: National nosocomial infections study, fourth quarter 1973, issued April 1974.

21. Centers for Disease Control: Nosocomial *Pseudomonas cepacia* bacteremia caused by contaminated pressure transducers, Morbid. Mortal. Weekly Rep. **23**:423, 1974.

22. Centers for Disease Control: Transducer associated bacteremia, Morbid. Mortal. Weekly Rep. **24**:295, 1975.

23. Centers for Disease Control: Primary bacteremia, Illinois, U.S.A., Morbid. Mortal. Weekly Rep. **25**:110+, April 1976.

24. Centers for Disease Control: Recommendations for the prevention of IV-associated infections, Atlanta, Aug. 1973 (reprinted May 1977), Bacterial Diseases Division, Bureau of Epidemiology, CDC.

25. Centers for Disease Control: Nosocomial pseudobacteremia, Morbid. Mortal. Weekly Rep. **29**:243-249, 1980.

26. Centers for Disease Control: Recall of contaminated intravenous cannulae—USA, Morbid. Mortal. Weekly Rep. **23**:57-58, 1974.

27. Chlorhexidine and other antiseptics: Med. Lett. Drugs. Ther. **18**:85-86, Oct. 1976.

28. Cleri, D.J., Corrado, M.D., and Seligman, S.J.: Quantitative culture of intravenous catheters and other intravascular inserts, J. Infect. Dis. **141**:781-786, 1980.

29. Clouse, M.E., et al.: Complications of long term transbrachial hepatic arterial infusion chemotherapy, Am. J. Roentgenol. **129**:799, 1977.

30. Cobbs, C.G.: IUD and endocarditis, Ann. Intern. Med. **78**:451, 1973.

31. Cobe, H.M.: Transitory bacteremia, Oral Surg. **7**:609-615, 1954.

32. Collins, R.N., et al.: Risk of local and systemic infection with polyethylene intravenous catheters, N. Engl. J. Med. **279**:340-343, 1968.

33. Cosentino, F.: The functions of personnel as a determinant of phlebitis rates, Am. J. IV Ther., pp. 35-60, April-May 1978.

34. Couchonnal, G., et al.: Complications with heparin-lock needles, J.A.M.A. **242**:2098-2100, 1979.

35. Crane, C.: Venous interruption for septic thrombophlebitis, N. Engl. J. Med. **262**:947-951, 1960.

36. Cross, A.S., and Steigbigel, R.T.: Infective endocarditis and access site infection in patients on hemodialysis, Medicine **55**:453-466, 1976.

37. Cruse, P.J., and Foord, R.: A five-year prospective study of 23,649 surgical wounds, Arch. Surg. **107**:206-209, 1973.

38. Daisy, J.A., Abutyn, E.A., and MacGregor, R.R.: Inadvertent administration of intravenous fluids contaminated with fungus, Ann. Intern. Med. **91**:563-565, 1979.

39. Dale, W.A., and Lewis, M.R.: Further experience with bovine arterial grafts, Surgery **80**:711-721, 1976.

40. Day, H.A., and Cho, C.T.: Barium enema septicemia, J.A.M.A. **227**:1258-1259, 1974.

41. Denton, C., et al.: Bacterial endocarditis following cardiac surgery, Circulation **15**:525, 1957.

42. DeSweit, M., Ramsay, I.D., and Rees, G.M.: Bacterial endocarditis after insertion of intrauterine contraceptive device, Br. Med. J. **3:**67, 1975.
43. Dillon, J.D., et al.: Septicemia and total parenteral nutrition: distinguishing catheter-related from other septic episodes, J.A.M.A. **223:**1341-1344, 1973.
44. Donowitz, L.G., et al.: *Serratia marcescens* bacteremia from contaminated pressure transducers, J.A.M.A. **242:**1749-1751, 1979.
45. Duma, R.J.: Thomas Latta, what have we done? The hazards of intravenous therapy, N. Engl. J. Med. **294:**1178-1180, 1976.
46. Ferguson, R., Hodges, G., and Barnes, W.: Complications with heparin-lock needles: a prospective evaluation of iodophor skin care, A.P.I.C. Journal **7:**22-25, March 1979.
47. Ferguson, R., et al.: Complications with heparin-lock needles: a prospective study, Ann. Intern. Med. **85:**583-586, 1976.
48. Fisher, G.W., et al.: Diminished bacterial defenses with intralipid, Lancet **2:**819-820, 1980.
49. Forscher, B.,K., editor: Immunopathology of inflammation: proceedings of a symposium sponsored by the international inflammation club, Augusta, Mich. June 1-3, 1970, Amsterdam, 1971, Excerpta Medica.
50. Garner, J.S.: Personal correspondence to Eileen Bren, Hospital Infection Branch, Centers for Disease Control, Oct. 7, 1980.
51. Gartenber, G., et al.: Hospital-acquired mucomycosis *(Rhizopus rizopodiformis)* of skin and subcutaneous tissue, N. Engl. J. Med. **299:**1115-1118, 1978.
52. Goldman, D., and Maki, D.G.: Infection control in total parenteral nutrition, J.A.M.A. **223:** 1360-1364, 1973.
53. Goldman, D.A., et al.: Guidelines for infection control in intravenous therapy, Ann. Intern. Med. **79:**848-850, 1973.
54. Greene, J.F., and Cummings, K.C.: Septic endocarditis and parenteral feeding, J.A.M.A. **225:** 315, 1973.
55. Greene, J.F., Fitzwater, J.E., and Clemmer, T.P.: Septic endocarditis and indwelling pulmonary artery catheters, J.A.M.A. **233:**891-892, 1975.
56. Guyton, A.C.: Textbook of medical physiology, ed. 4, Philadelphia, 1971, W.B. Saunders Co.
57. Haimov, M., et al.: Complications of arteriovenous fistulas for hemodialysis, Arch. Surg. **110:**708-712, 1975.
58. Haley, R.W., et al.: The SENIC Project: appendix E—algorithms for diagnosing infections, Am. J. Epidemiol. **3:**633-643, 1980.
59. Hanley, J.F., et al.: *Candida tropicalis* abscess following arterial puncture, West. J. Med. **130:**462-463, 1979.
60. Hoeprich, P., editor: Infectious diseases, ed. 2, New York, 1977, Harper & Row, Publishers, Inc.
61. Hoeprich, P.D., and Boggs, D.R.: Manifestations of disease. In Hoeprich, P.D., editor: Infectious diseases, ed. 2, New York, 1977, Harper & Row, Publishers, Inc.
62. Kreger, B.E., Craven, D.E., and McCabe, W.R.: Gram-negative bacteremia: reevaluation of clinical features and treatment in 612 patients, Am. J. Med. **68:**344-355, 1980.
63. Labet, C.G., and Roderick, M.A.: Infection control in the use of intravascular devices, Crit. Care Q. **3:**67-80, Dec. 1980.
64. Lapage, S.P., Johnson, R., and Holmes, B.: Bacteria from intravenous fluids, Lancet **2:**284-285, 1973.
65. Le Frock, J.L., et al.: Transient bacteremia associated with sigmoidoscopy, N. Engl. J. Med. **289:**467, 1973.
66. Le Frock, J.L., et al.: Transient bacteremia associated with barium enema, Arch. Intern. Med. **135:**835-837, 1975.
67. Le Frock, J.L., et al.: Transient bacteremia associated with percutaneous liver biopsy, J. Infect. Dis. **131:**S104-107, 1975.
68. Le Frock, J.L., et al.: Transient bacteremia associated with nasotracheal suctioning, J.A.M.A. **236:**1610-1611, 1976.
69. Maddox, R., John, Jr., J., and Brown, L.: Effect of in-line filtration on post-infusion phlebitis, Reprints of abstracts presented at Second International Conference on Nosocomial Infections, Atlanta, Aug. 1980.

70. Maki, D.G.: Growth properties of microorganisms in lipid for infusion and implications for infection control, Abstracts of original papers for Seventh Annual National Conference of the Association for Practitioners of Infection Control, San Francisco, June 22-26, 1980.
71. Maki, D.G., and Martin, W.T.: Nationwide epidemic of septicemia caused by contaminated infusion products: growth of microbial pathogen in fluids for intravenous infusion, J. Infect. Dis. **131**:267-272, 1975.
72. Maki, D.G., and McCormick, K.N.: Defatting in cutaneous antisepsis, Original paper abstracts of Seventh National Meeting of the Association for Practitioners of Infection Control, San Francisco, June 1980.
73. Maki, D.G., Drinka, P.J., and Davis, T.E.: Suppurative phlebitis of an arm vein from a "scalp-vein needle," N. Engl. J. Med. **292**:1116-1117, 1975.
74. Maki, D.G., McCormick, R.D., and Wirtenan, G.W.: Septic endarteritis from intro-arterial catheters for cancer chemotherapy, Presented at the Seventeenth Interscience Conference on Antimicrobial Agents and Chemotherapy, New York, Oct. 1977.
75. Maki, D.G., Weise, C.E., and Sarafin, H.: A semiquantitative culture method for identifying intravenous-catheter-related infection, N. Engl. J. Med. **296**:1305-1309, 1977.
76. Maki, D.G., et al.: Infection control in intravenous therapy, Ann. Intern. Med. **79**:867-887, 1973.
77. Maki, D.G., et al.: Nationwide epidemic of septicemia caused by contaminated intravenous products, Am. J. Med. **60**:471-484, 1976.
78. Mayer, M.M.: The complement system, Sci. Am. **229**:54-66, Nov. 1973.
79. McCloskey, R.V., and Gold, M.: Bacteremia after liver biopsy, Arch. Intern. Med. **102**:213-215, 1973.
80. McGowan, J.E.: Bacteremia at Boston City Hospital: occurrence and mortality during 12 selected years (1935-1972) with special reference to hospital-acquired cases, J. Infect. Dis. **132**:316-335, 1975.
81. McGowan, J.E., Parrott, P.L., and Duty, V.P.: Nosocomial bacteremia: potential for prevention of procedure related cases, J.A.M.A. **237**:2727-2729, 1977.
82. McGuckin, M.B., et al.: An outbreak of achromobacter xylosoxidans related to radiopharmaceuticals. Abstracts of original papers presented at Sixth National Conference of Association for Practitioners of Infection Control, Houston, May 1979.
83. Michael, L., et al.: Infection of pulmonary artery catheters in critically ill patients, J.A.M.A. **245**:1032-1036, 1981.
84. Michaels, I., and Ruebner, B.: Growth of bacteria in intravenous infusion fluids, Lancet **1**:772, 1953.
85. Mills, J.: Sepsis and septic shock. In Joseph, P., and Cooper, R., editors: Infectious diseases in clinical practice, Symposium presented in San Francisco, Jan. 27-Feb. 3, 1979.
86. Montgomerie, J.Z., and Edwards, J.E.: Association of infection due to Candida albicans with intravenous hyperalimentation, J. Infect. Dis. **137**:197-201, 1978.
87. Moran, J.M., Atwood, R.P., and Rowe, M.I.: A clinical and bacteriologic study of infections associated with venous cutdown, N. Engl. J. Med. **272**:554-559, 1965.
88. Munster, A.M.: Septic thrombophlebitis: a surgical disorder, J.A.M.A. **230**:1010, 1974.
89. Norden, C.W.: Application of antibiotic ointment to site of venous catheterization—a controlled trial, J. Infect. Dis. **120**:611-615, 1969.
90. Norden, C.W.: Septic thrombophlebitis. In Hoeprich, P.D., editor: Infectious diseases, ed. 2, New York, 1977, Harper & Row, Publishers, Inc.
91. O'Neill, J.A., et al.: Suppurative thrombophlebitis—a lethal complication of intravenous therapy, J. Trauma **8**:256-267, 1968.
92. Onorato, I.M., et al.: Fungal infections of dialysis fistulae, Ann. Intern. Med. **91**:50-52, 1979.
93. Pelletier, L.L., and Petersdorf, R.G.: Infective endocarditis: a review of 125 cases from the University of Washington Hospitals, 1963-72, Medicine **56**:287-313, 1977.
94. Petersdorf, R.G., and Dale, D.C.: Gram-negative bacteremia and septic shock. In Isselbacher, K.J., et al., editors: Harrison's principles of internal medicine, ed. 9, New York, 1978, McGraw-Hill, Inc.

95. Plouffe, J.F., et al.: Nosocomial outbreak of *Candida parapsilosis* fungemia related to intravenous infusions, Arch. Intern. Med. **137**:1686-1689, 1977.

96. Pollock, A.: Scalp-vein needle and infection, N. Engl. J. Med. **293**:560, 1975.

97. Price, P.B.: The bacteriology of normal skin: a new quantitative test applied to a study of the bacterial flora and the disinfection action of mechanical cleansing, J. Infect. Dis. **63**:301-318, 1938.

98. Pruitt, B.A., et al.: Intravenous therapy in burn patients: suppurative thrombophlebitis and other life-threatening complications, Arch. Surg. **100**:399-404, 1970.

99. Reyes, M.P., et al.: Pyrogenic reactions after inadvertent infusion of endotoxin during cardiac catheterizations, Ann. Intern. Med. **93**:32-35, July 1980.

100. Rhame, F.S., Maki, D.G., and Bennett, J.V.: Intravenous cannula-associated infections. In Bennett, J.V., and Brachman, P.S., editors: Hospital infections, Boston, 1979, Little, Brown & Co.

101. Rhame, F., et al.: Nosocomial *Pseudomonas cepacia* related to receipt of cryoprecipitate, Original paper abstracts presented at Seventh Annual National Conference of Association for Practitioners of Infection Control, San Francisco, June 22-26, 1980.

102. Rubin, S.J., Lyons, R.W., and Murcia, A.J.: Endocarditis associated with cardiac catheterization due to a gram-positive coccus designated micrococcus mucilaginosus incertae sedis, J. Clin. Microbiol. **7**:546-549, 1978.

103. Ryan, J.A., et al.: Catheter complications in total parenteral nutrition: a prospective study of 200 consecutive patients, N. Engl. J. Med. **290**:757-761, 1974.

104. Sanderson, I., and Deitel, M.: Intravenous hyperalimentation without sepsis, Surg. Gynecol. Obstet. **136**:577-585, 1973.

105. Scheckler, W.E.: Septicemia and nosocomial infections in a community hospital, Ann. Intern. Med. **89**:754-756, 1978.

106. Scheld, W.M., and Sande, M.A.: Endocarditis and intravascular infection. In Mandell, G.L., Douglas, R.G., and Bennett, J.E., editors: Principals and practice of infectious disease, New York, 1979, John Wiley & Sons, Inc.

107. Seropian, R., and Reynolds, B.M.: Wound infections after preoperative depilatory versus razor preparation, Am. J. Surg. **121**:251-254, 1971.

108. Serra, P., et al.: Synergistic treatment of enterococcal endocarditis, Arch. Intern. Med. **137**:1562, 1977.

109. Sharbaugh, R.J.: Suspected outbreak of endotoxemia associated with computerized axial tomography, Am. J. Infect. Control **8**:26-28, 1980.

110. Shawker, T.H., Kluge, R.M., and Ayella, R.J.: Bacteremia associated with angiography, J.A.M.A. **229**:1090-1092, 1974.

111. Shull, H.J., et al.: Bacteremia with upper gastrointestinal endoscopy, Ann. Intern. Med. **83**:212-214, 1975.

112. Smith, R.N.: Invasive pressure monitoring, Am. J. Nurs. **78**:1514-1521, 1978.

113. Stamm, W.E., et al.: Indwelling arterial catheters as a source of nosocomial bacteremia, N. Engl. J. Med. **292**:1099-1102, 1975.

114. Steere, A.C., et al.: *Pseudomonas* species bacteremia caused by contaminated normal human serum albumin, J. Infect. Dis. **135**:729-734, 1977.

115. Steere, A.C., et al.: Gram-negative rod bacteremia. In Bennett, J.V., and Brachman, P.S., editors: Hospital infections, Boston, 1979, Little, Brown, & Co.

116. Stein, J.M., and Pruitt, B.A.: Suppurative thrombophlebitis: a lethal iatrogenic disease, N. Engl. J. Med. **282**:1452-1455, 1970.

117. Sullivan, N.H., et al.: Clinical aspects of bacteremia after manipulation of genitourinary tract, J. Infect. Dis. **127**:49-55, 1973.

118. Tilkian, S.M., Conover, M.B., and Tilkian, A.G., editors: Clinical implications of laboratory tests, ed. 2, St. Louis, 1979, The C.V. Mosby Co.

119. Timms, R.M., and Harrell, J.H.P.: Bacteremia related to fiberoptic bronchoscopy, Am. Rev. Respir. Dis. **3**:555-557, 1975.

120. Tully, J.L., et al.: Clostridial sepsis following hepatic arterial infusion chemotherapy, Am. J. Med. **67**:707-710, 1979.

121. Watanakunakorn, C., and Baird, I.M.: *Staphylococcus aureus* bacteremia and endocarditis associated with infected intravascular device, Presented at the Sixteenth Interscience Conference on Antimicrobial Agents and Chemotherapy, October 1976.
122. Weinstein, R.A., and Young, L.S.: Other procedure related infections. In Bennett, J.V., and Brachman, P.S., editors: Hospital infections, Boston, 1979, Little, Brown & Co.
123. Weinstein, R.A., et al.: Pressure monitoring devices: overlooked source of nosocomial infection, J.A.M.A. **236:**923-938, 1976.
124. Wilson, W.R., et al.: Prosthetic valve endocarditis, Ann. Intern. Med. **82:**751-756, 1975.
125. Zinner, S.H., et al.: Risk of infection with intravenous catheters: effect of application of antibiotic ointment, J. Infect. Dis. **120:**616-619, 1969.

Genitourinary system

IMPORTANT ANATOMICAL CONSIDERATIONS

The genitourinary system includes the organs involved in reproduction and those responsible for the formation and excretion of body wastes. These organs are closely related, since some of the female and male reproductive organs and urinary structures originate from the same embryonic structure. During the birth process the genital and urinary systems share common passages.

Not all organs will be discussed in their entirety. Those characteristics that assist the infection control practitioner (ICP) in making an assessment will be highlighted.

Kidneys

The kidneys (Fig. 14-1) lie obliquely on the psoas major muscles of the posterior abdominal wall. The right kidney is slightly lower than the left because of the position of the liver. An adult kidney normally weighs about 150 gm. The closeness of the kidneys to other intraperitoneal organs explains why gastrointestinal tract symptoms may accompany genitourinary disease.[39]

Nephrons, the functioning units of the kidneys, do not regenerate. If one kidney is removed, the other one undergoes an enlargement because of an increase in the size of the nephron rather than an increase in the number of nephrons. Only 25% of total renal mass is necessary for survival.[22]

The kidneys have a rich blood supply from the renal artery, a branch of the aorta. It may divide before it reaches the kidneys. It then further divides, and from these vessels branches pass to the glomeruli.[39]

Ureters

The ureters extend about 25 to 30 cm from the kidneys to the posterior aspect of the urinary bladder. Contraction of the muscular layer initiates peristaltic waves from the pelvis to the bladder.

The musculature and anatomical angle at which the ureter enters the bladder is extremely important in terms of preventing vesicoureteral reflux.[24] If reflux does occur, bacteria that may be present in the bladder gain access directly into the kidneys.

Bladder

The bladder lies behind the pubic symphysis. When it is full, it rises well above the symphysis and can be readily palpated or percussed.

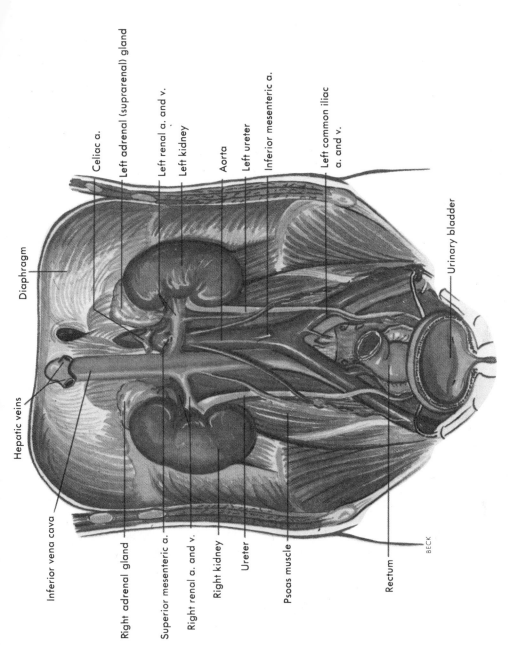

FIG. 14-1. Location of urinary system organs. (From Anthony, C.P., and Thibodeau, G.A.: Textbook of anatomy and physiology, ed. 10, St. Louis, 1979, The C.V. Mosby Co.)

The detrusor is the main muscle of the bladder. It is composed of three interconnected layers of muscle. The trigone muscle forming the base of the bladder is firmly attached to the detrusor. The trigone extends up into the ureters and down into the urethra.

The arterial supply to the bladder comes from the superior, middle, and inferior vesical arteries, which arise from the anterior trunk of the hypogastric artery. Smaller branches from the obturator and inferior gluteal arteries also reach the bladder.[39]

If the bladder becomes distended, these vessels become obstructed. This phenomenon was demonstrated in rats by Mehrotra[34] and in dogs by Finkbeiner and Lapides.[13] The increased pressure in the bladder predisposes it to infection by causing ischemia. Because of this decrease in blood flow, there are less polymorphonuclear leukocytes available to ward off infection.

Prostate gland

The prostate is a fibromuscular and glandular organ that surrounds the posterior urethra. There are epithelial glands embedded in the muscle fibers. These glands drain into the excretory ducts that open on the floor of the urethra.[39] Therefore bacteria present in the urine may in fact be seeded there from a focus in the prostate.

Male and female urethra (Fig. 14-2)

In the male the penis is composed of smooth muscle, erectile tissue, and vascular cavities. The prepuce is a layer of tissue that extends over the end of the penis. Prolonged retraction of the prepuce causes constriction of the blood vessels, edema, and, in time, necrosis.

The female urethra is from one third to one half the size of a male urethra, measuring approximately 3 to 4 cm in length. The distal end contains glands, the largest being the periurethral glands of Skene.

In both the male and female urethra there is an involuntary sphincter located proximally to the bladder. At the distal end is a sphincter composed of striated muscle that is under voluntary control.

The kidneys, ureters, and bladder are sterile. At the distal end of the urethra some bacteria are present, but ordinarily they do not invade deeper tissue. *Staphylococcus epidermidis*, α-hemolytic streptococci, *Bacteroides melaninogenicus*, and *Lactobacillus* species have been cited as normal inhabitants.[5,32]

Vagina

The vagina contains a large variety of bacterial flora. Larsen and Galask,[30] in a review of the literature, found documentation that the following microbes

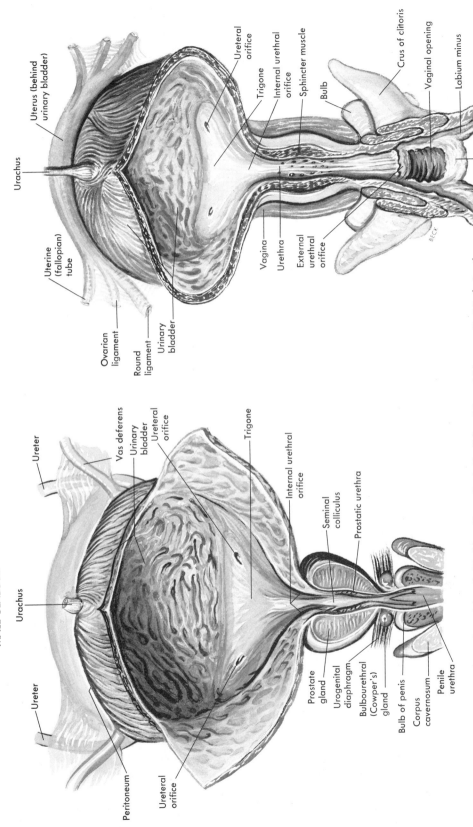

FEMALE BLADDER

- Uterus (behind urinary bladder)
- Urachus
- Uterine (fallopian) tube
- Ovarian ligament
- Round ligament
- Urinary bladder
- Ureteral orifice
- Trigone
- Internal urethral orifice
- Sphincter muscle
- Bulb
- Crus of clitoris
- Vaginal opening
- Labium minus
- Frenulum
- Vagina
- Urethra
- External urethral orifice

MALE BLADDER

- Ureter
- Vas deferens
- Urinary bladder
- Ureteral orifice
- Trigone
- Internal urethral orifice
- Seminal colliculus
- Prostatic urethra
- Urachus
- Ureter
- Peritoneum
- Ureteral orifice
- Prostate gland
- Urogenital diaphragm
- Bulbourethral (Cowper's) gland
- Bulb of penis
- Corpus cavernosum
- Penile urethra

FIG. 14-2. The male and female bladder. (From Beck. E., Gröer, M. and Monsen. H.: Mosby's atlas of concise functional human anatomy. St. Louis. 1982. The C.V. Mosby Co.)

have been present in the genital tracts of healthy premenopausal women:

- Lactobacilli
- Diphtheroids
- β-Hemolytic group B streptococci
- β-Hemolytic group D streptococci
- S. epidermidis
- Staphylococcus aureus
- Enterococci
- Escherichia coli
- Peptococcus species
- Bacteroides species

Lactobacilli and diphtheroids are associated with extremely low virulence. All of the other organisms are opportunistic and present a risk to the manipulated genital tract.

IMPORTANT PHYSIOLOGICAL CONSIDERATIONS
Micturition

Micturition is one of the most complex neuromuscular functions of the body. As the bladder fills, stretch receptors in the detrusor muscle cause minor fluctuations in the tone of the detrusor. The inhibitory impulses from the brain via the autonomic nervous system prevent a complete contraction. Instead, the detrusor gradually stretches to accommodate more urine.

When the bladder contents reach between 250 and 300 ml of urine, the stretch receptors react, and this is registered in the brain as discomfort. The detrusor then needs a conscious inhibitory impulse from the frontal lobe of the cerebral cortex before it will relax and allow more urine to be stored. Voiding can voluntarily be initiated at any stage of bladder filling, but when a capacity of 600 ml is attained, micturition becomes involuntary.

When voiding takes place, the trigone muscle contracts, pulling the ureter into the bladder and thus increasing ureteral occlusion.[39] This prevents reflux of urine into the kidneys. As urine enters the proximal urethra, the detrusor contracts. The bladder contents are forced out the urethra as the external sphincter fibers relax.

Neural supply

The reflexes controlling micturition are coordinated in various centers of the brain and spinal cord. The spinal center is located between S_2 and S_4. If an injury occurs above the conus medullaris (S_2, S_3, S_4), it is referred to as a central lesion or upper motor neuron lesion. It is characterized by hyperactivity of the deep tendon and muscular reflexes and skeletal muscle spasticity. Frequent involuntary voiding of small amounts of urine would be expected. If an injury is sustained peripherally to the conus medullaris, it is called a lower motor *neuron lesion.* This lesion is characterized by an absence of deep tendon or muscle reflex activity and skeletal flaccidity.[6] As a result, urinary retention and incomplete emptying of the bladder are common. The higher centers in the nervous system postpone voiding and allow the bladder to empty smoothly and completely.

Defense mechanism

The ability to empty the bladder completely is one of the best defense mechanisms the body has in preventing urinary tract infections. If bacteria enter the bladder through the urethra, they do not have an opportunity to multiply or invade tissue if the bladder is emptied completely during the voiding process.

The bladder itself has an intrinsic antibacterial capability. Some researchers believe that mucoprotein present on the mucosal surface of the bladder contributes to this defense mechanism.[38]

INFECTIOUS DISEASES THAT FREQUENTLY OCCUR IN THE GENITOURINARY SYSTEM
Urinary tract infection

Infection of the urinary tract includes microbial invasion of any portion of the urinary system: kidneys (pyelonephritis), bladder (cystitis), prostate (prostatitis), urethra (urethritis), or urine (bacteriuria). Once bacteria invade any portion, all other areas are at risk.

Urinary tract infections are the most commonly encountered infections in a hospital. There are many reasons for this. First, once a person has had a urinary tract infection, a recurrence or relapse is frequent. Second, it is a common practice that each patient admitted to a hospital has a urinalysis and/or urine culture performed. Therefore a urinary tract infection is easily detectable. Third, urinary tract instrumentation (i.e., by catheter or cystoscope) commonly used in diagnosis and treatment increases the risk of infection.

Urinary tract infection may be asymptomatic, whereby a patient has $\geq 10^5$ organisms per milliliter of urine without any other manifestations of infection. This is frequently referred to as asymptomatic bacteriuria or colonization. Urinary tract infection may be symptomatic, in which case in addition to $\geq 10^5$ organisms per milliliter of urine, clinical symptoms (e.g., fever, dysuria, backache) are present. Occasionally a patient may have symptoms and have less than 10^5 organisms. This occurs when a patient is well hydrated, which in turn will dilute the urine considerably, or it can also be observed at the onset of a urinary tract infection.

A community-acquired urinary tract infection is one in which the patient has a positive microscopic examination or culture on the day of admission. A nosocomial urinary tract infection is one in which a positive culture follows a negative microscopic or negative urine culture or one in which the pathogen has changed from the original pathogen that had been identified.

Endogenous sources. Two endogenous routes of transmission have been cited as causing urinary tract infection:

- Lymphatic system
- Vascular system

The fact that bacteria enter the urinary tract through the lymphatic system is rarely implicated. In infancy a hematogenous source of bacteria is important. The kidneys are well supplied by blood vessels, so any time there is a systemic infection present seeding to the kidney is possible. In adulthood staphylococcal bacteremia is commonly associated with spread to the kidneys. When S. *aureus* is found in the urine, another focus should be suspected. Seeding may be occurring from a perinephric abscess or osteomyelitis.

Exogenous sources

Urethral contamination. Entrance of bacteria through the urethra is undoubtedly the most common pathway leading to infection. The fact that urinary tract infections occur less frequently in males reinforces this theory. The longer urethra in the male is probably responsible for this.

Instrumentation. Instrumentation of the urinary tract predisposes to development of infection whether it be by a sound, cystoscope, or catheter.

Catheterization. Following a single catheterization, the occurrence of bacteriuria ranges from 0.5% to 22.8%, depending on the population.[7,40] Healthy ambulatory men and women are less susceptible than women undergoing a difficult obstetrical delivery.

Long-term indwelling catheterization through the urethra or suprapubically inevitably leads to bacteriuria. Incorporating aseptic technique at the time of insertion and maintaining a closed drainage system should delay the onset of bacteriuria for about 2 weeks.[27] Organisms in the perineal area enter the bladder around the catheter.[16]

Cross-contamination. E. *coli* and *Proteus*, enterococcus, *Pseudomonas*, *Klebsiella*, *Enterobacter*, *Serratia*, and *Candida* species are all common pathogens of the urinary tract. Many of these organisms are part of the normal endogenous bowel flora. Others are ubiquitous in nature. However, it is not uncommon for them to be acquired by cross-contamination from other patients, hospital personnel, contaminated solutions, or nonsterile equipment. Pathogens such as *Serratia marcescens* and *Pseudomonas cepacia* are not normal inhabitants of the intestines. Therefore their isolation from a catheterized patient suggests cross-contamination from an exogenous source.[25]

Signs and symptoms. Signs and symptoms of urinary tract infection are not always obvious. It is not uncommon for a patient to be asymptomatic and be found to have a urinary tract infection when having a general health checkup or participating in a screening survey or a preemployment examination.

Dysuria. Burning on urination is common in acute cystitis, prostatitis, and urethritis. It occurs during the voiding process and can be more marked at the beginning, middle, or end of micturition.

Hematuria. Hematuria in association with dysuria or frequency suggests urinary tract infection. However, by itself, it may be a symptom of a tumor of the bladder or kidneys.

Urgency and frequency. Urgency and frequency are usually suggestive of urinary tract infection. However, fecal impaction can cause frequency or involuntary micturition. Nervous tension is another noninfectious cause of urgency and frequency.

Pyuria. Only 50% of patients with bacteriuria have pyuria, the presence of five to ten polymorphonuclear leukocytes per high-power field. Cloudy urine is not always caused by polymorphonuclear leukocytes. Therefore pyuria does not always signify urinary tract infection. The urine may be cloudy because of its alkalinity, which causes precipitation of phosphate.

Fever and chills. Temperature varies widely in association with urinary tract infection. It may range from normal to 105° F.

Bacteria on microscopic examination. One organism per field is significant when a Gram stain is done of unspun urine and examined with an oil immersion lens. Robins et al.[37] found that they could detect bacteria without staining the urine and without centrifugation. Others use centrifugation. After pouring off the supernatant a drop of sediment is placed on a slide and examined. At least 20 organisms with or without polymorphonuclear leukocytes can be visualized in the presence of a urinary tract infection.

Positive urine culture. A urinary tract infection can be diagnosed when 10^5 or more organisms per milliliter of urine are cultured from a properly collected midstream urine specimen. Usually one organism dominates. The presence of several organisms is suggestive of an inadequately collected specimen. An organism numbering 10^4 per milliliter of urine is significant if the urine specimen is obtained by an aseptic catheterization. A finding of 10^2 or more organisms per milliliter cultured from a specimen obtained by suprapubic aspiration is diagnostic of a urinary tract infection.

Common hospital practices that cause nosocomial-induced urinary tract infections

Indiscriminate use of catheters. Catheters are sometimes inserted for convenience of the nursing staff when other alternatives could suffice. For example, external catheters can be used on male patients who are able to empty their bladders but who involuntarily urinate.

Lack of aseptic technique at the time of catheter insertion. Scrupulous cleansing of the perineum and care that the catheter does not inadvertently touch the bedding or patient are sometimes overlooked when busy staff members are assigned the extra task of inserting a catheter.

An iodophor that is effective against gram-positive and gram-negative bacteria and fungi is suggested for the prepping solution. The labia in the female should be separated with one hand during the cleansing process and until the catheter is inserted. In prepping the male the prepuce should be retracted, taking care to cleanse each fold of tissue thoroughly. The hand used to touch the labia or penis should not come in direct contact with the sterile catheter to be inserted.

The catheterization kit should be opened as close to the time of insertion as possible. It is important to check how long catheters are opened in the surgical suite before they are inserted.

Extended duration of catheter use. The catheter should be removed as soon as it is no longer needed. For example, if it is used to facilitate surgery, it should be removed immediately after surgery. Catheters can usually be removed within 24 hours after a cesarean section. The longer a catheter is left in place, the greater the risk of colonization.

Frequent change of indwelling catheters. If the catheter is needed and it is functioning adequately, it need not be changed.

Unnecessary change of urinary drainage bags. Each time a new drainage bag is attached, the closed system is interrupted, and the risk of introducing bacteria is increased.

Clamped and disconnected drainage bags. Drainage bags should remain attached to the catheter when the patient is up and out of bed, when he bathes, and when he goes to physical therapy, occupational therapy, or the x-ray department. The bag can be suspended on a string or gauze around the patient's waist but should remain below bladder level.

Use of leg bags. In an acute care facility, where the use of catheters is for short durations, leg bags are not necessary.

In an extended care facility the goal is to ensure unobstructed flow of urine. This can be accomplished with a leg bag when the patient is out of bed.

If leg bags are used, they should either be discarded after each use or washed well with soap and water. During the interim when the leg bag is not in use, the bag should be filled with about 50 to 100 ml of acetic acid (e.g., vinegar). Vinegar is effective in killing *Pseudomonas* organisms and other organisms resistant to antimicrobial agents. Before reusing the leg bag, the vinegar should be discarded.

Failure to secure catheter to thigh (or abdomen for immobile male). Movement of the catheter in and out of the urethra causes irritation at the meatal orifice. Bacteria on the exterior surface of the catheter may gain access into the bladder as the catheter is pulled or tugged.

Emptying of urine from drainage bags into a communal receptacle. Contamination of the drainage system can either occur from touching the receptacle to the drainage port or from contact with contaminated hands. It is advisable to have a separate container for each patient. Disposable paper cups are available.

Unnecessary bladder irrigations. The best bladder irrigation is accomplished by oral intake of fluids. This eliminates having to disconnect the catheter from the drainage tubing. Providing the patient does not have a fluid restriction, he should be encouraged to drink approximately 2500 ml of fluid every day.

If sediment accumulates and stagnates the flow of urine, a periodic irrigation may be necessary.

Reuse of irrigating sets. Once an irrigation set has been used, it is no longer sterile and should not be reused. If cost is a factor in using a new disposable set each time, then using a glass syringe that can be autoclaved between uses is an alternative.

Use of contaminated irrigants. Irrigants should be supplied in 100 to 150 ml amounts so that once the bottle is opened, the entire amount can be used instead of portions being saved. Unfortunately purchasing agents tend to buy 1000 ml bottles because large bottles cost nearly the same as small ones.

If all that is available is the large bottle, it may be possible for the pharmacy to divide the irrigant under a laminar flow hood, thus eliminating the problem of storage on the ward.

If leftover irrigants are stored on the wards, they should be refrigerated, and if not used within 48 hours, they should be discarded.

Indiscriminate use of antimicrobial agents to treat asymptomatic bacteriuria associated with an indwelling catheter. Patients who have indwelling catheters for longer than 2 weeks inevitably become colonized. Most of these patients remain asymptomatic. Although therapy may eradicate the organisms temporarily, the eventual outcome is recolonization with highly resistant organisms. It is recommended that antimicrobial agents be reserved for instances of symptomatic infection or sepsis.[26]

Surveillance techniques to detect urinary tract infections

Microbiological data. The following microbiological data should be checked:

- Urine cultures
- Urethral smears and cultures
- Prostatic secretions

All positive cultures, with an emphasis on those with a change in organism, should be followed up. Any urine cultures containing *S. marcescens* or *P. cepacia* should be noted because either usually indicates a nosocomial source.

Blood culture data. Any patients with positive urine cultures should be checked for positive blood cultures. It is not uncommon for a patient to develop bacteremia from an organism isolated out of the urine. This would make one wonder whether or not an invasive procedure was performed.

Ward rounds. The following items should be checked:

1. Did the patient have a negative urine culture before the positive one?
2. If the patient had a positive culture in the past, is the organism the same?
3. Was a catheterization done? When? By whom? How?
4. Did the patient have genitourinary surgery? When? By whom? The ICP should read the operative notes to assess if contamination may have occurred during the procedure.
5. How was the urine specimen collected? Clean catch? Catheterization? How long was it at room temperature before being cultured?
6. Do other patients on the same ward have the same organism? Have the same procedures been performed on them? By the same person?
7. If the patient has a catheter in place, is he in the same room with another catheterized patient?
8. What is the susceptibility pattern of the organism? Routine antimicrobial susceptibility testing on urine usually includes the following:

ampicillin	nalidixic acid
cephalothin	nitrofurantoin
gentamicin	sulfonamides
tetracycline	sulfamethoxazole/trimethoprim

   If the organism is resistant to many or all of the above, the nursing staff should be instructed to wear gloves when manipulating the catheter or handling urine.

9. What are the prescribed antibiotics? Occasionally the ICP will encounter an instance when the patient is being treated with an antimicrobial agent to which the urinary pathogen is resistant according to the susceptibility pattern, and from all indications his symptoms have disappeared. This is not unusual because some drugs reach the bladder in high enough concentrations to eliminate the organism in spite of the susceptibility results.

   Patients are usually given an antimicrobial agent for a 10- to 14-day course. It is important that the patient take the drug for this duration to prevent a relapse of infection.

Corrective measures to consider

Collection of urine specimens. To avoid overdiagnosis of urinary tract infections, it is important to collect an uncontaminated urine specimen.

CLEAN-VOIDED MIDSTREAM SPECIMEN. The least traumatizing method is to obtain a voided specimen. Clear, explicit instructions should be given to the patient. McGuckin[33] found a 20.2% incidence of contaminated urine specimens because patients could not understand the instructions, or they failed to clean

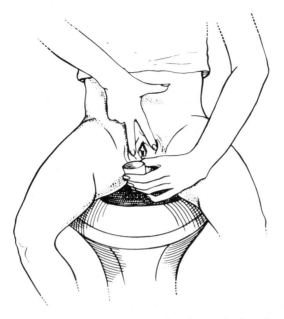

FIG. 14-3. Collecting clean-catch urine specimen. After thorough cleansing of urinary meatus, labia are held apart, and collecting receptacle is held so that it does not touch body. Sample is obtained while client is urinating. (From Billings, D.M., and Stokes, L.G.: Medical-surgical approaches throughout the life cycle, St. Louis, 1982, The C.V. Mosby Co.)

themselves properly because they had difficulty opening the towelette package. She advocates using diagrams and impregnated soap tissues.

In females it is important that the vulva be kept separated until the specimen is obtained (Fig. 14-3). To assist in holding the vulva separate, the female may sit on the toilet facing the back; this aids in keeping the legs separated. It is important to discard the first portion of urine, since it will contain organisms present in the distal urethra. The midstream portion should then be collected in a container.

The clean-voided midstream method should be used whenever possible. The reliability of one positive culture obtained from females is about 80%. This increases to about 90% when two consecutive specimens are positive and to 100% when all three specimens contain the same organism.[26]

CATHETERIZATION. Catheterization is not recommended for routine collection of urine specimens. It is an acceptable procedure, however, if a clean-voided midstream sample is impossible to obtain because the patient is bedridden, debilitated, uncooperative, or obese. Strict aseptic technique must be adhered to to ensure that bacteria are not inadvertently introduced into the bladder.

EXTERNAL CATHETER. If a male patient is incontinent of urine, an external cath-

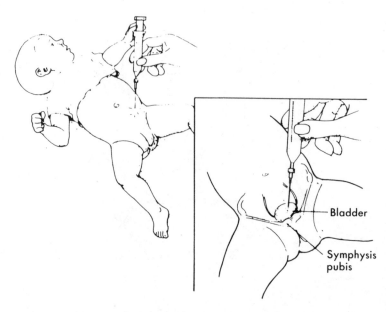

FIG. 14-4. Procedure for direct aspiration of bladder, using suprapubic approach. (From Abels, L.F.: Mosby's manual of critical care, St. Louis, 1979, The C.V. Mosby Co.)

eter may be applied to facilitate collection of a urine specimen. It is important that just before the time the sample is needed the perineum be cleansed, a new external catheter applied, and a sterile clean drainage bag attached. The drainage bag should be checked at 15-minute intervals for urine. As soon as urine enters the bag, it should be emptied into a specimen container.

SUPRAPUBIC ASPIRATION. This method is usually performed by a physician on infants and young children, but it can be useful in adults.[26] The procedure is performed when the bladder is palpable. Therefore it is important that the patient be well hydrated and that he has not voided recently. After introducing a local anesthetic, a 20-gauge needle is inserted directly into the palpable bladder just above the symphysis pubis. A specimen is aspirated using a 20 ml syringe (Fig. 14-4).

OBTAINING A URINE SPECIMEN FROM AN INDWELLING CATHETER. Urine specimens may be aspirated directly from a latex catheter distal to the bifurcation where the lumen leading to the balloon parallels the lumen opening into the bladder (Fig. 14-5). Care must be taken so that the lumen leading to the balloon is not punctured or the balloon will deflate and a specimen of water will be obtained. To avoid this the needle should be slanted toward the drainage tubing. The catheter is wiped off with an antiseptic. A 21-gauge needle is inserted at a slant to assure self-sealing of the latex, and urine is removed. Usually urine is present in the catheter when a specimen is needed because it is lying in a horizontal position.

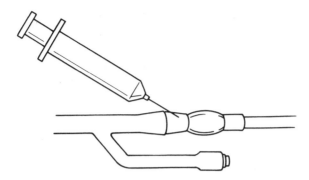

FIG. 14-5. A needle is inserted into a latex catheter, distal to the bifurcation where the lumen leading to the balloon parallels the lumen opening into the bladder.

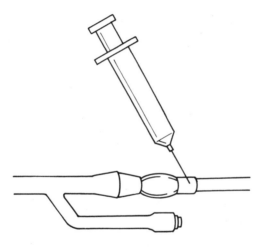

FIG. 14-6. A needle is inserted into a sampling of urinary drainage systems designed for specimen aspiration.

However, if this is not the case, the drainage tubing can be kinked and a rubberband applied. In approximately 15 minutes the drainage bag should be checked to see if urine has accumulated. The specimen should be aspirated before the rubber band is released.

Many drainage bags have a port in the tubing designed specifically for obtaining urine specimens (Fig. 14-6). This is very advantageous, since some of the silicone and plastic catheters do not self-seal. The actual procedure is similar to that of aspirating from the catheter. The port is cleansed. A 21-gauge needle is inserted perpendicular to the port. Most ports are made of a thick rubber diaphragm that can be punctured repeatedly without leaking.

Transportation of the specimen to the laboratory. All too frequently specimens are obtained promptly and carefully but then are set aside for hours until a laboratory runner or volunteer arrives to transport them to the laboratory. A system should be arranged to get the specimen to the laboratory immediately, or provisions should be made to refrigerate the specimen until it can be transported. Organisms are able to multiply in voided urine, and since the quantity of organisms is used to designate an infection it is important that an "infection" does not develop on the utility room counter.

In institutions where refrigeration of specimens is not possible or where a microbiology laboratory is not within the confines of the building, a dip slide method for culture may be useful. This eliminates the necessity for prompt transport, since the specimen is cultured at the bedside. The specimen is collected in any of the methods previously described. The dip slide, which is coated with an agar medium, is immersed in the urine. The slide is placed in its container, labeled, and incubated for 18 to 24 hours. Interpretation of the slide is accomplished by comparing the colony density to a photographic chart. The dip slide method has been shown to correlate well with the standard methods used in hospital laboratories.[12] If the count signifies infection, a colony may be subcultured directly from the slide and a susceptibility test performed.

Urinary catheterization practices. An outline of suggestions for basic urinary catheterization practices follows:

1. Limit use of urinary catheters to justifiable indications:
   a. To relieve retention
   b. To remove residual urine
   c. To facilitate surgical repair
2. Encourage the use of a sterile catheterization kit to avoid contamination.
3. Teach and/or review aseptic technique with medical and nursing staff and students.
4. Remove the indwelling catheter when it is no longer needed.
5. Avoid routine irrigations. Irrigations should be ordered only if the physician suspects obstruction.
6. Use a sterile irrigation set for each irrigation.
7. Use a sterile irrigant. Refrigerate the remainder. Discard if not used in 48 hours.
8. Maintain a "closed urinary system" by not disconnecting the catheter from the drainage tubing.
9. Avoid changing the catheter unnecessarily. The catheter should be changed:
   a. If obstruction is suspected
   b. If sandy particles are felt when the distal end of the catheter is rolled between the fingers

10. Change urinary drainage bags only as necessary. Valid reasons include the following:
    a. Accumulation of sediment
    b. Odor
    c. Leakage
    d. When the catheter is changed
11. Aspirate urine specimens from the sampling port or distal end of the catheter.
12. Secure catheter to the patient's thigh (or lower abdomen in the bed-ridden male patient) to eliminate unnecessary movement of the catheter within the urethra.
13. Use nonsterile gloves to handle urine from patients whose urine contains highly resistant organisms.
14. Geographically separate patients with indwelling catheters in an attempt to avoid colonization from other catheterized patients.

Alternatives to indwelling catheterization

Intermittent self-catheterization. Intermittent self–urethral catheterization is becoming a popular method of treatment for patients with neurogenic bladders. Sterile technique is used when hospital staff catheterize, but "clean" technique is used when patients perform the procedure.[1,29] This transition is often difficult for the nursing staff to make. One explanation for this is that because nursing staff members come in contact with so many patients, their hands are exposed to a number of organisms, many of which are resistant to antibiotics. Although they wash their hands, they cannot be sure that all of the organisms are removed. Resident microbial flora of a patient to be catheterized are usually nonpathogenic for that patient. Lapides[29] further explains that infection is a result of interaction between host resistance and bacteria. When patient immunity is adequate, microorganisms cannot invade tissue and cause damage.

Before intermittent self-catheterization is initiated the following criteria must be met:
- Patient acceptance
- Unobstructed urethra
- Continence between catheterizations

The primary goal in self-catheterization is frequent emptying of the bladder to ensure effective blood flow to the bladder.[28] Overdistention should be avoided.

The patient should begin self-catheterizing at 2-hour intervals to establish continence between catheterizations and then gradually increase the time span between catheterizations from 4 to 5 hours. The frequency of catheterizations should be increased if urine output exceeds 500 ml. Some patients can tolerate a 6- to 8-hour interval at night without self-catheterization.

Intermittent self-catheterization

Purpose
To provide a means of emptying the bladder and to eliminate the need for an indwelling catheter.

Equipment
Soap and water
Clean washcloth and towel
14 or 16 French rubber or plastic catheter
Lubricant
Container to collect urine
Clean receptacle to store catheter

Essential steps	Key points
1. Wash perineal area.	Soap and water may be used.
2. Wash hands.	
3. Lubricate tip of catheter approximately 2 inches down.	A water-soluble lubricant can be used. It is not necessary for females to lubricate catheter.
4. Hold penis up and extend. (Females should separate labia minora.)	The penis should be held on the sides so that the urethra is not pinched closed.
5. Insert catheter gently.	Direct catheter into receptacle (e.g., toilet).
6. Use gentle but firm pressure where catheter meets resistance (prostatic urethra).	Delay catheter insertion if erection occurs.
7. Insert catheter until urine flows.	If urine does not flow readily, use Credé method over bladder region.
8. Continue to introduce catheter a few more inches.	
9. Withdraw catheter slowly when urine ceases to flow.	If urine begins to flow as catheter is withdrawn, pause until all urine is drained.
10. Coil catheter in hand, holding tip up.	This prevents soiling of clothing.
11. Wash catheter with soapy water.	
12. Rinse catheter thoroughly and dry with clean towel.	
13. Place catheter in clean receptacle.	Covered cup, plastic bag, or towel may be used.
14. Wash hands.	

A procedure that can be given to the patient appears on opposite page.

External catheterization. The use of external catheters is often avoided because of the difficulty in application. Although the use of external catheters is not without some risk of infection,[21] it is a means to control urinary incontinence without subjecting the patient to instrumentation.

A procedure that can be used appears below.

Application of an external catheter on a male patient

Purpose
   To provide a dry environment for the patient who has the ability to empty his bladder but who does not have voluntary control.

Equipment
Washcloth, soap and water, and towel
External catheter
Strip with adhesive on both sides
Drainage bag with tubing

General information
A. The external catheter should be changed daily. Thorough, daily cleansing of the perineal area is imperative.
B. Urine specimens for culture may be obtained only after cleansing the penis and applying a new external catheter, drainage bag, and tubing.

Essential steps	Key points
1. Shave pubic hair an inch away from base of penis.	This prevents taping on the pubic hair.
2. Cleanse penis well with soap and water.	If prepuce is retracted, be sure to ease it back over glans before applying external catheter.
3. Dry penis well.	
4. Remove paper backing from one side of adhesive strip.	
5. Apply strip in a spiral manner around the penis, beginning just behind the glans.	
6. Remove paper backing from outside of strip.	
7. Apply external catheter over strip and press gently over tape.	
8. Attach drainage bag with tubing.	
9. Change external catheter daily.	Surgical lubricant can be used to remove residue from adhesive strip.

Sexually transmitted disease

Sexually transmitted disease (STD) encompasses an enormous number of diseases caused by protozoa, bacteria, and viruses (see box below). Although STD is frequently diagnosed and treated within a hospital, as a rule it is not nosocomially acquired. However, it is extremely important that the ICP be aware of all cases of STD for several reasons:

1. STD should be reported to the health department.
2. The ICP can assist the health department by initiating a contact interview in the hospital.
3. The ICP can discuss preventive measures, treatment modalities, and/or follow-up with the patient.

It is not possible in this chapter to discuss all of the sexually transmitted diseases. Thus I have selected those infections that may occur in the genital

---

Sexually transmissible diseases

Enteric infections

Protozoa
  Pathogenic
    Amebiasis, giardiasis, dientamebiasis, balantidiasis
  Nonpathogenic
    Entamoeba coli, Entamoeba hartmanni, Endolimax nanna, Iodamoeba bütschlii, Trichomonas hominis, Chilomastix mesnili, and other intestinal flagellates
Helminths
  Pinworms, *cysticercosis,* * strongyloidiasis*
Viruses
  Hepatitis A and B, poliomyelitis*
Bacteria
  Shigellosis, salmonellosis, others

Nonenteric infections

Classical venereal diseases
  Syphilis, gonorrhea, chancroid, lymphogranuloma venereum, granuloma inguinale
Others
  Genital herpes, condyloma acuminatum, molluscum contagiosum, *Candida* vaginitis, trichomoniasis, *Streptococcus* group B, *Corynebacterium* vaginitis, *Chlamydia* species, nongonococcal urethritis
Ectoparasites
  Scabies, *pediculosis* pubis

From Dritz, S.K., and Goldsmith, R.S.: Compr. Ther. **6:**35, 1980.
*Sexual transmission not expected in the United States, but could occur in areas of the world endemic for the disease.

tract of pregnant women and that may cause infection in neonates.

Genital herpes simplex infection. Genital herpes has been described as the most important sexually transmitted disease.[15] In a New England medical center it was seen seven times more frequently than primary syphilis.[8] It certainly deserves attention because its incidence is increasing, and it causes deleterious consequences in neonates.

It is a viral disease caused by either herpes simplex type I or type II. Reactivation of herpes genitalis has been noted within 12 hours following coitus, but the usual incubation period is from 2 to 5 days.

According to Nahmias[36] the overall risk of neonatal herpes in association with maternal infection occurring after 32 weeks was 10%, being higher in primary cases. If the virus is present at the time of delivery, this risk increases to at least 40% if the infant is delivered vaginally or if a cesarean section is not performed within 4 hours from the time the membranes rupture.

Endogenous sources. Patients who have a history of herpetic lesions may suffer a recurrence of latent infection at any time. The stimulus may be a febrile reaction, occurring during convalescence of another disease. It may follow physical shock, such as chilling, or a metabolic or hormonal disturbance, such as menstruation.[14] Usually the secondary lesions are less severe than the primary lesions because of the presence of herpes antibodies.

Babies delivered vaginally to mothers with active genital herpes lesions are at great risk for becoming infected.

Exogenous sources. Genital herpes is usually transmitted at the time of sexual intercourse. However, direct inoculation can occur from oral lesions. Herpes simplex type I usually causes lesions above the waist and type II below the waist. However, because the genital tract can become infected from the mouth and vice versa, either type I or type II can be the cause.

Signs and symptoms. Genital herpes is characterized by vesicular lesions that look like multiple ulcerations, containing a clear fluid and surrounded by an erythematous border. When they begin to heal, the lesions become crusted over.

Chang,[8] in his outpatient clinic in a New England medical center, describes the following accompanying features of genital herpes lesions:

- Dysuria
- Dyspareunia
- Pain
- Itching
- Inguinal lymphadenopathy
- Fever, headaches, and general malaise

A positive tissue culture is the most sensitive way to diagnose herpes simplex. Vesicular fluid can be collected in a tuberculin syringe, or ulcers can be swabbed, using a cotton tip and immersing it immediately in a tissue culture medium.

Neonatal herpes infection. Neonatal herpes infection is usually symptomatic and can be fatal. It can cause localized or disseminated disease. Symptoms to be aware of include the following:

- Irritability or seizures
- Respiratory distress
- Vesicular rash
- Central nervous system (CNS) involvement
- Ocular involvement

Recommendations for infected pregnant women at term. Every effort should be made to identify pregnant women who are at risk of having genital herpes:

- Are clinical signs present?
- Has she ever had a herpes infection?
- Is there a history of genital herpes in her sexual partners?

The recommendations for cesarean section at term in women with prior or concurrent herpes, as proposed by Kibrick,[23] are given in Table 14-1. Isolation measures include private room; gown and gloves worn for direct contact; and gown and gloves for contact with dressings or contaminated articles (e.g., bedding, diapers). Trash should be discarded in an impervious bag and incinerated.

Employee health considerations. An occupational hazard in caring for patients with a herpes infection is the development of herpetic whitlow.[11,19] This is an infection of the finger caused by either herpes simplex type I or type II.[18] A description of the syndrome and appropriate control measures is given in Chapter 17.

Syphilis. Syphilis is a complex disease that can express itself throughout the body in a variety of ways. It is the third most frequently reported communicable disease in the United States. The total number of cases increased 14.9% from 1978 to 1979.[41] Syphilis is caused by the spirochete *Treponema pallidum.* This disease is of particular interest to an ICP when an employee is accidentally punctured from a needle used on a syphilitic patient and when an infected mother is about to deliver her baby.

Endogenous sources. Congenital syphilis usually occurs transplacentally while the fetus is in utero. However, it is possible for the neonate to become infected as it passes through the birth canal.[31]

Exogenous sources. Syphilis is usually acquired by sexual contact but can be transmitted by kissing when oral lesions are present, by transfusion of contaminated blood, or by direct inoculation.[31]

Signs and symptoms. A chancre is characteristic of primary syphilis. This painless papule usually appears at the site of inoculation an average of 21 days from the time of contact. It may be tender to touch but usually does not contain an exudate.[31] The chancre usually heals in 3 to 6 weeks.

TABLE 14-1. Recommendations for cesarean section at term in women with genital herpes

Genital herpetic lesions present at term	Group	Primary genital lesions	Recurrent genital lesions (or genital reinfection)	Status of membranes*	Recommended route of delivery†	Isolation of mother	Isolation of newborn
Yes	1	+	—	Intact or ruptured <4 to 6 hr	Cesarean section	Yes	Yes
	2	+	—	Ruptured >4 to 6 hr	Per vaginam	Yes	Yes
	3	+	— or +	Baby has been delivered per vaginam	—	Yes	Yes
	4	—	+	Intact or ruptured <4 to 6 hr	Cesarean section	Yes	Yes
	5	—	+	Ruptured >4 to 6 hr	Per vaginam	Yes	Yes
No, but cervicovaginal culture or cytology is positive for herpes	6	—	—	Intact or ruptured <4 to 6 hr	Cesarean section	Yes	Yes
	7	—	—	Ruptured >4 to 6 hr	Per vaginam	Yes	Yes
No, but there is past history of genital herpes, presently inactive or status unknown	8	—	—	Intact or ruptured	Per vaginam	No	No
No, but nongenital herpes is present at term	9	—	—	Intact or ruptured	Per vaginam	Yes	No, at birth (yes, after newborn goes out to mother)
No, but there is past history of nongenital herpes	10	—	—	Intact or ruptured	Per vaginam	No	No

From Kibrick, S.: J.A.M.A. **243**:159, 1980. Copyright 1980, American Medical Association.
*The shorter the interval between rupture of the membranes and cesarean section, the less the risk of fetal infection. The critical period appears to be 4 to 6 hours.
†Dependent on evaluation of individual risks and benefits.

Secondary syphilis encompasses a wide variety of clinical manifestations:
- Maculopapular rash
- Oral or genital ulcers
- Fever, malaise, and anorexia
- Renal, gastrointestinal tract, or CNS involvement

Tertiary syphilis can affect any organ of the body.

There are a number of clinical signs of syphilis in neonates (Fig. 14-7):
- Stillborn
- Growth retardation
- Prematurity
- Failure to thrive
- Ascites
- Unexplained hydrops fetalis
- Rhinitis
- Rash
- Anemia
- Meningitis
- Delayed effects on the CNS, joints, teeth, and eyes

Transmission of the spirochete to the neonate occurs primarily during the last half of pregnancy. The risk of congenital infection is increased if the mother is in the early stages of disease.[3]

In a positive dark-field examination *T. pallidum* can be seen in transudate from a moist lesion or in saline aspirations from dry lesions. It is important that the saline be free of bacteriostatic additives.[31]

There are several serological tests for syphilis, thus making the interpretation very confusing. The reader is referred to Mandell's text[31] for explicit details.

The nontreponemal tests include the following:

1. *Venereal Disease Research Laboratory test (VDRL).* This is usually used to observe a patient's response to therapy.
2. *Rapid plasma reagin test (RPR)* and *automated reagin test (ART).* These are usually used for screening, since they have been found to be more sensitive than the VDRL.

The specific treponemal tests include the following:

1. *Treponema immobilization tests (TPI).* This is usually not used in hospitals because it requires replicating the spirochete in rabbits and determining the ability of antibody plus complement to immobilize *T. pallidum.*
2. *Fluorescent treponemal antibody-absorption test (FTA-ABS).* This test is usually used to verify the diagnosis of syphilis. Once positive, it is positive for life.

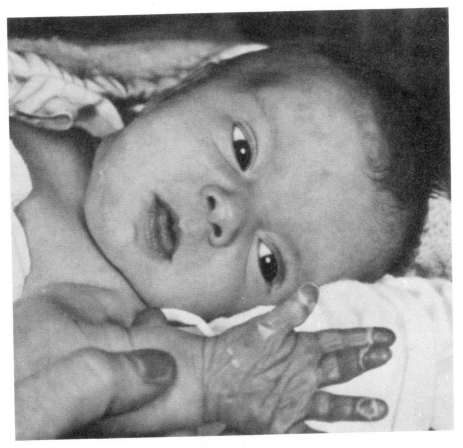

FIG. 14-7. This young infant has syphilis. The lesion shown here is a somewhat unusual cutaneous manifestation of congenital syphilis and may be classified as syphilitic paronychia and bullae. Note the shiny surface of the involved skin of the hand. Cutaneous symptoms occur in 70% of syphilitic infants and are analogous to those of early syphilis in adults. (From Wehrle, P.F., and Top, F.H.: Communicable and infectious diseases, ed. 9, St. Louis, 1981, The C.V. Mosby Co.)

3. *Treponema pallidum hemagglutination test (TPHA)*. This test is easier to perform than the FTA-ABS test and is more specific, but it is less sensitive during primary disease.

Recommendations for prevention and care. Good prenatal care is the best way of preventing congenital syphilis. If a child is born with congenital syphilis, gloves should be worn in handling the infant and his linen, blood, or saliva until 24 hours after the start of antibiotic therapy.[9] Syphilis can be transmitted percutaneously through a break in the skin.

Gonorrhea. Gonorrhea is the most frequently reported communicable disease in the United States. It is caused by a small gram-negative coccus called *Neisseria gonorrhoeae*. Since 1973, when federally assisted state and local programs were implemented to control gonorrhea, the reported number of cases has plateaued at about one million cases annually.[41]

It has been estimated that for every symptomatic case identified there are nine asymptomatic cases. In the female the mature squamous epithelium is relatively resistant to penetration by the gonococcus.[35] Many asymptomatic carriers are detected in prenatal clinics during routine screening.

Endogenous sources. Gonorrhea may be transmitted from infected mothers to neonates.[31]

Exogenous sources. Sexual contact is by far the most common means of acquiring gonorrhea. It has been estimated that approximately 50% of males or females having intercourse with an infected partner will acquire the disease. The disease is also transmitted by genital-oral contact, causing a pharyngitis. Transmission by fomites, including linens and towels, may cause epidemic spread of gonococcal vulvovaginitis in prepubescent girls living in a crowded environment.[31]

Signs and symptoms. Gonorrhea may be symptomatic or asymptomatic. The incubation period is 2 to 7 days. Usually patients have (1) urethral discharge, (2) dysuria, and (3) history of contact with an infected person.

A positive culture is diagnostic. The gonococcus is quite fastidious in that drying and/or ambient air temperatures can kill the organism. For this reason it is preferable to inoculate the agar at the bedside. If the specimen must be transported to the laboratory, Stuart's transport medium is considered to be most satisfactory.[14] For culture an infusion chocolate agar or modification, such as the Thayer-Martin medium, is used. The medium should be removed from the refrigerator at least 15 minutes before taking the culture. A calcium alginate swab is recommended to collect a urethral, vaginal, or cervical specimen. If another medium is inoculated in addition to the Thayer-Martin medium, the other medium should be inoculated first, since the Thayer-Martin medium contains inhibitory antimicrobial agents.

In the infant, gonococcal ophthalmia neonatorum can cause blindness. Not all states require the prophylactic measure of instillation of 1% silver nitrate into the conjunctivas of the newborn, so there may be an increase in this disease.

Recommendations for prevention and care. Gonococcal ophthalmia neonatorum results in an infant born to a mother who is infected with gonorrhea. A 1% silver nitrate instillation into the eyes of the newborn is one of the preventive measures widely used. Less than 2% of infants born to infected mothers become infected if this prophylaxis is used.[2]

Symptoms of ophthalmia usually manifest on the second or third day of life, at which time aggressive penicillin therapy is indicated. Secretion precautions are recommended until 24 hours after initiation of penicillin therapy.

Chlamydial infection. *Chlamydia trachomatis* can be responsible for a variety of clinical manifestations of infections: urethritis and epididymitis in the male; cervicitis, salpingitis, and urethral syndrome in the female; inclusion conjunctivitis and distinctive pneumonia syndrome in the infant.[31] The similarity to gonococcal infections is evident.

Endogenous sources. Chlamydial infections can be transmitted to newborns from maternal cervical chlamydial infections.

Exogenous sources. C. trachomatis infections in adults are most commonly spread by sexual transmission. The prevalence of cervical *C. trachomatis* infection, which ranges from 5% to 60% of women, is related to age, marital status, race, socioeconomic status, and sexual activity.[31]

Signs and symptoms. The signs and symptoms of chlamydial infections fall into two categories:
1. Urethritis
    a. Urethral discharge
    b. Itching
    c. Dysuria
    d. Meatal erythema
    e. Tenderness
2. Cervicitis
    a. Mucopurulent exudate
    b. Cervical erythema

Recommendations for prevention and care. To prevent neonatal complications, an effort must be made to diagnose and treat infected parents.

Group B streptococcal infections. Group B streptococcus continues to be the leading bacterial cause of serious infections in the neonate and young infant in the United States. A study of 93 pregnant women revealed that positive cultures were obtained from vaginal swab specimens on at least one occasion from 20.4% of the women. At the time of delivery 12.9% of the mothers were colonized with group B streptococcus. This colonization occurred in 41.7% of infants delivered from culture-positive mothers, in contrast to 1.2% of infants from culture-negative mothers.[42]

Endogenous sources. A major reservoir for group B streptococci seems to be the female genital tract. However, other sites include the throat and rectum.

Exogenous sources. Sexual transmission of group B streptococci is unknown. It has been found that 50% of men whose sexual partners are vaginally colonized with the organism do have the organism in their urethras.

Neonates become colonized from their mothers and from nosocomial- or community-acquired transmission.[42]

Signs and symptoms. There are two syndromes associated with group B streptococci described among neonates:

1. *Early onset (before sixth day of life).* Clinical manifestations consist of nonspecific findings associated with generalized sepsis.[31]
2. *Late onset (after fifth day of life).* Bacteremia and meningitis are common. Pulmonary symptoms are infrequent.[31]

Recommendations for prevention and care. Vertical spread of group B streptococcal colonization from mother to infant is quite common.[42] Therefore, if colonization is identified before delivery, special precautions in handling the baby should be emphasized. Wearing a gown and gloves seems reasonable.

Puerperal infection. The term puerperal infection includes all inflammatory processes that arise from bacterial invasion of the genital organs during labor or delivery. It is associated with a substantial mortality rate. Types of puerperal infection include vulvitis, vaginitis, endometritis, salpingitis and oophoritis, pelvic cellulitis, peritonitis, bacteremia, and thrombophlebitis.[20] Most puerperal infections should be considered nosocomial unless there is evidence of infection at the time of admission. In the case of endometritis the amniotic fluid may be infected at admission, thereby verifying a community-acquired infection.

Endogenous sources. The microorganisms responsible for puerperal infections may result from bacteria in the genital tract, from a distant site of suppuration by hematogenous spread, or from a contiguous inflammatory process, such as an appendiceal abscess.[20]

The most common manifestation of puerperal infection is endometritis. Organisms ascend into the endometrial cavity, invade the myometrium, extend beyond the uterus, and may even cause abscesses in adjacent organs.[4]

Exogenous sources. It is difficult to distinguish between endogenous sources and exogenous sources when addressing puerperal infections because of the great number of organisms in the normal vaginal flora. However, as with any operative procedure, infection can develop from contaminated equipment or from virulent bacteria from the nasopharynx or fingers of health care attendants.

Signs and symptoms. The signs and symptoms of puerperal infection can be divided into two phases[35]:

1. Phase of lymphatic spread
   a. Fever
   b. Leukocytosis
   c. Tachycardia
   d. Edema of uterus
   e. Pelvic tenderness
   f. Serosanguinous vaginal discharge

2. Phase of systemic spread
   a. Shaking chills
   b. Flushed cheeks
   c. Glassy eyes
   d. Euphoria
   e. Distended tympanic abdomen
   f. Absence of bowel sounds
   g. Bacteremia

Practices that can cause nosocomial infections

VAGINAL EXAMINATIONS. Several clinical studies have demonstrated that vaginal examination before delivery carried no greater infection risk than did rectal examination. However, Gibbs[17] found that the number of examinations was a definite risk factor for development of puerperal infection after cesarean section.

INTERNAL FETAL MONITORING. Controversy remains regarding the actual risk of internal fetal monitoring. It would seem reasonable that since the monitor is a foreign body, it would be associated with an infectious risk.

EPISIOTOMY. There seems to be a small but statistically significant risk when an episiotomy is performed.[17] However, the advantages of this procedure usually offset the slight risk.

FORCEPS DELIVERY. Forceps delivery is associated with a high risk of infection and bacteremia.[17] However, as Gibbs points out, the alternatives, prolonged labor or cesarean section, also carry risks of infection.

SUMMARY

Exogenous infections are primarily responsible for causing problems in the genitourinary system. Microorganisms reside near the entrance of this system, and some individuals seem to be more prone to the development of infection than others.

Any manipulative procedure (catheterization, cystoscopy, forceps delivery) increases the risk of infection. The duration of the procedure and the trauma that it creates are also significant variables.

The urinary catheter is cited as causing most of the nosocomially acquired urinary tract infections. It is definitely a valuable instrument but should only be used when clearly indicated, for only as long as necessary, and under aseptic conditions.

REFERENCES

1. Altshuler, A., Meyer, J., and Butz, M.K.J.: Even children can learn to do clean self-catheterization, Am. J. Nurs. 77:97-101, 1977.
2. Armstrong, J.H., Zacarias, F., and Rein, M.F.: Ophthalmia neonatorum, a chart review, Pediatrics 57:884-892, 1976.

3. Avery, G.B.: Neonatology-pathophysiology and management of the newborn, Philadelphia, 1975, J.B. Lippincott Co.
4. Bennett, J.V., and Brachmann, P.S.: Hospital infections, Boston, 1979, Little, Brown & Co.
5. Bowie, W.R., et al.: Bacteriology of the urethra in normal men and women with nongonococcal urethritis, J. Clin. Microbiol. **6:**482-488, 1977.
6. Boyarsky, S.: Neurogenic bladder, Baltimore, 1967, The Williams & Wilkins Co.
7. Brumfitt, W., Davies, B.I., and Rosser, E.: Urethral catheter as a cause of urinary tract infection in pregnancy and puerperium, Lancet **2:**1059-1062, 1961.
8. Chang, T.W., Fiumara, N.J., and Weinstein, L.: Genital herpes: some clinical and laboratory observations, J.A.M.A. **229:**544-545, 1974.
9. Cloherty, J.P., and Stark, A.R.: Manual of neonatal care, Boston, 1980, Little, Brown & Co.
10. Dritz, S.K., and Goldsmith, R.S.: Sexually transmissible, protozoal bacterial and viral enteric infections, Compr. Ther. **6:**34-40, 1980.
11. Dunbar, C.: Herpetic whitlow: an occupational hazard for nursing personnel, Heart Lung **7:**654-656, 1978.
12. Ellner, P.D., and Papachristos, T.: Detection of bacteriuria by dipslide: routine use in a large general hospital, Am. J. Clin. Pathol. **63:**516-521, 1975.
13. Finkbeiner, A., and Lapides, J.: Effect of distension on blood flow in dog's urinary bladder, Invest. Urol. **12:**210-212, 1974.
14. Freeman, B.A.: Burrows' textbook of microbiology, ed. 21, Philadelphia, 1979, W.B. Saunders Co.
15. Gardner, H.L.: Herpes genitalis: our most important venereal disease, Am. J. Obstet. Gynecol. **135:**553-554, 1979.
16. Garibaldi, R.A., et al.: Meatal colonization and catheter-associated bacteriuria, N. Engl. J. Med. **303:**316-318, 1980.
17. Gibbs, R.S.: Clinical risk factors for puerperal infection, Obstet. Gynecol. **55**(5 suppl.):178S-184S, 1980.
18. Glogau, R., Hanna, L., and Jawetz, E.: Herpetic whitlow as part of genital virus infection, J. Infect. Dis. **136:**689-692, 1977.
19. Greaves, W.L., et al.: The problem of herpetic whitlow among hospital personnel, Infect. Control **1:**381-385, 1980.
20. Greenhill, J.P., and Friedman, E.A.: Biological principles and modern practice of obstetrics, Philadelphia, 1974, W.B. Saunders Co.
21. Hirsh, D.D., Fainstein, V., and Musher, D.M.: Do condom catheter collecting systems cause urinary tract infection? J.A.M.A. **242:**340-341, 1979.
22. Jacob, S.W., Francone, C.A., and Lossow, W.: Structure and function in man, Philadelphia, 1978, W.B. Saunders Co.
23. Kibrick, S.: Herpes simplex infection at term: what to do with mother, newborn, and nursery personnel, J.A.M.A. **243:**157-160, 1980.
24. King, L.R., et al.: Vesicoureteral reflux, J.A.M.A. **203:**169-174, 1968.
25. Krieger, J.N., et al.: A nosocomial epidemic of antibiotic-resistant *Serratia marcescens* urinary tract infections, J. Urol. **124:**498-502, 1980.
26. Kunin, C.M.: Detection, prevention and management of urinary tract infections, ed. 3, Philadelphia, 1979, Lea & Febiger.
27. Kunin, C.M., and McCormack, R.C.: Prevention of catheter-induced urinary tract infections by sterile closed drainage, N. Engl. J. Med. **274:**1156-1161, 1966.
28. Lapides, J.: Tips on self-catheterization, Urol. Dig., pp. 11-13, July, 1977.
29. Lapides, J.: Mechanisms of urinary tract infection, Urology **14:**217-225, 1979.
30. Larsen, B., and Galask, R.P.: Vaginal microbial flora: practical and theoretical relevance, Obstet. Gynecol. **55**(5 suppl.):100S-113S.
31. Mandell, G.L., Douglas, Jr., R.G., and Bennett, J.E.: Principles and practice of infectious diseases. I & II, New York, 1979, John Wiley & Sons, Inc.
32. Marrie, T.J., Harding, G.K.M., Ronald, A.R.: Anaerobic and aerobic urethral flora in healthy females, J. Clin. Microbiol. **8:**67-72, 1978.

33. McGuckin, M.B.: Getting better urine specimens with the clean-catch midstream technique, Nurs. 81 **11**:72-73, Jan. 1981.
34. Mehrotra, R.M.L.: Experimental study of vesical circulation during distension and in cystitis, J. Path. Bact. **66**:79-89, 1953.
35. Monif, G.R.G.: Infectious diseases in obstetrics and gynecology, New York, 1974, Harper & Row, Publishers, Inc.
36. Nahmias, A.J., et al.: Perinatal risk associated with maternal genital herpes simplex virus infection, Am. J. Obstet. Gynecol. **110**:825-837, 1971.
37. Robins, D.G., et al.: Urine microscopy as an aid to detection of bacteriuria, Lancet **1**:476-478, 1975.
38. Shrom, S.H., Parsons, C.L., and Mulhalland, S.G.: Role of urothelial surface mucoprotein in intrinsic bladder defense, Urology **9**:526-533, 1977.
39. Smith, D.R.: General urology, ed. 10, Los Altos, Calif., 1981, Lange Medical Publications.
40. Turck, M., Goffe, B., and Petersdorf, R.G.: The urethral catheter and urinary tract infection, J. Urol. **88**:834-837, 1962.
41. U.S. Department of Health and Human Services: Annual summary—1979, Morbid. Mortal. Weekly Rep. vol. 28, no. 54, Sept. 1980.
42. Yow, M.D., et al.: The natural history of group B streptococcal colonization in the pregnant woman and her offspring, Am. J. Obstet. Gynecol. **137**:34-38, 1980.

Gastrointestinal system

Infections of the gastrointestinal tract include a variety of syndromes and infectious agents. The significant morbidity and mortality associated with nosocomial hepatitis and gastroenteritis require consideration of prevention and control measures by the infection control practitioner (ICP).

ANATOMICAL AND PHYSIOLOGICAL CONSIDERATIONS
Structure and function

The gastrointestinal system includes the alimentary canal (mouth, esophagus, stomach, and small and large intestine) and accessory organs (teeth, salivary glands, liver, gallbladder, and pancreas). The mouth and the esophagus are the only organs that lie outside the abdomen (Fig. 15-1). The remaining organs are located within a cavity bounded ventrally by the abdominal muscles, dorsally by the vertebral column and lumbar muscles, caudally by the plane of the pelvic inlet, and cranially by the diaphragm.

Starting at the level of the esophagus, the organs of the alimentary canal are composed of four layers:

1. The mucous layer (mucosa) consists of epithelial cells. The surface of this layer extends from the mouth to the anus. The epithelium rests on a thin layer of areolar tissue called the *lamina propria*.
2. The submucous layer (submucosa) is composed of loose connective tissue containing blood, lymph vessels, and nerves. The submucosa is a flexible base that adjusts to movement and changes in size of the canal as digestion occurs.
3. The muscular coat (muscularis externa) consists of an inner circular layer and an outer longitudinal layer to promote peristaltic action.
4. The serous layer (serosa) forms the outer layer of the alimentary canal. The serosa, absent in the esophagus, is continuous with the mesentery. It contains blood and lymph vessels.

The primary function of the gastrointestinal tract is the digestion and assimilation of nutrients. Through a series of mechanical and chemical processes, ingested food is reduced to soluble, absorbable substances. Usable portions are absorbed; indigestible or waste materials are eliminated. This system also possesses complex, sophisticated mechanisms that prevent the invasion of microorganisms.

Digestion of food, heavily contaminated with pathogenic and nonpatho-

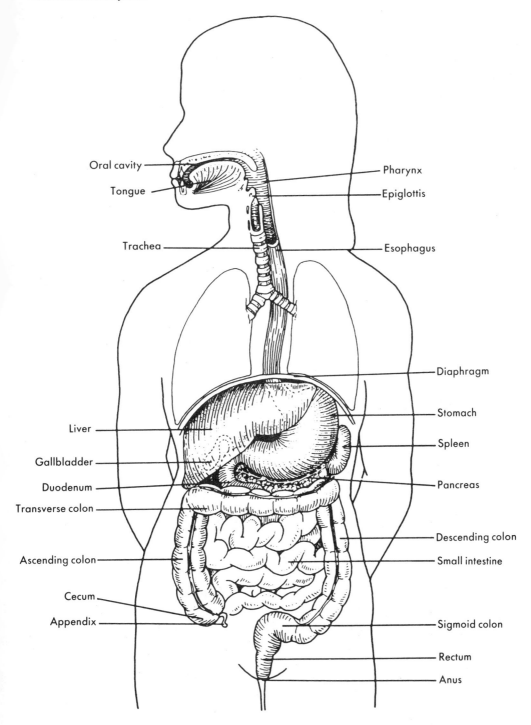

FIG. 15-1. Alimentary canal, including primary and accessory organs. (From Broadwell, D.C., and Jackson, B.S., editors: Principles of ostomy care, St. Louis, 1981, The C.V. Mosby Co.)

genic agents, begins with mastication. Food is ground in the mouth into fine particles; this action increases the total surface area of food exposed to intestinal secretions and also prevents excoriation of the mucosal surfaces. The food bolus then moves from the mouth, through the esophagus, and into the stomach.

The stomach is responsible for storage and modification of food substances into chyme and for the delivery of chyme in proper amounts and proper state to the duodenum. The normal gastric acid barrier (pH < 4) prevents the majority of ingested bacteria from reaching the intestines. Furthermore, vomiting removes certain ingested poisons or toxins.

Once food enters the duodenum, it is mixed with bile and pancreatic juices by contractions that occur at regularly spaced segments, giving the appearance of a chain of sausage. The next contraction occurs at a new point, moving the chyme and mixing it with new secretions from the intestinal wall.

There are two basic types of movement that occur within the gastrointestinal tract: (1) mixing movements that keep the intestinal contents thoroughly mixed and (2) propulsive movement. The basic propulsive movement is peristalsis, a wavelike contraction that moves material toward the anus. The usual stimulation for peristalsis is distension.

The normal motility of the intestines also has a role in preventing potentially serious intestinal infections in two ways. First, peristalsis maintains a normal distribution of microflora; thus it prevents stasis and bacterial overgrowth. Second, direct, intense irritation of the intestinal mucosa by organisms or their by-products or extreme distension of the intestine secondary to increased secretion of fluid can elicit a peristaltic rush—a powerful peristaltic wave begins at the duodenum and passes the entire distance of the small intestine to the ileocecal valve in a few minutes to empty the irritant into the colon. This action may prevent disease caused by enteric pathogens.

Once the chyme has moved through the small intestine, it passes through the ileocecal valve into the large intestine where sodium and water absorption occurs. Numerous bacteria present in the colon play a twofold role. The bacteria aid digestion by acting on cellulose, which becomes part of the dietary residue, forming substances such as certain vitamins. In addition, the normal microflora prevent infection by attaching to the intestinal epithelial surface and producing volatile, short-chained fatty acids that inhibit the reproduction of enteric pathogens.[9]

The final aspect of host defense mechanisms in the alimentary canal is the immunity bestowed by phagocytic, humoral, and cell-mediated elements. A dynamic equilibrium between the host and potentially pathogenic microorganisms is maintained by the activity of neutrophils, macrophages, and lymphocytes within the lamina propria, the specific humoral immunity associated with formation of IgA in plasma cells, and the direct bactericidal effects of IgM and IgG antibodies.

In addition to the organs of the alimentary canal, the accessory organs of the gastrointestinal tract also aid digestion and, to a lesser degree, provide protection.

Liver. Approximately one million hepatic lobules form the principal mass of the parenchyma of the liver and are considered its anatomical unit. Each lobule consists of hepatic cells in irregular, radiating columns with blood channels or sinusoids sandwiched in between. These sinusoids differ from capillaries in that they lack a definitive cell wall but instead contain a lining of phagocytic cells with some nonphagocytic cells of modified epithelium. These phagocytic cells, known as *Kupffer cells*, have the ability to engulf bacteria. Also located between the hepatic cells are minute bile capillaries. All blood that enters the liver, whether by the hepatic artery or the portal vein, passes through the sinusoids to empty into the central veins of the lobules. After cleansing, it passes into the central veins of the lobules and continues its circuit through the body.

The bile capillaries form a network through the liver and eventually join to form the left and right hepatic ducts. These ducts merge with the cystic duct of the gallbladder to form the common bile duct. A summary of the important functions of the liver follows:

Storage
Glycogen
Vitamins
Iron

Circulatory
Blood transfer
Blood volume regulation

Metabolic
Carbohydrates
Proteins
Lipids
Vitamins A, D, and K
Iron
Steroids

Detoxification
Drugs
Endotoxins
Alkaloids

Phagocytic
Kupffer cells

Excretion
Bile salts
Bile pigments
Heavy metals and dyes

Gallbladder. The function of the gallbladder is to concentrate and store bile, which enters it through the cystic duct from the common hepatic duct. Bile is forced out by contraction of the gallbladder when cholecystokinin is secreted by the duodenal mucosa.

Pancreas. The function of the pancreas is to secrete digestive enzymes, insulin, and glucagon.

Normal flora of the gastrointestinal tract
Escherichia coli *Enterococcus* species *Bacteroides* species *Streptococcus viridans* *Clostridium perfringens* *Peptostreptococcus* species *Peptococcus* species *Klebsiella* species *Proteus* species *Candida* species

Alteration of host defenses

Alteration of the normal host defense mechanisms can occur through disease or iatrogenic means.

Gastric acidity. The normal gastric pH (<4) is highly effective in controlling the bacterial load present in food. Hypochlorhydria or achlorhydria permits the survival and entry of potential pathogens into the small intestine. These conditions can be induced by ingestion of antacids; surgical alteration, such as gastric resection or vagotomy; fasting; or aging.

Intestinal motility. The normal peristaltic movement that maintains even distribution of microflora and prevents epithelial attachments of pathogens can be altered by the administration of anticholinergic agents or opiates. The hospitalized patient may be at higher risk for decreased motility because of prolonged bed rest, decreased food intake, and development of an ileus secondary to surgery or disease states.

Microflora. Antibiotic administration may alter the normal gastrointestinal flora. Opportunistic and resistant microorganisms may emerge as more susceptible bacteria are killed off. In addition, newborns are particularly at risk for nosocomial disease before acquisition of normal, enteric flora (see box above).

Specific immunity. The phagocytic, humoral, and cell-mediated aspects of specific intestinal immunity can be altered through aging, malignancy, or immunodeficient states. Intestinal antibodies, or coproantibodies, appear to play a significant role in regulation of intestinal flora.

MAJOR INFECTIONS

Although a variety of infectious agents produce diseases of the gastrointestinal system, this chapter will focus on the major bacterial and viral causes of gastroenteritis and viral hepatitis.

Gastroenteritis

The term gastroenteritis is used to describe a complex of syndromes characterized by a combination of the following classical symptoms: nausea, vomiting, diarrhea, abdominal cramping or pain, fever, malaise, anorexia, and weakness.

Three primary mechanisms are responsible for this clinical entity:

1. Toxogenic agents, such as cholera and enterotoxigenic Escherichia coli, elaborate an enterotoxin that acts on the small intestine to produce a secretory diarrhea.

2. Invasive microbes penetrate the epithelium of either the small or large intestine, with subsequent disruption of the mucosal integrity. Because of the invasion of submucosal layers, diarrheal stools frequently contain leukocytes and erythrocytes. Shigella and Campylobacter organisms are examples of invasive agents.

3. Epithelial diarrheas are caused by agents, including rotavirus, that destroy cells of the intestinal villi and result in malabsorption of electrolytes and fats in the small intestine.

Infectious agents associated with gastroenteritis

Campylobacter species. Campylobacter fetus, previously known as Vibrio fetus, has been recognized as a pathogen in animals since the turn of the century. However, with the development of selective culture techniques by DeKeyser, Gossuin-Detrain, and Butzler[24] the true significance of Campylobacter species as a human pathogen is now being appreciated.

C. fetus is divided into three subspecies: fetus, intestinalis, and jejuni; the latter two are associated with disease in humans. The exact pathogenesis is unknown. Guerrant et al.[33] were unable to demonstrate enterotoxin production. However, the presence of blood and leukocytes in diarrheal stools suggests an invasive mechanism. Recently Duffy, Benson, and Rubin[26] reported a case study that supports this hypothesis. Direct invasion of the colonic mucosa was confirmed by rectal biopsy in a 14-year-old boy suffering from Campylobacter gastroenteritis.

Blaser et al.[10] reported on the clinical course of 35 patients with Campylobacter enteritis. The disease was characterized by an abrupt onset of abdominal pain, frequently associated with malaise, fever, headache, myalgias, and arthralgias. Diarrhea ensued within 24 hours of the abdominal pain. The stools, initially watery or mucoid and later bloody, usually diminished within 2 to 4 days and resolved in 1 week. The diagnosis is confirmed by identification of C. fetus on selective culture media. In most individuals the disease is self-limited, but in protracted or severe cases antibiotic therapy with erythromycin may be helpful. The efficacy of antibiotics has not been established by controlled studies.

A fecal-oral mode of transmission has been postulated. The known reservoirs of dogs and farm animals have been implicated as sources, but often animal contact is not demonstrated in the epidemiology of individual cases. Contaminated water, unpasteurized milk, and contaminated food have also been incriminated as vehicles for transmission. Recently, based on two epidemiological investigations, person-to-person spread has been suggested.[11]

Escherichia coli. Three clinical syndromes are produced by *E. coli*: infantile diarrhea caused by enteropathogenic strains, acute diarrheal illness in older children and adults secondary to enterotoxigenic strains, and acute dysentery-like disease related to invasion of the intestinal mucosa.

Enteropathogenic *E. coli* (EPEC) produces a self-limited diarrheal illness of 1 to 2 weeks' duration in children under the age of 2 years; 80% of the cases occur in infants less than 6 months old.[42] Lethargy and poor feeding are the heralding symptoms, followed by watery, yellow-green, or "pea soup" stools. Vomiting is infrequent, and fever, if present, is low grade.

The unusual susceptibility of newborns may be traced to the lack of acquired normal microflora and lack of specific intestinal immunity. Breast-fed infants may be at less risk for the disease because of the ability of human colostral cells to phagocytize *E. coli* and the presence of IgA to enterotoxin in human milk.[64] If the illness is severe, excessive fluid and electrolyte loss may ensue because of immature homeostatic mechanisms and minimal fluid and electrolyte reserves.

Transmission is thought to be fecal-oral. Nosocomial disease may occur in nurseries where overcrowding and short staffing leads to decreased observance of aseptic practices such as handwashing and individualized equipment.

In outbreak situations serotyping may be helpful in identifying the etiological agent. Serotypes are based on classification by three major antigens: the O, or somatic, antigen; the K, or capsular, antigen; and the H, or flagellar, antigen. Two separate investigators,[28,30] however, have reported little correlation between classical serotypes of EPEC and demonstrated enteropathogenicity in animal models and tissue culture assay. Therefore routine serotyping, a time-consuming and costly laboratory procedure, should not be employed in the evaluation of sporadic cases but may be useful in identifying an epidemiological marker in outbreaks caused by a single organism.

Enterotoxigenic *E. coli* (ETEC) is frequently associated with travel in adults and older children. So-called *traveler's diarrhea*, or *turista*, ranges from a mild illness with no fever to a more severe form with acute onset of diarrhea (up to 20 stools per day), accompanied by nausea, vomiting, abdominal cramps, chills, and fever.[42] This cholera-like syndrome is induced by the elaboration of a heat-labile and/or a heat-stable toxin.

The incubation period of 1 to 2 days is followed by a self-limited illness lasting 7 to 10 days. Food and water contaminated by fecal material are usually incriminated as the vehicles.

Invasive *E. coli* gastroenteritis is secondary to certain strains that invade the intestinal mucosa.[27] Signs and symptoms of fever, malaise, tenesmus, abdominal cramping, and diarrhea appear 12 to 24 hours after exposure and last 7 to 10 days. Stools may have leukocytes or erythrocytes unlike those associated with EPEC or ETEC.

Salmonella species. Four clinical syndromes are associated with *Salmonella* infections caused by over 1700 serotypes classified into 5 groupings (A through E):

1. Acute *gastroenteritis* begins within hours of ingesting contaminated food or water. The reservoir may be animals, birds, reptiles, or humans. Symptoms include nausea, vomiting, abdominal cramping, and numerous watery stools that may contain blood, pus, or mucus (rare in adults). Occasionally organisms invade the lymphatic system and produce metastatic lesions in distant organs.
2. *Enteric fever* is caused by *Salmonella typhi* or *Salmonella paratyphi.* Onset is usually gradual with fever, headache, malaise, and anorexia. An elevated temperature with a corresponding low pulse rate is characteristic if the fever is not masked with antipyretic agents. Diarrhea may be present, but often the patient complains of constipation. Bacteremia is more likely to occur with typhoid fever than with acute gastroenteritis.
3. *Septicemia* may be accompanied by localized infection. This syndrome is typically characterized by intermittent fever, anorexia, and weight loss. Stool cultures may be negative; the diagnosis is confirmed by positive blood cultures.
4. Individuals with *inapparent infection* or *carrier state* frequently have no history of prior disease or known exposure. The carrier state is estimated at 0.2% of the normal population; approximately 50% have had prior gastroenteritis.[42]

The ingested *Salmonella* organisms penetrate the epithelial cells of the small intestine and lodge in the lamina propria. Large inocula of 100,000 organisms or more[9,42] are necessary to induce the inflammatory response that produces gastroenteritis. While phagocytosis by polymorphonuclear leukocytes and macrophages ensues, these cells may not be able to destroy the organisms. This phenomenon may be responsible for the development of the carrier state.[42]

Treatment for salmonellosis is generally supportive by correction of fluid and electrolyte imbalances. There is some evidence that antibiotic therapy in the treatment of acute gastroenteritis or inapparent infection may prolong the shedding of *Salmonella* organisms in the stool. Specific treatment of enteric fever and septicemia depends on the clinical course of the patient.

Control measures are aimed at minimizing exposure through adherence to proper hygienic measures and food processing techniques. Turkey, chicken, pork, beef, unpasteurized milk, and egg products have all been associated with outbreaks. Inadequate heating of foods to temperatures high enough to destroy the organisms or cross-contamination of cooked foods by utensils used to prepare raw foods are problematic areas. Several hospital outbreaks have been traced to the use of carmine dye in performing examinations of the gastrointestinal tract. *Salmonella cubana* was recovered from bottles of the dye, which was used as a fecal marker.

Shigella species. In contrast with *Salmonella* gastroenteritis, the infective dose for *Shigella* gastroenteritis may range from 10 to 200 organisms.[9] Disease is induced by the penetration and multiplication of organisms in mucosal cells of the terminal ileum and colon. The subsequent destruction of cells leads to ulceration. Bloody stools result either from erosion of blood vessels or leakage of red blood cells through damaged tissues into the bowel.

The incubation period ranges from 1 to 4 days and results in mild to severe forms of the disease. Symptoms include fever, abdominal pain, tenesmus, and diarrheal stools containing pus, blood, and mucus. Antibiotic therapy is usually reserved for more moderate to severe cases.

The host is human, and there is a fecal-oral mode of transmission. Outbreaks in health care settings like homes for the mentally retarded or elderly are usually traced to contaminated food or water, as well as person-to-person spread. The latter mode occurs when poor hygienic habits of patients result in contamination of the environment. The low infecting dose of *Shigella* organisms probably accounts for the ease of person-to-person transmission.

Staphylococcus species. Staphylococci produce two separate clinical entities in humans: enterocolitis and food poisoning.

ENTEROCOLITIS. Staphylococci, although normal inhabitants of the bowel, are usually present in small numbers. The pathogenesis of enterocolitis is felt to be related to two distinct mechanisms, both associated with administration of broad-spectrum antimicrobial agents. First, antimicrobial therapy encourages the emergence of resistant staphylococci capable of producing enterotoxin, and second, broad-spectrum coverage suppresses normal bowel flora with subsequent overgrowth of staphylococcal organisms.

These two factors produce a *pseudomembranous* enterocolitis characterized by fever, nausea, vomiting, abdominal distension, and severe, watery diarrhea. In severe cases the patient may be confused and go into shock; death occurs occasionally. Smears of stool reveal large numbers of polymorphonuclear leukocytes and clusters of gram-positive cocci; cultures yield a heavy growth of *Staphylococcus aureus*. Treatment includes isolation of the patient, discontinuation of broad-spectrum antibiotics, and, in severe forms of the disease, administration of antistaphylococcal agents.

FOOD POISONING. In contrast, staphylococcal food poisoning is the result of ingesting food containing the *preformed* enterotoxin. Staphylococcal organisms may be recovered from food samples but not from stool. The diagnosis is thus made on epidemiological grounds.

This syndrome is characterized by the explosive onset of nausea, vomiting, severe abdominal cramps, and diarrhea 1 to 6 hours after consumption of contaminated food. The clinical course seems to depend on both the dose of enterotoxin and the host's susceptibility. Supportive therapy of analgesics and fluids usually suffices as the patient improves within 24 hours. Ham, poultry, fish, meat, egg products, and cream-filled pastry have been the source of outbreaks when improper refrigeration has occurred.

Viral agents. Recent advances in negative-contrast stain electron microscopy (EM) have led to the recognition of several viral agents as important causes of gastroenteritis.

ROTAVIRUS. This virus, also known as orbivirus, reovirus-like agent, and duovirus, has been established as the primary etiological agent for infantile gastroenteritis during winter months.[48] Tallet et al.[60] studied 610 children admitted with acute diarrhea between November 1974 and April 1975. A total of 176 (29%) had enteritis secondary to human rotavirus (HRV), whereas only 28 (5%) were found to be affected by bacterial or protozoal agents. The ubiquitous nature of this illness is appreciated in the findings of Kapikian et al.[38] In a sample population in Washington, D.C., 90% of children over the age of 2 had detectable HRV antibody.

Typically the disease occurs in children younger than 2 years of age. The incubation period of 24 to 72 hours is followed by the onset of fever, vomiting, and diarrhea. It is postulated that the virus invades the epithelium of the jejunum and ileum, causing a diarrhea lasting from 5 to 8 days. Viral excretion peaks at day 3 or 4 of the illness. Respiratory tract symptoms are also frequently noted, but the virus has not been recovered from nasopharyngeal secretions. Fecal-oral transmission is felt to be the predominant mode of spread.

Occasionally adults will contract the disease, usually after close exposure to an infected child. This factor may be significant in newborn and pediatric outbreaks. In one study[53] none of the 34 nursery personnel had reovirus-like agent diarrhea, although 4 did report diarrheal disease. However, Tallett et al.[60] documented seroconversion in 10 of 27 (37%) parents of children with HRV infection, suggesting that infection may be subclinical.

NORWALK AGENT. The Norwalk agent, so named for its association with an outbreak in Norwalk, Ohio,[1] is a virus resembling a parvovirus. The disease is characerized by a sudden onset of nausea, vomiting, fever, myalgias, headache, and, less frequently, diarrhea. Primarily older children and adults are affected by this agent, which runs its clinical course in 24 to 48 hours. Although peak viral shedding occurs in the first 24 hours, prolonged excretion of up to 6 weeks has been documented. Modes of transmission include ingestion of contaminated water and person-to-person spread.

ADENOVIRUS. The role of adenovirus in the development of gastroenteritis is controversial. Virus has been demonstrated in similar numbers in stools obtained from ill subjects, as well as controls. Recent data support the hypothesis that adenovirus affects long-stay patients. Observing pediatric patients with sequential episodes of diarrhea over extended hospitalizations, Middleton, Szmanski, and Petric[48] noted that the first bout was usually associated with rotavirus, followed by a second bout related to adenovirus excretion.

Yersinia enterocolitica. *Yersinia enterocolitica* is one of three species of the genus *Yersinia.* Although the organism has been well recognized as a pathogen in animals, there has been a recent increase in the reported incidence of human disease; this increase is probably a result of increased awareness of diagnosticians and improved laboratory techniques for recovery of the organism.

Most infections are sporadic, but a foodborne outbreak was reported by Black et al.[8] Over 200 children were involved in an epidemic traced to contaminated chocolate milk. Person-to-person transmission has not been documented; animal-to-person spread has been presumed but not proven.

The pathogenesis of *Y. enterocolitica* involves the ingestion of the organism with subsequent ulceration of the mucosal layer of the terminal ileum. Clinical manifestations range from acute enterocolitis, acute mesenteric adenitis and ileitis, to septicemia. The classical syndrome is enterocolitis characterized by fever, diarrhea, and abdominal pain. Stools may contain leukocytes. Young children (younger than 5 years old) are predominantly affected. Since the symptoms of acute mesenteric adenitis mimic those of acute appendicitis, the differential diagnosis is often difficult. In Black's study[8] 16 children underwent appendectomies.

Enteroviral infections

Several viruses, rarely associated with diarrhea, naturally inhabit the human gastrointestinal tract. Spread primarily by fecal-oral transmission, these agents cause a spectrum of clinical syndromes but display a predilection for the central nervous system.

Poliomyelitis. Poliomyelitis is a highly contagious disease ranging from inapparent infection to paralytic disease. The ingested virus, type 1, 2, or 3, moves from the alimentary canal to the lymph nodes, blood, and finally the central nervous system and neural pathways. The significance of this disease has markedly decreased with the availability of effective immunization. Salk vaccine, used from 1955 to 1962, is an injectable solution containing inactivated virus. Sabin vaccine, containing live, attenuated virus, has been used since 1962; it is generally felt to be more advantageous for three reasons[42,]

- Ease of administration (oral)
- Resistance to reinfection through induction of secretory IgA in the gastro-intestinal tract
- Antigenic potency

Disease caused by wild virus is almost nonexistent in countries observing a high standard of hygiene and maintaining a high level of immunity in children. The risk of vaccine-induced poliomyelitis is 1 in 3.6 million doses of trivalent Sabin vaccine.[42]

Coxsackievirus. Groups A and B coxsackievirus cause the following syndromes:

1. *Herpangina*. The self-limited disease manifests itself by the sudden onset of fever, vomiting, sore throat, and the appearance of vesicles or ulcerations on the areola and tonsillar fauces. The lesions caused by group A coxsackievirus are frequently confused with herpes simplex.

2. *Pleurodynia*. The acute onset of severe, paroxysmal chest pain is characteristic of pleurodynia. The self-limited course incubates for 2 to 12 days and lasts approximately 1 week. Other symptoms include headache, fever, and malaise.

3. *Aseptic meningitis* (see Chapter 18). There is no clinical distinction between viral meningitis secondary to poliomyelitis, ECHO virus, or coxsackievirus. Fever, headache, nuchal rigidity, and cerebrospinal fluid pleocytosis are characteristic signs and symptoms.

4. *Exanthema*. Rashes frequently accompany coxsackievirus infections.

5. *Pericarditis* and *myocarditis*. The infection of heart tissue manifests in fever, electrocardiogram changes, and leukocytosis.

The agent is found in both oropharyngeal secretions and feces. Control of the spread of illness can usually be achieved by observing careful disposal of secretions and feces along with good handwashing techniques.

ECHO virus. ECHO virus causes aseptic meningitis, transient paralysis, encephalitis, an acute febrile illness accompanied by a rash, and mild respiratory tract infection. The infection is usually self-limited, although occasionally disease in neonates may be severe enough to cause death.

Necrotizing enterocolitis

The syndrome of neonatal necrotizing enterocolitis (NEC) has been attributed to both infectious and noninfectious causes. Although mild forms undoubtedly occur, this fulminant syndrome is characterized by abdominal distention, an increased volume of gastric secretions, apneic spells, and vomiting. Bloody stools may or may not be present. Roentgenographic examination may demonstrate air in the intestinal wall (pneumatosis intestinalis), venous portal system, or peritoneal cavity. Frequently complications include intestinal necrosis and perforation, peritonitis, and bacteremia. The mortality rate may exceed 70%.[32]

The pathogenesis of NEC focuses on alteration of the intestinal mucosa. Presumably because of this alteration, feedings are poorly tolerated, and normal intestinal flora produce gas that dissects through the friable mucosa.[62] Theories concerning the initial damage to the mucosa include congenital deficiency of the bowel wall, fetal hypoxia in utero or at birth, trauma secondary to umbilical catheters, maternal infections, plasticizers from polyvinylchloride blood bags, and bacterial, fungal, and viral agents. NEC has been associated with the recovery of *Salmonella* species, *E. coli*, *Klebsiella* species, group B coxsackievirus, and *Clostridia* species.[40]

Recent outbreaks of NEC in neonatal intensive care units have prompted epidemiological investigations to ascertain the etiological agents and preventive measures. Virnig and Reynolds[62] reviewed their experience with 21 cases of NEC in 2423 admissions to a newborn intensive care unit over an 8-year period. The investigation was prompted by the occurrence of five cases in a 3-week period in August 1971. No transmissible viral, fungal, or bacterial agent was identified. Although *E. coli* was frequently isolated from the infants' stools, serotyping revealed a different type for each patient. More recently Book et al.[13] demonstrated the interruption of an outbreak of NEC through the institution of infection control measures despite the lack of a common, identifiable, etiological agent. The presumed mode of transmission was fecal-oral spread. Control measures used included enteric isolation for known or suspected cases, cohorting of sick infants, strict handwashing with an iodophor preparation, institution of a primary care nursing system, and exclusion of all staff with signs and symptoms of gastrointestinal disease. This protocol, coupled with an aggressive screening program to permit early diagnosis, led to the reduction of NEC incidence.

Pseudomembranous colitis

Pseudomembranous colitis (PMC) is a severe gastrointestinal disease antedating the advent of antimicrobial agents. Although it was previously associated with a variety of risk factors (e.g., gastrointestinal tract surgery, intestinal ischemia, obstruction), the focus of the past 40 years has been on PMC related to the use of antibiotics.

The pseudomembrane that forms on the colonic mucosa is composed of epithelial cells, fibrin, and white blood cells. Evidence now suggests that antibiotics alter the normal bowel flora, allowing the emergence of resistant microorganisms that produce cytotoxins. As mentioned earlier, *S. aureus* has been linked to this syndrome. More recently *Clostridium difficile* has been isolated from patients with PMC.[63] Chloramphenicol, tetracycline, ampicillin, and clindamycin are among antibiotics associated with the development of PMC.

The clinical presentation of antibiotic-associated PMC is variable. Virtually all patients have diarrhea. Fever, leukocytosis, and abdominal pain may also be noted. Onset is usually abrupt after patients receive antibiotics for 4 to 9 days.[32] The diagnosis is confirmed on proctoscopic examination of the colon by the presence of characteristic raised, whitish yellow plaques over an erythematous mucosa. Early diagnosis and prompt discontinuance of the drug usually results in the spontaneous resolution of the condition. However, continuation of the drug may cause prolonged diarrhea, resulting in electrolyte imbalance and protein loss.

PREVENTION AND CONTROL

Diagnostic measures. The clinical and laboratory workup of enteric symptoms is determined by both patient factors and available support facilities. Both infectious and noninfectious causes must be given careful consideration.

The clinical assessment of the patient includes eliciting an accurate history and performing a thorough physical examination. Age, sex, travel history, underlying conditions, drug therapy, and severity and duration of illness are factors that guide the clinician in making the appropriate diagnosis.

Specific laboratory tests and diagnostic procedures are determined by the results of the clinical assessment and the limitations of services and equipment.

Stool specimen. Examination of a freshly passed stool is helpful in determining the cause of diarrhea. On gross examination the stool may be characterized by color, consistency, and odor. Microscopically the stool should be examined for fecal leukocytes, erythrocytes, undigested food, and fat.

Stool specimens uncontaminated by urine are preferable to rectal swabs in assessing an infectious agent. Fresh, warm stool is required for identification of ova and parasites. For culture of enteric pathogens specimens should be inoculated onto media as soon after collection as possible. When this is not possible, a non–nutrient-holding medium to prevent drying and normal flora overgrowth should be employed. If, from the clinical history, a fastidious or unusual organism is suspected, the laboratory should be informed to ensure the use of selective media and provision of appropriate growth conditions. Specimens for viral isolation are usually not practical because of the limited availability of electron microscopy and tissue culture facilities. If performed, a rectal swab can be transported in a viral culture medium (Hank's).

Proctoscopy. Although proctoscopic examination is not a routine procedure in the workup of diarrhea, it can be helpful when inflammatory colitis is present. Crohn's disease, shigellosis, amebiasis, ulcerative colitis, and pseudomembranous colitis caused by antibiotic use all produce distinctive lesions that assist in making a diagnosis.

Rectal biopsy. Biopsy of the rectal mucosa may also differentiate between certain infectious and noninfectious causes.

Roentgenographic examination. X-ray studies are of limited use in diagnosing infectious causes of diarrhea. If barium studies are considered, stool specimens for microbes should be completed before performing these procedures, since barium renders stool useless for microscopic examination.

Isolation procedures. The types of infection control precautions are based on the mode of transmission of the disease. Entities presumed to be animal-to-human spread or that are the result of ingesting preformed enterotoxins require excretion precautions: the observance of scrupulous handwashing techniques and careful disposal of feces and urine. Conditions known to be transmitted person-to-person through fecal-oral spread necessitate the use of enteric precautions, which include excretion precautions and the use of gown and glove technique. Private rooms are important for children and incontinent patients.

All patients admitted to the hospital with acute-onset diarrhea should be placed on enteric precautions until an infectious cause is disproven or until stool cultures no longer reveal the pathogen. Guidelines for isolation are outlined in Table 15-1.

Proctoscopes and endoscopes. Since patients harboring pathogenic organisms may or may not be symptomatic, it is imperative that hospital personnel recognize the potential for spread of enteric infection through contaminated proctoscopic and endoscopic equipment. Routine disinfection of this equipment is discussed in the section on hepatitis.

Employee health. Employees who prepare or serve food or who provide direct patient care should not work when they have diarrhea. Acute-onset diarrhea lasting more than 2 days requires a clinical evaluation and a stool culture to rule out bacterial pathogens.

Some local or state health departments mandate preemployment and annual stool cultures for dietary personnel. This practice is of questionable cost/benefit value. A more practical method of infection control places emphasis on early recognition and follow-up of diarrheal illness and education of employees regarding food, personal hygiene, and handwashing techniques.

Reportable diseases. Notifying the local health authority is an important control measure. The reporting mechanisms serve as a means of initiating follow-up and investigation of potential community outbreak situations. Prompt recognition and reporting of diarrheal illness may identify a common source of exposure and avert new cases within the community. Local and state requirements vary in defining which pathogens are reportable. The role of the ICP in this responsibility should be defined in the job description.

Nosocomial gastroenteritis. Nosocomial gastroenteritis is defined as clinically symptomatic gastroenteritis that was not present or incubating on admission to the hospital and that is associated with a positive culture for a recognized pathogen or a viral cause assessed by epidemiological data suggesting cross-infection.[16]

Although the majority of hospitalized patients suffering from acute gastro-

TABLE 15-1. Pathogenesis and epidemiological features of acute bacterial gastroenteritis

Agent	Incubation period	Mechanism	Intestinal site	Reservoir	Mode of transmission	Isolation	Duration of isolation
Campylobacter species	2 to 10 days	Invasion	Colon	Animal or human	Water, milk, and food; fecal-oral (?)	Enteric	Duration of illness
E. coli							
Enteropathogenic	4 to 24 hr	Unknown	Small bowel (?)	Human	Fecal-oral	Enteric	Three consecutive negative cultures; off antibiotics
Enterotoxigenic	1 to 2 days	Toxin	Small bowel	Human	Food and water	Enteric	Duration of illness
Invasive	12 to 24 hr	Invasion	Small bowel and colon	Human	Food (?)	Enteric	Duration of illness
Salmonella species	8 to 72 hr	Invasion	Small bowel and colon	Animal or human	Food and water; fecal-oral	Enteric	Three consecutive negative cultures; off antibiotics
Shigella species	1 to 3 days	Invasion	Small bowel and colon	Human	Food and water; fecal-oral	Enteric	Three consecutive negative cultures; off antibiotics
Staphylococcus species							
Enterocolitis	Variable	Invasion	Colon	Human	Alteration of normal flora	Enteric	Culture negative; off antibiotics
Food poisoning	1 to 6 hr	Toxin	Colon	Human	Food and pre-formed toxin	Excretion	Duration of illness
Yersinia species	Unknown	Invasion	Unknown	Animal or human	Food and water (?); fecal-oral	Enteric	Duration of illness

enteritis will be classified as those who have community-acquired disease, a small proportion of patients will develop nosocomial infections. Data from the National Nosocomial Infections Study for 1979[22] concerning the incidence of hospital-acquired nosocomial gastroenteritis give an indication of the relative frequency of this disease:

Service	Rate*
Medicine	0.4
Surgery	0.4
Obstetrics	0.0
Gynecology	0.0
Pediatrics	11.9
Nursery	3.3
All services	1.4

The rate for documental gastrointestinal infections was 1.4 per 10,000 discharges from all services. The highest rates occurred on pediatrics and nursery services, with the lowest incidence on obstetrics and gynecology services.

Three mechanisms may lead to sporadic cases or outbreaks of nosocomial gastroenteritis:
- A common food or water source
- Person-to-person transmission
- Laboratory exposure

The first step in evaluating a patient with suspected nosocomial gastroenteritis is the careful assessment of the clinical condition. Noninfectious causes, varying from drug-induced diarrhea to underlying endocrinological, oncological, or mechanical abnormalities, must be considered.

The occurrence of nosocomial gastrointestinal infections requires consideration of individual control measures (as described for isolation precautions) and an assessment of the epidemiological implications. A single case of nosocomial salmonellosis or shigellosis requires a prompt evaluation of possible sources (e.g., an improperly isolated index case or unusual food source). Generally, a cluster of two or more cases of hospital-acquired gastroenteritis caused by the same organism and occurring within a 1- or 2-week interval warrants an investigation. The search for human or environmental reservoirs will depend on the epidemiological factors of the etiological agent (Table 15-1).

Common food and water sources. Campylobacter, enterotoxigenic E. coli, Salmonella, and Shigella infections are usually associated with community outbreaks traced to contaminated food and water sources. However, person-to-person transmission has also been documented.

Within the hospital, newborn nursery outbreaks of salmonellosis have been

*Per 10,000 discharges.

traced to contaminated formula[56] and pooled breast milk.[52] A combined common-source and person-to-person outbreak has been reported by Steere et al.[57] Thirty-two people were affected. Within a 6-day period, eighteen patients developed nosocomial gastroenteritis secondary to ingestion of eggnog contaminated with *Salmonella typhimurium*. Subsequently, six patients and eight employees became ill, presumably through person-to-person spread. The outbreak was controlled through isolation of infected patients and elimination of the use of raw eggs in dietary supplements.

Person-to-person spread. Although occasional cases of person-to-person transmitted gastroenteritis occur in adult populations of hospitalized patients, the majority arise in the pediatric, neonatal, and newborn nursery units.

In April 1970 an outbreak of *Salmonella newport* infections occurred in the newborn and premature nurseries of an acute care community hospital.[15] The index case was a premature male who developed sepsis and died. Postmortum examination revealed a brain abscess that was culture positive for the organism. Subsequently, five more infants, three manifesting symptoms after discharge from the hospital, were infected. The source of this epidemic was identified as the mother of the second infected infant; it was postulated that the infant was colonized at birth, and transmission occurred through hand contact by personnel.

Multiple reports of *E. coli* gastroenteritis in newborn populations have been published. Boyer et al.[14] reported on 21 cases of diarrhea occurring among 56 infants in a high-risk nursery over a 7-month period. The epidemic strain was isolated from the hands of five personnel, suggesting person-to-person spread from personnel to infants. Vigorous control measures, including closure of the nursery to new admissions, oral antibiotic therapy for infected infants, and wearing of disposable gloves by all personnel engaged in direct patient care, were necessary to control the outbreak.

Ryder et al.[53] evaluated the significance of nosocomial transmission of viral infections in a controlled, prospective study during a community outbreak in January and February of 1976. In their study 10 of 60 children (17%) admitted to the pediatric unit without diarrhea subsequently developed reovirus-like agent gastroenteritis. Age and room location were the only significant factors in this person-to-person spread disease. Cohorting children by age, a typical pediatric practice, may actually increase the likelihood of nosocomial disease.

Control measures to prevent person-to-person transmission can be categorized into management of individual and multiple cases.

1. Individual cases
   a. Prompt recognition of gastroenteritis and institution of appropriate isolation techniques for infants and toddlers

b. Careful screening of maternity patients for diarrheal disease; use of rooming-in or isolation techniques for the newborn

c. Scrupulous handwashing and individual equipment and toys observed by staff and visitors for all patients

2. Multiple cases (outbreaks)
   a. Closure of nursery or room to new admissions
   b. Institution of enteric precautions
   c. Cohorting (by common nursing personnel) of all infected and exposed patients
   d. Early discharge for uninfected and infected patients whenever clinically possible
   e. Careful surveillance for new cases
   f. Microbiological culturing appropriate to the known or suspected causative agent
   g. Terminal disinfection of the environment

Laboratory-associated infections. Laboratory-associated gastroenteritis can be attributed to hand-to-mouth activities during the processing of specimens and cultures. Nineteen cases of laboratory-associated typhoid fever were reported to the Centers for Disease Control (CDC) between January 1977 and November 1979.[18] The exposures varied: 11 individuals performed proficiency exercises to identify unknown organisms; 4 persons were involved in laboratory accidents; although direct contact was not documented, three persons worked in laboratories where co-workers had been processing cultures with S. typhi as an unknown. Strict adherence to safety procedures in processing all laboratory specimens should prevent these infections.

Viral hepatitis

In typical viral hepatitis the major clinical symptoms and findings are caused by an inflammatory process in the liver and associated disturbances in bilirubin pigment excretion. Hepatic cell necrosis also occurs. These changes in liver function manifest in several ways, with a systemic, influenza-like illness predominating in the early phase of typical viral hepatitis. In addition, more specific symptoms include jaundice, dark urine, clay-colored stools, anorexia, fever, liver enlargement, nausea, vomiting, abdominal pain, and generalized fatigue. Subclinical disease is common, especially among children, and jaundice occurs in less than one third of all cases.

There are at least three etiologically separate forms of viral hepatitis: hepatitis type A, hepatitis type B, and non-A, non-B hepatitis. The latter is thought to be caused by more than one antigenically distinct agent. The viral markers and terms associated with each virus are presented on pp. 384 and 385.

Clinical syndromes. Although it is difficult to distinguish between the types of viral hepatitis on clinical grounds, there are some characteristic differences.

Hepatitis type A. Hepatitis A is characterized by the abrupt onset of symptoms. Many cases are asymptomatic and thus escape detection. Fatality rates are low, with a recovery rate exceeding 98%.

The hepatitis A virus (HAV) is transmitted primarily by the fecal-oral route and usually requires ingestion of the virus to infect. There have been case reports of parenteral transmission of hepatitis A through blood transfusion, but this route of transmission is extremely rare. Common-source outbreaks have been associated with contaminated water supplies and with food handlers who have prepared food for numbers of people without adequate attention to hygienic habits and handwashing. Consumption of raw foods, such as salads, and shellfish, such as raw oysters, have often been implicated in these outbreaks, since the virus is killed by adequate cooking.

HAV has consistently been demonstrated in the stools of infected persons, with peak viral excretion occurring during the late incubation and early prodromal phases of illness. The period of maximal infectivity and disease communicability occurs during the 2-week period before the onset of jaundice and before the person becomes clinically ill. Infectivity and viral excretion decline rapidly after onset of jaundice. A chronic fecal or blood carrier state for HAV has not been demonstrated. Viremia is transient but occurs briefly during the late incubation period and early acute phase, usually before hospitalization.[41,51]

Hepatitis type B. The clinical presentation for hepatitis B is similar to that of hepatitis A, except that the onset is usually insidious rather than acute. Patients with hepatitis B may also be asymptomatic, and the illness can occur with or without jaundice. Anicteric hepatitis is two to three times more common than the icteric form. Rash and joint symptoms occur in about 10% of patients. Hepatitis B appears to be a more serious disease than hepatitis A. It may manifest in chronic forms of liver disease or primary hepatocellular carcinoma.[12] The hepatitis B virus (HBV) is found in blood, saliva, and semen and has most often been associated with transmission through blood, such as by blood transfusion, shared needles, and needles-stick accidents. There is no evidence that HBV is in the stool.

Before the availability of testing donor blood for HBsAg, transfusion-associated hepatitis B was fairly common. Now over 80% of transfusion-associated hepatitis is caused by non-A, non-B hepatitis.[2] The major risk today is from commercial clotting concentrates prepared from thousands of units of plasma from commercial donors. Testing for HBsAg appears ineffective in detecting the virus. Attack rates from these materials exceed 50% in susceptible individuals.[49] Studies of hepatitis B antigen have closely linked hepatitis B infectivity with presence of the e antigen (HBeAg) in the blood.[4,61]

The mechanisms of HBV transmission can occur in a variety of epidemio-

Standard nomenclature and definition of terms associated with viral hepatitis

Hepatitis A virus

HAV — *Hepatitis A virus:* a 27-nm* virus. Detectable in stool as early as 2 weeks after exposure and prior to onset of disease.

Anti-HAV — *Antibody to hepatitis A virus:* May be detected at onset of disease and before onset of jaundice. Peak levels reached 1 to 2 months later; appearance of anti-HAV in serum coincides with disappearance of HAV in stool. Remains detectable in serum for many years and apparently confers lifelong immunity to reinfection.

Hepatitis B virus

HBV — *Hepatitis B virus:* A 42-nm, double-shelled virus, originally known as the "Dane particle."

HBsAg — *Hepatitis B surface antigen:* The antigen found on the surface of the virus, and on variable-length tubular and spherical particles (22 nm in diameter) accompanying HBV. Usually detected within 30 days of exposure, although the time interval varies with the size of inoculum and type of exposure. Hepatitis B surface antigen may persist up to 3 months after onset of jaundice. Persistence beyond this period is usually associated with a carrier state.

HBcAg — *Hepatitis B core antigen:* The antigen found within the core of the virus.

HBeAg — *The e antigen (closely associated with hepatitis B infectivity):* Usually detectable several days after appearance of HBsAg. A soluble antigen found in sera containing HBsAg; associated with presence of many circulating HBV particles, high levels of anti-HBc, and DNA polymerase activity. Usually disappears by the time jaundice is noted.

Anti-HBs — *Antibody to hepatitis B surface antigen:* Usually detectable 1 to 2 months after HBsAg is no longer detectable. Found in about 80 per cent of patients who eventually become HBsAg-negative.

Anti-HBc — *Antibody to hepatitis B core antigen:* Detectable shortly after onset of jaundice, may be closely associated with hepatitis B infectivity.

Anti-HBe — *Antibody to the e antigen:* Detection in HBV carriers indicates a relatively low degree of infectivity.

From Jackson, M.M.: Nurs. Clin. North Am. **15**:730-731, 1980; modified from Krugman, S., and Gocke, D.J.: Viral hepatitis, Philadelphia, 1978, W.B. Saunders Co.
*nm = nanometer (one millionth of a millimeter).

Hepatitis non-A, non-B	A "candidate" virus, 27 nm in diameter, has been visualized; studies are in progress to establish the specific association of this candidate virus with hepatitis non-A, non-B.
DNA polymerase activity	An indicator of active virus replication.
AST (SGOT)	*Aspartate aminotransferase (serum glutamic oxaloacetic transaminase):* An indicator of liver damage when present in an excessive amount.
ALT (SGPT)	*Alanine aminotransferase (serum glutamic pyruvic transaminase):* An indicator of liver damage when present in an excessive amount. Increased levels of AST and ALT denote hepatocellular necrosis; elevated during clinical disease and period of jaundice in all forms of viral hepatitis.
Serum bilirubin	An indicator of the extent of liver dysfunction. Values are abnormal during the period of jaundice in all forms of viral hepatitis.

logical settings. Favero et al.[29] enumerated them in order of efficiency of disease transmission:

1. Direct percutaneous inoculation by needle of contaminated serum or plasma (e.g., blood transfusion, needle stick)
2. Percutaneous transfer of infective serum or plasma in the absence of overt needle puncture (e.g., through cuts, abrasions, or other lesions)
3. Contamination of mucosal surfaces by infective serum or plasma (e.g., by mouth pipetting, accidental splashes of blood in eyes or mouth)
4. Contamination of mucosal surfaces by infective secretions other than serum or plasma (e.g., through saliva and semen during sexual activities)
5. Transfer of infective material through vectors or inanimate environmental surfaces (e.g., through shared toothbrushes or surfaces of hospital equipment, such as in hemodialysis units)

Non-A, non-B hepatitis. Clinically, non-A, non-B hepatitis closely resembles hepatitis B but appears to be a milder disease. Chronic forms of liver disease have also been documented. The non-A, non-B hepatitis viruses are thought to be similar to hepatitis type B and to be transmitted by the same routes.

Hepatitis B and non-A, non-B hepatitis are the types of hepatitis most commonly associated with the hospital setting. This is largely because transmission of these agents is most efficient through blood, and there are a great many

TABLE 15-2. Comparison of clinical and epidemiological characteristics of viral hepatitis

Characteristic	Type A hepatitis	Type B hepatitis	Non-A, non-B hepatitis
Incubation period (days)			
Range	15 to 48	28 to 180	10 to 180
Usual	25 to 30	70 to 75	50 to 60
Usual type of onset	Acute	Insidious	Insidious
Fever	Common; precedes jaundice	Less common	Less common
Jaundice	Rare in children; more common in adults	Same as in type A	Same as in type A
Abnormal AST or ALT	Transient (1 to 3 weeks duration)	Prolonged (may be elevated 1 to 8+ months)	Prolonged
Age group affected	Usually children and young adults	All age groups	All age groups
Virus in feces	Present during late incubation period and acute phase	No direct evidence of presence	Unknown
Virus in blood (viremia)	Present during late incubation period and *early* acute phase	Present during late incubation period and acute phase; may persist for months or years	Probably similar to type B
Virus in urine	Very low level or negative	Low level	Low level likely but unproved
Virus transmitted by saliva	Unlikely	Yes, but direct transfer probably necessary	Unknown
Usual mechanism(s) of transmission	Fecal-oral route	Percutaneous; oral-oral route	Percutaneous (especially via transfused blood); possibly oral-oral route
Carrier state	No	Yes	Evidence suggests yes

From Jackson, M.M.: Nurs. Clin. North Am. **15**:735, 1980; modified from Krugman, S., and Gocke, D.J.: Viral hepatitis. Philadelphia, 1978, W.B. Saunders Co., and Mosely, J.W.: Epidemiology of viral hepatitis, and Control and prevention of viral hepatitis. In Barrett-Connor, E., et al., editors: Epidemiology for the infection control nurse, St. Louis, 1978, The C.V. Mosby Co.

patient care activities in which blood contamination or exposure can occur. In addition, it is known that a long-term carrier state can persist for hepatitis B and occurs in as many as 10% of patients infected with HBV. It has also been documented that a carrier state exists for non-A, non-B hepatitis.[35,59] These carriers provide a reservoir of individuals who may be clinically without symptoms but capable of transmitting the infection to others through their blood that is positive for the infective antigen.

Table 15-2 outlines additional clinical and epidemiological characteristics of the three types of hepatitis.

Laboratory tests. Laboratory tests are required to determine with accuracy the type of hepatitis manifested by the patient. The tests are specific for hepatitis A and B but are not yet available for non-A, non-B hepatitis. Accordingly, a diagnosis of non-A, non-B hepatitis is often a diagnosis of exclusion.

A patient who comes to the hospital with acute hepatitis will have several tests ordered. A test for serum bilirubin is ordered to note the extent of liver dysfunction. The serum aminotransferase levels, AST and ALT, will denote the amount of hepatocellular necrosis. The hepatitis B surface antigen test (HBsAg) is ordered to determine if the clinical hepatitis is hepatitis B. The viral markers for hepatitis B appear in the blood at different times during the course of the patient's illness (Fig. 15-2). Correlation of laboratory values and clinical symptoms is important in determining the course of the infection in the patient.

If the clinician suspects that the patient may have hepatitis A, a serological test to measure for anti-HAV can be done by most laboratories.[20] If the anti-HAV test is positive, it indicates that the individual has antibody to the HAV. How-

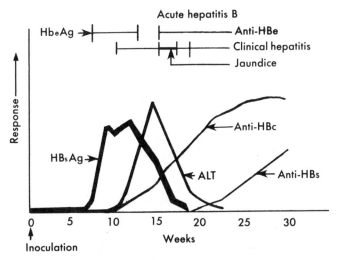

FIG. 15-2. Clinical correlation of laboratory values and viral markers in acute hepatitis type B.

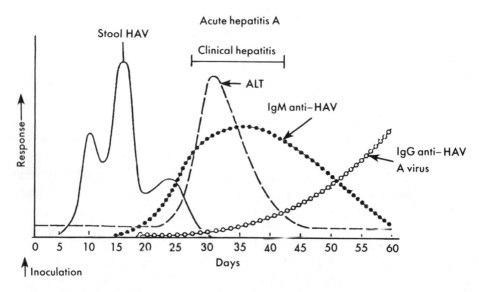

FIG. 15-3. Clinical correlation of laboratory values and viral markers in acute hepatitis type A.

ever, it does not determine with certainty that the present infection is hepatitis A. A second test to differentiate between IgG and IgM antibody is necessary to make this determination. If the second test is positive for IgM, it indicates current infection; if it is negative for IgM, then the hepatitis A infection occurred sometime in the past. Fig. 15-3 presents the relationship between time of inoculation with HAV and measurable levels of IgM and IgG in the blood. The IgM level drops rapidly after the peak of illness and usually disappears from the blood within 3 to 4 months. The IgG antibody persists for years. In fact many patients with acute hepatitis B will also be IgG anti-HAV positive, indicating an earlier infection with HAV. Over half of the U.S. adult population has had a hepatitis A infection, but a much smaller proportion of the population recalls being ill with hepatitis A. This is because many cases are asymptomatic and occur during early childhood.

Theoretically risk reduction for HBV in the hospital setting could be focused on identifying all HBsAg- and HBeAg-positive patients. This is neither realistic nor cost-effective. HBsAg testing is done in most commercial laboratories but is not done on a daily basis. This means that a determination of a patient's antigen status requires at least 1 or more days. Testing for HBeAg is done in a few commercial laboratories, but it is a test that is run infrequently. Both tests are fairly costly. Rather than attempting to test the entire population entering the hospital, certain high-risk patient groups have been defined. Personnel and patients in hemodialysis, oncology, and transplantation units are at special risk because exposure to blood and blood fractions is common and because patients on these wards have a greater likelihood of being carriers and/or asymptomatic than do other patients, partly because of their exposure to immunosuppressive drugs. Other patients for whom an increased index of suspicion is appropriate include those with acute, unconfirmed viral hepatitis, patients institutionalized with Down's syndrome, persons of Asian birth, male homosexuals, and users of illicit, intravenous drugs.[21]

Implications for infection control

Isolation procedures. The modes of transmission of the hepatitis viruses are different and determine the precautions necessary in the hospital setting to reduce risk to personnel and other patients. In 1979 Favero et al.[29] of the CDC published guidelines for the care of patients hospitalized with viral hepatitis. The guidelines include these major features:

1. *Room assignment.* Patients need not be put in a private room unless they are fecally incontinent, as with small children, and the type of hepatitis is unknown or has been shown to be non-B hepatitis.
2. *Hands.* Hands must be washed before or after direct contact with a patient or with items in contact with a patient's blood or feces.
3. *Gloves.* Persons having direct contact with the patient's feces or blood or articles contaminated with blood or feces or using instruments for vascular access must wear gloves. Persons who have dermatitis should wear gloves for all patient contact.
4. *Gowns.* Persons should wear gowns when they have contact with a patient's blood or feces, when carrying out procedures in which excessive blood spills or spatters may occur, or when using instruments on a patient in such a manner that excessive fecal or blood contamination can be expected, such as proctoscopy.
5. *Linen.* No special precautions are needed with linens unless they are visibly contaminated with feces or blood, in which case they should be put in a laundry bag in the patient's room and carefully placed into washing machines without being sorted; the bags must be washed or discarded.
6. *Clothing and personal effects.* No special precautions are needed for these items unless there is visible contamination with feces or blood.
7. *Dishes.* No special precautions are needed.
8. *Visitors.* No special precautions are required.

If the type of hepatitis is known to be hepatitis B, personnel can concentrate on blood precautions and use care when suctioning oral secretions, such as wearing gloves on both hands.

If the type of hepatitis is known to be hepatitis A, personnel can concentrate on careful handling of stool. Fig. 15-3 delineates the time of stool-HAV excretion and shows clearly that by the time the patient is clinically ill, the amount of HAV in the stool is relatively small. These patients are most infectious in the 2 weeks before the onset of clinical illness and during that time have possibly transmitted hepatitis A to close household contacts. It is important for these contacts to be counseled about the need for immune serum globulin (IG) to reduce their risk of developing hepatitis A. Personnel are at very little risk of contracting hepatitis A from the patient hospitalized with that disease.

The CDC recommends several methods for cleaning, disinfecting, and sterilizing HBV-contaminated items.[17] It is hypothesized that the same agents would be effective for HAV and non-A, non-B virus contamination although such studies have not been done.

Whether or not an item needs sterilization, high-level disinfection, or low-level disinfection is based partly on how and where the item is to be used. Guidelines for making these determinations have also been published by the CDC.[19]

In general, concurrent and terminal cleaning of the patient's room can be done according to routine cleaning procedures for other areas of the hospital; however, special attention should be given to areas or items grossly soiled with feces or blood. Gloves should be worn by cleaning personnel while cleaning these areas with a detergent or disinfectant known to be effective against hepatitis viruses. A freshly prepared solution of sodium hypochlorite (0.05 to 0.5% solution of commercial household bleach prepared by adding about one-fourth cup of 5.25% sodium hypochlorite to a gallon of water) is an effective cleaning agent, as are various strengths of formaldehyde, iodophors, and alkalinized glutaraldehyde.

The processing of flexible, fiberoptic endoscopes for examination of the gastrointestinal tract should include the following[34]:

1. Scrupulous mechanical cleaning of the insertion tube and channels is necessary to remove organic material. A detergent solution should be used.
2. Inspection of the equipment for damage should be done.
3. Disinfection of the insertion tube and channels is performed by using 0.5% iodophor solution or 2% glutaraldehyde (follow manufacturer's instructions).
4. Disinfection is followed by a thorough rinsing and drying of the equipment.
5. Accessories (biopsy forceps and cytology brushes) should be thoroughly cleaned and terminally sterilized with steam or ethylene oxide.

Hemodialysis units. Hemodialysis units have been studied extensively for risk of HBV transmission because of a number of serious outbreaks of hepatitis type B before the availability of HBsAg testing. Since the early 1970s, hemodialysis units have used routine serological screening programs for both patients and personnel to maintain awareness of the hepatitis B antigen and antibody status of both groups and have developed effective control measures to separate antigen-positive patients from other patients receiving hemodialysis. Specific recommendations from the CDC Hepatitis Laboratories Division were published in 1977[17] and are summarized in the following sections.

SEROLOGICAL SCREENING. The purpose of serological screening is to determine the immune status of patients and staff. This assessment identifies individuals who are:

- HBsAg positive (potential sources of infection)
- anti-Hbs positive (immune)
- HBV seronegative (at risk for disease)

Initial screening of dialysis candidates and prospective employees should be performed to establish baseline status and screening intervals.

1. Patient screening
   a. Seronegative status (HBsAg and anti-HBs negative): monthly testing for HBsAg and AST and/or ALT; quarterly testing for anti-HBs
   b. Anti-HBs positive: annual testing for anti-HBs to verify immunity
   c. HBsAg positive: quarterly testing for HBsAg (more frequently if clinically or epidemiologically indicated)
2. Staff surveys
   a. Seronegative staff (HBsAg and anti-HBs negative): testing every 2 or 3 months for HBsAg and anti-HBs
   b. Anti-HBs positive: annual testing
   c. HBsAg positive: quarterly testing for HBsAg

Patients and staff who are anti-HBs or HBsAg positive are placed on the regular screening schedule if two consecutive tests are confirmed as positive. Individuals who are HBsAg positive should not be tested for anti-HBs until they become antigen negative.

PREVENTION AND CONTROL MEASURES

Staffing assignments and sound, consistent environmental control measures minimize the risk of cross-infection.

1. Patients who are HBsAg positive should be isolated or spatially segregated from seronegative patients.
2. Staff members who are HBsAg positive or anti-HBs positive should care for HBsAg-positive patients. Ideally these staff members should not care for both seropositive and seronegative patients in the same shift. If this is impossible, they must change gloves and laboratory coats and wash their hands between seeing patients.
3. All patients should have assigned dialysis stations and individual supply trays, linen, and diet trays.
4. If possible, dialysis equipment used for HBsAg-positive patients should not be used for seronegative patients.
5. Gloves should be worn by staff members when handling patients, dialy-

sis equipment, or blood specimens. Scrub suits and gowns should be worn on the unit; a laboratory coat should be worn over the uniform when leaving the patient care area within the unit.

6. Staff members should not smoke, eat, or drink in patient care or laboratory areas.
7. Blood spills should immediately be sponged up and the area cleaned with a disinfectant.
8. Specimens from HBsAg-positive patients should be clearly labeled.

Laboratories. Another area of the hospital where there is clearly increased risk is in the clinical laboratory where blood is handled. A study of environmental contamination in clinical laboratory areas suggested that transmission of HBV in the clinical laboratory was subtle and mainly by hand contact with contaminated items during the various steps of blood processing through inapparent breaks in skin and mucous membranes.[43] This is another area where scrupulous prevention techniques, such as frequent handwashing and adequate cleaning of surfaces and equipment, need to be emphasized and enforced.

Maternity and newborn care. Questions frequently arise about the risk of hepatitis in infants born to mothers who have active disease during pregnancy or are chronic carriers for HBsAg or non-A, non-B hepatitis. Tong et al.[61] recently completed a study in which they observed infants born to 83 pregnant women with acute icteric hepatitis during pregnancy (Table 15-3). Six women had acute hepatitis A; however, there was no evidence of hepatitis A in their infants during follow-up. Sixty-five pregnant women had acute hepatitis B during pregnancy or in the immediate postpartum period. Transmission to infants often occurred when both maternal HBsAg and HBeAg were positive at delivery and postpartum. Fig. 15-2 shows clearly that HBsAg and HBeAg are present before clinical symptoms and could thus be transmitted during the

TABLE 15-3. Frequency of viral agents in pregnant women and neonatal outcome

| Viral agent | Number | Neonatal outcome | | Total |
		Clinical symptoms	Laboratory evidence	
Hepatitis A	6	0	0	0
Hepatitis B	65	2	23	25 (38%)
Hepatitis non-A, non-B	12	0	6*	6 (50%)

Modified from Tong, M.J., et al. Gastroenterology **80**:999-1004, 1981.
*As indicated by elevated serum alanine aminotransferases (ALT).

preclinical phase of illness. A majority of the infants born to mothers with hepatitis B never developed jaundice, have remained persistently HBsAg positive, and have had periodic serum enzyme elevations during follow-up. The risk to the infant of developing hepatitis B was strongly correlated with the trimester in which the mother experienced the HBV infection (Table 15-4).

Twelve women had acute non-A, non-B hepatitis during pregnancy. Infants born to six of these women near term had transient elevations of serum enzyme values at 4 to 8 weeks of age, suggesting maternal transmission of the non-A, non-B virus to the infant.

It has also been shown that neonates infected at birth are at high risk of becoming long-term chronic carriers of HBV. Such carriers are prone to develop serious chronic sequelae of HBV infection, such as chronic active hepatitis, cirrhosis, and primary hepatocellular carcinoma.[12] It has also been shown that prompt use of hepatitis B immune globulin (HBIG) can prevent the development of the chronic carrier state in the majority of infected infants.[7] As a result of these findings, the Advisory Committee on Immunization Practices (ACIP) recommendations of September 1981 include treating all infants born to HBsAg-positive mothers with HBIG immediately after birth and at 3 and 6 months.[21]

Other questions that frequently arise are can the infant be with the mother during the time they are in the hospital and can the infant breast-feed? During delivery the infant is exposed to large amounts of blood; therefore separating him from his mother after delivery is pointless. Although HBsAg has been detected in some samples of breast milk, the concentration has been shown to be very low. Studies in Taiwan have shown that breastfed infants of carrier

TABLE 15-4. Maternal-infant transmission of HBV in mothers with acute hepatitis B during pregnancy

Number of mothers	Clinical hepatitis during trimester of pregnancy	Number of HBsAg-positive infants
16	First	0
17	Second	1 (6%)
24*	Third	16 (67%)
8	Postpartum (up to 6 wk)	8 (100%)
TOTAL 65		25 (38%)†

Modified from Tong, M.J., et al.: Gastroenterology **80**:999-1004, 1981.
*21 of 24 mothers were HBsAg positive at time of delivery.
†Only one infant was HBsAg positive at birth; the other 24 became HBsAg positive within 4 to 16 weeks after delivery.

mothers are not more likely to be infected at 1 year of age than are infants for whom breast-feeding is withheld.[6] Exposure of the infant to HBV through breast milk appears insignificant when compared with the intensive exposure during the birth process.

Employee considerations

HBsAg carriers. An area of concern and controversy is the management of health care professionals who are HBsAg carriers. Mosley[49] suggests that an estimated 1% or more of this group may have chronic antigenemia. This estimate exceeds the prevalence in blood donor populations, which ranges from 0.1% to 1.0%.[41]

Alter et al.[3] prospectively studied 228 patient contacts of health care workers who were acutely or chronically positive for HbsAg. No exposed or control patient acquired clinical hepatitis or developed antigenemia.

Similarly, Meyers et al.[47] followed the clinical and serological courses of 30 of 49 patients undergoing operative procedures in 2 months preceding the acute onset of hepatitis B in an orthopedic surgeon. Five patients were seropositive for anti-HBs, and one was found to have asymptomatic antigenemia. It was not clear whether these results were caused by exposure or represented prior infection.

A statement by the American Hospital Association summarizes the current recommendation: "On the basis of presently available data, otherwise healthy carriers should be allowed to work in the hospital without restrictions. As with all personnel who have patient care responsibilities, they should be advised to practice strict personal hygiene and to exercise care in preventing their blood or secretions from contacting other individuals."[5] Restrictions should be placed only when epidemiological evidence suggests transmission of disease to patients.

Needle sticks. Outside of these clearly defined high-risk areas, the most frequent exposure to potentially infectious blood occurs as a result of an accidental needle stick. In a study conducted at the University of Wisconsin Hospitals 316 reported needle-stick injuries that occurred in hospital employees over a 47-month period were reviewed. Housekeeping employees (127.0 cases per 1000 employees annually) and laboratory personnel (104.7/1000) experienced the highest incidence of injuries, followed by registered nurses (92.6/1000). Most injuries occurred during disposal of used needles (23.7%), administration of parenteral injections or infusion therapy (21.2%), drawing of blood (16.5%), recapping of needles after use (12.0%), or handling of linen or trash containing uncapped needles (16.1%). The authors recommended installation of a needle disposal system that would provide for needle disposal in the patient rooms and at the nursing stations. Based on the findings of the study, they also developed formal guidelines for the prevention of needle sticks and a protocol for management of the injuries by the employee health service.[46]

Prophylaxis with immune serum globulins. In the hospital the risk of clinical hepatitis B following exposure to blood known to contain HBsAg is approximately 5%, or 1 in 20. If the blood is of unknown HBsAg status, the risk is 100 times lower, or about 1 in 2000. Risk increases in direct proportion to the likelihood that blood is HBsAg positive.[20] These odds are based on the results of several cooperative studies[31,36,54,55] and form the basis for the current recommendations for immunoprophylaxis for needle-stick injuries presented by the ACIP.[21] At the time of a needle-stick injury in an employee two decisions are involved: whether to test for HBsAg in the donor and which IG to give. Because these decisions relate both to the relative probability that the source will be HBsAg positive and to the inherent delay in obtaining test results, the ACIP has developed specific guidelines, as presented in Table 15-5.

Recent studies have shown that (1) IGs can greatly reduce risk of hepatitis B

TABLE 15-5. Summary of prophylaxis after acute exposures to HBV

Exposure	HBsAg testing	Recommended prophylaxis
HBsAg positive	—	HBIG* (0.06 ml/kg) immediately and 1 month later
HBsAg status unknown Source known High risk†	Yes‡	IG§ (0.06 ml/kg) immediately: if test positive, HBIG (0.06 ml/kg) immediately and 1 month later; if test negative, nothing
Low risk‖ HBsAg status unknown	No	Nothing or IG (0.06 ml/kg)
Source unknown	No	Nothing or IG (0.06 ml/kg)

Modified from Centers for Disease Control: Morbid. Mortal. Weekly Rep. **30:**433, 1981.
*Hepatitis B immune globulin prepared from plasma preselected for high titer anti-HBs. In the United States HBIG has an anti-HBs titer of >1:100,000 by radioimmunoassay. Currently the price of a dose of HBIG is more than 20 times that of IG.
†Patients with acute, unconfirmed viral hepatitis; patients institutionalized with Down's syndrome; patients on hemodialysis; persons of Asian origin; male homosexuals; users of illicit, intravenous drugs.
‡If results can be known within 7 days of exposure.
§Immune globulin prepared from plasma that is not preselected for anti-HBs content. Since 1977 all lots tested have contained anti-HBs at a titer of at least 1:100 by radioimmunoassay.
‖The average hospital patient.

in certain settings and generally indicate that HBIG is the IG of choice after percutaneous (needle stick) or mucous membrane exposure to blood containing HBsAg; (2) IG appears to have some effect in preventing clinical hepatitis B; and (3) the more rapidly either is given after exposure, the better.[39,44,55]

Hepatitis B vaccine. The hepatitis B vaccine is made from human plasma obtained from healthy persons who are persistent carriers of HBsAg. The virus is inactivated during preparation.[65] Clinical trials have shown that 75% to 90% of adults developed antibody (anti-HBs) after two doses, and over 90% developed anti-HBs after the third dose. Among vaccine recipients, clinical hepatitis B or HBV infection developed in 1.4% to 3.4%, compared to 18% to 27% of the placebo groups.[58]

In June of 1982 the ACIP published recommendations intended as initial guides for immunization practice.[23] These guidelines are based in part on serological surveys of various population groups. Table 15-6 denotes the preva-

TABLE 15-6. Expected hepatitis B virus prevalence in various population groups

Risk	Prevalence of serological markers of HBV infection	
	HBsAg (%)	All markers (%)*
High		
Immigrants and refugees from areas of high HBV endemicity	13	70 to 85
Clients in institutions for the mentally retarded	10 to 20	35 to 80
Users of illicit parenteral drugs	7	60 to 80
Homosexually active males	6	35 to 80
Household contacts of HBV carriers	3 to 6	30 to 60
Patients of hemodialysis units	3 to 10	20 to 80
Intermediate		
Prisoners (male)	1 to 8	10 to 80
Staff of institutions for the mentally retarded	1	10 to 25
Health care workers Frequent blood contact	1 to 2	15 to 30
Low		
Health care workers No or infrequent blood contact	0.3	3 to 10
Healthy adults (first-time volunteer blood donors)	0.3	3 to 5

From Centers for Disease Control: Morbid. Mortal. Weekly Rep. **31**:318, 1982.
*Includes presence of HbsAg, anti-HBs, HBeAg, and others.

lence of serological markers of HBV infection. These surveys demonstrate that although HBV infection is uncommon among adults in the general population, it is highly prevalent in certain groups. For example, immigrants and refugees and their descendants from areas of high HBV endemicity are at high risk of HBV infection because of the proportion of the population that is HBsAg positive and thus a reservoir for HBV. Surveys of health care workers with frequent blood contact have found this group to be seropositive for one or more HBV markers 15% to 30% of the time, whereas health care workers with none or infrequent blood contact are only slightly more likely (3% to 10%) to be positive for one or more HBV markers than the healthy adult population (3% to 5%). These personnel are no more likely to be HBsAg positive than the healthy adult population (3 HBsAg positive per 1000 screened). These data were used by the ACIP in determining groups at highest risk of HBV infection, and thus groups for whom the hepatitis B vaccine would confer the most benefit.

Studies are also underway to establish the role that hepatitis B vaccine may play in the prevention of perinatal transmission of HBV. The optimal timing for vaccination in conjunction with HBIG administration has not been established; however, pending additional information, it is recommended that vaccination begin at 3 months of age or shortly thereafter.[23]

For health care workers the degree of risk is proportional to the amount of contact with blood from infective patients. Employment in a hospital without exposure to blood carries no greater risk than for the general population. However, certain medical and dental workers and related laboratory and support personnel who have frequent blood contact are at increased risk. In developing specific immunization strategies hospitals should use available published data about the risk of infection[25,45,50] and, in addition, wish to evaluate their own clinical institutional experience with hepatitis B. Health care workers (medical, dental, laboratory, and support groups) who are deemed by the hospital to be eligible for hepatitis B vaccine because of the risks of exposure to HBV in their jobs should be vaccinated as soon as possible after beginning work in a high-risk environment, ideally during the period of training.[23]

SUMMARY

The majority of nosocomial infections involving the gastrointestinal system can be divided into two distinct clinical entities: gastroenteritis and hepatitis. Although neither occurs in large numbers, both can produce significant morbidity in both patient and employee populations. Basic infection control measures include early recognition of infection, appropriate isolation of infected individuals, and careful handling of specimens and potentially contaminated equipment. The most important issue facing ICPs concerning hepatitis prevention and control is the development of a rational, pragmatic protocol for hepatitis B vaccine administration.

REFERENCES

1. Adler, J.L., and Zickl, R.: Winter vomiting disease, J. Infect. Dis. **119:**668-673, 1969.
2. Alter, H.J., et al.: Clinical and serological analysis of transfusion-associated hepatitis, Lancet **2:**838-841, 1975.
3. Alter, H.J., et al.: Health-care workers positive for hepatitis B surface antigen: are their contacts at risk? N. Engl. J. Med. **292:**454-457, 1975.
4. Alter, H.J., et al.: Type B hepatitis: the infectivity of blood positive for e antigen and DNA polymerase after accidental needle exposure, N. Engl. J. Med. **295:**909-913, 1976.
5. American Hospital Association: Hepatitis B antigen carriers, Chicago, 1975, The Association.
6. Beasley, R.P., et al.: Evidence against breastfeeding as a mechanism for vertical transmission of hepatitis B, Lancet **2:**740-741, 1975.
7. Beasley, R.P., et al.: Hepatitis B immune globulin (HBIG) efficacy in the interruption of perinatal transmission of hepatitis B virus-carrier state, Lancet **2:**388-393, 1981.
8. Black, R.E., et al.: Epidemic *Yersinia* enterocolitica infection due to contaminated chocolate milk, N. Engl. J. Med. **298:**76-79, 1978.
9. Blacklow, N.R., et al.: Acute infectious nonbacterial gastroenteritis: etiology and pathogenesis, Ann. Intern. Med. **76:**993-1008, 1972.
10. Blaser, M.J., et al.: *Campylobacter* enteritis: clinical and epidemiological features, Ann. Intern. Med. **91:**179-185, 1979.
11. Blaser, M.J., et al.: Outbreaks of *Campylobacter* enteritis in two extended families: evidence for person-to-person transmission, J. Pediatr. **98:**254-256, 1981.
12. Blumberg, B.S., and London, T.W.: Hepatitis B virus and prevention of primary hepatocellular carcinoma, N. Engl. J. Med. **304:**782-784, 1981.
13. Book, L.S., et al.: Clustering of necrotizing enterocolitis: interruption by infection-control measures, N. Engl. J. Med. **297:**984-986, 1977.
14. Boyer, K.M., et al.: An outbreak of gastroenteritis due to E. *coli* 0142 in a neonatal nursery, J. Pediatr. **86:**919-927, 1975.
15. Centers for Disease Control: *Salmonella newport* outbreak in a NNIS community hospital nursery, Atlanta, 1970, CDC.
16. Centers for Disease Control: Outline for surveillance and control of nosocomial infections, Atlanta, 1976, CDC.
17. Centers for Disease Control: Hepatitis—control measures for hepatitis B in dialysis centers, Viral Hepatitis Investigations and Control Series, Atlanta, Nov. 1977, CDC.
18. Centers for Disease Control: Laboratory-associated typhoid fever, Morbid. Mortal. Weekly Rep. **28:**521-522, 1979.
19. Centers for Disease Control: Guidelines for the prevention and control of nosocomial infections: guidelines for hospital environmental control, Atlanta, issued Feb. 1981, CDC.
20. Centers for Disease Control: Hepatitis Surveillance Report, no. 46, Atlanta, issued March 1981, CDC.
21. Centers for Disease Control: Immune globulins for protection against viral hepatitis, Morbid. Mortal. Weekly Rep. **30:**423-428+, 1981.
22. Centers for Disease Control: National Nosocomial Infections Study report: annual summary— 1979, Atlanta, March 1982, CDC.
23. Centers for Disease Control: Inactivated hepatitis B vaccine, Morbid. Mortal. Weekly Rep. **31:**317-322+, 1982.
24. DeKeyser, P., Gossuin-DeTrain, M., and Butzler, J.P.: Acute enteritis due to related vibrio: first positive stool cultures, J. Infect. Dis. **125:**390-392, 1972.
25. Dienstag, J.L., and Ryan, D.M.: Occupational exposure to hepatitis B virus in hospital personnel: infection or immunization, Am. J. Epidemiol. **115:**26-39, 1982.
26. Duffy, M.C., Benson, J.B., and Rubin, S.J.: Mucosal invasion in *Campylobacter* enteritis, Am. J. Clin. Pathol. **73:**706-708, 1980.
27. DuPont, H.L., et al.: Pathogenesis of *Escherichia coli* diarrhea, N. Engl. J. Med. **285:**1-9, 1971.
28. Echeverria, P.D., Chang, C.P., and Smith, D.: Entero-toxigenicity and invasive capacity of enteropathogenic serotypes of *Escherichia coli*, J. Pediatr. **89:**8-10, 1976.

29. Favero, M.S., et al.: Guidelines for the care of patients hospitalized with viral hepatitis, Ann. Intern. Med. **91**:872-876, 1979.
30. Goldschmidt, M.C., and DuPont, H.L.: Enteropathogenic *Escherichia coli*: lack of clinical correlation of serotype with pathogenicity, J. Infect. Dis. **133**:153-156, 1976.
31. Grady, G.F., et al.: Hepatitis B immune globulin for accidental exposures among medical personnel: final report of a multicenter controlled trial, J. Infect. Dis. **138**:625-638, 1978.
32. Guerrant, R.L.: Inflammatory enteritides. In Mandell, G.L., Douglas, R.G., Jr., and Bennett, J.E., editors: Principles and practice of infectious diseases, New York, 1979, John Wiley & Sons, Inc.
33. Guerrant, R.L., et al.: Campylobacteriosis in man: pathogenic mechanisms and review of 91 blood stream infections, Am. J. Med. **65**:584-592, 1978.
34. Hedrick, E.: Cleaning and disinfection of flexible, fiberoptic endoscopes (ffe) used in gastrointestinal endoscopy, A.P.I.C. Journal **6**:8-9, 1978.
35. Hoofnagle, J.H., et al.: Transmission of non-A, non-B hepatitis, Ann. Intern. Med. **87**:14-20, 1977.
36. Hoofnagle, J.H., et al.: Passive-active immunity from hepatitis B immune globulin: reanalysis of a Veterans Administration Cooperative Study of needle-stick hepatitis, Ann. Intern. Med. **91**:813-818, 1979.
37. Jackson, M.M.: Viral hepatitis, Nurs. Clin. North Am. **15**:729-746, 1980.
38. Kapikian, A.Z., et al.: Human reovirus-like agent as the major pathogen associated with "winter" gastroenteritis in hospitalized infants and young children, N. Engl. J. Med. **294**:965-972, 1976.
39. Klein, H.G., Alter, H.J., and Holland, R.V.: Post-exposure immunoglobulin prophylaxis of hepatitis B: a comparison of two dosage schedules. In Vyas, G.N., Cohen, S.N., and Schmid, R., editors: Viral hepatitis, Philadelphia, 1978, The Franklin Institute Press.
40. Kosloske, A.M., Urlich, J.A., and Goffman, H.: Fulminant necrotizing enterocolitis associated with *chostridia*, Lancet **2**:1014-1016, 1978.
41. Krugman, S., and Gocke, D.J.: Viral hepatitis, Philadelphia, 1978, W.B. Saunders Co.
42. Krugman, S., and Katz, S.L.: Infectious diseases of children, ed. 7, St. Louis, 1981, The C.V. Mosby Co.
43. Lauer, J.L., et al.: Transmission of hepatitis B virus in clinical laboratory areas, J. Infect. Dis. **140**:513-516, 1979.
44. Maynard, J.E.: Passive immunization against hepatitis B: a review of recent studies and comment on current aspects of control, Am. J. Epidemiol. **107**:77-86, 1978.
45. Maynard, J.E.: Viral hepatitis as an occupational hazard in the health care profession. In Vyas, G.M., Cohen, S.N., and Schmid, R., editors: Viral hepatitis, Philadelphia, 1978, The Franklin Institute Press.
46. McCormick, R.D., and Maki, D.G.: Epidemiology of needle-stick injuries in hospital personnel, Am. J. Med. **70**:928-932, 1981.
47. Meyers, J.D., et al.: Lack of transmission of hepatitis B after surgical exposure, J.A.M.A. **240**:1725-1727, 1978.
48. Middleton, P.J., Szymanski, M.T., and Petric, M.: Viruses associated with acute gastroenteritis in young children, Am. J. Dis. Child. **131**:733-737, 1977.
49. Mosley, J.W.: Hepatitis, type B. In Wehrle, P.F., and Top, F.H., editors: Communicable and infectious diseases, ed. 9, St. Louis, 1981, The C.V. Mosby Co.
50. Pattison, C.P., Epidemiology of hepatitis B in hospital personnel, Am. J. Epidemiol. **101**:59-64, 1975.
51. Rakela, J., and Mosley, J.W.: Fecal excretion of hepatitis A virus in humans, J. Infect. Dis. **135**:933-938, 1977.
52. Ryder, R.W., et al.: Human milk contaminated with *Salmonella kottbus*: a cause of nosocomial illness in infants, J.A.M.A. **238**:1533-1534, 1977.
53. Ryder, R.W., et al.: Reovirus-like agent as a cause of nosocomial diarrhea in infants, J. Pediatr. **90**:698-702, 1977.
54. Seeff, L.B., and Hoofnagle, J.H.: Immunoprophylaxis of viral hepatitis, Gastroenterology **77**:161-182, 1979.

55. Seeff, L.B., et al.: Type B hepatitis after needle-stick exposure: prevention with hepatitis B immune globulin, Ann. Intern. Med. **88:**285-293, 1978.

56. Silverstrope, L., et al.: An epidemic among infants caused by S. muenchen, J. Appl. Bacteriol. **24:**134-142, 1961.

57. Steere, A.C., et al.: Person-to-person spread of *Salmonella typhimurium* after a hospital common-source outbreak, Lancet **1:**319-322, 1975.

58. Szmuness, W., et al.: Hepatitis B vaccine: demonstration of efficacy in a controlled clinical trial in a high-risk population in the United States, N. Engl. J. Med. **303:**833-841, 1980.

59. Tabor, E., et al.: Transmission of non-A, non-B hepatitis from man to chimpanzee, Lancet **1:**463-465, 1978.

60. Tallett, S., et al.: Clinical, laboratory, and epidemiological features of a viral gastroenteritis in infants and children, Pediatrics **60:**217-222, 1977.

61. Tong, M.J., et al.: Studies on the maternal-infant transmission of the viruses which cause acute hepatitis, Gastroenterology **80:**999-1004, 1981.

62. Virnig, N.L., and Reynolds, J.W.: Epidemiological aspects of neonatal necrotizing enterocolitis, Am. J. Dis. Child. **128:**186-190, 1974.

63. Viscidi, R.P., and Bartlett, J.G.: Antibiotic-associated pseudomembranous colitis in children, Pediatrics **67:**381-386, 1981.

64. Wilson, R.: Enteric infections. In Wehrle, P.F., and Top, F.H., editors: Communicable and infectious diseases, ed. 9, St. Louis, 1981, The C.V. Mosby Co.

65. Zuckerman, A.J.: Hepatitis B: its prevention by vaccine, J. Infect. Dis. **143:**301-304, 1981.

CHERYL R. COX

Respiratory system

Surveillance data collected for more than a decade by the Centers for Disease Control (CDC)[13] document that 13% to 14% of nosocomial infections are associated with the respiratory tract. This percentage has remained relatively constant from the early National Nosocomial Infection Studies (NNIS) of 1970 to 1973 to the more recent Study on the Efficacy of Nosocomial Infection Control (SENIC) Project report of 1980.[20] In light of this reported constancy it is reasonable to assume that the respiratory tract as a site of nosocomial infection will remain as a persistant problem in the coming years.

Nosocomial respiratory tract infection is one of the more elusive infections for the infection control practitioner (ICP) to document. This is a result, in part, of the inability to achieve a consensus of opinion on criteria for these infections and the difficulty in interpretation of the presenting patient data (e.g., radiographic interpretations, microbiology of sputum specimens, patient history). In an attempt to clarify some of these problems a discussion of respiratory tract infections, including a review of defense mechanisms of the respiratory tract and practical infection control practices, is presented.

DEFENSE MECHANISMS OF THE RESPIRATORY TRACT

The defense mechanisms of the "normal" healthy individual prevent most microorganisms and foreign objects from entering the lungs. When these defenses are unable to withstand invasion, infection may occur. The inability to withstand the invading agent may be caused by impairment of host defenses or characteristics of the invading agent, such as virulence or the quantity of organisms present (dose relationship).

The offending agent can reach the alveolar level of the lungs by aspiration or inhalation or through the vascular system. Of these routes, the hematogenous pathway is the least common.[2]

The respiratory system may be divided into two sections: the upper respiratory, or conducting portion (i.e., the nose, pharynx, larynx, and trachea) and the lower respiratory portion, whose major function is the exchange of oxygen and carbon dioxide in the bronchioles and the alveoli (Fig. 16-1). All aspects of the respiratory system from the portal of entry of air through the nares to the alveoli are designed to provide maximal defense against any agent that might interfere with this prime function.

The conducting portion of the respiratory system is continuously exposed

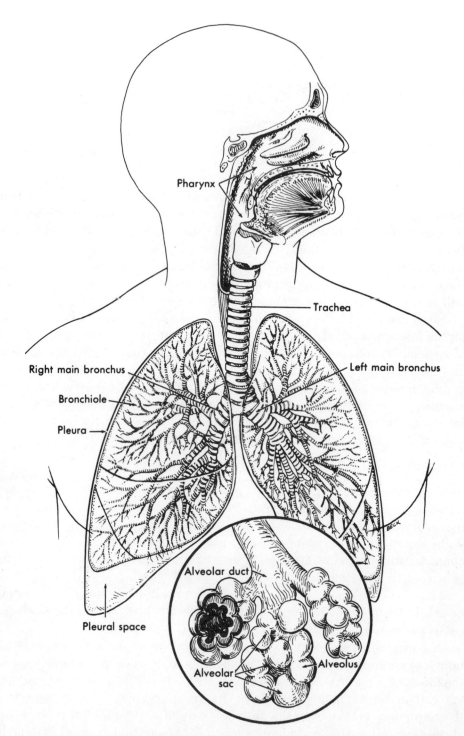

FIG. 16-1. The pharynx, trachea, and lungs. The inset shows the grapelike alveolar sacs where air and blood exchange oxygen and carbon dioxide through the thin walls of the alveoli. (From Anthony, C.P., and Thibodeau, G.A.: Textbook of anatomy and physiology, ed. 10, St. Louis, 1979, The C.V. Mosby Co.)

to a wide variety of dust particles and microorganisms. It is, however, endowed with several defense mechanisms, including the cilia of the epithelial lining in both the upper and lower respiratory tracts, the goblet cells located in the mucosa, mucus-excreting glands, the elastic fibromusculature of the bronchial wall, lymphocytes, macrophages, granular leukocytes, the glottis, the larynx, and cough and sneeze reflex actions.

On inhalation turbulence and filtration of large particles take place by the vibrissae located just inside the nares. The air is warmed and humidified as it progresses toward the lung field. A mucociliary transport system extends from the posterior two thirds of the nasal cavity to the nasopharynx and from the larynx to the terminal bronchioles and consists of cilia and mucus. Cilia are hairlike projections (approximately 200 cilia per ciliated cell) that protrude into the lower level of the mucous blanket and beat in recurrent waves, propelling mucus and trapped particles toward the pharynx. Mucus is released from the mucous cells by rupture of the goblet through the cell surface. The mucous blanket that coats the celia consists of two layers: a liquid layer next to the cilia and a gel layer on which particles are trapped. The surface of the mucous layer provides bactericidal activity by the presence of immunoglobulins, especially secretory IgA and lysozyme. Secretory IgG and IgM are present in small amounts. Their importance, however, becomes more evident when an infecting agent penetrates the mucosal wall.[33] Working in concert, the mucus and cilia provide an effective mucociliary escalator that carries entrapped particles to the nasopharyngeal area where they are either expectorated or, as most often occurs, swallowed (Fig. 16-2).

Droplet nuclei, small enough (0.2 to 6 μm in diameter) to bypass all defense mechanisms and penetrate the alveolar spaces, may contain microorganisms. These droplet nuclei can, however, acquire moisture from the upper respiratory tract where they are quickly enlarged through absorption of moisture, making them susceptible to control by the cilia. It has been estimated that 90% of the inhaled particles of 10 μm or greater are removed by entrapment and the action of the mucociliary system. In addition the activities of these mechanical defenses, nasal secretions also contain antimicrobial elements such as IgA antibody, phagocytes, and lysozyme. The normal resident flora of the nasopharyngeal area offer defense in their ability to prevent colonization of potential pathogens by *bacterial interference*. Bacterial interference is a process whereby transient bacteria, especially gram-negative, are prevented or inhibited from attaching to the epithelial cells, thus preventing colonization from taking place. Bacterial interference may be the result of any or all of the following mechanisms: (1) production of a change in the physiological environment (such as pH) that the potential invading organisms cannot tolerate, (2) depletion of essential nutrients (vitamins), or (3) production of an antibiotic substance.[35] Alteration of any of these mechanisms increases the potential of col-

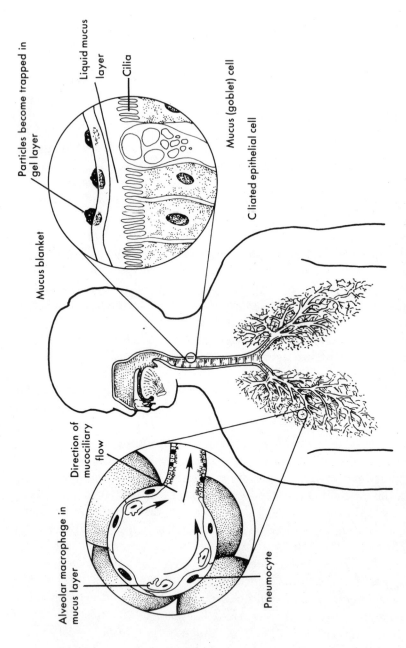

Particles become trapped in gel layer

Liquid mucus layer

Cilia

Mucus blanket

Mucus (goblet) cell

Ciliated epithelial cell

Direction of mucociliary flow

Alveolar macrophage in mucus layer

Pneumocyte

FIG. 16-2. Anatomy of the mucociliary escalator (*right*) and the alveolar clearing mechanism (*left*).

onization. Of all the bacterial species in the oropharyngeal area, streptococci appear to have the greatest inhibitory activity.[35]

Working in concert with bacterial interference is the process of selective adherence of bacteria to the epithelial cell surface. This adherence process is known as a *recognition mechanism*. The surface of the epithelial cell contains molecular structures called *receptors*. These receptors are sparsely located in the oropharyngeal area. The surface of bacteria contains a molecular structure known as a *ligand*. For bacteria to adhere to the epithelial lining, the ligand of the bacteria and the receptor of the epithelial cell must recognize each other.[35] This recognition mechanism with its resulting attachment of bacteria to the epithelial lining is the first step in the process of colonization. The complex and dynamic interaction between bacterial interference and the recognition mechanism factor is collectively called the *cellular inhibitory defense mechanism*.[35]

Unlike the upper respiratory tract, which contains normal resident flora, the lower respiratory tract is normally sterile. However, like the upper respiratory tract, the lower respiratory tract has both mechanical and antimicrobial activity. Protection is given to the lower respiratory tract through the expulsive action of sneezing and coughing or by the use of the gag reflex and the mucociliary escalator. The gross motor activities, stimulated by receptors in the nose or the parasympathetic and sympathetic fibers innervated in the bronchi, are facilitated by the elastic musculature of the bronchial wall. In the terminal air spaces of the lung the alveolar macrophages play a primary role. Macrophages are responsible for physical removal of inhaled particles from the alveoli. The mucociliary transport system then carries them upward. Macrophages may be activated or armed in an infectious process to increase their capability in bactericidal activity, or they may be nonspecific (nonactivated). Once activated, macrophages have an increased lysosomal enzyme level, are more phagocytic, and possess greater bactericidal activity. The activated macrophages can display a non–antigen-specific capacity to ingest and digest organisms. When the primary infecting organism disappears from the alveolar tissue, the activated macrophages rapidly decline in number.[34] It is suggested that in infection secretory IgA promotes phagocytosis of the alveolar macrophages. Other immunoglobulins, IgG and IgM, are also activated during infection. During the resting or noninfected state of the lungs, the macrophage is the primary defense mechanism that offers bactericidal activity.

The intact, healthy defense mechanisms of the respiratory tract offer exceptional protection to the individual host. As a result of these factors, the terminal or alveolar section of the respiratory system distal from the first bronchial division is ordinarily free from demonstrable, viable microorganisms. Of all the defense mechanisms, the intact mucous membrane is the most important.

POTENTIAL DISRUPTIONS OF THE NORMAL DEFENSE MECHANISMS

In spite of an impressive defense system alterations in these defenses can and do occur, resulting in an increased risk for infection. These disruptions may be temporary, leaving no residual damage, or they may be permanent, with damage to one or more parts of the defense system. Several types of disruption will be discussed.

Obstruction. Obstruction can occur anywhere in the respiratory tract. Obstruction can be caused by a foreign body, such as food obstructing the epiglottis; by trauma to the trachea, resulting in edema; by an increase in the tenacity of mucous secretions in response to infection, as with cystic fibrosis, causing mucous plugs in the bronchi or alveoli; or by other factors, such as malignancies or defects in cartilage development.

Alteration of mucus. Dehydration of the host can alter respiratory tract defense mechanisms by decreasing the viscosity or quantity of mucus production, which in turn affects entrapment and removal by the cilia. Damage or hypertrophy of the mucosal glands, as in chronic bronchitis, can result in a change in viscosity and quantity of mucus production. Alteration by increasing the liquid characteristic of the mucus may increase the spread of microorganisms by the pooling of secretions in the lung.

Alteration of the cilia. Successful functioning of the cilia directly depends on the proper amount and quality of mucus production. Cilia may be altered or destroyed. Chemical irritation, such as smoking, can alter the function of the cilia. Certain bacterial agents, such as *Staphylococcus aureus* and *Pseudomonas* organisms, are known for the necrotizing and destructive nature of their infections, which destroy not only the cilia but the entire ciliated cell. Once destroyed, the ciliated cells are replaced by squamous epithelium. Squamous epithelium does not support regeneration of ciliated cells.

Alteration of the musculature. Trauma and anesthesia are examples of occurrences that interfere with the peristaltic action of the muscular lining of the trachea and may result in an impaired lung function. Alteration in the gag or cough reflex may allow aspiration of foreign particles or microorganisms, resulting in aspiration pneumonia. Postoperative patients, alcoholics, and patients with central nervous system disorders that result in coma have potential for this type of alteration. In many cases of lung abscess a temporarily impaired gag reflex allows large quantities of secretion to pool in a dependent location in the lung. This leads to proliferation of entrapped bacteria, which may result in destruction of the intact alveoli.

Alteration of macrophage activity. The alveolar macrophage can be depressed when a person inhales toxic particles, such as asbestos. After viruses are ingested the macrophage has a decreased ability to phagocytize secondary bacterial invaders.[34]

Bypass. Mouth breathing or mechanical bypasses, such as the use of endotracheal tubes or tracheostomies, rob the patient of the vital defenses provided by the nasopharyngeal area. Eliminating the function of the nasal hairs and the warming and moisturizing of air before it reaches the lungs can have a negative effect on mucociliary activity.

Medications. Medications that alter the function of the respiratory system and affect the mucous lining or the cough center in the medulla include anticholinergic drugs (scopolamine or atropine), bronchodilators, bronchoconstrictors, antitussives, expectorants, narcotics, and respiratory tract stimulants.

The altered function of the respiratory system may also be a side effect of other therapy. Examples of side effects of drug therapy are alteration of the immune response from corticosteroids and cytotoxic drugs, alteration of normal resident flora from antibiotics, alterations of the gag reflex from the use of anesthetics, and a drying effect on the mucous lining as a result of Pro-Banthine or oxygen therapy.

Alteration of normal flora. Alteration of the normal resident flora of the oropharyngeal area in the chronically ill or severely ill hospitalized patient by gram-negative bacteria takes place within the first days of hospitalization. The complex process of new organisms becoming a part of the endogenous flora of an area is called *colonization*. Colonization takes place as a result of the host's interaction with the new environment and is influenced by drug therapy (e.g., antibiotics, cytotoxic or immunosuppressive drugs). This alteration increases the potential for lower respiratory tract infections by bacteria with different characteristics (e.g., resistance to antibiotics, altered virulence). A summary of the conditions that may influence or predispose the host to colonization follows:

- Impairment of pharyngeal clearing mechanism*
- Depression of local inhibitory activity at the cellular level*
- Age (advancing with debility)
- Alcoholism
- Antibiotic therapy
- Length of hospitalization
- Diabetes mellitus
- Surgical procedures
- Underlying disease entities
- Use of nasogastric or ventilatory apparatus
- Contact transmission of bacteria via hands of personnel

Prevention of respiratory tract infection depends on an active, healthy defense system. Any alteration or disturbance of these mechanisms can compromise the ability of the host to resist infection. A summary of the defense mechanisms and alterations of these defenses is presented on p. 408.

*Primary consideration.

**A composite of the defense mechanisms of the respiratory tract and
potential alterations of these defenses**

Defense mechanisms	Potential alterations of defense mechanisms
Nasal hairs; warming and moisturization of air	Alteration of cellular inhibitory defenses: bacterial interference; recognition mechanism
Intact surfaces	
Mucociliary escalator	Depression of alveolar macrophage
Reflexes: gag, cough, and sneeze	Obstruction
Lymphatic system	Depression of reflex actions
Lymphocytes	Bypass: mouth breathing; endotracheal or tracheostomy tubes
Macrophages	
Polymorphonuclear leukocytes	Alteration of production or characteristics of mucus
Immunoglobulins: IgA, IgG, and IgM	Colonization by gram-negative bacilli
	Medications

The dynamic interrelationship of the intactness and health of the host's defense mechanisms versus the number (quantity) of invading organisms, the duration of the contact with the invading organisms, and the virulent characteristics of the organisms determines the health status of the host. An alteration of any one of these factors can upset the balance of health, and disease can occur.

INFECTIONS OF THE RESPIRATORY TRACT

Acute respiratory tract infection is listed as the number one reason for patients seeking medical attention in the private office.[25] It has been estimated that more than 90% of these cases are upper respiratory tract infections caused by 100 or more distinct rhinoviruses. Among hospitalized patients, excluding deliveries and births, all respiratory tract infections involving pneumonia ranked fourth in the frequency of admission diagnosis. In 1975 acute upper respiratory tract infection (URI) ranked twentieth, acute bronchitis thirty-first, chronic bronchitis forty-fifth, and influenza ninety-second. When combining these diagnoses with emphysema, it is clear that respiratory tract illness is one of the major causes of hospitalization.[2,14]

It is therefore beneficial for the ICP to be aware not only of the incidence and severity of URIs in the community but also of the number of patients admitted as a result of unresolved or advanced respiratory tract infections. These data can be useful when developing policies and practices of patient placement and employee health, as well as considerations for visitor restriction during the peak respiratory tract infection season.

A more in-depth discussion of infection control measures will be presented in the latter part of this chapter.

Terminology

The terminology used by lay and medical personnel regarding respiratory tract infections is often confusing. Terms such as *flu, URI, strep throat, bronchitis, laryngitis, pneumonia,* and *pneumonitis* are used freely and often interchangeably. The etiology of these infections may be viral, bacterial, protozoal, or fungal. Infections caused by viruses are usually self-limiting, benign, and not responsive to treatment with antimicrobial agents. Bacterial infections usually require identification of the offending organisms and appropriate antimicrobial and other symptomatic therapy. When the ICP is documenting nosocomial or community respiratory tract infections, an appropriately obtained history, in addition to observation of clinical symptoms, will assist in accurately identifying the site of the infection. A brief description of commonly used terms and their frequently used synonyms is presented to assist with clarification:

upper respiratory tract infection (URI) This term is used synonymously with *flu, influenza,* or *head cold.* URIs are usually viral in etiology and are characterized by nasal congestion with a watery mucus discharge and general malaise. There is usually no fever, and there is an absence of cough (cough is a symptom of a lower respiratory tract infection). Complications are otitis media with secondary bacterial infection and progression to a lower respiratory tract infection (LRI).

pharyngitis This term is used interchangeably with *sore throat* or *strep throat.* Of these infections, 95% are of viral etiology. Of the remaining percentage, group A β-hemolytic streptococci are the most significant microorganisms. The diagnosis of viral versus streptococcal sore throat cannot be made by clinical observation alone. Diagnosis is made by clinical observation and culture. The significance of group A streptococcal infection is its potential role in the etiology of rheumatic heart disease and its sequelae. Prompt and effective treatment of these organisms is a key issue in the management and prevention of this disease. Because group A β-hemolytic streptococci are the most significant of the upper respiratory tract pathogens (excluding pertussis and diphtheria), microbiology laboratories usually culture only for these organisms when handling routine throat cultures.

laryngitis The etiology of laryngitis can be an extension of infections of the nose or throat. These infections are predominantly viral, are self-limiting, and are not life threatening. Laryngitis can also be caused by improper use of the throat (prolonged shouting), or it may be associated with systemic disease, such as measles. It may also be a symptom of a disease of the larynx. The characteristic symptoms are hoarseness or loss of voice and cough.

bronchitis Bronchitis can be divided into two categories: acute and chronic. The term bronchitis has been used interchangeably with *chest cold* because of the close proximity of the larynx to the bronchi and the similarity in symptoms. Acute bronchitis is rarely an infection in and of itself. The etiology can be viral or bacterial and is usually seen as an extension of an upper respiratory tract infection. The circuitous relationship of edema—congestion—cough is characteristic of bronchitis. Edema of the bronchial mucosal lining results in narrowing of the airway, general congestion, and a decrease in ciliary activity. The distended mucous glands may contain purulent material, resulting in a productive cough. A persistent cough causes further irritation and edema; with increased edema a continuing cycle is established. Bronchitis is an obstructive infection of the lower respiratory tract. Bacterial complications do not always occur in these patients if they are otherwise healthy and are promptly treated. When complications of bronchitis do occur, they are (1) a development of chronic bronchitis, which can result in significant bacterial infections, and (2) progression or extension of the infection to the interstitial tissue and/or alveolar spaces of the lungs resulting in pneumonia.

pneumonia Pneumonia has been described as an inflammation of and exudation into the alveolar and supportive interstitial tissue, resulting in an abnormal density of the chest roentgenogram.[47] In contrast to URIs, which are 90% viral in origin, pneumonias are 50% bacterial.[47] Pneumonias may be classified specifically by anatomical location, by cause, or, for purposes of gross data collection, as community or nosocomial. The general characteristic symptoms of pneumonia are fever, productive cough (a result of an increase or alteration of the lower respiratory tract's normal mucociliary escalator and secretion production), respiratory chest pain, and radiographic changes.

Classification by anatomical location. Frequently used terms in descending anatomical sites are *bronchopneumonia, patchy pneumonia, lobar pneumonia,* and *interstitial pneumonia.* The significance of location to the ICP is that specific bacteria are frequently associated with each site.[2,47] When the epidemiological significance of nosocomial infection is being evaluated, these sites take on new meaning. In addition to the epidemiological information, treatment can be more specific while awaiting bacteriological results.

Classification by cause

Primary versus secondary pneumonia. Most authors agree that a primary pneumonia is an infection of the lower respiratory tract, usually of the alveoli, in a previously uninfected site.[25] A more restrictive definition would add that a primary pneumonia is one that occurs in patients whose immune system has not been compromised.[47] Secondary pneumonias are infections of the lower respiratory tract that are the result of a previous or resolving infection or the result of an alteration in the normal defense mechanisms of the respiratory system. These alterations allow pathogenic microorganisms and organisms of normally low virulence to overwhelm the host, creating a new infectious process. Examples of secondary pneumonias are those (1) secondary to infections elsewhere in the body, such as staphylococcal endocarditis, which embolizes to the lung; (2) secondary to a mechanical or physical event, such as pneumonia after drowning or aspirations; (3) secondary as a complication of surgery, such as postoperative pneumonia; (4) secondary as a complication of medications, such as chemotherapy in malignancy like leukemia; and (5) secondary to a disease entity or a varicella or protozoal infection (*Pneumocystis*).

Secondary pneumonias can be referred to as "opportunistic" infections. Nosocomial respiratory tract infections are, for the most part, secondary opportunistic infections. These respiratory tract infections may be either endogenous or exogenous.

Endogenous versus exogenous. Endogenous respiratory tract infections, or those infections resulting from the patient's own flora, can be acquired by two major modes of transmission: as a direct extension of colonization of the upper respiratory tract through aspiration or inhalation or by the hematogenous pathway. Theoretically, any bacteremia that has a primary focus of infection can shower septic emboli to the lower respiratory tract, causing infection. The greater the depression or alteration of the defiense mechanisms of the alveolar spaces, the greater the chance for these infections to occur. Hematogenous sources of pneumonia on serial chest roentgenograms are seen as increasing, numerous, diffuse sites and almost always involve both right and left lung fields.[47] The term *aspiration pneumonias* has been used to describe those pneumonias that follow aspiration of oral secretions, nasopharyngeal secretions, or gastric contents. The majority of these pneumonias are caused by aspiration from the upper respiratory tract. Aspiration results in localization of the pneumonia into a dependent pulmonary lobe. Because the patient is usually in the supine position, aspirated material tends to flow into the posterior segment of the right upper lung. However, either lung may be involved, depending on the position of the patient at the time of aspiration.

Exogenous sources of infection, or those brought to the patients, are acquired by inhalation, by contact with personnel, or by the use of contaminated equipment. It is possible that any bacteria could be transmitted by the airborne method. However, with the exception of only specific organisms, such as *Mycobacterium tuberculosis* and S. *aureus*, few pneumonias are known to be caused by this method. On chest x-ray film inhaled microorganisms that result in pneumonia appear as a diffuse infiltrate usually involving one lung and are often described as patchy, fluffy, or alveolar infiltrates.[2,27]

Numerous outbreaks of respiratory tract infections caused by contaminated respiratory positive pressure equipment were reported in the 1960s.[29,31,36,38] With the institution of strict infection control measures and the common use of products, such as bacterial filters on the driveline of this high-risk equipment, few outbreaks have recently been attributed to this source of contamination. A description of these infection control measures will be discussed later. Specific techniques and manipulations of the respiratory tree, such as tracheostomy or endotracheal tubes, lend themselves to exogenous contamination.

The transmission of bacteria from an exogenous source to the endogenous state is a step-by-step process. It is apparent that bacteria are transmitted to the patient by hand contact of personnel or by inhalation. The invading bacteria multiply in the oropharyngeal area where they then become endogenous to the host. Contamination of the lower lung field may then take place by aspiration or by inhalation of the endogenous flora. It is imperative to understand that the status of the host has a direct and significant relationship to acquisition or prevention of nosocomial respiratory tract infection. This includes the integrity of all aspects of the defense mechanisms and the lack of iatrogenic factors, such as the use of corticosteroids and antibiotics, surgery, or manipulation of ventilatory tubes.

Viral versus bacterial. Viral nosocomial infections have long been recognized. However, well-defined criteria that can be applied to community hospitals, which for the most part, are lacking diagnostic viral laboratories have not been developed. This may be one reason why the NNIS report of 1978[13] reflects only a 0.2% incidence of viral infection. Another study[44] reported a higher rate of 5% and gave evidence that this type of nosocomial infection is greatly underestimated. In this study 75% of nosocomial viral infections were found to be associated with the respiratory tract. The significance of this cause of respiratory tract infection to the ICP is the ease of transmission to a confined, yet susceptible, population. Viral respiratory tract infection in the hospitalized patient may have two distinct outcomes. In the healthy subject it may be self-limiting and only an inconvenience. In the chronically ill, immunosuppressed, or otherwise compromised host a viral respiratory tract infection may result in significant morbidity.

Increased incidence of pneumonia during influenza epidemics has been documented in various studies. Type A influenza appears to result in a greater incidence of pneumonia than does type B influenza.[16,44] Studies also indicate that type A influenza is a more common nosocomial infection among pediatric patients. This patient population can, therefore, be considered a high-risk group for nosocomial acquisition.[16,43,44] Other viral agents frequently seen in nosocomial respiratory tract infection include parainfluenza viruses, adenoviruses, influenza viruses, respiratory syncytial viruses, and cytomegalovirus. Cytomegalovirus has been associated with disease in immunologically compromised patients and can cause extensive interstitial pneumonia.

The most common cause of epidemic viral respiratory tract infections in the community is the adenovirus. Respiratory syncytial virus (RSV) is responsible for a major number of bronchopneumonias in infants and in the pediatric population. In one study[17] 34% of LRIs in children were caused by RSV. Other viruses that are frequently seen as causative agents in URIs and LRIs are listed in Table 16-1. Specific respiratory tract viruses tend to produce fairly well-defined clinical symptoms, although each is capable of producing any of the respiratory tract symptoms. Acquisition of the disease depends on the resistance of the host and the virulence/dose relationship of the organism. It should be pointed out that some of these viruses may also be manifested in syndromes that involve body sites other than the respiratory tract.

Agents responsible for LRIs frequently give clinical clues about their identity. The significance of these clues is that they allow the physician to initiate therapy based on patient history and clinical judgment while awaiting diagnostic test results. For example, Streptococcus pneumoniae is the most common cause of community-acquired bacterial pneumonia. Mycoplasma pneumoniae, a small, unique bacterium, is also a source of community-acquired infection and a common cause of pneumonia in otherwise healthy young adults.[17,42,47] Table 16-2 presents the striking characteristic differences of pneumonia caused by these two organisms.

Three bacterias account for almost all of the community-acquired LRIs: S. pneumoniae (frequently referred to as pneumococcus) causes 90% of community-acquired pneumonias; type B Haemophilus influenzae causes 1% to 5% of LRIs; and Klebsiella pneumoniae (also known as Friedländer's bacillus) is responsible for 1% to 5% of community-acquired pneumonias.[47]

S. pneumoniae, a gram-positive, lancet-shaped encapsulated diplococcus usually arranged in chains of varying lengths or in pairs on the Gram stain, is frequently found as part of the normal oropharyngeal flora. Transmission to the lower respiratory tract is by aspiration of these oropharyngeal secretions or droplet spread from a carrier to a susceptible host. It is estimated that 20% to 70% of the population are streptococcal carriers.[47] Pneumococcal infections usually occur in winter and early spring.

There are in excess of 80 serotypes of S. pneumoniae. The virulence of the organism appears to depend on the specific serotype of the organisms' polysaccharide capsular material. The age of the patient and the geographical location also tend to be related to the serotype acquired. Adults are more commonly affected by serotypes 8, 4, 3, 1, 7, and 12, whereas children are infected by serotypes 13, 14, 19, 3, 6, and 1.[43,46,47] Pneumococcal pneumonia is frequently an infection of the extremes; that is, it affects children under age 5 and adults over age 50. Crowded living conditions appear to increase the risk of infection. Mortality occurs mainly in the older patient with underlying disease, such as a history of lung disease or a previous episode of pneumonia. It is common for pneumococcal pneumonia to be preceded by a URI caused by a virus. For this reason it is recommended that persons over 50 years of age receive pneumococcal vaccine specifically when influenza is expected to be epidemic in the area. A polyvalent vaccine is currently available for this high-risk population. Epidemics of pneumococcal pneumonia, either nosocomial or community acquired, are rare. Patients with pneumococcal pneumonia are less likely to spread the organism than are those who are nasopharyngeal carriers. Adequate antimicrobial therapy results in rapid resolution of the infection. Complications of lung abscess or empyema are rarely seen. Isolation of patients with pneumococcal pneumonia is not recommended.

H. influenzae is a small gram-negative pleomorphic rod. It is a common

TABLE 16-1. Viral respiratory tract infections

Virus	Infection	Major target population	Transmission	Season	Incubation	Comments
Influenza (classified into groups A, B, C, and D)						
Group A	URI (commonly seen in epidemics)	Age 5 through adulthood	Droplet	Throughout year (more common in winter months)	24 to 48 hr	Has remarkable ability to mutate; *complications:* suprainfection by pneumococcus, *H. influenzae,* and staphylococcus; takes place 2 weeks after initial viral infection; pneumonia as a complication is rare (less than 2%); when it occurs, it has a rapid onset with increased mortality; seen in patients with underlying disease
Parainfluenza (classified as types I, II, and III)	Croup Acute bronchitis Pneumonia Pharyngitis Tonsillitis	Infants Children Adults	Droplet	Winter	24 to 72 hr	In adults URI is mild and self-limiting
Respiratory syncytial virus (RSV)	Bronchitis	Infants and small children	Droplet	Winter and early spring	3 to 5 days	Prior infection appears to offer immunity

Coxsackievirus (classified as group A or B) Group A 21 & 24	URI	All ages	Droplet	Summer and early fall		Pneumonia is rare
ECHO (enteric cytopathic human orphan) virus	LRI	Infants; especially premature or compromised neonates		Any season		
Adenovirus	URI	All ages	Droplet	Summer and fall	4 to 5 days	Most common cause of acute respiratory tract infections; common cause of epidemics in military population; frequently results in pneumonia
Cytomegalovirus (CMV)	LRI	Neonates or small infants; Adults with underlying reticuloendothelial diseases; those with immunological deficiencies; those receiving immunosuppressive therapy, organ recipients	Contact occurs as a consequence of passage through birth canal			Latent virus that is triggered by the previously listed predisposing factors

TABLE 16-2. Differential diagnostic features of pneumonia

Feature	Pneumococcal lobar pneumonia	Mycoplasmal pneumonia
Onset	Sudden	Gradual
Rigors	Single chill	"Chilliness"
Facies	"Toxic"	Well
Cough	Productive	Paroxysmal; nonproductive
Sputum	Purulent (bloody)	Mucoid
Herpes	Frequent	Rare
Temperature	103° F to 104° F	103° F
Pleurisy	Frequent	Rare
Consolidation	Frequent	Rare
White blood cell and differential count	15,000; immature neutrophils	15,000; normal
Gram stain (sputum)	Neutrophils; cocci	Mononuclear cells; mixed flora
Chest x-ray film	Defined density	Nondefined infiltrate

From Youmans, G.P., Paterson, P.Y., and Sommers, H.M.: The biologic and clinical basis of infectious diseases, ed. 2, Philadelphia, 1980, W.B. Saunders Co.

inhabitant of the oropharyngeal area. Infection usually starts as a URI with progression to the lower respiratory tract. These LRIs are usually associated with children and are caused by H. influenzae serotype B. In some children the URI can be severe and may rapidly develop into severe epiglottitis and laryngeal obstruction, requiring immediate emergency tracheostomy.

K. pneumoniae, a gram-negative bacillus, may be a part of the normal resident oropharyngeal flora. Unlike S. pneumoniae and H. influenzae, K. pneumoniae usually causes secondary infections and frequently occurs in patients with underlying lung disease or illness that lowers or alters the normal defense mechanisms of the respiratory tract. Alcoholics are frequently plagued by this type of LRI. Unlike the other two organisms, K. pneumoniae causes destruction of the alveolar spaces where abscess formation and bronchial obstruction commonly occur.

The term *compromised host* is frequently associated with nosocomial respiratory tract infections. A commonly accepted definition of a compromised host is one whose underlying disease or treatment of a disease alters his ability to fight infection.[48] The host impairment may be the result of affected humoral or cellular mechanisms involved in immunity or a reduction in the number and bactericidal capabilities of polymorphonuclear neutrophils, leukocytes, and macrophages. It may also be a result of antimicrobial or steroid therapy that alters nasopharyngeal and gastrointestinal flora, or it may be a consequence of treatment by cytotoxic drugs that may alter gastrointestinal mucosa, permitting portals of entry for bacteria and fungi.[5,8] It becomes clear then that a large number of hospitalized patients can become compromised.

When evaluating nosocomial pneumonias in relation to the impaired host, it is, then, more understandable that these infections can be caused by organisms that do not usually affect the general population. This is true of the gram-negative bacteria, fungi, and viruses. The etiological agents of pneumonias resulting from the ubiquitous fungi in immunologically altered patients are *Aspergillus* species in patients with cardiac transplants, *Candida* species in patients with neoplasms or renal transplants, and mucormycosis in patients with leukemia or malignant lymphoma. A protozoan that is increasingly a cause of infection in patients with altered immunity is *Pneumocystis carinii*.[5] Of the gram-negative bacteria, *Proteus* species, *Enterobacteriaceae*, *E. coli*, *Pseudomonas* species, and *Klebsiella* species are frequently the organisms identified in nosocomial pneumonias. *S. aureus* is the primary gram-positive organism causing LRIs. Pneumonias caused by any of these organisms are transmitted to the lower respiratory tract primarily by microaspiration or macroaspiration. They are also transmitted in lesser amounts by secondary bacteremias that have primary foci of infection in the genitourinary tract, gastrointestinal tract, or other major sites of infection.

As previously mentioned, colonization of these bacteria in the oropharyngeal area occurs after hospitalization. The exact method or conditions that promote colonization are not known. Factors that influence colonization are listed on p. 407. From studies of outbreaks of respiratory tract infections it is hypothesized that colonization takes place from the patient's gastrointestinal tract or through contact transmission by the hands of personnel.[2,4] Other studies indicate that colonization increases as the severity of illness increases. One study suggests that age affects the rapidity of colonization. For independent residents (over 65 years of age) in a retirement facility the colonization rate was about 9%, but this rate increased dramatically to 60% in the acute areas of the hospital.[42] Evidence by researchers suggests that the major determinant of colonization with gram-negative bacilli is the underlying disease itself with resulting impairment of normal pharyngeal clearance mechanisms. Prior or concurrent antibiotic therapy and the presence of nasogastric tubes and ventilatory apparatus further impair the normal defense mechanisms, thus facilitating colonization.[15] In the compromised, susceptible host colonization precedes the majority of nosocomial pneumonias.

Although much has been said regarding pneumonias in compromised patients, it would be inappropriate to assume that these take place only in medical areas of the hospital. The NNIS reports indicate that pneumonia rates in surgical areas are very similar to those in medical areas.[13]

Of great concern with pneumonias caused by gram-negative organisms is their ability to advance to abscess formation and/or empyema, their destructiveness to the respiratory tract, their resistance to antimicrobial agents, and the high mortality rate (see Table 16-3). The complication of lung abscess can be defined as a necrotic lesion in the lung parenchyma that contains purulent material. Abscesses can be caused by aspiration, necrotizing LRIs, or a secondary infection to lung disease or malignant lesions. Pneumonias or lung abscesses can extend to involve the pleural space and cause empyema. The major predisposing factor to abscess formation appears to be aspiration from the oropharyngeal area. Aspiration is usually caused by an altered state of consciousness with temporary loss of gag and cough reflex action. This may occur during anesthesia, trauma, and medical emergencies such as cerebrovascular accident or seizure disorders, or it may be self-induced, as in alcoholism or drug intoxication.

The frequency of lung abscess and pleural empyema has decreased markedly over the last several decades. A noted pediatric problem 40 years ago, lung abscess currently is rare in children and adolescents but continues to be an important and serious disease among adults.[28,40] When lung abscesses do occur in children, it is not uncommon to find periodontal disease.[6] The most common causative microorganisms of lung abscesses are (1) certain anaerobes, such as *Bacteroides melaninogenicus*, *Bacteroides fragilis*, and *Fusobacterium nucleatum*; and (2) those aerobes that cause necrotizing infections, such as *K. pneumoniae*, *S. aureus*, and *Pseudomonas* species.[6,28] A large number (40%) of patients with lung abscesses have mixed cultures of both aerobes and anaerobes.[28]

PRACTICAL IMPLICATIONS
Specimen collection

Specimens can be obtained by several methods: expectorations, transtracheal aspiration (TTA), bronchial washings, suctioning from endotracheal or tracheostomy tubes, empyema fluid aspirates, transthoracic lung aspirations, tissue removed during surgical procedures, and blood cultures. Any method that either bypasses or greatly reduces contamination of the oropharyngeal resident flora is a preferred specimen. Each of these methods is not without

TABLE 16-3. Common bacterial pneumonias—a composite review

Infecting organism	Person-to-person transmission	Common modes of transmission	Pneumonic infiltrate	Complications
Anaerobic organisms *Bacteroides* species *Fusobacterium nucleatum*	—	Endogenous aspiration of oropharyngeal flora or bacteremia from pelvic or GI source	Segmental pneumonia	Lung abscess and necrotizing cavitary pneumonia with large recurring empyema
Enterobacter species	Uncommon	Endogenous aspiration of oropharyngeal flora or bacteremia from extrapulmonary source	Bronchopneumonia	Rare
Escherichia coli	Uncommon	Endogenous aspiration of oropharyngeal flora or bacteremia from extrapulmonary source	Bronchopneumonia (often lower lobe)	Empyema (common) and abscess
Haemophilus influenzae type B	Rare	Endogenous aspiration of oropharyngeal flora	Bronchopneumonia or lobar consolidation	Abscess and empyema
Klebsiella pneumoniae	Rare	Endogenous aspiration of oropharyngeal flora	Lobar pneumonia	Abscess (common) and empyema
Proteus species	Uncommon	Endogenous aspiration of oropharyngeal flora	Lobar or segmental consolidation	Multiple abscesses (often upper lobe)
Pseudomonas aeruginosa	Uncommon	Bacteremia from extrapulmonary source or by aspiration: exogenous—contaminated nebulizer reservoir; endogenous—from oropharyngeal flora	Nodular bronchopneumonia	Coalescing microabscess
Streptococcus pneumoniae	Common	Endogenous aspiration of oropharyngeal flora or by droplet spread from carriers	Defined density	Rare

potential complications or risks in either the procedure required to obtain the specimen or in the interpretation of the culture data.

The indigenous microflora of the orpharyngeal area (extending down to the level of the larynx) include approximately 200 different species of aerobes, facultative anaerobes, and obligatory anaerobes. The concentration of the bacteria has been estimated at 10^8 per milliliter of saliva.[3] Because of the potential for human error in specimens acquired by expectoration, the quantity of resident flora, and the rapidity with which these organisms reproduce, it is not surprising that 75% of the specimens submitted to the microbiology department at the Mayo Clinic and 60% of the specimens submitted at several Philadelphia hospitals were unsatisfactory for culture.[22,30] These same results of unacceptability can be reproduced in most hospital laboratories. However, even in the presence of these obstacles, an adequate specimen can be obtained. These specimens can give objective data that can assist in the initial and concurrent plan of therapy for the patient.

Acquisition of sputum for laboratory analysis should be accomplished before initiation of antimicrobial therapy. Antimicrobial agents rapidly alter cultivable flora. Presumptive diagnosis and treatment of pneumonia usually begin immediately on completion of the patient's history. Roentgenograms assist in defining the location and extent of lung involvement with suggestion as to cause. Gram stains of sputum can give further clues about the presence of an inflammatory process. Culture results can provide confirming identification of the etiological agent or misleading information, depending on the adequacy of the specimen collection. Treatment based on poorly obtained specimens can result in a lesser quality of patient care. It is interesting to note that the choice of antimicrobial therapy is frequently based on culture results. It is even more interesting to note the indifference with which personnel and patients respond to collection of this most important diagnostic tool.

Sputum obtained by fiberoptic bronchoscopy results in a specimen relatively free of oropharyngeal contamination. However, in the process of passage of the bronchoscope, contamination from the upper respiratory tract is introduced to the lower respiratory tract. Bronchial brushings are preferred over bronchial washings, since the washing greatly dilutes the specimen. In addition, topical anesthetics and lubricants can further alter the specimen. Specimens obtained from bronchial brushing or biopsy will result in more objective specimens. Bronchial washings or brushings are not valid specimens for anaerobic cultures.

Transtracheal aspirations (Fig. 16-3) have become more popular in the past decade as a reliable method of obtaining specimens that are demonstrably free of contamination. In this procedure a large-bore intravenous catheter is inserted through the cricothyroid membrane into the trachea. The catheter is advanced and the needle carefully withdrawn. The specimen is acquired by

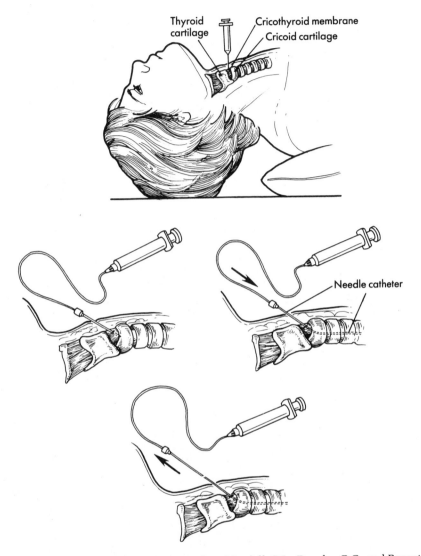

FIG. 16-3. Transtracheal aspiration. (Redrawn from Mandell, G.L., Douglas, R.G., and Bennett, J.E., editors: Principles and practices of infectious disease, New York, 1979, John Wiley & Sons, Inc.)

applying suction to the catheter. Because of the method of acquisition, these specimens are valid for determination of anaerobic infections. Transtracheal aspirations (TTA) (also known as translaryngeal aspiration) are especially meaningful when an acutely ill patient fails to respond to therapy. This method is recommended when (1) other methods are inconclusive, (2) infection is sufficiently severe to merit the risk of the procedure, (3) there is a suspected anaerobic infection, or (4) infection is present in a compromised host (e.g., necrotizing pneumonia of obscure cause, or chronic infiltrates). This procedure is not without limitations or complications. It is limited in that it may only assess the microbiological flora of the larger airways, but it may not be able to identify the condition of the alveolar spaces, especially if obstruction occurs proximal to the infected lung site. Complications of the procedure are rare. When they do occur, they may include pneumothorax, hemorrhage, and mediastinal or subcutaneous emphysema. Two reasons for not using the TTA as a means of specimen collection are the risk of complications and the physical condition of the patient (e.g., known abnormal clotting factor). TTA procedures are primarily done in teaching facilities. These procedures have yet to be fully accepted as an alternative method of obtaining specimens in the community hospital. With the exception of anaerobic culture, this may be a result of the fact that bronchial brushings or an appropriately obtained expectorated sputum specimen can yield results that are equal to that of TTA.[3,18,32]

Aspiration from tracheostomy or endotracheal tubes through a Luken tube provides for a quick and easy acquisition of a specimen. It should be noted that within 24 hours after insertion of a tracheostomy tube colonization occurs from flora of the upper respiratory tract. Histological studies of tracheostomy sites show inflammation at the site of the tube, which is thought to be caused by the device, not lung infection. When the specimen results of Gram stain and culture are interpreted, the alterations resulting from the device must be taken into account. During insertion of the endotracheal tube resident flora of the upper respiratory tract are carried to the lower tract. This contamination may result in misinterpretation of the culture data.[3]

As noted in Table 16-3, nosocomial pneumonia can be caused by bacteremias from extrapulmonary sites. Positive blood cultures from a patient with evidence of pneumonic infiltrates on roentgenogram and clinical symptoms of pneumonia constitute a positive confirmation of the cause of the pneumonia regardless of what the sputum culture may yield.[2] Bacteremias occur in approximately 21% of the gram-negative bacillary pneumonias.[10]

The most common method used to obtain sputum for laboratory analysis is by expectoration. Expectorated specimens are delegated specimens. The physician delegates by the written order; the nurse delegates to the aide, who in turn delegates to the patient. The majority of delegated specimens are obtained with little training given to the patient. However, when properly obtained, these specimens can give adequate information, especially when qualitatively evaluated for adequacy of the specimen. Basic principles of when and how to obtain the specimen would avoid many of the problems associated with inadequate specimen collection. The majority of patients with LRIs have a productive cough. Early morning specimens are preferred because they are usually free of gross contamination by oral and nasal secretions, and the hours of rest have allowed pooling of sputum to take place in the lung. If early morning is not possible, the next acceptable time is when the cough is productive, representing lung, not pharyngeal, secretions. Oropharyngeal contamination of an expectorated specimen is unavoidable. One can, however, reduce the level of contamination with some basic principles. The specimen should be obtained *before* starting antibiotic therapy. The specimen should not be taken immediately after the patient eats, chews gum or tobacco, brushes his teeth, or does any activity that increases oral or nasal secretions. If he is able, the patient should be encouraged to rinse his mouth with clear tap water to remove gross saliva before attempting to cough. If the patient has difficulty in coughing, a simple but effective method can be applied. The patient should take a deep breath and hold it as long as possible. On the next inhalation he should attempt to cough. During the period of apnea with the lung expanded the bronchial secretions are allowed to pool, thus triggering the cough mechanism. A deep cough at this time may result in productivity. If a patient cannot elicit an expectorated specimen, assistance of the respiratory care department can be beneficial. Ultrasonic nebulization with 10% saline with a positive pressure treatment frequently stimulates a productive cough. Respiratory care technicians are well versed in techniques for obtaining sputum and can be an invaluable resource. Many hospitals use this method of obtaining quality expectorated specimens. Postural drainage has also been an effective tool.

During the process of acquiring an expectorated specimen it is imperative that the delegates know three facts. First, knowing the difference between saliva and sputum is vital. An expectorated sputum is characteristically different from saliva. Saliva is a relatively clear, watery, frothy secretion originating from the oropharyngeal area. It yields no useful information regarding potential pathogens in the lower respiratory tract.[3,4,26] Sputum is purulent, frequently tenacious, and may be yellow or varying shades of green. It may also be bloody. If the infection is from anaerobic bacteria, sputum may have a foul odor. Second, the delegate must know methods to reduce oropharyngeal and nasal contamination. Third, the delegates should be aware of the importance of time loss. A potentially good quality sputum specimen may be rendered invalid if too much time elapses between acquisition and plating in the microbiology laboratory. Normal pharyngeal flora reproduce with great rapidity and can overgrow a more delicate pathogen or alter the pathogen/oral flora ratio. Inordinate delays can be reduced by assignment of key personnel to take specimens to the laboratory and avoiding a system that involves using the messenger service or waiting until there is a lull in ward routine.

Gram stains on sputum specimens sent to the microbiology laboratory have two specific benefits. First, they act as a screening method to determine the quality of the specimen and its adequacy for culture, and second, they can give initial objective data to the physician in preliminary diagnosis and treatment of the LRI. Several methods of evaluating Gram stains have been reported using scoring systems. It is generally accepted that after viewing the slide a stain with 10 or more squamous epithelial cells per low-power visual field (×100) is unacceptable for culture and should result in a request for a repeat specimen. Gram stains of saliva reveal many epithelial cells and a variety of both gram-positive and gram-negative bacteria that represent the normal pharyngeal flora. Few, if any, neutrophils will be seen. Gram stains of sputum give evidence of numerous neutrophils, few if any epithelial cells, and one to four potential pathogens. The greater the number of squamous cells, the more indicative it is of contamination from oropharyngeal secretions and the less likely to give information that will assist in patient treatment. The converse is also true. The fewer the number of squamous cells and the greater the number of neutrophils, the more indicative it is of information that will assist in patient treatment. The presence of white cells (pus) is indicative of an inflammatory process and can be an indication of LRI.

The ICP has an important role in assisting the microbiology department in adopting the practice of taking Gram stains of all submitted sputum specimens. This will not only assist the laboratory in improving quality outcome and eliminating routine culture of inappropriate specimens, but it can also act as a teaching tool for personnel who obtain these specimens. The ICP can influence the quality of a specimen through the education of personnel in the proper procedure of acquiring a specimen and the importance of prompt transportation to the microbiology laboratory.

Throat swabs of the pharyngeal area are obtained and must be done in such a manner to prevent contamination by the tongue, teeth, and oral secretions. Recovery of group A streptococci is the primary purpose of these cultures. Nasopharyngeal swabs are used in an attempt to recover either pertussis or diphtheria.

Swabs with holding medias are available from several manufacturers. Their purpose is to protect fragile organisms. However, the use of a holding medium does not negate the need for prompt, rapid transport of the specimen to the microbiology laboratory.

Surveillance

The purpose of surveillance is to detect and record infections in a consistent, systematic, and practical manner. The critical issues with respiratory tract infections are establishment of criteria for determining the presence of infection, selecting the population to survey, and deciding the method and frequency of surveillance. (See Chapter 7 for surveillance procedures.)

Investigators vary in their approaches to the determination of the presence of a respiratory tract infection. One approach is to classify the infection as *probable infection* or *definite infection*, with criteria established for each group.[4] Another approach is to identify the infection by radiological, clinical, and bacteriological data.

As established earlier, it is usually the critically ill or the compromised host who contracts nosocomial respiratory tract infections. Because of the acuity of the illness, the host may not be able to verbally communicate symptoms, resulting in little subjective data noted in physician, nursing, or respiratory care progress notes. Even with well-established criteria, the underlying host factor and therapy given to the host (e.g., antibiotics, steroids, chemotherapy) may mask or cloud the initial symptoms. This masking of symptoms increases the confusion when an attempt is made to evaluate clinical symptoms against hard laboratory or radiological data in the chart. For these reasons the decision of whether or not a nosocomial infection is present must be based on all sources of information, not just on culture and radiological reports.

It is the responsibility of the infection control committee to establish the criteria of respiratory tract infection to be used by the ICP. In development of the criteria several questions must be addressed:
1. Should surveillance be just for LRIs, or should it include both URIs and LRIs?
2. What are the anatomical sites involved in each of these divisions?
3. Should surveillance be for "definite" infections, or should it be graded into "probable" and "definite" categories?
4. What are the criteria for each infection by site and cause?
5. Should documentation concern only bacterial infections, or should viral infections also be identified?
6. If in the process of surveillance there is a discrepancy about whether or not a respiratory tract infection exists, who is responsible for and has the authority to make these decisions?

Other questions that are institution specific may arise, but the criteria that are established must be objective, practical for all areas of the hospital, and easily interpreted by the ICP.

Because of the wide acceptance of the CDC criteria for respiratory tract infections, they are included below*:

1. *Upper respiratory infections.* This category includes clinical manifest infections of the nose, throat or ear (singly or in combination). The signs and symptoms vary widely and depend on the site or sites involved. Coryzal syndromes, streptococcal pharyngitis, otitis media and mastoiditis are all included in this category; though these diverse entities have been grouped together, the specific diagnosis should be entered on the line listing form to allow separate analysis, if desired. The majority of

*From Centers for Disease Control: Outline for surveillance and control of nosocomial infections, Atlanta, 1972, U.S. Department of Health, Education, and Welfare, Public Health Service.

these infections will be viral or of uncertain etiology. Careful attention must be paid to the incubation period in order to separate community-acquired infections that develop after admission and nosocomial infections.

2. *Lower respiratory infections.* Clinical signs and symptoms of a lower respiratory infection (cough, pleuritic chest pain, fever and particularly purulence) developing after admission are regarded as sufficient evidence to diagnose respiratory infection, whether or not sputum cultures or chest x-rays are obtained. When there is evidence of both upper and lower respiratory infections, concomitantly entries should be made for both sites on the line listing form.

    Other conditions which may result in similar signs or symptoms (congestive heart failure, post-operative atelectasis, pulmonary embolism, etc.) may often be differentiated by the clinical course of the patient. However, even if such entities are suspected to be present, the diagnosis of lower respiratory infection is made in the presence of one or more of the following: purulent sputum (with or without recognized pathogen on sputum culture) or suggestive chest x-ray. Supra-infection of a previously existing respiratory infection may result in a new nosocomial infection when a new pathogen is cultured from sputum and clinical or radiologic evidence indicates that the new organism is associated with deterioration in the patient's condition. Care must be used in distinguishing supra-colonization from supra-infection.

Criteria for viral respiratory tract infections have been documented and are based on usual incubation periods of the different viruses. If the patient develops symptoms compatible with a viral illness and has been hospitalized for as long or longer than the incubation period, the infection is considered nosocomial. For URIs the symptoms are cough, sore throat, and/or nasal discharge after 3 days or more of hospitalization.[44]

Once the criteria have been established, a decision of who should be surveyed must be answered. Much time can be spent on total house surveillance with resulting data representing the different medical disciplines and areas of the institution. When the ICP is evaluating the characteristics of those who are more likely to contract nosocomial respiratory tract infections versus the time required to do total house surveillance, evidence suggests that concentration of efforts on the high-risk areas is more meaningful and productive. There are, however, benefits to both approaches, total house versus area specific. The decision of who to survey depends on the purpose of the surveillance, the intended use of the data, and the number of personnel available. In general, an area-specific approach to a high-risk population is more beneficial. It should be noted that the determination of the population to survey may change when the purpose for surveillance changes (e.g., during a high influenza season a prevalence or short-term concurrent surveillance of the total house may be done to give indications of nosocomial acquisition and for purposes of visitor restrictions). Once the purpose for which surveillance was instituted is complete, it is discontinued.

Equipment used in association with the respiratory tract

For ease of identification and clarification the equipment used in association with the respiratory tract can be divided into three categories: those used for diagnostic purposes, those used in maintenance of airways, and those used for ventilatory assistance.

Diagnostic. Two pieces of equipment used in diagnostic procedures are the rigid and the flexible fiberoptic bronchoscope (FFB). Little documentation is available on the infection rates associated with either of these pieces of equipment. The potential for infection, however, does exist. Outbreaks and pseudoepidemics from FFB use have been reported.[1,24,45] These outbreaks have usually been attributed to human error in following directions for disinfection. The major difference between these two pieces of bronchoscopy equipment in reference to infection control is the method applied in terminal cleaning. Rigid bronchoscopes can be autoclaved; flexible fiberoptic equipment is as delicate as it is expensive and cannot tolerate autoclaving. Flexible fiberoptic equipment can tolerate gas sterilization with ethylene oxide (ETO), using the cool cycle. However, coiling the equipment too tightly or frequently using gas sterilizations tends to break or damage the fragile optics and render them inoperable. The down-time required for gas sterilization and aeration decreases the frequency with which most institutions wish to use the equipment. Flexible fiberoptic equipment can be adequately disinfected if the manufacturer's recommendations are followed carefully. The use of povidone-iodine is suggested as part of the disinfection procedure.[24,45] It would be appropriate to reiterate the importance of close adherence to procedure when using disinfection as a means of terminal cleaning. Contamination during the process of disinfection or an improperly carried out procedure is usually the incriminating factor in pseudoepidemics or actual epidemics. After use with a known infectious case (e.g., patient with tuberculosis) many institutions terminally clean with gas sterilization. Anytime disinfection is used in preference to sterilization the ICP must be alert to the potential for nosocomial infection.

Maintenance of airways. Two types of equipment are used in maintaining airways: endotracheal tubes and tracheostomy tubes. There are numerous types of tracheostomy tubes on the market that are made from various materials, ranging from polyethylene to stainless steel or silver.

Studies of intubations in adults, children, and infants indicate that a significant percentage of these populations become colonized by gram-negative bacilli within 48 hours after intubation. Furthermore, colonization, as discussed earlier, is frequently a predisposition to LRI or systemic infection.[7,21]

Local irritation and inflammation may occur at the site where the distal end of the tracheostomy cannula rubs against the tracheal wall. Although rare, cannula-induced tracheitis with severe morbidity has been reported.[38] Colonization at the site of the cannula is common and occurs within 24 hours of the tracheostomy.[39] Because the tracheostomy and endotracheal tubes bypass the normal humidification offered by the upper respiratory tract, external high humidification is recommended to prevent drying of the mucous membrane of the lower respiratory tract. If drying does occur, it can result in alteration of the mucociliary escalatory activity of the lower respiratory tract.

Both endotracheal tubes and tracheostomies increase the potential for LRI. In addition to the compromised state of the critically ill patient who requires these procedures, there are other inherent complications associated with the presence of the devices and their care. These include bypassing the upper respiratory tract defense mechanism, colonization by gram-negative bacteria, care of the devices (suctioning and cleaning), and use of respiratory care equipment such as humidifiers, intermittent positive pressure breathing (IPPB), or continuous respiratory assistance with the MA-1 or the BEAR respirator.

Infection control intervention can minimize the potential for acquisition of nosocomial LRI associated with these devices. The establishment of tracheostomy care as a sterile procedure is the basis from which other procedures can be developed. The infection control committee, as well as other appropriate medical staff committees, must establish guidelines for the use of endotracheal tubes, such as duration (limitation) of use of an endotracheal tube before a tracheostomy should be considered, proper suctioning techniques, and routine humidification procedures. Questions to be asked regarding care and use of tracheostomy tubes are the same as with endotracheal tubes but may also address procedures such as cleaning of the inner cannula (if present), frequency of change of the outer cannula, and maximal time for inflation of the cuff.*

When patients with these devices are monitored, care must be taken to prevent culture reports with possible indication of colonization at the tracheostomy site from being interpreted as an LRI or as an infection at the tracheostomy site. Colonization and infection can be two separate entities. A patient may have colonization of the lower respiratory tract without an LRI. A patient may also have colonization at the site of the tracheostomy without presence of infection at that site. However, when infection is present in the lungs, colonization also occurs at the tracheostomy site.

Ventilatory assistance. There are numerous types of equipment used for ventilatory assistance. All of these can be divided according to three basic

---

*Reprints on current recommendations for care of the patient with a tracheostomy are available on request from the CDC.[9]

functions: (1) those used in the delivery of oxygen, (2) those used in humidification, and (3) those using positive pressure, either intermittent or continuous.

Oxygen equipment (tank or wall outlet) with humidification as a source of infection has not been documented. This may be caused in part by the humidification process (Fig. 16-4). Humidification does not produce water droplets. The water source can, however, become contaminated. A recovery room study of multiple-use oxygen humidification bottles as potential infectious sources gave evidence that these bottles are not high-risk pieces of equipment, since contamination greater than that of the room air was not observed.[32] Changing of the oxygen tubing with each patient, a part of the routine procedure, may have had an impact on the results of the study. In lieu of disposables procedures must be established that would not allow refilling of water containers. When the water supply is depleted, a fresh bottle should be attached and the empty one sent for terminal cleaning.

The most common method of delivering high humidification to the patient is the use of cold mist. Cold mist can be used with or without a Child Adult Mist Tent. If the water well in these units does not employ a closed system, there is potential for contamination because of the tendency to add to the fluid level.

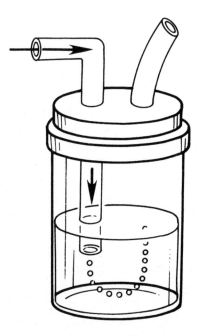

FIG. 16-4. A humidifier bubbles gas through water, enabling gas to pick up water vapor (molecules) but not actual droplets. (Redrawn from Castle, M.: Hospital infection control: principles and practice, New York, 1980, John Wiley & Sons, Inc.)

Routine cleaning and handling procedures must be developed to ensure hygienic standards and prevention of contamination.

Equipment that uses positive pressure has been implicated in a significant number of nosocomial respiratory tract infections in the 1960s.[30,31,36,38] Sporadic outbreaks do, however, continue to occur but at a greatly reduced rate. The nebulizer on the machine has been identified as the source of this morbidity. A nebulizer is a device that breaks up solutions and suspends them in a gas (air). Nebulizers create aerosols. The droplets in the aerosol are not uniform in size. The larger particles either settle quickly in the corrugated tubing of the machine or they are trapped in the upper respiratory tract and are physically removed by the mucociliary escalator. The smaller particles are forced under positive pressure into the alveolar spaces of the lung. Because of the size of the aerosols that reach the alveoli (approximately 2 μm), they arc easily assimilated. The purpose of aerosolization is to instill a medication, such as a bronchodilator; to prevent drying of the mucous membrane; or to break up thick secretions and increase the effectiveness of the cilia. Unfortunately, bacteria of the same size can be carried with the aerosol into the lung. The potential for infection then exists.

There are three methods of creating an aerosol in nebulizers: the spinning disk, ultrasonic energy, and the Venturi jet principle.[19] The spinning disk produces aerosols by releasing liquids onto a rapidly rotating disk, which is then dispersed into small droplets (Fig. 16-5, A). Most humidifiers use this principle. Ultrasonic energy produces aerosols by a vibrating object with frequencies above audible sound waves (Fig. 16-5, B). A Cough-a-lator is an example of equipment using this method of aerosolization. In the Venturi jet principle a rapid flow of air creates a partial vacuum (Fig. 16-5, C). The flow of air over a capillary tube, submerged in a reservoir of fluid, will draw fluid in the reservoir upward into the air flow where the aerosol is produced. This principle is used in the nebulizer of Bird and Bennett IPPB equipment and in continuous ventilatory equipment such as the MA-1 or the BEAR.

The problem that arises with nebulizers is contamination. If the nebulizer reservoir becomes contaminated, the potential to introduce large quantities of pathogens into the alveolar spaces is great. During the 1960s frequent outbreaks of nosocomial respiratory tract infections were documented, and the majority implicated a contaminated nebulizer as the source of infection.

The aim of prevention of infection in respiratory care equipment is either to eliminate the microbial contamination or reduce it to a very low level. The source of contamination usually involves the "patient breathing circuit." This is the tubing that attaches to the main driveline of the machine and extends to the mouthpiece, which includes the small nebulizer where medication or water is placed for each treatment.

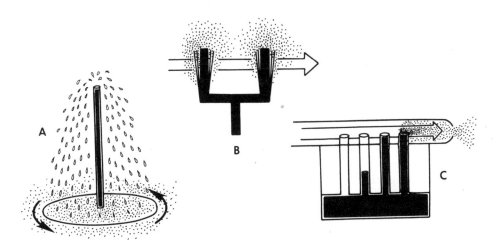

FIG. 16-5. A, Rapidly spinning disk produces aerosol when solution is poured onto it, creating large and small droplets. B, Solution is vibrated by ultrasonic energy, thereby breaking up solution into small droplets. C, Venturi jet nebulizer draws solution into stream of gas that passes rapidly over tube immersed in reservoir. (From Castle, M.: Hospital infection control: principles and practice, New York, 1980, John Wiley & Sons, Inc.; redrawn from Malecka-Griggs, B., and Reinhardt, D.J.: Fundamentals of nosocomial infections associated with respiratory therapy, Upper Montclair, N.J., 1981, Healthscan.)

Methods of terminal cleaning. Studies have been conducted to determine the level of terminal cleaning to which respiratory equipment should be submitted. There are four methods of terminal cleaning: sterilization, disinfection, pasteurization, or use of disposable equipment.

Sterilization. Sterilization can be accomplished by steam autoclaving or exposure to ETO. If the equipment can tolerate autoclaving, this is the recommended method because it is the most efficient, nontoxic, and economical method available. Few respiratory equipment devices fall into this category. ETO is recommended for sterilization of all nonautoclavable items. The disadvantages of ETO are cost and the time required for aeration. When ETO is used for patient breathing circuits, a large inventory must be maintained to allow for time used in the sterilization and aeration process.

Disinfection. When disinfection is chosen as the method of terminal cleaning, care must be given in choosing the correct agent. Only the buffered glutaraldehydes are recommended for use on respiratory equipment. Currently there are two: the acid-activated dialdehyde and the alkaline-activated dialdehyde. Discard dates must be carefully watched, and neither solution should be used after the specified time limit. Sterile water should be used for rinsing off the toxic germicides. Unfortunately, this is usually not practiced, and tap water is substituted. This is a poor practice because many municipal water supplies are contaminated with large numbers of nonenteric, gram-negative bacteria, including *Pseudomonas* species. Should material be rinsed in this manner, the items must be dried in a heated, ultrafiltered drying chamber, using an air flow through tubing to ensure drying. Solutions that contain quaternary ammonium compounds, phenols, and hexachlorophene are not recommended as disinfectants for respiratory care equipment.

Pasteurization. Pasteurization is a process of mechanically washing the equipment in a heat-controlled water bath. Pasteurization equipment uses the principle of a washing machine. Recontamination can frequently occur during the machine's drying cycle; therefore separate drying chambers are recommended. Pasteurization equipment and drying chambers are commercially available.

Use of disposable equipment. A wide variety of disposable equipment is available for most respiratory therapy procedures. Many institutions are now using this method, since most insurance companies will accept charges for disposable breathing circuitry. It is an accurate method of assuring noncommunicability of bacteria by contaminated equipment. Disposable equipment is to be disposed of after use. Under no circumstances should an attempt be made to disinfect or sterilize these materials for reuse. The material used in disposable equipment is different from that used in reusable equipment even though both may be produced by the same manufacturer. When disposables are submitted to sterilization by ETO or to a disinfectant, the material used may act or react: toxins may be absorbed by the equipment; a chemical reaction may take place; leaching or permeation may occur; or there may be an alteration in the physical properties.

The method of terminal cleaning selected by the institution must be based on need, type of equipment used, and budgetary considerations.

Prevention

Recommendations for prevention of nosocomial infection associated with respiratory care equipment have been published by the CDC[11]:

1. *Use sterile medications.* Multidose vials and bottles can become contaminated with reuse. Open medications, if used, should be kept at 4° C. Several manufacturers now provide for single-use vials of sterile water and commonly used medications in nebulizers.
2. *Use sterile distilled or deionized water.* The water must be dispensed aseptically. Unused portions should be discarded after 24 hours.
3. *Do not add to fluid levels.* Sterile water should not be added to replenish half-filled nebulizers or humidifiers. If additional fluid is needed, the reservoir should be emptied first, then refilled. When not in use, the containers should be emptied, cleaned, and dried before storage.
4. *Use sterile, adequately disinfected, or disposable patient breathing circuits.* This includes any accessory that has contact with the respiratory tract.

5. *Use ultra–high-efficiency filters.* These filters have a stated efficiency of 99.7% for a particle 0.3 μm. Large filters are used on the main-flow driveline, thereby giving protection from anything proximal to the filter. The machine can be protected from contamination by the patient's exhaled air through the use of smaller filters placed on the medication nebulizer.

6. *Replace the patient breathing circuit regularly.* Continuous assisted or controlled ventilation (e.g., MA-1 or BEAR) requires that the circuit be changed every 24 hours. Removal of fluid buildup in the corrugated tubing should be performed frequently. A safe method is to insert a T tube at the lowest point of the tube closest to the patient. By turning the valve in the T tube, fluid can be removed without accidental "dumping" of large amounts of fluid into the patient's lungs.

7. *Replace patient circuitry on intermittent therapy regularly.* It is recommended that patient circuitry be replaced every 24 hours. Care should be taken to ensure that there is no contamination during storage between use during the 24 hours.

8. *Fill water reservoirs at the time needed.* Reservoirs should not be filled in advance of use.

Another method of infection control practice has been the use of copper sponges (Chore Girl) placed in the reservoirs of nebulizers and humidifiers. This procedure has been said to decrease contamination of the water, but it has received questionable reviews.[4] With the current availability of other methods, the use of copper sponges is not recommended.

Home care programs. A large number of patients with chronic lung disease continue the use of respiratory therapy in their homes. The equipment they use is either rented or purchased with little or no education given in the proper maintenance of the equipment or infection control practices regarding the breathing circuitry. The responsibility of infection control does not stop once the patient is discharged. Self-induced pulmonary infections can occur through the use of equipment contaminated by the patient's own environmental or endogenous flora. Patient education on the care and use of this equipment is part of the total responsibility of patient care. Some hospitals with an outpatient respiratory therapy department have established programs for periodic cleaning of home units for their outpatients at little or no cost. Teaching of proper cleaning of the breathing circuitry is also stressed. Many persons with chronic lung disease are long-standing patients of the hospital; therefore this service may be a benefit to the hospital and the patient.

Employee health

Considerations for employee health in relation to respiratory tract infections are primarily those of prevention. The key to success is administrative support for the development and enforcement of employee health policies. Hospitals without an employee health clinic can have an effective preventive program using the service of their emergency room physician or other physician designee. The following should be considered when establishing employee health policies:

1. Exposure to disease by the airborne route during employment; tuberculosis (TB), meningococcal meningitis, and childhood disease; laboratory accidents with organisms such as *Coccidioides* species.

2. Prevention of disease transmitted by the airborne mode of transmission by vaccination (e.g., rubella vaccine, annual influenza vaccination); if vaccination is considered to be a part of the employee health program, is the vaccine recommended or required? Who is financially responsible, the employee or the institution?

3. Routine skin testing for TB should be considered for preemployment, annual physicals, and known exposure any time during employment.

4. Employee education to increase awareness of proper procedure when handling secretions of persons not deemed necessary to have isolation precautions (e.g., respiratory syncytial virus, cytomegalovirus).

5. Employees working with respiratory tract infection: If employees are allowed to work, may they have patient contact? How much contact? May these employees work in high-risk areas such as pediatrics and ICU or with oncology patients receiving cytotoxic drugs? Similar concerns relate to the health of food handlers.

Authorities have varied opinions regarding the questions just listed. These and other associated questions concerning patients, employees, and visitors with respiratory tract infections must be addressed by the individual hospital infection control and employee health committees. Regardless of the number or sophistication of the hospital policies, the key to infection control among employees is enforcement of these policies.

Tuberculosis control. Every hospital should have an employee TB surveillance program. There is evidence of TB increasing in certain geographical areas within the United States where a high population of immigrants exists. Before reviewing recommendations for a TB testing program, it is essential to review the difference between TB infection and TB disease. TB infection refers to the presence of TB bacilli in the body with subsequent development of a positive purified protein derivative (PPD) skin test. Disease refers to a TB infection developing into a disease process with the resulting symptoms of the disease. Following are recommendations for a TB skin testing program.[12]

Initial testing. A PPD skin test should be given to all employees at the time of hire using the two-step method (booster effect). If the reaction to the first test is less than 10 mm of induration, a second test is given at least 1 week and no more than 3 weeks after the first test. The result of the second test is the baseline for that employee. This two-step method will identify otherwise "false-positive" converters at a later date. Once a person becomes infected by tubercle bacilli or other *Mycobacterium* species, he develops a delayed hypersensitivity to the organism. Over a period of time, if repeated skin tests are not done, this delayed hypersensitivity may wane. When a person is skin tested after this waning period, a negative or doubtful reaction may occur. However, the skin test does boost the immune recognition by the bone marrow, spleen, and reticuloendothelial system. A repeat skin test applied 1 to 3 weeks later will result in a positive reaction in the employee who is infected. The result of the "booster" to the immune system will be a more accurate description of the employee's TB status. If the initial skin test is positive, a chest x-ray examination is recommended.

Repeat skin testing. Repeat skin testing should be done (1) in conjunction with the annual physical and (2) after known significant exposure to a recently diagnosed nonisolated patient.

When maintaining records of a TB testing program, it is imperative that the results of the PPD be measured and written in millimeters of induction, not in reference to positive or negative. If possible, the number of persons administering and interpreting skin tests should be limited. This will greatly improve the reliability of the test data.

Guidelines must be established by the institution on methods of preventive treatment. Some institutions exclusively use workman's compensation, whereas others have accepted the assistance of local public health offices in the treatment of employees with known PPD conversion.

Problem solving

Identification of potential outbreaks of respiratory tract infections is accomplished through comparative data review. The identification can be a new organism, an unusual sensitivity pattern, or an increase in the gross rate or rates by service or area. When a suspected outbreak of respiratory tract infection has been identified, specific areas must be evaluated concurrently; changes or variations in the method of terminal cleaning of equipment, patient care procedures (e.g., tracheostomy care, a new product), employees, type of patient population, host factors, diagnostic procedures, or therapy. An alteration in any of these may affect whether or not a true increase in infection can be considered epidemic. The process of evaluating each area can be accomplished by using the epidemiological model outlined in Chapter 7.

Culturing is a common method of evaluation in an attempt to identify a potential source of the proposed outbreak. However, cultures of personnel and/or equipment should only be undertaken when there is a high index of suspicion that these will reveal the source. When culturing respiratory equipment is indicated, several methods can be employed:

1. When using a swab for culturing equipment, a greater yield will result if the swab is moistened before obtaining the culture. If a transport medium is provided in the culture package, this should be used. If sterile swabs are made up by the laboratory, the swab may be dipped in broth before swabbing and achieve similar results. Swabbing should be reserved for easy access or flat areas.

2. Room or background air may be tested by using settle plates or an air sampler. The culture media used and the exposure time of the settle plates or the length of time the air sampler is on will vary.

3. Testing for potential contamination of an aerosol can be done with the assistance of an air sampler. Variation may occur in the exposure time, culture media, flow rate of the effluent gas, and the method of adapting the exit port of the equipment being tested to the air sampler intake. The effluent gas may also be tested by direct exposure to a Petri plate. There are one-stage and two-stage environmental sampler kits available that are specifically manufactured to adapt to respiratory therapy and anesthesia equipment. The type of medium to be used in conjunction with these kits, exposure time, and flow rate may vary.

4. Solutions may be tested by obtaining an aliquot (i.e., 1 ml) of the fluid using aseptic technique with a needle and syringe.

5. Tubing or other articles of equipment with hollow centers that will allow water to flow through can be easily cultured using the rinse method. Using a known amount of sterile water or saline (i.e., 100 ml) the internal side of the equipment should be rinsed, and care should be taken not to contaminate by putting fingers into openings or splashing water over the sides. If the tubing is corrugated, the tubing should be stretched while rinsing and each end lowered alternately to assure a thorough rinse. The rinse is then poured into the upper chamber of a Millipore filter. With the use of negative pressure, the solution should be pulled through into the lower chamber of the filter unit. Care must be taken when disassembling the unit to prevent contamination of the filter located between the upper and lower chambers. The type of medium the filter is placed on will vary as to the anticipated outcome.

6. Small pieces of equipment may be dropped directly from their package into a sterile bath. After gentle agitation the solution is then poured through a Millipore filter as described above.

Environmental culturing can provide data to assist in an epidemiological survey. Before initiating any environmental culturing, it is important to establish what is being cultured for, the methods that will be used, and the procedural guidelines for obtaining the culture. Decisions relating to the selection must be made before obtaining the culture (e.g., culture media, exposure time).

A key factor in the epidemiological investigation is the interpretation of the culture data. This can be a most difficult and confusing task. A good understanding of the who, when, where, and what of the suspected epidemic will assist in the interpretation and conclusion that will be drawn from the environmental review.

Nosocomial respiratory infections caused by contaminated respiratory therapy equipment are uncommon because of current standards of infection control and the degree of adherence to these practices. Therefore routine in-use environmental monitoring of respiratory equipment is not recommended.

SUMMARY

Nosocomial respiratory tract infections can affect all hospital patients. They are, however, frequently associated with patients who have underlying disease, acute illness, and other compromised factors that lower their defense mechanisms. High standards of infection control practices in all areas that influence the respiratory tract may minimize risks to the patient. Because of the complexity of medical problems associated with these patients, nosocomial respiratory tract infections will continue to plague medical practice and all who work in this field. Through continued observation and monitoring of these infections, additional insight will be gained, and new methods of control will be developed. The responsibility of searching for and developing new controls belongs to those who work in the field of infection control.

REFERENCES

1. Aeolny, Y., and Finegold, M.S.: Serious Infections Complications after flexible fiberotic bronchoscopy, West. J. Med. **131**:327-333, 1979.
2. Barrett-Connor, E., et al., editors: Epidemiology for the infection control nurse, St. Louis 1978, The C.V. Mosby Co.
3. Bartlett, J.G., Brewer, N.S., and Ryan, K.J.: Laboratory diagnosis of lower respiratory infections, CUMITECH-7, Washington D.C., 1978, American Society for Microbiology.
4. Bennett, J.V., and Brachman, P.S.: Hospital infections, Boston, 1979, Little, Brown & Co.
5. Black, N., Castellino, R.A., and Shaw, V.: Radiographic aspects of pulmonary infections in patients with altered immunity, Radiographic Clin. North Am. **11**:176, April 1973.
6. Brook, I., and Finegold, S.: Bacteriology and therapy of lung abscess in children, J. Pediatr. **94**:10-12, 1979.
7. Bryant, L.R., et al.: Bacterial colonization profile tracheal intubation and mechanical ventilation, Arch. Surg. **104**:647, 1972.
8. Burke, J.F., and Hildick-Smith, G.Y., editors: The infection-prone hospital patient, Boston, 1978, Little Brown & Co.
9. Centers for Disease Control: The control of pulmonary infections associated with tracheostomy, Atlanta, 1972, U.S. Department of Health, Education, and Welfare, Public Health Service.
10. Centers for Disease Control: Outline for surveillance and control of nosocomial infections, Atlanta, 1972, U.S. Department of Health, Education, and Welfare, Public Health Service.
11. Centers for Disease Control: Recommendations for decontamination and maintenance of inhalation therapy equipment, Atlanta, 1975, U.S. Department of Health, Education, and Welfare, Public Health Service.

12. Centers for Disease Control: Guidelines for prevention of T.B. transmission in hospitals, Atlanta, 1979, U.S. Department of Health, Education, and Welfare, Public Health Service.
13. Centers for Disease Control: National Nosocomial Infection Study (NNIS), annual reports for year 1972, Atlanta, 1974, CDC.
14. Commission on Professional and Hospital Activities: Length of stay in PAS hospitals in the United States, Chicago, 1975, The Commission.
15. Eickhoff, T.C.: Pulmonary infections in surgical patients, Surg. Clin. North Am. **60**:175-183, Feb. 1980.
16. Foy, H.M., et al.: Rates of pneumonia during influenza epidemics in Seattle, 1964-1975, J.A.M.A. **241**:253-258, 1979.
17. Fraser, R.G., and Pare, J.A.: Diagnosis and disease of the chest, vols. 1 and 2, Philadelphia, 1970, W.B. Saunders Co.
18. Geckler, R.W., Gremillion, D.H., and McAllister, C.K.: Microscopic and bacteriologic comparison of paired sputa and transtracheal aspirates, J. Clin. Microbiol. **6**:396-399, 1977.
19. Grigg, B.M., and Reinhardt, D.J., Fundamentals of nosocomial infection associated with respiratory therapy, ed. 2, New York, 1976, Projects in Health Inc.
20. Haley, R.W., and Emori, T.E.: SENIC report, Presented at the Second International Conference on Nosocomial Infection, Aug 1980, Atlanta.
21. Harris, H., Wirtschafter, D., and Cassady, G.: Endotracheal intubation and its relationship to bacterial colonization and systemic infections of newborn infants, Pediatrics **56**:816-822, 1976.
22. Heineman, H.D., Chawla, J.K., and Lofton, W.M.: Misinformation from sputum cultures without microscope examination, J. Clin. Microbiol. **6**:518-527, 1977.
23. Johanson, W.B., et al.: Nosocomial respiratory infection with gram negative bacilli: the significance of colonization of the respiratory tract, Ann. Intern. Med. **77**:701, 1972.
24. Kellerhals, S.: A pseudoepidemic of *Serratia marcescens* from a contaminated fiberbronchoscope, A.P.I.C. Journal **6**:5-9, Dec. 1978.
25. Junin, C.M., and Edelman, R.: The impact of infections on medical care in the United States: problems and priorities for future research, Ann. Intern. Med. **89**:737-868, 1978.
26. Lerner, A.M.: The gram-negative bacillary pneumonias, Disease-a-month, Chicago, 1980, Year Book Medical Publishers, Inc.
27. Little, J.W., and Smith, L.H.: Pulmonary aspiration—medical conference, University of San Francisco, West. J. Med. **131**:122-129, Aug. 1979.
28. Lung abscess: West. J. Med. **124**:475-482, 1976.
29. McGuckin, P.A., et al.: Disposable humidifiers in a recovery room—a microbiological evaluation, A.P.I.C. Journal **7**:20-22, Sept. 1979.
30. Mentz, J.J., Scharer, L., and McClement, J.H.: A hospital outbreak of *Klebiella* pneumonia from inhalation therapy with contamination aerosol solutions, Am. Rev. Respir. Dis. **95**:454-460, 1967.
31. Moffett, H.L., and Williams, T.: Bacteria recovered from distilled water and inhalation equipment, Am. J. Dis. Child. **114**:7-12, 1969.
32. Murray, P.A., and Washington, J.A.: Microscopic and bacteriologic analysis of expectorated sputum, Mayo Clinic. Proc. **50**:339-334, 1975.
33. Newhouse, M., Sanchis, J., and Bienenstock, J.: Lung defense mechanisms, part I, N. Engl. J. Med. **295**:990-996, 1976.
34. Newhouse, M., Sanchis, J., and Bienenstock, J.: Lung defense mechanisms, part II, N. Engl. J. Med. **295**:1045-1050, 1976.
35. Penn, R.G., Sanders, W.E., Jr., and Sanders, C.C.: Colonization of the oropharynx with gram-negative bacilli: a major antecedent to nosocomial pneumonia, Am. J. Infect. Control **9**:25, 1981.
36. Pierce, A.K., and Sanford, J.P.: Treatment and prevention of infections associated with inhalation therapy, Mod. Treat. **3**:1171-1174, 1966.
37. Reeder, G.S., and Gracey, D.R., Aspiration of intrathoracic abscesses, J.A.M.A. **240**:1156-1159, 1978.

38. Reinarz, J.A., et al.: The Potential Role of inhalation therapy equipment in nosocomial infections, J. Clin. Invest. **44:**831-839, 1965.
39. Reinarz, J.A., et al.: Tracheostomy care and control of colonization with gram-negative bacteria, Clin. Res. **16:**334-335, 1968.
40. Schachter, E.N., Kreisman, H., and Putman, C.: Diagnostic problems in supportive lung disease, Arch. Intern. Med. **136:**167-171, 1976.
41. Teplitz, C., et al.: Necrotizing tracheitis induced by tracheostomy tube, Arch. Pathol. **77:**14-19, 1964.
42. Valenti, W.M., Trudell, R.G., and Bentley, D.W.: Factors predisposing to oropharyngeal colonization with gram-negative bacilli in the aged, N. Engl. J. Med. **298:**1108-1111, 1978.
43. Valenti, W.M., et al.: Nosocomial viral infections. I. Epidemiology and significance, Infect. Control **1:**33-37, 1980.
44. Valenti, W.M., et al.: Nosocomial viral infections. II. Guidelines for prevention and control of respiratory viruses, herpes viruses and hepatitis viruses, Infect. Control **1:**154-178, 1980.
45. Webb, S.F., and Vall-Spinosa, A.: Outbreak of *Serratia marcescens* associated with the flexible fiberbronchoscope, Chest **58:**703-708, 1975.
46. Werhle, P.F., and Top, F.H., editors: Communicable and infectious diseases, ed. 9, St. Louis, 1981, The C.V. Mosby Co.
47. Youmans, G.P., Patterson, P.Y., and Sommers, H.M.: The biologic and clinical basis of infectious diseases, ed. 2, Philadelphia, 1980, W.B. Saunders Co.
48. Young, L.S.: The impaired host, Proceedings of the 1976 Association for Practitioners of Infection Control Educational Conference, St. Paul, Minn. 1977, pp. 31-48.

Integumentary system

The integument, or skin, is the largest organ of the body. The complexity of this system is appreciated by reviewing its five primary functions:

- Protection of underlying tissues from physical, chemical, electrical, thermal, or biological injury
- Regulation of heat and water loss in response to environmental stimuli
- Assistance in the excretory process through perspiration
- Perception of sensations, such as pain, touch, temperature, and pressure
- Production of vitamin D

This chapter will address the major cutaneous infections occurring in hospitalized patients through the examination of etiological agents, predisposing factors, surveillance techniques, and prevention and control methodology.

ANATOMICAL AND PHYSIOLOGICAL CONSIDERATIONS
Structure and function

The integumentary system consists of the skin and its derivatives (Fig. 17-1). Providing a protective covering over the entire body, the skin is composed of the epidermis and dermis.

The epidermis, or outermost component, contains four layers of varying thickness of stratified squamous epithelium; the basal layer (stratum germinativum) lies adjacent to the dermis and is the only layer containing epidermal cells capable of reproduction through mitosis. Thus if the stratum germinativum is destroyed through trauma or burns, regeneration of the epidermis cannot occur. As daughter cells are continuously pushed upward, they die from lack of tissue fluid, and a chemical transformation occurs. The once soft protoplasm of the cell becomes keratinized or cornified, resulting in layers of horny, waterproof cells that prevent dehydration.

The dermis, also called the corium, is a strong, flexible, elastic layer of connective tissue. Numerous, small, conelike elevations, the papillae, serve to attach the dermis to the epidermis. Ridges formed by these papillae are most noticeable on the palms and soles of the feet and are characteristically known as hand and foot "prints." The corium is well supplied with blood and lymph vessels that are critical for both temperature regulation and nourishment of tissue. Interference with the blood supply results in necrosis and ulceration, as in the formation of decubiti from pressure.

Cutaneous sense organs are also present in this layer. Impulses from corium

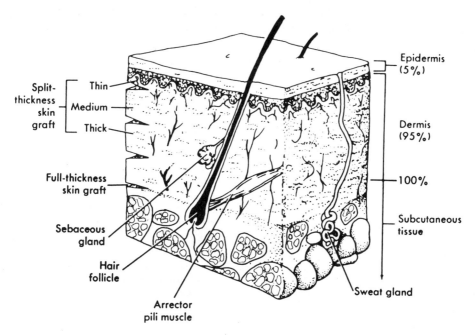

FIG. 17-1. Diagram of the layers of the skin. (From, Graab, W.S., and Smith, J.W.: Plastic surgery, ed. 3, Boston, 1979, Little, Brown & Co.)

receptors are carried on afferent nerve fibers to register touch, pressure, pain, and temperature, while efferent fibers transmit impulses to blood vessels, smooth muscles, and glands.

Derivatives of skin include sweat, sebaceous, ceruminous, and mammary glands; hair and hair follicles; and nails. Of these derivatives, two glands are important in keeping the skin's bacterial flora under control:

1. Sweat (sudoriferous) glands are coiled, tubular structures that produce sweat, which is composed of water, salt, and urea. Besides playing a vital role in temperature regulation, these glands excrete lysozyme, or muramidase. This enzyme lyses the cell wall of gram-positive organisms.
2. Sebaceous glands secrete an oily substance called sebum, which contains fatty acids that have antifungal and antibacterial properties.

Although the specific antimicrobial properties of skin have not been well delineated, two additional protective mechanisms are suggested. First, the acid pH (5 to 6) inhibits the growth of most pathogenic organisms. Second, the presence of indigenous skin flora (p. 442) may prevent or retard colonization by other species. This phenomenon, termed *bacterial interference,* may result from preferential attachment to specific receptors between bacteria and epithelial cells.

Normal flora of skin	
Staphylococcus epidermidis	*Bacillus* species
Staphylococcus aureus	*Enterobacteriaceae*
Peptococcus species	*Mycobacterium* species
Streptococcus species	*Pseudomonas* species
Diphtheroids	*Acinetobacter* species
Corynebacterium species	*Candida* species
Propionibacterium acnes	

TABLE 17-1. Potential disruption of the anatomical barrier of skin

Type	Example
Before hospitalization	
Traumatic wounds	Abrasions, lacerations, ulcerations, punctures, and amputation
Thermal injuries	Burns and frostbite
Chemical injuries	Burns and dermatitis
After hospitalization	
Traumatic wounds	Radiation burns and decubitus ulcers
Diagnostic and therapeutic measures	Biopsies, aspirations, surgical incisions, debridement, cannulations (dialysis, intravenous therapy, hemodynamic monitoring), and injections
Chemical injuries	Dermatitis secondary to irrigations and drugs

Potential disruption of anatomical barriers

The skin presents an effective mechanical barrier to the penetration of underlying body structures by microorganisms. Hospitalized patients are often at high risk for the development of infection through the skin in two ways: (1) the continuity of the skin is breached by trauma or injury before the patient enters the hospital, and (2) the integrity of the anatomical barrier is compromised through diagnostic and therapeutic procedures (Table 17-1).

The healing process

Once the integrity of the skin and tissue has been breached, the process of healing begins.

Types of wound healing. Tissue may heal by one of three ways: primary, secondary, or tertiary intention. Most surgical wounds heal by primary intention. The incision is a clean, straight line, and all layers of tissue are approximated by suturing. Wounds such as ulcers or burns are characterized by tissue loss. These have edges that cannot be approximated, and healing occurs through filling in of the wound by granulation tissue over a larger area. This is healing by secondary intention. Healing by tertiary intention (also known as delayed primary intention) occurs when there is a delay between injury and suturing.

Four-stage process. Carpenter, Gastes, and Williams[17] describe the healing process in four classic phases: hemostasis, acute inflammation, repair, and consolidation/reconstruction. This process begins at the time of tissue injury and may take as long as 2 years for completion. At best the tensile strength of healed tissue is only 80% of undamaged, intact integument.

Hemostasis. The first phase of the healing process is characterized by the constriction and retraction of blood vessels. Blood and fluid leak into the damaged tissues, increasing tension and compressing the vessels. This mechanical action is assisted on a microscopic level by platelets that adhere to subendothelial collagen. Fibrin strands appear and hold the platelet mass together. This platelet "plug" occludes the blood vessel to stop the flow of blood.

Acute inflammation. As soon as tissue injury occurs, the second phase is initiated. Damaged tissue releases amines, polypeptides, and acidic lipids that stimulate the body's inflammatory response. Vasodilation of the vascular bed, accompanied by increased permeability of capillaries and venules, allows plasma and neutrophils to enter the wound. This action permits the dilution and neutralization of toxins, formation of a network of fibrin strands, ingestion of bacteria, and phagocytosis and enzymatic digestion of necrotic tissue and clots.

Repair. Through the revascularization process, in which new capillaries form, fibroblasts manufacture collagen, which replaces the more fragile fibrin network. These fibroblasts also produce "ground substance," which cements the collagen fibers together, thus lending elasticity and resiliency to the new structure. Contraction, or the reduction in the size of the wound, begins in this third phase.

Consolidation/reconstruction. The fourth and final phase of healing is consolidation, also known as remodeling. Although the mechanism of this phase is not well understood, the healing tissue increases in strength, with a corresponding decrease in both vascularity and hypertrophy of the scar.

Factors influencing healing. Many factors influence the body's ability to regenerate tissue.

Age is an important factor. The very young and very old are classically at higher risk of infection because of a decreased ability to mount an adequate inflammatory response, an integral part of the healing process. Infants, because of immaturity, have sluggish endocrine functions and limited reserves of fat, glycogen, and extracellular water. At the other extreme, the elderly are also affected by altered function of the cardiovascular, renal, pulmonary, and musculoskeletal systems because of chronic disease or degeneration. In addition, there is some evidence of decreased cellular or humoral immune mechanisms beginning at age 25.[53]

Malnutrition in the forms of malnourishment and obesity affects wound healing. The undernourished individual has diminished carbohydrate and fat reserves; consequently, body protein, necessary for wound healing, is used to provide energy necessary for basic metabolic functions. The resultant nitrogen imbalance depresses fibroblastic synthesis of collagen, the connective tissue essential for scar formation,[17,41] and may suppress antibody response.[53] Vitamin C deficiency also affects fibroblast function.[41] Each of these factors delays wound healing.

Obesity also presents several risk factors. Excessive force or traction on adipose tissue may be required to achieve adequate visualization of or access to the surgical site; this in turn increases the potential for trauma and devitalization. In addition, the relative avascularity of adipose tissue promotes wound separation and inhibits healing.

Abnormalities in *endocrine function* adversely influence the healing process. In diabetic ketoacidosis sluggish phagocytic function alters the host's ability to mount an inflammatory response. Chronic vascular changes may also prevent an adequate blood supply to the traumatized tissues. Corticosteroid therapy depresses antibody formation and phagocytic activity, suppresses new capillary formation and fibrogenesis, and alters reactivity to irritants.[53] Hence the reparative sequence of healing is interrupted.

The decreased hemoglobin levels associated with *anemia* result in tissue hypoxia, which alters the synthesis of collagen and epithelialization.[41] The effects of mild anemia are minimized by the normal physiological compensatory mechanisms, such as increased circulation. However, if the hematocrit falls below 20%, the lower oxgen tension in the tissues can disrupt local metabolism for cell regeneration.[17]

Immunosuppression arising from administration of chemotherapeutic agents, pregnancy, or diseases affecting the immune system is characterized by an alteration in the body's inflammatory response, a critical phase of wound healing. Manifestations of this alteration include quantitative or qualitative defects in leukocyte function, decreased production of immunoglobulins, or depressed collagen synthesis for tissue repair.[17,41]

The presence of a *foreign body* in a wound alters healing by serving as a nidus for infecting microbes or by preventing granulation of tissue. The use of cardiovascular or orthopedic prostheses enhances the ability of a relatively small number of pathogenic or opportunistic microorganisms to cause serious infection. The relationship between the infecting dose and a foreign body has been demonstrated in experimental studies; the presence of suture material greatly reduces the number of *Staphylococcus aureus* organisms required to produce an abscess in otherwise normal hosts. Sutures also may induce problems if they are tied too tightly. The subsequent increased mechanical tension at wound edges disrupts the collagen network, compromises tensile strength, alters contraction, and increases the width of the final scar.[41]

The healing process can also be affected by two other factors. The avascular nature of necrotic and edematous tissues lowers the oxygen tension around fibroblasts and alters collagen synthesis. The altered blood flow also prevents access by phagocytes and penetration by systemic antibiotics, and thus increases the risk of infection. Infection is further enhanced by the collection of blood and serum in tissues—both excellent media for bacterial growth.

The final significant factor in wound healing is the local "climate" of the wound. Regeneration of the epithelium is strongly influenced by the temperature and humidity at the wound site. The migration of epidermal cells in the first 48 to 72 hours after injury is the most important factor in restoration of the dermis. If the denuded dermis is exposed to air, dehydration causes a crust to form; this crust serves as a mechanical barrier to migration.[41]

MAJOR INFECTIONS

The infection control practitioner (ICP) is frequently called on to assist in the assessment of a variety of skin lesions and advise on the implementation of appropriate control measures. Fig. 17-2, *A, B,* and *C,* depict common skin lesions and their related causes.

This section will address significant cutaneous infections, or infections with skin manifestations, encountered in the hospital environment.

Viral etiology

Although the primary mode of transmission for some of the following diseases is not direct inoculation of the skin, the cutaneous manifestations may be the definitive factor in making the diagnosis of a communicable disease of importance to the ICP.

Chickenpox (varicella) and herpes zoster. Varicella-zoster (V-Z) virus is highly communicable, leading to high attack rates of exanthematous chickenpox among healthy, susceptible children. A small proportion of adults escape childhood infection and remain susceptible. The incidence of complications, such as pneumonia and encephalitis, is higher in adults, but rare. A more virulent form of the infection is known as *progressive varicella* and occurs primarily in children whose susceptibility is enhanced by immunosuppression. In this state visceral involvement, including the lungs, liver, and brain, is not uncommon with resultant fatality.

Chickenpox is characterized by fever and a disseminated, vesicular rash erupting first on the scalp and trunk and extending to the periphery. The

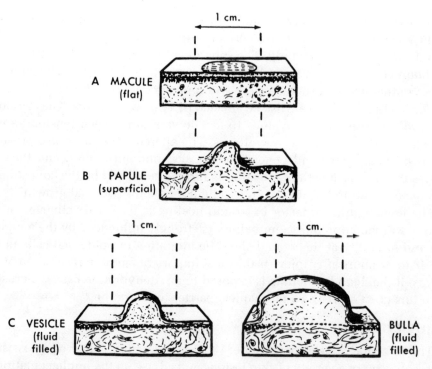

FIG. 17-2. A, Macule. A circumscribed area without elevation or depression of the surface relative to the surrounding skin. Appears in various colors, sizes, and shapes. B, Papule. A solid red circumscribed lesion, generally less than 1 cm in diameter and elevated above the plane of surrounding skin. C, Vesicle (bulla). A circumscribed, elevated lesion containing fluid (serum, lymph, blood). (From Stewart, W.D., Danto, J.L., and Maddin, S.: Dermatology: diagnosis and treatment of cutaneous disorders, ed. 4, St. Louis, 1978, The C.V. Mosby Co.)

incubation period is 2 to 3 weeks, commonly 13 to 17 days. The period of communicability begins 2 to 5 days before eruption of the vesicles and lasts for approximately 3 days after the appearance of the last crop of vesicles. The primary V-Z infection typically bestows a lifelong immunity; recurrence is extremely rare.

Herpes zoster, or *shingles*, is a local manifestation of "recurrent," "recrudescent," or "reactivation" infection with the V-Z virus. Although primary herpes zoster occasionally occurs from direct inoculation of the virus into the skin, most disease manifests in individuals who have had chickenpox on a previous occasion. The precise mechanism of reactivation is not well understood. However, it is hypothesized that the virus remains latent at the site of dorsal root ganglia, travels down the nerve, and produces vesicles with an erythematous base. Lesions appear in crops in an irregular fashion along a nerve pathway, are usually unilateral, and affect from one to three dermatomes. Severe pain and paresthesias are common. Herpes zoster may recur and has been associated with advancing age, Hodgkin's disease, irradiation, and immunosuppressive therapy.

The mode of transmission of V-Z virus has not been unequivocally determined. Epidemiological evidence, primarily the apparent communicability before the onset of the exanthem, suggests that airborne transmission may play an important role in the spread of chickenpox. However, V-Z virus has been isolated from oropharyngeal secretions of a patient with chickenpox on only one occasion; it has never been isolated from the respiratory tracts of patients with herpes zoster lesions.[20,54] Desquamated epithelial cells from fresh, infected lesions are known to contain virus particles. Contact with lesions from both patients with chickenpox and herpes zoster is thought to be a significant mode of spread. The role of airborne dissemination from lesions has been considered to be important in chickenpox but less so in herpes zoster.[20]

Isolation procedures recommended by the Centers for Disease Control (CDC)[28] are based on the epidemiological evidence of spread and the presumed high level of immunity in the adult population. For chickenpox and disseminated herpes zoster, strict isolation is advised. This technique employs the use of a private room, masks for susceptible individuals, and gowns and gloves for all individuals entering the isolation room. Identical mask, gown, and glove techniques are recommended for the care of patients with localized herpes zoster lesions, and a private room is considered desirable (wound and skin precautions). Whenever possible, it is preferable not to assign susceptible hospital staff to care for these patients. The hospital's policy governing isolation precautions for patients with herpes zoster or chickenpox should be carefully considered in light of three high-risk populations: pediatric, immunosuppressed, and neonatal patients.

Pediatrics. Because of the high degree of susceptibility in the pediatric population, all patients with chickenpox and herpes zoster should be placed in strict isolation. Patients with uncomplicated chickenpox remain in isolation for 7 days after the eruption first appears in a normal host.[20] Isolation is continued for patients with herpes zoster until the lesions are dry and crusted.

A sound, preventive measure is to screen all pediatric admissions for recent exposure to chickenpox or herpes zoster. If such an exposure has occurred in the previous 3 weeks and the child is thought to be susceptible, the admission should be postponed. When the child's clinical condition precludes this postponement, strict isolation measures are instituted for the duration of the communicable period.

In the event that the onset of chickenpox or herpes zoster occurs in a hospitalized child the ICP will need to institute a prompt investigation to avoid secondary or tertiary cases. The index case should be isolated immediately

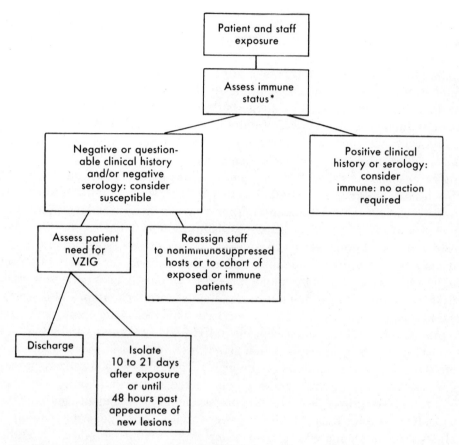

*1. 98% of adults who were exposed in childhood to siblings with chickenpox have positive titers regardless of a clear-cut clinical history.

2. Individuals with antibody titer of ≥ 1:8 by fluorescent antibody or radioimmunassay technique are considered immune.

FIG. 17-3. Management of nosocomial varicella-zoster exposures.

using strict isolation technique. Next, a clinical history for chickenpox must be assessed for every child reasonably exposed to the disease. Exposed children should be cohorted by relocation to a geographical area and assignment of immune and exposed staff. Children who have had chickenpox previously may also be included in the cohort. Susceptible patients who have not been exposed or are newly admitted comprise a second cohort. Any exposed, susceptible child who was unable to be discharged should be placed in strict isolation on the tenth day after the first exposure. If disease has not developed by the twenty-second day, isolation precautions may be discontinued (Fig. 17-3).

Oncology units. Morens et al.[52] described an outbreak of V-Z infection at the National Cancer Institute. In their retrospective analysis they postulated that the epidemic represented two epidemiologically distinct diseases: zoster as an endogenous reactivation infection and varicella as an exogenously acquired disease. The first entity occurred in patients who were basically in a remission phase of their malignancy and were not receiving chemotherapy; epidemiological evidence suggested sporadic occurrence of cases without relation to contact or airborne transmission. In contrast, the varicella group had pronounced time-space clustering. The patients were characteristically in relapse, receiving chemotherapy, and had disseminated lesions.

Morens et al. commented that other descriptions of zoster as a transmittable disease in oncology patients may instead have been varicella. They hypothesized that immunoincompetence related to disease, disability, or chemotherapy may have rendered these patients susceptible because of low or absent circulating neutralizing antibody. Therefore patients who have a history of chickenpox may experience exogenous reinfection.

Because V-Z infection in immunosuppressed patients can be a devastating event, strict isolation may be a necessary control measure on nursing units caring for these types of patients.

Neonates. Neonatal varicella infections occur in infants whose mothers develop chickenpox either during the first trimester or near the time of delivery. Congenital varicella syndrome, associated with maternal infection in the early months of pregnancy, is characterized by low birth weight, cicatricial skin lesions, hypotrophic extremities, brain damage, mental retardation, eye conditions (e.g., chorioretinitis, optic atrophy, cataracts), and immunodeficiencies.[49] The occurrence of maternal varicella less than 5 days before or within 48 hours following delivery can result in serious or fatal neonatal disease. Infants with congenital and neonatal varicella require strict isolation techniques.

In addition to appropriate isolation techniques, passive immunization in selected patient populations may be an important control measure for varicella infection. Although pooled immune serum globulin (ISG) is ineffective, prophylactic administration of varicella-zoster immune globulin (VZIG) has been shown to prevent disease in normal hosts and to modify the disease in immunosuppressed patients. Because VZIG is in short supply, its intended use is for susceptible immunodeficient patients, especially children, who have had significant exposure to chickenpox or zoster.[21] These children are generally under 15 years of age and have primary immunodeficiency disorders or neoplastic diseases, are recipients of immunosuppressive therapy, or are at risk for neonatal varicella. VZIG must be administered within 96 hours of exposure. The following outline summarizes the Food and Drug Administration's guidelines for administration of VZIG for the prophylaxis of chickenpox*:

1. One of the following underlying illnesses or conditions
   a. Leukemia or lymphoma
   b. Congenital or acquired immunodeficiency
   c. Under immunosuppressive treatment
   d. Newborn of mother who had onset of chickenpox 5 days before delivery or within 48 hours after delivery
2. One of the following types of exposure to chickenpox or zoster patient(s)
   a. Household contact
   b. Playmate contact (1 hour play indoors)
   c. Hospital contact (in same 2- to 4-bedroom or adjacent beds in a large ward)
   d. Newborn contact (newborn of mother who had onset of chickenpox 5 days before delivery or within 48 hours after delivery)
3. Negative or unknown prior history of chickenpox
4. Age of <15 years, with administration to older patients on an *individual* basis
5. Time elapsed after exposure is such that VZIG can be administered within 96 hours

Herpes simplex virus. Herpes simplex virus (HSV) produces a common viral illness principally affecting the skin and mucous membranes. Lesions commonly are seen at first as single or grouped clusters of small, clear vesicles on an erythematous base. These may erode to form ulcerations. Although HSV is usually a benign and self-limited disease, severe and even fatal infections may occur in premature neonates, in infants born to mothers with active genital lesions, and in individuals with dermatitis, burns, severe malnutrition, or immunodeficiencies. In these high-risk patients the disease may progress to severe, chronic mucocutaneous lesions or to dissemination with muliple-organ involvement. The rare complication of herpes encephalitis is discussed on pp. 522-524.

HSV (herpesvirus hominis) is a member of the herpesvirus group, which includes V-Z, cytomegalovirus, and Epstein-Barr (EB) viruses. Two distinct subgroups of HSV have been identified. Both types cause primary infection, often asymptomatic in nature, and recurrent disease. Table 17-2 compares and contrasts V-Z and HSV infections.

Primary HSV-type 1 (HSV-1) infection is characterized by the onset of fever and sore throat. The resultant gingivostomatitis and pharyngitis are manifested in small, rapidly ulcerating vesicles on the oral and pharyngeal mucosa. The self-limited disease usually occurs in children and runs its course in 10 to 14

*From Centers for Disease Control: Morbid. Mortal. Weekly. Rep. **30:**22, 1981.

TABLE 17-2. A comparison of clinical manifestations of herpesvirus infections

Factors	Chickenpox (varicella)	Herpes zoster	Herpes simplex
Etiological agent	Varicella-zoster virus	Varicella-zoster virus	Herpesvirus hominis type 1 and type 2
Signs and symptoms	Fever, malaise, and maculopapular-to-vesicular rash predominantly on trunk and scalp	Vesicular rash; distributed along nerve pathways; pain and paresthesia at site	Superficial, clear vesicles on an erythematous base
Incubation period	10 to 21 days	Unknown	HSV-1: 2 to 12 days HSV-2: 2 to 7 days
Communicable period	2 days before rash to 5 to 6 days after last crop of lesions	Duration of draining vesicles	Usually duration of illness
Mode of transmission	Direct, person-to-person contact; droplet; airborne; scabs are not infectious	Direct, person-to-person contact; droplet; airborne (?); scabs are not infectious	Direct contact with saliva (type 1) or secretions from lesions; venereal transmission (type 2)
Isolation	Strict until all lesions have crusted; do not use room for immunosuppressed patient for 24 hours after terminal cleaning	Strict until all lesions have crusted; do not use room for immunosuppressed patient for 24 hours after terminal cleaning	Discharge precautions (strict for disseminated disease)

days with no significant sequelae. HSV-1 may also cause conjunctivitis that spontaneously heals in 2 to 3 weeks. However, if systemic symptoms appear along with signs of stromal involvement, healing may be delayed.[43] After primary infection the latent virus resides in nerve ganglia. Reactivation of HSV-1 results in herpes labialis, a recurrent infection producing painful vesicles on the lips. Prodromal symptoms of pain, burning, tingling, or itching precede the appearance of lesions for 6 to 24 hours. Within the first 2 days the vesicles progress to ulceration and crusting with healing within 7 to 10 days.

Isolation of patients with herpetic gingivostomatitis or herpes labialis is rarely necessary. Discharge precautions and the careful handling and disposal of oropharyngeal secretions are usually adequate. Hospital personnel with these lesions should not be assigned to care for neonates, pediatric patients under the age of 12, or immunosuppressed patients.

Although hospital personnel must be considered as the possible source of infection for high-risk patients, they may also be at risk for nosocomial herpes simplex infections after exposure to patients secreting the virus. Greaves et al.[38] reported sporadic incidence of hospital-personnel developing nosocomial herpetic whitlow after direct contact with oral, pharyngeal, and/or tracheal secretions of patients with herpes simplex labialis. Exposed personnel developed painful, deep-seated vesicles on the paronychial or volar aspects of the distal phalanx 5 to 8 days after contact with secretions. Adams et al.[2] documented occurrence of two additional herpesvirus syndromes after similar exposure. These included acute gingivostomatitis and acute diphtheria-like membranous pharyngitis.

Herpes whitlow can be mistakenly diagnosed as pyogenic paronychia. Diagnosis can be confirmed by carefully aspirating fluid from the vesicle. In herpetic whitlow it is serous rather than purulent. No bacteria or neutrophils are seen on Gram stain, and the viral culture is usually positive within 24 to 48 hours.[38] Treatment is supportive, including analgesics or immobilization of the digit. Surgical incision and drainage is contraindicated. Greaves et al.[38] reported two such cases involving surgical intervention that led to excessive morbidity and disability.

Specific control measures for caring for patients with known or suspected active HSV disease include the following:

1. Identify patients with active HSV infections. Particular caution must be observed when hospital personnel have skin abrasions or cuts.
2. Wear gloves on both hands when there is direct contact with oral or pharyngeal secretions from patients with active HSV disease (e.g., suctioning).
3. Identify personnel with active herpetic whitlow disease and exclude them from direct patient care. This can be accomplished by removing personnel from the patient care area for the duration of their infection[2] or

by requiring them to wear a glove on the involved hand during patient contact. When using the gloved hand method, personnel should be excluded from maternal-neonatal areas, burn units, immunosuppressed patients, patients with eczema, or patients with open skin lesions.[38]

HSV type 2 (HSV-2) is usually associated with lesions of the genital tract. The epidemiology and significant clinical features of these infections are described in Chapter 14.

Measles. Measles (rubeola) is an acute, highly communicable viral disease characterized by a generalized maculopapular rash appearing on the fourth day of illness. After an incubation period of 10 to 14 days the appearance of fever and malaise is followed by coryza, conjunctivitis, and cough. Approximately 24 to 48 hours before the onset of the generalized rash Koplik's spots may be seen on the buccal mucosa opposite the molars; this manifestation is pathognomonic of measles. The duration of the exanthem, which begins at the hairline and spreads downward to the face, neck, upper extremities, and trunk, seldom exceeds 5 to 7 days. Complications can include otitis media, mastoiditis, pneumonia, and central nervous system involvement.

Transmission of measles is primarily by droplets and by contact with respiratory tract secretions or articles freshly contaminated by nose and throat secretions. The virus is shed from the respiratory tract during the prodromal period and for up to 5 days after the appearance of the rash. The virus invades the epithelium of the respiratory tract and possibly the conjunctivae.

When a person with known or suspected measles is hospitalized, respiratory isolation is instituted.[28] This technique includes a private room and masks for susceptible individuals entering the room. Fortunately, since the licensure of measles vaccine in 1963, aggressive immunization programs have resulted in a 99% reduction in the reported incidence.[3] Currently a single injection of the live measles virus vaccine confers immunity in at least 95% of susceptible children over the age of 15 months.

In the rare instance that hospital exposures may occur the ICP should be aware of active and passive immunization as one control measure.[3] If measles vaccine is administered to a susceptible host within 72 hours of exposure, it may prevent the disease. Certain conditions preclude the administration of a live virus vaccine: pregnancy, allergies and altered immune states induced by malignancy, chemotherapy or irradiation, and deficits in cell-mediated immunity. If susceptible patients in this latter group are exposed, passive immunization with ISG is indicated as soon after exposure as possible. The efficacy of prophylaxis with ISG is variable.

One aspect of concern to the ICP is the documentation of a severe atypical type of measles characterized by high fever, pneumonitis, pleural effusion, edema of the extremities, and an unusual rash. The rash, unlike that in classic measles, begins peripherally and may be urticarial, maculopapular, hemorrhagic, and/or vesicular in nature.[48] These patients universally give a history of immunization with inactivated (killed) vaccine, which was removed from the market in 1968. Hypersensitivity to the wild measles virus is thought to be the pathogenesis of this syndrome in individuals with partial immunity.[35] Consequently, this disease will be seen in adolescents and adults who received inactivated measles vaccine between 1963 and 1967.

Rubella. Rubella, or German measles, is a mild, febrile illness characterized by a diffuse macular rash. Minimal or absent prodromal symptoms of fever, malaise, and anorexia appear 14 to 21 days after exposure. The most prominent features of the syndrome are adenopathy and rash. The lymph nodes of the posterior auricular, posterior cervical, and suboccipital chains are most often involved.[36] The rash, which lasts 3 to 5 days, begins on the face and spreads rapidly downward to the rest of the body. Many cases of rubella, however, are asymptomatic.

Transmission of the virus is through droplets of infected respiratory tract secretions. Respiratory isolation techniques, as with measles, are employed for these patients.[28]

Since the introduction of rubella vaccine in 1969, the chief significance of rubella infections lies in the occurrence of congenital rubella syndrome (CRS). CRS occurs in up to one fourth of infants born to women who acquired primary rubella during the first trimester of pregnancy. The syndrome is manifested in fetal death, premature delivery, and congenital anomalies, such as cataracts, microphthalmia, microencephaly, deafness, patent ductus arteriosus, thrombocytopenic purpura, hepatosplenomegaly, and bone defects. A detailed list of manifestations follows*:

Growth retardation (low birth weight)
Eye defects
    Cataracts
    Glaucoma
    Retinopathy
    Microphthalmia
    Cloudy cornea
    Severe myopia
Hearing loss
Cardiac defects
    Patent ductus arteriosus
    Ventricular septal defect
    Pulmonary stenosis and coarctation
    Myocardial abnormalities

*Modified from Gershon, A.A.: Rubella virus (German measles). In Mandell, G.L., Douglas, R. G., and Bennett, J.E., editors: Principles and practices of infectious diseases, New York, 1979, John Wiley & Sons, Inc.; Krugman, S., and Katz, S.L.: Infectious diseases in children, ed. 7, St. Louis, 1981, The C.V. Mosby Co.

Central nervous system defects
  Psychomotor retardation
  Microencephaly
  Meningoencephalitis
  Spastic quadriparesis
  Mental retardation
Central language disorders
Seizure disorders
Degenerative brain disease (progressive panencephalitis)
Hepatosplenomegaly
Hepatitis
Thrombocytopenic purpura
Bone lesions
Interstitial pneumonitis
Diabetes mellitus
Behavior disorders
Thyroid disorders
Precocious puberty
Cryptorchidism
Dermatoglyphic abnormality
Generalized lymphadenopathy
Hemolytic anemia

The spectrum of CRS manifestations may relate to the gestational age at the time of the infection; generally, the younger the fetus, the more severe the sequelae.

Protection of the susceptible pregnant woman from rubella infection presents two issues for consideration by the ICP. The first is the management of patients with CRS. Since these children excrete virus in respiratory tract secretions and urine, strict isolation is recommended for all suspected and known infants with this syndrome.[28] In addition, staff should be assigned based on immune and childbearing status. In one hospital a susceptible nurse had a single 8-hour exposure, and in spite of appropriate isolation techniques during this interval she developed rubella.[22] Since these infants may shed virus for variable periods after birth, some hospitals isolate children who are readmitted with CRS up to the age of 18 to 24 months.

In addition to the personal risk for female employees in the childbearing age group, hospital staff of either sex may develop rubella and expose patients. In 1978 several health care professionals exposed 56 susceptible pregnant women in a prenatal and family planning clinic.[34] Two women subsequently developed rubella and delivered uneventfully. This outbreak and others[51,58] have prompted recommendations for rubella screening and immunization programs from the Public Health Service Advisory Committee on Immunization Practices

(ACIP),[59] the American Hospital Association,[9] the American Academy of Pediatrics,[7] and the American College of Obstetricians and Gynecologists.[8]

These recommendations have touched off a debate among administrators, attorneys, physicians, and other health care workers. Key points of discussion are cost/benefit ratios, employee-union relations, safety, and implementation methods. To develop and administer an effective rubella screening and immunization program, the following issues must be addressed by the ICP in consultation with administrative and clinical staff:

- Identification of staff to be screened and/or immunized
- Establishment of a mechanism for serological testing and, when necessary, vaccine administration
- Provision of funds for the program
- Support and approval of the hospital administration, including legal counsel
- Establishment of a record keeping system
- Determination of disciplinary action for noncompliant staff
- Evaluation methodology of program objectives

The appendix at the end of the book is a sample protocol from Stanford University Hospital. This program has been in effect since 1980. During this time there have been no severe or permanent sequelae from immunization or has disciplinary action been necessary. The success of the program lies in careful planning and the emphasis on education of hospital staff.

Bacterial etiology

Surgical wound infections. Surgical wound infections (SWIs) rank second as the most frequent cause of nosocomial infections, accounting for one quarter of the total number.[61] The significance of these infections is staggering when evaluated in terms of patient morbidity, mortality, and expense.

Although the incidence of SWIs has decreased with the introduction of aseptic practices and advancement of surgical technology, the cause remains unclear. Three major factors that influence the risk of infection have been identified[61]:

- The amount and type of microbial contamination of the wound at the time of closure
- The condition of the wound at the termination of the procedure
- The host factors affecting susceptibility and resistance

Microbial contamination. Contamination of the operative site with microorganisms is a critical factor in the development of SWI. Such contamination occurs primarily at the time of surgery and may arise from both endogenous and exogenous sources. A multitude of control measures have been recommended; some of these measures are based on well-controlled studies, whereas others have evolved from anecdotal experience. In this latter group the cost must be weighed against the potential benefits before developing elaborate infection control protocols that are difficult to eradicate once established as the "norm" or "standard" of practice.

In a classic study performed under the auspices of the National Academy of Sciences, National Research Council,[53] a classification system of surgical procedures was used to identify sources of contamination and estimate the potential risk for infection. The four classes ranged from "clean" wounds, which predictably had the lowest infection rates, to "dirty" or known infected wounds, in which the highest rates were predicted (Table 17-3).

ENDOGENOUS SOURCES. The causative agents (p. 458) of SWIs frequently arise from patients' own microbial flora. The following discussion identifies these sources and suggests potential control measures.

REMOTE INFECTION. In addition to the presence of microbes in the actual operative field, a coexisting, active infection at a remote site increases the risk of SWIs twofold to fourfold.[12,30,53] The specific mechanism is unclear, but it is postulated that the remote infection may (1) represent a general, increased host susceptibility, (2) decrease the patient's resistance by taxing the immune re-

TABLE 17-3. Classification of surgical wounds

Classification	Description of wound	Anticipated infection rate
Class I—clean	Nontraumatic; no inflammation encountered; no break in technique; respiratory, alimentary, or genitourinary tracts or oropharyngeal cavities not entered; elective, primary closure, and undrained	1% to 5%
Class II—clean-contaminated	Respiratory, alimentary, or genitourinary tracts entered without unusual contamination; minor break in technique; mechanically drained	8% to 11%
Class III—contaminated	Gross spillage from gastrointestinal tract; fresh traumatic wounds; major break in technique; acute, nonpurulent inflammation	15% to 17%
Class IV—dirty	Old traumatic wounds; perforated viscus; clinical infection	≥27%

Based on data from Simmons, B.: Infect. Control 3(suppl.):187-196, 1982.

Pathogens isolated from nosocomial surgical wound infections			
Gram-positive		**Gram-negative**	
Staphylococcus aureus	14.8%	Escherichia coli	13.4%
Staphylococcus epidermidis	4.7%	Klebsiella species	5.2%
Streptococcus pneumoniae	0.1%	Enterobacter species	4.3%
Streptococcus, group A	0.6%	Proteus and Providencia species	6.1%
Streptoccus, group B	2.1%		
Streptococcus, group D	9.2%	Pseudomonas aeruginosa	5.9%
		Pseudomonas, other species	0.6%
Other		Serratia species	1.6%
Bacteroides fragilis	3.2%		
Candida species	0.8%		
Other fungi	0.3%		
Other pathogens	12.6%		
No culture or pathogen isolated	14.5%		

Modified from Centers for Disease Control: National Nosocomial Infections Study—annual summary, 1979, Atlanta, issued March 1982, CDC.

sponse, and/or (3) promote autogenous seeding of the operative site.[53] It is imperative that all patients undergoing elective surgery be carefully evaluated and treated for urinary tract, respiratory tract, and soft tissue infections before surgery.

PREOPERATIVE STAY. Although the duration of hospitalization before surgery has not been assessed in a controlled study, this variable has been associated with higher rates of infection. Cruse and Foord[27] found that patients hospitalized for 1 day before surgery had an infection rate of 1.2%; the rates increased to 2.1% with a 1-week preoperative stay and to 3.4% if the patient had been in the hospital longer than 2 weeks. Similarly, Haley et al.[39] found that, except for patients operated on on the day of admission, rates increased with prolonged hospitalization. The increased rates associated with surgery performed on the day of admission are related to the higher number of emergency procedures in this category. The lowest rates occurred in patients undergoing surgery after only 1 day in the hospital; thereafter the risk gradually increased up to approximately fivefold for patients hospitalized for 10 or more preoperative days.

SKIN PREPARATION. The preparation of skin surfaces before transecting this natural barrier includes two aspects of minimizing endogenous flora: antiseptic cleansing and hair removal.

Measures to promote skin antisepsis include general body bathing and operative site cleansing. In one series of patients preoperative showering with regular soap had no effect on the subsequent incidence of SWIs; however, the use of a hexachlorophene compound was found to be a significant factor in lower rates.[27] Many surgeons employ the use of antiseptic solutions for showering or bathing as a safe and inexpensive intervention. The efficacy of this practice has not, however, been subjected to evaluation by a controlled study. Beyond this general approach the operative site is prepared immediately before surgery in the operating room. After skin debris and superficial microorganisms are removed through cleansing with a detergent solution an antiseptic scrub is performed to minimize the flora residing in deeper recesses of the epidermis. Both tincture of chlorhexidine and iodophor solutions possess a broad spectrum of antimicrobial activity and are used for this purpose.

Removal of hair adjacent to the operative site is a controversial practice, seemingly more grounded in aesthetics than in infection control. Evidence suggests that, depending on the methodology, hair removal not only may have little benefit but also may actually increase the risk of infection. Seropian and Reynolds[60] reviewed infection rates in 406 patients who underwent either shaving or depilatory preparation. The former group experienced a 5.6% rate, compared to 0.6% in the depilatory group. Furthermore, the interval between the time of skin preparation with a safety razor and the time of the surgical procedure was critical. If the preparation was done immediately before surgery, the rate was 3.1%; if the preparation was performed within 24 hours, it was 7.1%. However, the rate soared to 20% if the interval exceeded 1 day. Cruse and Foord[27] documented similar findings and also found no difference in infection rates when depilatory preparation was compared with no hair removal. The reason for the increase in rates may be explained by microscopic nicks and cuts induced through shaving, which provide bacterial access into injured tissue.[40] If shaving the operative site is employed, it should be performed immediately before surgery either on the nursing unit or in a holding area within the operating room suite.

PROPHYLACTIC ANTIBIOTICS. The prophylactic use of antibiotics in selected operative procedures may be useful in reducing the level of bacterial contamination in tissues and hence in reducing the risk of postoperative wound infection.[11,57,65] The efficacy of this practice depends on sufficient concentration of the antibiotic in tissue at the time of bacterial challenge, the general condition of the wound, and the host immune defenses.

The judicious selection and use of prophylactic antimicrobial agents includes a thoughtful assessment of the nature of the surgical procedure and the microorganisms usually associated with infection at that site. Prophylaxis is generally not indicated in class I—clean procedures, since contamination is usually minimal. However, in orthopedic, cardiovascular, or neurological procedures involving prosthetic implants or grafts where postoperative infection could result in significant morbidity or mortality, prophylaxis may be indicated. Generally, antibiotics may be most useful in patients undergoing class II—clean-contaminated procedures.

The appropriate route, dosage, and timing of administration of prophylactic antibiotics are critical factors in practice. With the exception of oral agents administered for gastrointestinal tract decontamination, the intravenous route is the preferred mode of administration. Intravenous administration of the antibiotic in a small volume of diluent in a 30- to 60-minute period provides serum and tissue fluid levels that are superior to those achieved with continuous intravenous infusion or intermittent intramuscular injection.[55] The dosage should be calculated to achieve adequate blood and tissue levels.

Bernard and Cole[11] performed an elegant, prospective, randomized, double-blind study that demonstrated the effectiveness of prophylaxis in patients undergoing potentially contaminated abdominal procedures. A critical feature was the administration of drugs *before* the start of the operation. Stone et al.[65] studied the timing factor as well. When prophylactic antibiotics were initiated 1 to 4 hours postoperatively, the incidence of infection was almost identical to that in a control group that received no antibiotics; no benefit was found in extending administration beyond the time in the recovery room. Generally, prophylaxis should be initiated within 1 hour of surgery and discontinued within a maximum of 24 to 48 hours. This schedule promotes therapeutic drug levels in wound tissue and body fluids while minimizing the risks of toxicity or selection of resistant strains of bacteria. This latter risk is present both on a microenvironmental (individual patient) and a macroenvironmental (hospital-wide) level.

Antibiotics have also been incorporated into irrigation solutions used to lower bacterial contamination of the operative site. The efficacy of this practice has not been compared with administration of parenteral antibiotics in a controlled study. If such solutions are used, caution must be exercised in the selection of the agent to avoid local or systemic toxicity.[61]

EXOGENOUS SOURCES. The operating team and the operating room environment may contribute to the development of SWIs by introduction of exogenous organisms into the wound. To a lesser degree, the staff and environment of the nursing unit may also play a role.

PREOPERATIVE SCRUB. Similar to the preparation of the operative site, the preoperative scrub by the surgical team is intended to remove or destroy resident skin bacteria. All jewelry must be removed before the scrub. Antiseptics such as chlorhexidine, iodophors, and hexachlorophene have been used. Scrubs may be either timed or performed by a prescribed number of strokes on each surface of the hands, fingers, and forearms. The superiority of a 10-minute scrub over a 5-minute scrub has not been demonstrated.[29]

GLOVES. Once the preoperative scrub is completed, sterile gloves are worn by the team. It has been hypothesized that since bacteria multiply rapidly under the gloves, glove punctures constitute a significant source of wound contamination. However, Cruse and Foord[27] found that while 11.6% of gloves used in 1209 operations were punctured at the end of surgery, no wound infections occurred as a result of the glove punctures.

BARRIER TECHNIQUE. The use of gowns, hoods, caps, high-efficiency masks, shoe covers, and drapes represents a general barrier technique to prevent microorganisms shed by the operating room staff from contaminating the operative site. Although these measures are recognized as the backbone of aseptic techniques in the operating suite, policies governing personnel scrub apparel are often the source of conflict and noncompliance. Any policy developed should be carefully considered for its infection control, practical, and financial considerations. Most important, it must be consistently enforced among all disciplines.

The use of natural versus synthetic and woven versus nonwoven fabrics has received considerable attention in the selection of gowns and drapes. In one series the use of adhesive plastic drapes was associated with higher infection rates.[25] Gowns should be made of impermeable fabric or tightly woven cotton, treated with a water repellent on areas most vulnerable to exposure to body fluids.

AIRBORNE CONTAMINATION. Simple to elaborate measures have been employed to minimize wound contamination by airborne routes in the operating suite. Basic measures include limiting the number and movement of individuals present during surgery, keeping conversations to a minimum, and instituting "traffic control" in and out of the room during the procedure.

Beyond these routine procedures the role of air handling systems is a topic of enduring controversy. In 1964 the National Research Council[53] published the results of a random, double-blind study of the influence of ultraviolet irradiation on the incidence of postoperative wound infection. This collaborative study evaluated approximately 15,000 operations performed in five institutions over a 2-year period. Although the use of ultraviolet irradiation markedly reduced the levels of airborne contamination in the operating room, this reduction produced virtually no effect on the overall infection rates (7.4% versus 7.5% in nonirradiated rooms). A marginal effect was demonstrated in clean-refined procedures (2.9% versus 3.8%). These minimal findings, coupled with the problems associated with the safety and maintenance of ultraviolet lights, have engendered little acceptance of this control measure.

Currently, unidirectional or laminar air flow systems are receiving great attention. The efficacy of these expensive units, which deliver near sterile air, has yet to be demonstrated by controlled, well-designed research. Proponents of laminar flow recommend it for clean-refined surgery, particularly when placing a prosthetic implant. However, others have pointed out that similar infection rates can be achieved in rooms with standard ventilation systems (Hill Burton recommendation of 25 air exchanges per hour[61]) coupled with strict adherence to sterile techniques.

ENVIRONMENTAL DISINFECTION. Standard cleaning methods between cases—consistently performed by the operating room staff—minimize the potential for cross-infection between patients. Routine procedures should be designed to ensure thorough decontamination after treatment of *all* patients, which negates the need for scheduling "dirty" procedures at the end of the day. The use of devices, such as "tacky" mats, for environmental control has not been shown to reduce infection rates.[61]

LOCAL WOUND CARE. Once the patient leaves the operating room, the major factors influencing the potential for an SWI have been determined. However, management of the wound in the postoperative period may also affect the healing process and the development of infection:

1. *Dressings.* Sterile dressings serve several purposes: protection from trauma and contamination, absorption of drainage, immobilization and support, compression to aid in homeostasis and minimize edema, application of topical medications, and debridement.

The initial postoperative dressing is usually occlusive to minimize air exposure. By limiting tissue death and maintaining hydration, epidermal migration is enhanced, and the formation of a crust in the denuded dermis is avoided.[41] Within 18 to 24 hours the incision is effectively sealed. Unfortunately, occlusive dressings also trap wound exudate, which becomes a culture medium. The ideal dressing, yet to be developed, would be semipermeable, providing a moist surface to promote epithelialization while allowing drainage or absorption of tissue fluids.[41]

Sterile or "no touch" technique should be employed for all dressing changes regardless of the condition of the wound. All dressings and equipment should be placed in impermeable bags at the bedside before disposal.

2. *Irrigations.* Irrigation solutions vary in composition and purpose. Multiple-use bottles should be dated, refrigerated when not in use, and discarded 24 hours after opening. Solution should be poured from the larger container into smaller reservoirs for use. All equipment should be sterile and used only once.

Condition of the wound. The condition of the wound at the time of incisional closure is a seocnd major determinant of SWI. Minimization of trauma to tissue, achievement of homeostasis, and approximation of tissue edges to reduce dead space are all important variables directly attributable to the skill of the surgeon.[27,44] A fourth variable also linked to surgical technique is the length of the operation. The longer the procedure, the greater the propensity for devitalized tissue secondary to trauma or dehydration and the greater the potential for contamination, which result in higher rates of SWIs.[27,31,53]

The presence of a foreign body in the wound has also been associated with higher infection rates. Specifically, the use of drains to promote evacuation of blood, pus, and body fluids from operative sites in an effort to reduce the risk of infection may actually have the opposite effect. Cerise, Pierce, and Diamond,[23] using an experimental rabbit model, demonstrated the ability of micro-organisms to migrate down a Penrose drain into the peritoneal cavity. The clinical application of this finding was established in a retrospective analysis of splenectomized patients. A fourfold increase in the incidence of subphrenic abscess and inflammation was observed in the group who had drains placed. Alexander, Korelitz, and Alexander[5] suggest that when abdominal drainage is indicated, the use of closed suction drainage is superior to silastic or latex drains. The infection risk may be further reduced by placing the drain through a separate stab wound adjacent to the incision rather than bringing it through the primary incision itself.[26] Additional benefit may be gained in class IV—dirty procedures by using delayed primary closure rather than primary closure accompanied by a drain.[26,67]

Host factors. The final critical determinant in operative wound infection is the adequacy of host defense mechanisms. The factors influencing the host response to a bacterial challenge have been outlined earlier in the chapter. Whenever possible, these factors should be considered before the surgical procedure:

1. Anemia should be corrected by transfusion or iron supplements.
2. Diabetes should be well controlled with insulin or oral hypoglycemic agents.
3. Obesity should be addressed through diet and exercise.
4. Malnourishment should be corrected through enteral or parenteral therapy.
5. Immunosuppression should be reduced by tapering or discontinuing drug or radiation therapy.

Cruse and Foord[26] find that the incidence of clean wound infections significantly increases from 1.8% to 10.7% with uncontrolled diabetes, 13.5% with obesity, and 16.6% with malnutrition. Ultimately the risks of these concomitant conditions must be weighed against the predicted benefits and risks of surgery in determining the urgency of the operation.

Table 17-4 summarizes the factors and control measures for surgical wound infections using the CDC category structure.

Neonatal staphylococcal infections. Neonates, particularly premature infants, represent another high-risk population within the hospital. Although the risks of nosocomial infection vary with the nature of the underlying disease and corresponding diagnostic and treatment intervention, the skin and soft tissue manifestations of staphylococcal disease are a major infection control concern.

TABLE 17-4. Infection control measures for the prevention of surgical
wound infections

Factor	Category I	Category II	Category III
Preoperative preparation	Treatment of remote infections	Enteral or parenteral hyperalimentation of severely malnourished	Short preoperative hospitalization
	Cleansing of the operative site with a detergent, then antiseptic solution (tincture of iodine or chlorhexidine, iodophor); use of sterile drapes	Removal of hair adjacent to the operative site immediately before procedure	Bathing or showering with an antiseptic soap
Personnel practices	Attire for all persons entering operating room (high-efficiency mask, cap or hood, shoe covers)		
	Preoperative scrub of arms and hands with chlorhexidine, iodophor, or hexachlorophene solution 5 min at start of day and between surgical procedures	Hexachlorophene solution contraindicated for pregnant women	Scrubs between consecutive surgical procedures (2 to 5 min)
Personnel	Sterile gowns worn by surgical team	Fabric of disposable or reusable gowns impermeable to bacteria	
	Sterile gloves worn; replaced if glove puncture occurs	Double gloves worn for open bone and orthopedic implant procedures	
	Procedure performed efficiently and gently to minimize devitalized tissue, prevent bleeding, and eradicate dead space in wound		

Based on guidelines from the Centers for Disease Control: Infect. Control **3**(suppl.):194-196, 1982.

TABLE 17-4. Infection control measures for the prevention of surgical wound infections—cont'd

Factor	Category I	Category II	Category III
Environ-mental controls	All doors remain closed during procedure and traffic kept to a minimum; operating room ventilation: minimum of 25 air changes per hour (all air filtered); establish procedures for cleaning operating room between surgical procedures daily and weekly; routine environmental culturing *not* done; tacky or antiseptic mats *not* used		
Wound care	"Dirty" wounds closed by secondary or delayed primary intention; drainage, when necessary, performed by closed suction system through an adjacent stab wound; handwashing performed by personnel before and after wound care; sterile gloves worn for dressing changes if open wound; "no touch" technique for sealed wound; prompt changing of saturated dressings with inspection of wound; suspected infections cultured and smeared for Gram stain		

Continued.

TABLE 17-4. Infection control measures for the prevention of surgical
wound infections—cont'd

Factor	Category I	Category II	Category III
Prophylactic antibiotics	Parenteral prophylactic antibiotics for high-risk procedures	Value of specific antibiotic demonstrated in randomized, prospective, controlled studies	
	Administration of antibiotics 2 hr before, during, and up to 48 hr after procedure; oral antibiotics for colorectal operations limited to 24 hr before operation		
Surveillance	Wounds classified as clean, clean-contaminated, contaminated, or dirty at time of procedure	Classification recorded in medical record	
	Computation of classification-specific attack rates done every 6 to 12 mo	Computation of procedure-specific attack rates done every 6 to 12 mo	Follow-up of discharged patients performed within 30 days of operation

The spectrum of disease secondary to S. aureus in neonates includes pyoderma, omphalitis, mastitis, conjunctivitis, otitis media, and, in severe cases,
bacteremia. The frequency of the superficial infections varies with the site;
pyoderma or *pustulosis* occurs most often (48%), with omphalitis, characterized by inflammation and purulence at the umbilical stump, accounting for
27%. Conjunctivitis, associated with purulent drainage and inflammation of
the conjunctival sac, often occurs (21%) as a concomitant infection with the
other two lesions.[63] Maternal mastitis has also been associated with infant
morbidity.

Disseminated staphylococcal disease is less common than in the past. However, on occasion, more severe cutaneous manifestations are seen. Certain
strains of S. aureus elaborate an exfoliative exotoxin, which in turn can produce a scarlatiniform, "sandpaper" rash or extensive bullous impetigo, also
known as pemphigus neonatorum, Ritter's disease, or scalded skin syndrome.

The latter condition is characterized by generalized erythema, fever, and the subsequent appearance of large, flaccid bullae. These bullae are filled with clear fluid and eventually rupture to reveal a moist, erythematous, glistening surface similar to a burn or scalded skin. Since the apparent pathophysiology is related to the effects of exotoxin on the epidermis, staphylococcal organisms are not recovered from the bullae or skin surface itself.[32]

The source of staphylococcal infections is often unclear. Colonization of the infant occurs in the first few days of life. S. aureus can be recovered from the umbilicus, nares, groin, or circumcision site, representing acquisiton of maternal or hospital flora. Actual transmission of organisms occurs by the hands of personnel or through exposure to an asymptomatic carrier or an infected individual. Disease may occur on a sporadic or epidemic basis.

Pandemics of newborn staphylococcal disease of the mid-1950s and early 1960s were instrumental in the development of infection control programs both wthin the nursery and the hospital as a whole. Measures included the identification and treatment of staphylococcal carriers among the hospital staff. Unfortunately, routine screening programs do not yield epidemiologically significant data. Many individuals are consistently or intermittently colonized with S. aureus yet do not transmit the organism. Although the ability to shed or disseminate staphyloccal organisms cannot be determined by a qualitative culture, dissemination has been associated with the presence of large numbers of organisms in the anterior nares, dermatitis, and viral upper respiratory tract diseases or hay fever. Outbreaks have also been traced to infected individuals with superficial pyodermas, paronychia, or styes.[63]

Transmission via unwashed hands is probably the most significant mode of spread, the airborne route playing a minor role. Current control measures based on the epidemiology of neonatal disease include patient placement systems, isolation procedures, handwashing, personnel practices, patient care procedures, and environmental maintenance.

Patient placement. One means of controlling potential exposure to infection, particularly in larger nurseries, is the use of a cohort system. Establishment of the cohort occurs by admitting all infants born within a 24- to 48-hour period to one room of the nursery. When the room is full, no further admissions are accepted until all infants from the cohort are discharged and terminal cleaning has been performed.[19] In the event that an infant becomes ill or must remain longer than other infants in the cohort, a separate room is necessary. For a cohort system to work effectively nursery personnel must be assigned to only one cohort per work shift. Cohorts are impractical in a neonatal intensive care environment.

In addition to the cohort system, many hospitals are employing "rooming-in" procedures for newborns. After a short observation period the infant and mother are roomed together on the nursing unit; general care for the infant is then provided by the mother. If the infant is to be returned to the nursery on a regular or as needed basis, care must be exercised not to intermingle equipment and supplies from the obstetrical unit and the nursery.

Regardless of the system used, it is imperative that adequate space be provided for the bassinet and individual equipment and supplies of each infant. Overcrowding and inadequate staff/patient ratios are two highly significant factors in the occurrence of staphylococcal disease.

Isolation procedures. Prompt identification and isolation of infected infants is a key element in the infection control program. Under most circumstances patients with superficial staphylococcal infections can be managed within the nursery or intensive care unit by instituting wound and skin precautions.[28] Although the value of incubators or isolettes in preventing airborne spread of infection has not been confirmed by studies, they can be a useful means of barrier technique relating to contact transmission.

Handwashing. All visitors and personnel within the nursery must observe scrupulous handwashing practices. For all individuals who will have direct patient contact a 2- to 3-minute scrub with either an iodophor or hexachlorophene compound should be performed on entering the nursery.[64] Recently chlorohexidine solutions have also been used. All others need to thoroughly cleanse their hands for 15 seconds. Thereafter, all individuals are required to perform a 15-second handwash before and after contact with each infant and after handling equipment or supplies.

Personnel practices. Much of the ritualistic behaviors surrounding masks, caps, and beardbags have been eliminated from nursery practice; however, these measures are recommended when invasive procedures requiring sterile techniques are performed. Many nurseries provide short-sleeved scrub attire for personnel involved in direct patient care. Cover gowns are worn by anyone holding or examining an infant and are changed after each task.

Individuals with active infections—acute respiratory tract infection, gastroenteritis, skin lesions, or nonspecific febrile illness—must be removed from direct patient contact for the duration of the illness.

Patient care procedures. Routine infant bathing with hexachlorophene preparations was widely advocated as a means of controlling staphylococcal disease in the newborn nursery.[37,62] Despite clinical studies demonstrating the prophylactic value of this practice, the Food and Drug Administration, in conjunction with the American Academy of Pediatrics, recommended modification of hexachlorophene use in December 1971.[19] The statement, based on clinical and experimental studies suggesting neuropathogenic toxic side effects after exposure to hexachlorophene, recommended discontinuing routine newborn bathing with hexachlorophene preparations and substituting either dry skin care or plain soap and water. Hexachlorophene was not eliminated for personnel handwashing.

The subsequent staphylococcal outbreaks that occurred following implementation of the new recommendation prompted further evaluation, and a subsequent recommendation was issued.[6] Currently hexachlorophene preparations should be considered as an adjunct measure in the control of a staphylococcal outbreak. Short-term, prophylactic bathing with a 3% hexachlorophene solution once per day offers potential benefits that must be weighed against possible toxicity.[19]

Topical antiseptics applied to the umbilical stump have also been suggested as a means to reduce colonization. Bacitracin and alcohol have both been used for this purpose without apparent toxic effects.[45] Triple dye solution (brilliant green, proflavine, and crystal violet) has been painted on the cord and approximately 1 inch of surrounding skin, but the efficacy and safety of this practice has not been well studied.[6,63]

Environmental maintenance. Daily housekeeping procedures to maintain a clean environment should be performed at times when infants are removed from the nursery; this, of course, is impossible in a neonatal intensive care setting. It is preferable to have a regular housekeeper assigned to the nursery.

Individual linen packets and other supplies should be stored at the bedside and used only for the care of a single infant to prevent cross-infection. Bassinets and incubators should be thoroughly cleaned and disinfected between use. Porthole cuffs, most easily contaminated in routine care, should be replaced or cleaned on a daily basis.[6]

Burns. Management of the burn victim is one of the greatest challenges in infection control. Despite advances in the physiological and metabolic management of these patients, sepsis remains a leading cause of morbidity and mortality. The focus of this discussion will be the infection control implications of altered host defenses, burn wound management, and the burn unit environment.

Altered host defenses. The most immediate and obvious alteration of the host defense mechanisms is the destruction of the protective integument. Both the severity and extent of the burn wound influence the patient's subsequent susceptibility to infection (Table 17-5).

The pathophysiological changes associated with burns affect the patient's ability to withstand bacterial challenges. Both humoral and cellular defense mechanisms are reduced either qualitatively or quantitatively in the first 2 weeks after the burn injury.[56] Decreased circulating immunoglobulins and complement, coupled with defects in the chemotaxic, phagocytic, and killing abilities of white blood cells, inhibit the inflammatory response. In addition; the avascular nature of the wound itself prohibits the delivery of phagocytes and antibodies and leads to colonization and infection of the burn.

Burn wound management. To reduce fluid and protein losses and minimize the level of bacterial contamination, efforts are first directed at debridement of

TABLE 17-5. Characteristics of burn wounds*

First degree	Second degree	Third degree
Superficial layer of epidermis affected	Whole epidermis and varying depths of dermis involved	All dermal elements destroyed
No blistering	Blisters present	No blistering
Pain and erythema	Pain	No pain
Subsequent epithelial slough ("peeling")	Healing through epithelial regeneration through viable dermal remnants	Healing only through skin grafting
Healing without treatment		

Modified from Heimbach, D.M.: A.P.I.C. Journal **6**:6-11, 1978.
*Moderate burns: second-degree burns involving more than 10% but less than 20% total body surface (TBS); if third degree, up to 5% TBS; serious burns: second-degree burns involving more than 20% TBS; if third degree, greater than 5% TBS.

necrotic tissue and subsequent grafting. Necrotic tissue, or eschar, may be removed in three ways. Mechanical debridement, often used in conjunction with hydrotherapy, is achieved through the use of scissors, forceps, and/or wet-to-dry dressings. Enzymes have also been employed but are not widely accepted. Surgical excision for removal of eschar can be performed by scalpel, electrocautery, or laser for full-thickness excision; tangential excision has been used in both second- and third-degree injuries.[4]

Aggressive debridement, accompanied by the use of topical antimicrobial agents, minimizes the proliferation of microorganisms on the burn surface. The ideal agent is bactericidal, nontoxic, gentle to tissues, nonantigenic, easily applied, and inexpensive. In addition, it should permeate the burn eschar, reduce pain, prevent emergence of resistant microbes, and permit adequate observation of the burn surface. None of the agents in current use fulfills all these criteria; Table 17-6 summarizes the advantages and disadvantages of each.

Systemic antibiotics are generally discouraged, with the exception of two specific instances: short periods of decreased host resistance and established infection.[13] Prophylactic antibiotic administration is intended to supplement the patient's innate ability to fight infection during the immediate period of lowered resistance and potential contamination. Examples of these times are the first few days after burn injury, in which penicillin may be used to prevent group A streptococcal infection, and during surgical procedures. Guidelines for prophylaxis in burn patients mirror the recommendations for general surgical prophylaxis. The agent is chosen for the suspected organism. In this instance previous cultures of the burn with corresponding antibiograms are critical to the selection process. Administration is begun immediately before the operation to achieve adequate serum and tissue levels, and the drug is

TABLE 17-6. Comparison of antimicrobial agents: advantages and disadvantages

Features		Neomycin	Iodophor Betadine	Silver nitrate	Mafenide acetate Sulfamylon	Silver sulfadiazine Silvadene	Gentamicin Garamycin	Nitrofurazone Furacin
				Topical antimicrobial agent (generic and trade name)				
Preparations		1% solution	0.5% solution; ointment	0.5% aqueous solution	5% solution; 10% cream	1% cream	0.1% solution	0.2% ointment
Antimicrobial spectrum		Limited	Broad	Broad	Broad	Broad	Broad	Limited
Eschar penetration		Rapid	Slow	Slow	Rapid	Slow	Rapid	Rapid
Toxicity								
	Local tissue	Low	Low	Possible	Possible	Low	Low	Low
	Systemic	Eighth nerve; renal	Elevated protein-bound iodine	Electrolyte imbalance and methemoglobinemia	Metabolic acidosis and pulmonary complications	Bone marrow and cytotoxicity (suspected)	Eighth nerve; renal	Renal (suspected)
Pain on application		No	Occasional	Occasional	Yes	No	No	Yes
Hypersensitivity		Rare	Rare (contact)	7% (rash)	Rare	Rare	Rare	Rare
Occlusive dressings required		Yes	Yes	Yes	No	No	Yes	Yes

Modified from Pierson, C.L.: Crit. Care Q. 3:81-92, 1981.

discontinued after stabilization of vital signs and recovery from anesthesia. Prolonged administration only enhances emergence of resistant microorganisms.

The line between colonization and actual infection of the burn wound is often obscure. After the initial edematous, hyperemic phase of injury when aerobic, gram-positive organisms pose the greatest threat, the burn becomes ischemic, and gram-negative organisms proliferate in the devitalized tissue.[47] Alexander and MacMillan[4] devised a system for categorizing burn wound infections based on clinical, microbiological, and histological grounds. *Noninvasive* infection is characterized by mild to moderate systemic symptoms, including fever and leukocytosis. Although quantitative cultures reveal 10^6 organisms or more per gram of eschar or drainage, biopsies of healthy tissue reveal less than 10^5 organisms per gram of tissue and no histological evidence of bacterial invasion. *Invasive* infections, however, are ascertained by demonstration of bacterial counts greater than 10^5 organisms per gram of tissue; it is not uncommon for counts to reach 10^{10} or 10^{11} organisms per gram. Clinically, formerly healthy granulation tissue becomes pale and edematous and fails to bleed briskly when abraded. Invasion of tissue is demonstrated on frozen sections of biopsy specimens. Fever or subnormal temperatures, progressive leukocytosis with a left shift, and alteration in mental status accompany the local symptoms. Failure to stem this process may "convert" a partial thickness wound into a full-thickness injury because of destruction of the epithelium and thrombosis, which extends necrosis into deeper subcutaneous tissues. A further insult may occur with the development of sepsis through bacterial invasion of the lymphatic system or blood vessels. Invasive infection requires aggressive antimicrobial therapy selected for the etiological agent.

In addition to early debridement and antimicrobial treatment of the burn wound, grafting plays an important role in minimizing the risk of infection and promoting healing. Grafts are biological "dressings" that reduce bacterial counts and prevent water and protein losses. Previously contaminated wounds become sterile within hours of successful grafting.[47] Grafts may be accomplished through the application of human cadaver skin (allograft or homograft), skin from another species (heterograft or porcine [pig] xenograft), or the patient's own skin (autograft). Only the autograft is a permanent means of resolving the injury.

Burn unit environment. The final aspect of infection control management of the burn patient addresses the patient care environment. Burn units provide a concentration of highly trained staff and specialized technology that is countered by a concentration of high-risk patients in a potentially contaminated environment. Measures to control or reduce cross-infection include isolation or barrier technique, personnel practices, and environmental disinfection.

Isolation or barrier technique varies in complexity from the use of single room or open ward isolation to laminar flow units. The value of protective isolation has not been clearly demonstrated. Paradoxically, the burn wound places the patient at high risk for infection while serving as a reservoir for potential cross-infection to others. Mounting evidence that the patient's endogenous fecal flora gives rise to colonization and infection suggests that elaborate isolation protocols may be expensive and ineffective. Elaborate isolation techniques employing a private room, sterile gowns, gloves, and masks may only be necessary for severely and extensively burned patients. For smaller burns sterile technique may be required only for direct burn treatment.[56] Infected patients should be segregated and isolation techniques observed.

Personnel caring for the burn patient may serve as both the source of and vector for infection. Strict adherence to handwashing technique cannot be overemphasized as a basic control measure. Any staff member with an active infection should be excluded from direct patient care. The issue of protective clothing is controversial. In some units scrub uniforms are worn within the general burn unit and cover gowns employed for direct patient care. Minimally, staff should wear sterile gloves for local wound care; the value of masks, caps, and shoe covers is unknown. When providing hydrotherapy treatments, personnel should wear waterproof aprons and elbow-length gloves for both patient and employee protection.

Minimizing potential environmental reservoirs requires the development of regular, effective cleaning procedures. Patient care areas should be designed with adequate storage facilities and constructed from materials that readily withstand frequent applications of germicides. Particular attention must be given to disinfection of equipment used between treatment of patients, such as gurneys, wheelchairs, IV poles, and to handling of contaminated trash, linen, and supplies.

A critical area of potential cross-infection is the hydrotherapy area. The high-volume, short turnaround time adds to the ever-present problem of the warm, moist environment as a breeding ground for bacteria. The design of the equipment itself poses a major infection control problem; agitators and filling hoses are extremely difficult to adequately disinfect. The tub surfaces should be mechanically cleaned with a germicide between treatment of patients. Agitators should be run during the disinfection process or may actually be removed from the equipment. In the latter situation the tub is lined with a single-use plastic liner for each patient treatment. Compressed air forced through channels in the bottom of the liner provides the necessary agitation.[50] A final approach used in some burn centers to prevent cross-infection is the addition of hypochlorite or iodophor solutions to hydrotherapy water; the effectiveness of this practice has not been well studied. All means of disinfection are not a substitute for sound, aseptic technique by personnel.

Ectoparasitic infestations

Two ectoparasitic infestations, pediculosis and scabies, occasionally cause nosocomial outbreaks.

Pediculosis. Three species of the family Pediculidae are important causes of human disease: *Pediculus humanus* var. *corporis* is the human body louse; *Pediculus humanus* var. *capitis* is the human head louse; and *Pthirus pubis* is the pubic louse, colloquially known as "crabs." Although these infestations are viewed as a nuisance and embarrassment, body lice are also vectors for epidemic typhus fever, trench fever, and epidemic relapsing fever.[68]

Body lice are thought to be transferred by close personal contact or contact with fomites, such as infested clothing. Head and pubic lice also require close personal contact; sexual intercourse is a major factor in the transmission of pubic lice.

Transmission occurs through the transfer of nymphs or adult lice. The mature, fertilized female louse lays eggs that are firmly attached to hair shafts or fibers of the host's clothing. Within 7 to 10 days these nits, or small oval capsules, hatch into nymphs. Communicability through fomites is limited: nits or eggs require a higher temperature than ambient room temperature for incubation; nymphs and adult lice must have a source of human blood for frequent feeding.[46] Intense itching and subsequent pyoderma are chief complaints of infestation.

Isolation of the hospitalized patient is not necessary after treatment with an effective pediculicidal agent, such as gamma-benzene hydrochloride (Kwell) or crotamiton (Eurax). Personal clothing may be dry-cleaned or washed in hot water (60° C).[46]

Scabies. Scabies is an infestation of the skin caused by a scab or itch mite (*Sarcoptes scabiei* var. *hominis*). The adult female burrows beneath the skin to the stratum granulosum and lays her eggs in the resultant tunnels. The eggs hatch in 3 to 4 days. The distribution of lesions is fairly classic. The hands, particularly in the web between fingers, and the arms are the most common sites. The male genital area and female breasts are also characteristic sites in adults. The diagnosis is confirmed by demonstrating the presence of mites in skin scrapings under microscopic examination. Itching is the primary symptom; often the intensity is greater at night. In the primary infestation the onset of itching may be delayed for several weeks and is the result of a hypersensitivity or allergic reaction.[15]

Transmission is thought to occur with direct, close contact, although clothing may also be a vehicle. Several outbreaks among hospital staff caring for patients with unrecognized disease have been reported.[10,16,69] Infection control intervention is similar to the management of pediculosis. Gown and glove technique should be observed until the first application of gamma-benzene hydrochloride or crotamiton.

INFECTION CONTROL CONSIDERATIONS
Specimen collection

The definitive diagnosis of infection depends on both clinical signs and symptoms confirmed by laboratory findings. Successful confirmation relates to the appropriateness of the tissue or fluid obtained, the methods of collection and transport, and, finally, the laboratory techniques employed. More sophisticated methodology for identification of bacterial and viral isolates is available through local, state, or federal health agencies.

Bacterial infections. Under ideal conditions purulent material of sufficient quantity should be aspirated by needle and syringe and transported immediately to the laboratory for processing. Often this is impractical, and swabs are used. For all cutaneous lesions, superficial drainage, which may be colonized by skin flora, should be carefully removed with a sterile gauze wipe. The swab is then firmly but gently pressed into the infected tissue and inoculated into transport media. In the presence of scant purulent or serous drainage the swab can be premoistened with saline or culture media. Cellulitis without external drainage can be cultured by injecting a small amount of saline intradermally (into the advancing edge of the cellulitic area) and aspirating the fluid. A Gram stain of all specimens should be done before culture.

If an anaerobic infection is suspected, special transport and culturing conditions must be met. Most hospitals purchase commercially prepared transport systems: small "gassed-out" vials for aspirates or tubes for swabs and tissue. The manufacturer will provide specific directions for use, but a general guideline is to hold the container upright to prevent the loss of carbon dioxide, introduce the specimen, and cap the tube as rapidly as possible to avoid exposure to ambient air.

Accurate assessment of a burn wound poses a particularly difficult problem. As previously discussed, the burn eschar is devitalized tissue that supports the proliferation of bacteria. Methodology may be aimed at quantitative or qualitative analysis of bacterial levels in the wound.

Swabs and contact plates used to quantify the numbers of bacteria on the surface of the wound provide little information concerning the degree of invasive infection. Incisive biopsy of burn wound tissue has been suggested as a solution. A specimen is obtained from deep wound tissue, examined histologically for invasive bacteria or fungi, and subjected to weighing, grinding, and quantitation by a tube dilution method.[42] Although this method yields a far more objective assessment, it is not routinely performed for practical and economic reasons.

Routine qualitative cultures are a more pragmatic means of monitoring potential pathogens and their antibiograms. Moistened sterile swabs of more than one burn are obtained several times per week, preferably after the burn is cleansed during dressing changes, after debridement, or following hydrotherapy.

Viral infections. Diagnosis of viral infections based on clinical manifestations may be confirmed by a variety of laboratory techniques:

- Cultivation of a virus in tissue culture
- Measurement of serum antibody levels
- Demonstration of viral antigens in lesions
- Examination of stained fluid or tissue under electron microscopy

A clinical history including signs and symptoms, the suspected agent, and the date of onset and/or exposure should accompany the specimen. Rapid transportation of specimens is critical. If transport of fluids or tissue for culture cannot be accomplished within 30 minues of collection or within 2 hours if placed on wet ice, the specimen should be frozen at −70° C.

Depending on the suspected etiological agent, one or more of the following specimens should be obtained for viral studies:

Blood. A 10 cc tube of clotted blood is collected during the acute and convalescent (14 to 21 days after onset) phases of the illness. A fourfold rise in specific antibody titers suggests recent infection.

Urine. A clean-catch midstream specimen should be collected; the specimen should not be frozen.

Throat washings and throat or nasopharyngeal swabs. The patient should gargle with appropriate transport media and expectorate into a sterile container. Swabs are passed firmly over the nasopharynx to remove the superficial layer of cells. The tip of the swab is broken off into a tube of transport medium containing antibiotics to inhibit bacterial growth.

Vesicle scrapings. The fresh vesicle should be opened with a sterile scalpel or needle. If a culture is desired, the base of the lesion should be swabbed. The swab is placed in a vial of medium. Slides may be prepared for fluorescent antibody examination by scraping the epithelial cells lining the lesion with the wooden end of a sterile applicator. The scraping is streaked on two clean glass slides and allowed to air dry.

Body fluids. Two to three ml of fluid is placed in a sterile container.

Isolation procedures

Barrier technique for cutaneous infections depends on the infecting agent and the degree of potential contamination based on the drainage from the lesion. Small wounds in which the drainage can be adequately contained by a dressing usually require no more than discharge precautions.[28] This technique includes careful handling and disposal of all dressings and strict adherence to handwashing procedures.

Conversely, extensive wounds that are difficult to cover or wounds in which large amounts of drainage saturate dressings necessitate the use of wound and skin precautions.[28] A private room is desirable, and gown and glove technique is observed for all individuals having direct patient contact. Masks are generally worn only during dressing changes. Occasionally a patient will develop extensive lesions secondary to S. *aureus* or group A streptococcus and will require strict isolation techniques.[28]

Unfortunately, far too many patients with minor skin lesions are overisolated, resulting in increased costs and personnel time, often to the detriment of patient care. The ICP, as an educator and consultant, must evaluate the patient's clinical condition and laboratory findings and recommend the maximal appropriate precaution at minimal disruption to routine patient care.

Surveillance of SWI

Despite the recent skepticism about the value of routine infection surveillance, documentation of SWIs has been advocated as a quality assessment mechanism.[24,25,33] Several authorities have suggested that infection rates, particularly clean wound rates, reflect the technique and skill of the surgeon. Publication of collective and individual infection rates sensitizes all staff to the need for constant vigilance in infection control measures.

To develop an accurate, reliable data base, the ICP must devise a system that ensures appropriate numerator and denominator data.

Numerator data. Complete and accurate identification of the number of infected patients is essential for the calculation of meaningful infection rates. The first consideration in this process is the endorsement of definitions of infection. Criteria for SWIs range from simply the presence of purulent material in the incision to a more sophisticated algorithm that distinguishes between incisional and deep SWIs (pp. 478 and 479). Regardless of the definition used, it must be consistently applied in all cases, and it must be agreed on by the surgeons, the members of the infection control committee, and the ICP.

A second aspect of collecting accurate numerator data is adequate follow-up of patients at risk. Confining the review to inpatient populations may grossly underestimate the true incidence of SWIs. Cruse reported that 11.3% of SWIs became evident only after discharge. Burns and Dippe[14] evaluated 1271 patients undergoing surgical procedures; of 49 patients with postoperative wound infections identified, 26 (53%) manifested symptoms after discharge from the hospital. The significance of postdischarge review will become more important as economic pressures encourage shorter hospital stays and same-day or outpatient procedures. Collection of these data requires the cooperation of clinic or physician office staff to report infections to the ICP.

Denominator data. Accurate assessment of infection rates depends on two aspects of denominator data: identification of the population at risk and comparison of surgical procedures with similar risks of infection.

Calculations of most nosocomial infection rates by service are performed

Criteria for diagnosis of surgical wound infections

Pertinent definitions

Surgical wound infections are subdivided into two categories on the basis of anatomical location: (1) incisional surgical wound infection (ISWI) and (2) deep surgical wound infection (DSWI)

Criteria for infection

Incisional Surgical Wound Infection (ISWI)
Any one of the four criteria may be met:
1. Physician's definite diagnosis of ISWI and no previous diagnosis of ISWI at the same anatomical site
2. Purulent drainage from operative wound site and no previous diagnosis of ISWI at the same site
3. Nonpurulent drainage from operative site, fever, no previous diagnosis of ISWI at the same site, and either of the following:
   a. Redness (erythema) or separation of wound edges
   b. Positive wound culture
4. Physician's diagnosis of stitch abscess and incision not healed within 3 days after sutures removed and no previous diagnosis of ISWI at the same site

Deep Surgical Wound Infection (DSWI)
Any one of the three criteria may be met:
1. Physician's definite diagnosis of any of the following conditions and no previous diagnosis of DSWI at the same site:
   a. Meningitis following neurosurgery or ear, nose, and throat surgery
   b. Pleural empyema following thoracic surgery
   c. Abdominal abscess following abdominal surgery
   d. Endocarditis following cardiac surgery
   e. Septic arthritis or osteomyelitis after bone or joint surgery
   f. Vaginal cuff abscess following hysterectomy
   g. Endometritis following cesarean section or other gynecological surgery
   h. Pelvic abscess after abdominal or pelvic surgery
2. Purulent drainage from a drain, fistula, or a natural body opening and no previous diagnosis of DSWI at the same site
3. Pus encountered at reoperation at or near the surgical field of a previous operation and no previous diagnosis of DSWI at the same site

Signs
1. Purulent drainage from wound or from drain or fistula
2. Nonpurulent drainage (e.g., serous, sanguineous)
3. Redness (erythema) of wound edges
4. Separation of wound edges
5. Stitch abscess
6. Delayed wound healing
7. Pus encountered at reoperation

Modified from Centers for Disease control: Am. J. Epidemiol. **111**:642-643, 1980.

Positive Wound Culture
Culture of surgical wound drainage with isolation of any pathogen except the following:
  1. *Bacillus* species
  2. *Candida* species
  3. *Corynebacterium* species
  4. *Staphylococcus epidermidis*
  5. Unidentified gram-negative rod
  6. *Micrococcus* species
  7. Any unidentified organism

Nosocomial versus Community-Acquired Status
SWIs are hospital acquired if the surgery was performed during the admission being reviewed. SWIs of operations performed in a previous admission to the index or another hospital are considered community acquired.

using the number of admissions, discharges, or patient days during a given time interval. This figure is far too general to produce a meaningful index of SWIs. Only patients actually undergoing a surgical procedure that requires an incision are at risk and hence are included in the denominator.

A further refinement of these rates is achieved by classifying the procedures by potential risk of infection based on the level of wound contamination. This classification system, described earlier in Table 17-3, provides a more sensitive measure of the quality of care and fosters a more realistic approach to control measures. Significant differences in the incidence of infection within these four categories suggest that overall rates for services and surgeons are difficult to interpret and may, in fact, be misleading.

Implementation of the classification system depends on the internal procedures of each institution. However, the assessment is best made by a member of the operating room team who has directly observed both the wound and the surgical technique. The class of the wound should be recorded in all procedures and may be noted on the anesthesia or nursing record at the time of incisional closure. Reliance on retrospective chart review to determine the classification is less accurate, since key information may be omitted and results in misleading denominator data. Fig. 17-4 is a suggested format for reporting surveillance data.

Surveillance of neonatal staphylococcal disease

Monitoring the true incidence of staphylococcal infections in the normal newborn population is difficult because of increasingly shorter hospital stays. Often infections in the inpatient population represent "the tip of the iceberg";

Department of surgery

Infection·rate

Number of admissions _____

Number of hospital-associated infections _____   %
Number of community-acquired infections _____   %

                                                     Number   Percent

Respiratory tract
Urinary tract
Cutaneous
Bacteremia
Other
Operative wounds*

   Classification

I _____ = %
II _____ = %
III _____ = %
IV _____ = %

*Number of infections
─────────────────────────────── = Attack rate expressed as a percent
Number of patients undergoing surgery

Services

General surgery   Orthopedic surgery

I _____ = %   I _____ = %
II _____ = %   II _____ = %
III _____ = %   III _____ = %
IV _____ = %   IV _____ = %

Surgeon A   Surgeon C

I _____ = %   I _____ = %
II _____ = %   II _____ = %
III _____ = %   III _____ = %
IV _____ = %   IV _____ = %

Surgeon B   Surgeon D

I _____ = %   I _____ = %
II _____ = %   II _____ = %
III _____ = %   III _____ = %
IV _____ = %   IV _____ = %

FIG. 17-4. Suggested format for reporting SWI rates.

consequently, even small numbers of infections are considered presumptive evidence of an epidemic. The occurrence of two or more simultaneous cutaneous infections or a single case of mastitis in either an infant or nursing mother warrants prompt investigation.[19]

Two particular aspects of continuous surveillance are controversial in a cost/benefit evaluation. The first is the performance of routine surveillance cultures. Although colonization generally precedes infection in staphylococcal disease and high rates of colonization have been associated with outbreaks of infection, the potential value of routine sampling of infants by umbilical and nares cultures has not been well documented as an effective control measure. Routine culturing of nursery personnel is not an effective means of identifying sources of infection and is discouraged.[18]

The second consideration is postdischarge surveillance. This time-consuming, expensive process is beneficial only with cooperation of the pediatricians responsible for reporting infections in infants seen in their offices. Both telephone and written surveys have been performed.

At Stanford University Hospital a simple yet effective system has been used for over 10 years. At the time of discharge the parents are provided with a letter and a pink-colored, preaddressed, stamped postcard (Fig. 17-5). The letter, signed by the medical director of the nurseries, explains to the parents and the

---

Addressograph

Discharge date _____

Examining physician _____

Date of examination _____

Evidence of infection in mother _____

Culture results _____

Evidence of infection in infant _____ Site _____

Culture results _____

Comments/description

Lab work by _____ Date _____

Parents—Please note:

Did brothers or sisters visit your new baby in your room in the hospital?

Yes_____ No_____

If no, did other mothers in the same room have visits by children?

Yes_____ No_____

FIG. 17-5. Postcard for surveillance of newborns after discharge.

pediatrician that the hospital performs a continuous assessment of the incidence of staphylococcal disease in infants discharged from the newborn nursery. The parents are requested to complete the information concerning sibling visitation during hospitalization and to take both the card and letter to the initial office visit. The pediatrician completes the clinical information portion and mails the card back to the hospital where data are reviewed and statistics are calculated on a monthly basis. To encourage laboratory confirmation of the infections, physicians are encouraged to obtain cultures, which are processed by the hospital at no charge.

Problem solving

Recognition of potential outbreaks of cutaneous infections is based on a comparative review of infection rates or the occurrence of an unusual organism or antibiogram. A detailed description of epidemiological principles used in an investigation is provided in Chapter 7. However, a few salient concepts relating to bacterial infections of the integument follow.

Identification of reservoirs. The potential reservoir of bacteria is frequently defined by the type of infecting organism. Whereas endogenous flora consisting of both gram-negative and gram-positive organisms give rise to sporadic or endemic infections, exogenous sources of outbreaks can be differentiated by animate and inanimate reservoirs. In general, gram-positive organisms such as S. aureus and group A or group B streptococcus are related to human sources. An asymptomatic carrier or an infected individual may serve as the source of the infecting organism, which in turn is spread by contaminated hands or fomites.

Outbreaks of cutaneous infections secondary to aerobic gram-negative bacilli have been reported less frequently.[1] Human reservoirs have been implicated, but most often such epidemics are traced to environmental sources: contaminated irrigation equipment, disinfectants or antiseptics, hand lotions, or patient care supplies (Table 17-7).

If a specific microorganism is suspected of causing a "cluster" or outbreak of infections, isolates should be saved for future typing. Additional surveillance cultures of the environment or personnel should be obtained only when there are strong epidemiological implications for a specific source or reservoir; widespread, "shotgun" culture surveys are expensive and time consuming and may result in unnecessary confusion and anxiety if results are misinterpreted.

Control measures. Efforts to control an outbreak focus on primary and secondary levels. Primary efforts include the removal of the epidemiologically implicated individuals from patient care until appropriate treatment has been provided. If an inanimate reservoir is identified, the source is either adequately disinfected, sterilized, or discarded, as in the case of contaminated solutions. Control measures initiated on a secondary level include both short-term and

TABLE 17-7. Epidemiological considerations in outbreak management of cutaneous infections

Organism	Source or reservoir	Mode of transmission	Culture sites	Epidemiological markers	Intervention
Staphylococcus aureus	Human—active infection or carrier state; fomites (usually not primary reservoir)	Direct and indirect contact; airborne less significant	Anterior nares; skin or groin dermatitis	Bacteriophage typing	Appropriate isolation procedures (wound and skin or strict precautions); identification and treatment of individuals with overt infection and carriers; removal of epidemiologically implicated staff from patient care; initiation of cohort system for patients and staff
Group A streptococcus	Human—active infection or colonization	Airborne or direct contact	Anus or rectum; vagina; nares and pharynx	Serological typing for M and T strains	Appropriate isolation procedures (wound and skin or strict precautions); identification and treatment of infected individuals and carriers; removal of epidemiologically implicated staff from patient care
Aerobic gram-negative bacillus	Inanimate—vehicles include solutions, hand lotions, creams, and antiseptics; human—skin and gastrointestinal colonization	Direct or indirect contact	Suspected reservoir	Biotype, antibiogram, and R factors; serotype (E. coli); capsular serotype (Klebsiella species); serotype, pyocin type, and bacteriophage (Pseudomonas species)	Wound and skin isolation; appropriate treatment of infected cases; removal of reservoirs

long-term considerations. Appropriate isolation of infected patients will prevent further spread; wound and skin precautions are initiated for gram-negative bacilli infections and minor staphylococcal or streptococcal disease. Strict isolation may be required for extensive infections caused by staphylococci or streptococci.[28]

Other short-term measures may include cohorting both infected and colonized patients with accompanying staff restrictions; treating infected and colonized individuals; restricting the use of specific antimicrobial agents when resistant organisms are involved; reviewing patient care procedures; using continuous, intensive surveillance to search for additional cases; and, on occasion, closing a unit to admissions when all other efforts fail.

Once the initial outbreak is under control, consideration should be given to long-term measures to prevent future outbreaks. Revision of patient care procedures, changes in products, equipment, or supplies, renovation of hospital facilities, and modification of staffing ratios are all potential areas for review in light of the epidemic experience. The ICP plays a central role in both control and prevention of outbreaks. An understanding of both the human and microbiological factors is critical to successful resolution of the problem with minimal disruption of patient care.

SUMMARY

The integument provides an effective mechanical barrier against the invasion of microorganisms into the body. The hospitalized patient is at high risk for cutaneous infections secondary to diagnostic and therapeutic procedures that breach this barrier.

Infection control policies and procedures must be developed to prevent the occurrence of nosocomial infections from bacterial, viral, and ectoparasitic causes. Special consideration must be given to newborn, pediatric, surgical, oncological, and burn patient populations.

REFERENCES

1. Aber, R.C., and Garner, J.S.: Postoperative wound infections. In Wenzel, R.P., editor: CRC handbook of hospital acquired infections, Boca Raton, Fla., 1981, CRC Press.
2. Adams, G., et al.: Nosocomial herpetic infections in a pediatric intensive care unit, Am. J. Epidemiol. 113:126-132, 1981.
3. Advisory Committee on Immunization Practices: Measles prevention, Morbid. Mortal. Weekly Rep. 31:217-224+, 1982.
4. Alexander, J.W., and MacMillan, B.G.: Infections of burn wounds. In Bennett, J.F., and Brachman, P.S., editors: Boston, 1970, Little, Brown & Co.
5. Alexander, J.W., Korelitz, J., and Alexander, N.S.: Prevention of wound infections: a case for closed suction drainage to remove fluids deficient in opsonic proteins, Am. J. Surg. 132:59-66, 1976.
6. American Academy of Pediatrics: Standards and recommendations for hospital care of newborns, Evanston, Ill., 1977, The Academy.

7. American Academy of Pediatrics Committee on Infectious Diseases: Revised recommendations on rubella vaccine, Pediatrics **65:**1182-84, 1980.
8. American College of Obstetricians and Gynecologists Committee on Technical Bulletins: Rubella clinical update, A.C.O.G. Tech. Bull., no. 62, July 1981.
9. American Hospital Association Advisory Committee on Infections Within Hospitals: Recommendations for the control of rubella within hospitals, Chicago, May 1981, The Association.
10. Axnick, K.J., and Cherry, J.D.: Scabies outbreak in a pediatric unit, A.P.I.C. Newsletter **4:**4-6, 1976.
11. Bernard, H.R., and Cole, W.: The prophylaxis of surgical infection: the effect of prophylactic antimicrobial drugs on the incidence of infection following potentially contaminated operations, Surgery **56:**151-156, 1964.
12. Brachman, P.S., et al.: Nosocomial surgical infections: incidence and cost, Surg. Clin. North. Am. **60:**15-25, 1980.
13. Burke, J.F.: Burns. In Mandell, G.L., Douglas, R.G., and Bennett, J.E., editors: Principles and practices of infectious diseases, New York, 1979, John Wiley & Sons, Inc.
14. Burns, S.J., and Dippe, S.E.: Postoperative wound infections detected during hospitalization and after discharge in a community hospital, Am. J. Infect. Control **10:**60-65, 1982.
15. California State Department of Health: Diagnosis and control of scabies, Calif. Morbid., no. 4, Feb. 6, 1976.
16. California State Department of Health: Scabies outbreaks—recommendations for management, Calif. Morbid., no. 6, Feb. 15, 1980.
17. Carpenter, H.H., Gastes, D.J., and Williams, H.T.G.: Normal processes and restraints in wound healing, Can. J. Surg. **20:**314-324, 1977.
18. Centers for Disease Control: Approach to the staphylococcal nasal carrier, Atlanta, 1970, CDC.
19. Centers for Disease Control: Control of nursing-acquired staphylococcal disease: present status of the use of hexachlorophene, Atlanta, revised 1973, CDC.
20. Centers for Disease Control: Isolation precautions for patients infected with varicella-zoster virus, Atlanta, 1974, CDC.
21. Centers for Disease Control: Varicella-zoster immune globulin, United States, Morbid. Mortal. Weekly Rep. **30:**20-23, 1981.
22. Centers for Disease Control: Nosocomial rubella, National Nosocomial Infections Study Report—annual summary, 1979, Atlanta, issued 1982, CDC.
23. Cerise, E.J., Pierce, W.A., and Diamond, D.L.: Abdominal drains: their rate as a source of infection following splenectomy, Ann. Surg. **171:**764-769, 1970.
24. Committee on Control of Surgical Infections, American College of Surgeons: Definitions and classifications of surgical infections, Manual on Control of Infections in Surgical Patients, Philadelphia, 1976, J.B. Lippincott Co.
25. Cruse, P.J.E.: Infection surveillance: identifying the problems and the high-risk patient, South Med. J. **70:**4-8, 1977.
26. Cruse, P.J.E., and Foord, R.: A five year prospective study of 23,649 surgical wounds, Arch. Surg. **107:**206-210, 1973.
27. Cruse, P.J.E., and Foord, R.: The epidemiology of wound infection: A ten year prospective study of 62,939 wounds, Surg. Clin. North. Am. **60:**27-40, 1980.
28. Department of Health, Education, and Welfare: Isolation techniques for use in hospitals, ed. 2, Washington, D.C., 1975, Superintendent of Documents.
29. Dineen, P.: An evaluation of the duration of the surgical scrub, Surg. Gynecol. Obstet. **129:**1181-1184, 1969.
30. Edwards, L.D.: The epidemiology of 2056 remote site infections and 1966 surgical wound infections occurring in 1865 patients, Ann. Surg. **184:**758-766, 1976.
31. Ehrenkranz, N.J.: Surgical wound infection occurrence in clean operations: risk stratification for interhospital comparisons, Am. J. Med. **70:**909-914, 1981.
32. Elias, P.M., Fritsch, P., and Epsteen, E.H., Jr.: Staphylococcal scalded skin syndrome, Arch. Dermatol. **113:**207-218, 1977.

33. Emori, T.G., Haley, R.W., and Garner, J.S.: Techniques and uses of nosocomial infection surveillance in U.S. hospitals, 1976-1977, Am. J. Med. **70**:933-940, 1981.

34. Fliegel, P.E., and Weinstein, W.M.: Rubella outbreak in a prenatal clinic: management and prevention, Am. J. Infect. Control **10**:29-33, 1982.

35. Gershon, A.A.: Measles (rubeola) virus. In Mandell, G.L., Douglas, R.G., and Bennett, J.E., editors: Principles and practices of infectious diseases, New York, 1979, John Wiley & Sons, Inc.

36. Gershon, A.A.: Rubella virus (german measles). In Mandell, G.L., Douglas, R.G., and Bennett, J.E., editors: Principles and practices of infectious diseases, New York, 1979, John Wiley & Sons, Inc.

37. Gezon, H.M., et al.: Control of staphylococcal infections and disease in the newborn through the use of hexachlorophene bathing, Pediatrics **51**(suppl.):331-434, 1973.

38. Greaves, W.L., et al.: The problem of herpetic whitlow among hospital personnel, Infect. Control **1**:381-385, 1980.

39. Haley, R.W., et al.: Nosocomial infections in U.S. hospitals, 1975-1976: estimated frequency by selected characteristics of patients, Am. J. Med. **70**:947-958, 1981.

40. Hamilton, H.W., Hamilton, K.R., and Lone, F.J.; Preoperative hair removal, Can. J. Surg. **20**:269-275, 1977.

41 Harris, D.R.: Healing of the surgical wound II: factors influencing repair and regeneration, J. Am. Acad. Dermatol. **1**:208-215, 1979.

42. Heimbach, D.M.: Burn wound infection, A.P.I.C. Journal **6**:6-11, 1978.

43. Hirsch, M.S.: Herpes simplex virus. In Mandell, G.L., Douglas, R.G., and Bennett, J.E., editors: Principles and practices of infectious diseases, New York, 1979, John Wiley & Sons, Inc.

44. Hunt, T.K.: Surgical wound infections: an overview, Am. J. Med. **70**:712-718, 1981.

45. Johnson, J.D., et al.: A sequential study of various modes of skin and umbilical care and the incidence of staphylococcal colonization and infections in the neonate, Pediatrics **58**:354-361, 1976.

46. Juranek, D.D.: The nuisance diseases: Pediculosis and scabies, A.P.I.C. Newsletter **4**:1-5, 1976.

47. Krizek, T.J., and Robson, M.C.: Evolution of quantitative bacteriology in wound management, Am. J. Surg. **130**:579-584, 1975.

48. Krugman, S., and Katz, S.L.: Measles (rubeola). In Krugman, S., and Katz, S.L.: Infectious diseases in children, ed. 7, St. Louis, 1981, The C.V. Mosby Co.

49. Krugman, S., and Katz, S.L.: Varicella-zoster infections. In Krugman, S., and Katz, S.L.: Infectious diseases in children, ed. 7, St. Louis, 1981, The C.V. Mosby Co.

50. Mayhall, C.G.: Infections in burn patients. In Wenzel, R.P., editor: CRC handbook of hospital acquired infections, Boca Raton, Fla., 1981, CRC Press.

51. McLaughlin, M.C., and Gold, L.H.: The New York rubella incident: a case for changing hospital policy regarding rubella testing and immunization, Am. J. Public. Health. **69**:287-289, 1979.

52. Morens, D.M., et al.: An outbreak of varicella-zoster virus infection among cancer patients, Ann. Intern. Med. **93**:414-419, 1980.

53. National Academy of Sciences–National Research Council: Post-operative wound infections: the influence of ultraviolet irradiation of the operating room and various other factors, Ann. Surg. **160**(suppl.):1-192, 1964.

54. Nelson, A.M., and St. Geme, J.W.: On the respiratory spread of varicella-zoster virus, Pediatrics **37**:1007-1009, 1966.

55. Nichols R.L.: Techniques known to prevent post-operative wound infection, Infect. Control **3**:6-9, 1982.

56. Pierson, C.L.: Infection control in burn care facilities, Crit. Care Q. **3**:81-92, 1981.

57. Polk, H.C., Jr., and Lopez-Mayor, J.F.: Perioperative prophylactic antibiotics in abdominal surgery: a prospective study of determinant factors and prevention, Surgery **66**:97-103, 1969.

58. Polk, B.F., et al.: An outbreak of rubella among hospital personnel, N. Engl. J. Med. **303**:541-545, 1980.

59. Public Health Service Advisory Committee on Immunization Practices: Rubella prevention, Morbid, Mortal. Weekly Rep. **30**:37-47, 1981.

60. Seropian, R., and Reynolds, B.M.: Wound infections after preoperative depilatory versus razor preparation, Am. J. Surg. **121:**251-254, 1971.
61. Simmons, B.P.: CDC guideline for prevention of surgical wound infections, Infect. Control **3**(supl.):187-196, 1982.
62. Simon, H.J., Yaffe, S.J., and Geuck, L.: Effective control of staphylococi in a nursery, N. Engl. J. Med. **265:**1171-1176, 1961.
63. Stamm, W.E., Steere, A.C., and Dixon, R.E.: Selected infections of the skin and eye. In Bennett, J.V., and Brachman, P.S., editors: Hospital infections, Boston, 1979, Little, Brown & Co.
64. Steere, A.C., and Mallison, G.M.: Handwashing practices for the prevention and control of nosocomial infections, Ann. Intern. Med. **83:**683-690, 1975.
65. Stone, H.H., et al.: Antibiotic prophylaxis in gastric, biliary, and colonic surgery, Ann. Surg. **184:**443-452, 1976.
66. Stone, H.H., et al.: Prophylactic and preventive antibiotic therapy: timing, duration, and economics, Ann. Surg. **189:**691-698, 1979.
67. Verrier, E.D., Bossart, K.J., and Heer, F.W.: Reduction of infection rates in abdominal incisions by delayed wound closure techniques, Am. J. Surg. **138:**22-28, 1979.
68. Weary, P.E.: Lice (pediculosis). In Mandell, G.L., Douglas, R.G., and Bennett, J.E., editors: Principles and practices of infectious diseases, New York, 1979, John Wiley & Sons, Inc.
69. Werdegar, D., and Atlas, E.: Scabies outbreak in a community hospital, A.P.I.C. Newsletter **4:**7-8, 1976.

Central nervous system

Infections of the central nervous system (CNS) can produce devastating outcomes for individuals and society. At one extreme death may be the outcome, and in the case of certain acute bacterial infections this extreme is almost a certainty in the absence of prompt diagnosis and therapy. More often, however, the impact is on people's adjustment to life through temporary or permanent alterations in the conscious or unconscious perception of their environment and their reaction to it. Destruction of neuronal tissue as a result of CNS infection may cause any number or combination of neurological defects that interfere with maximal perception or reaction (e.g., blindness, paralysis, deafness, and palsies) or result in impairment of intelligence and psychiatric disturbances. The resulting socioeconomic traumas are severely felt by patients, their families, and the community. The need for long-term counseling, custodial care, and rehabilitation for these unfortunate individuals is well documented in neurological literature.

At the very minimum, nosocomial CNS infections can result in exorbitant cost to the patient and family through prolonged hospitalization, antibiotic use, additional diagnostic and therapeutic procedures, and consultation fees.

Minimizing the risks of hospital-acquired CNS infections and their devastating outcomes through effective prevention and control programs is the major goal of both the infection control practitioner (ICP) and all concerned health professionals. The challenge can be great, for infections originating in almost any other body system can result in invasion of the brain or its surrounding structures. Although a wide variety of microorganisms can invade the CNS by various routes, the most common route for both bacterial and viral infections is the hematogenous route. The most common nosocomial route for bacterial invasion is through invasive surgical and diagnostic procedures.

This chapter will present anatomical and physiological considerations of the CNS pertinent to the understanding of the development of infections; identify and discuss major infections of the CNS, including the clinical characteristics most frequently demonstrated; and review the principal invasive routes of the major acute infections. Emphasis will be placed on recognition of factors that predispose to the development of infections and recommendations for recognition and control of risks.

ANATOMICAL AND PHYSIOLOGICAL CONSIDERATIONS

The CNS consists of the brain and spinal cord, of which the neuron is the functional and anatomical unit (Figs. 18-1 and 18-2).[19] Each neuron is capable of individual activity and forms circuits to integrate functions in the CNS.[97] The neuron receives stimuli, interprets them at various conscious and unconscious levels, and transmits them for action.[21]

Millions of individual neurons make it possible for the brain to store information, generate thoughts, create ambition, and determine reactions (conscious and subconscious) that the body performs in response to sensations. Appropriate signals are then transmitted by these neurons through the motor portion of the CNS to carry out the person's desires.[43]

At the subconscious level the autonomic system, another closely integrated segment of the CNS, controls many involuntary functions of the internal organs, including action of the heart, movement of the gastrointestinal tract, and secretion by different glands.[43]

The CNS is a sterile, closed system. Structures and mechanisms that protect the CNS from infections and maintain the sterile system can be identified as either internal or external to the CNS.

Internal protective structures

Glial cells. Glial cells surround the neuron, providing structural support and nourishment. In response to infection or injury glial cells can provide some protection for the neuron by dividing and becoming phagocytes, clearing, to a limited extent, particulates from the neural environment.[94,97]

Blood-brain and blood-cerebrospinal fluid (CSF) barriers. The CNS and its fluids are protected against bloodborne contaminants by the restrictive phenomena of the blood-brain and blood-cerebrospinal fluid (CSF) barriers. The absolute nature of these barriers is as yet unproven; however, their importance to CNS infection and therapy continues to be a focus of considerable research.

Anatomically, the blood-brain and blood-CSF barriers exist in the choroid plexuses and in essentially all areas of the brain parenchyma except the hypothalamus.[43] Virtually all materials that pass from the blood into the brain must pass through these barriers: from capillaries into the extracellular space or from capillaries by way of the choroid plexuses into CSF, from which a small amount may pass into the brain tissue.[21] The blood-brain and blood-CSF barriers restrict passage of unwanted and potentially toxic biochemical substances into the extracellular environment of the neuron.

The barriers are highly permeable to water, oxygen, carbon dioxide,[43] and other metabolically important substances, such as glucose and some amino acids.[69] Penetration of these substances occurs by active cellular transport mechanisms and not mere transudation.[6]

The blood-brain and blood-CSF barriers are essentially impermeable to a

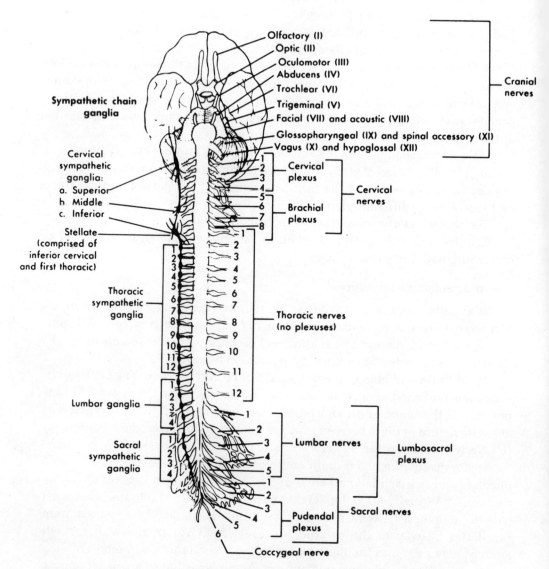

FIG. 18-1. Anterior view of brain and spinal cord. *Right,* Spinal nerves; *left,* sympathetic chain. Note that sympathetic chain of ganglia includes all regions even though cells of origin are only in thoracolumbar area. (From Conway-Rutkowski, B.L.: Carini and Owens' neurological and neurosurgical nursing, ed. 8, St. Louis, 1982, The C.V. Mosby Co.)

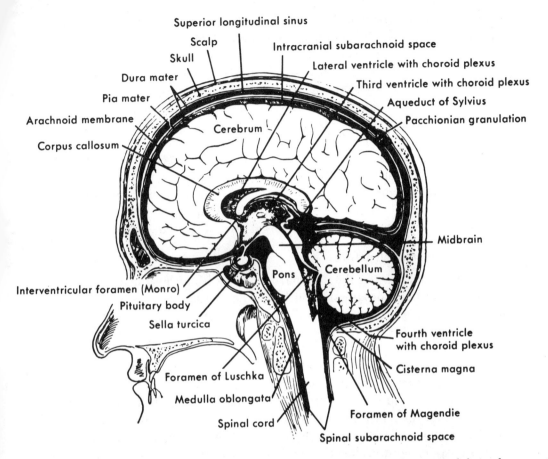

FIG. 18-2. Diagram of sagittal section of head, showing cerebrospinal fluid spaces and their relationship to venous circulation and principal subdivisions of the brain and its coverings. (From Conway-Rutkowski, B.L.: Carini and Owens' neurological and neurosurgical nursing, ed. 8, St. Louis, 1982, The C.V. Mosby Co.)

large molecular substance, such as plasma proteins,[43] and to some hydrophilic substances even as small as sodium ions.[69] The low permeability of these barriers has been explained by recent electron microscope findings that demonstrate the endothelial cell membranes of capillaries to be almost fused with each other, or, in other words, joined by so-called "tight junctions."[21,43]

The restrictive nature of the blood-brain and blood-CSF barriers is also important to drug therapy in CNS infection. For example, these barriers restrict penetration of most antimicrobial drugs into the brain and CSF. It is almost impossible to achieve effective concentrations of some drugs in the CSF and brain parenchyma even if they are administered intravenously or intramuscularly.[43,101] Research conducted with clinically well human volunteers and experimental animals has shown that drug concentrations in the CSF and parenchyma are approximately 1:200 to 1:500 those in the serum.[101] Exceptions to the rule are sulfonamides, chloramphenicol, cycloserine, isonicotinic acid, hydralazide, and 5-fluorocytosine, which have all been shown to readily penetrate the blood-brain and blood-CSF barriers.[45] Inflammation involving the CNS materially enhances drug penetration (e.g., penicillin); however, this facilitating effect will naturally decrease with effective treatment.[45] Intrathecal and intraventricular injections are alternate, and sometimes concomitant, routes used to accomplish effective drug levels in the brain.[74]

The protective function of the blood-brain and blood-CSF barriers can also have a detrimental effect on CNS infection by restricting transport of antibody and complement components from the intravascular compartments to the CNS.[101] Opsonizing antibody with or without C3 represents an important host defense mechanism in combating bacterial infections (see Chapter 13).

External protective structures

Meninges. Examining the external structures from those nearest the brain and spinal cord and progressing outward, the first is the meningeal covering, the pia mater. The pia mater is a very thin membrane that closely adheres to the entire surface of the brain and spinal cord, dipping into sulci and following contours exactly.

The next layer of the meningeal covering is the arachnoid, which has many threadlike connections to the pia mater. The compartment between the pia mater and arachnoid is called the subarachnoid space. Within this space CSF circulates over the entire surface of the CNS. The protective function of CSF is to act as a shock absorber, thus reducing the force of external impact on the brain and spinal cord.[21] The arachnoid also forms the structural mechanism for absorption of CSF: pacchionian or arachnoid granulation.

Together the pia mater and arachnoid serve as the roadbed for the vascular system of the cerebral cortex.[21] The veins lie in the subarachnoid space, and the cortical arteries are carried with the pia mater into the cortex.

The dura mater, the final layer of meninges, is a leathery, tough membrane that is firmly attached to the skull but has no attachment to vertebrae.[21] Unlike the spinal dura mater, which has only one layer, the cranial dura mater has two layers that separate in places to form venous sinuses into which draining veins deliver venous blood.[97]

The meninges separate one part of the brain from another (i.e., the two cerebral hemispheres) and the cortex from the cerebellum. They also serve as structural supports for both the spinal cord and brain.

Bones. The bones of the skull and vertebral column and the skin coverings provide the final external protection. The skull, a thick, rigid compartment of numerous bones fused together (after about 12 to 18 months of age), contains an opening at the base, called the foramen magnum, through which the brainstem passes and is continuous with the spinal cord. There are also many smaller openings in the skull that allow cranial nerves and blood vessels to pass through to the periphery of the face.[97]

Supporting the head and protecting the spinal cord are the bones of the vertebral column, which consists of 7 cervical, 12 thoracic, and 5 lumbar vertebrae, as well as the sacrum and coccyx.

Immunocompetency

Corticosteroid therapy can severely affect host defense mechanisms by depressing the inflammatory response and by suppressing cell-mediated immune mechanisms.[67] Other drugs that can suppress the immune response are alkylating agents, folic acid antagonists, purine analogs, and antilymphocyte globulin.[67]

A recent report[20] of an outbreak of group Y *Neisseria meningitidis* among oncology patients at Yale-New Haven Hospital emphasizes the potential risk of nosocomial meningitis in this patient population. The investigators speculated that the infected patients were unable to mount a response because they had malignancies and were immunosuppressed.

MAJOR INFECTIONS
Bacterial etiology

Acute bacterial meningitis. Acute bacterial meningitis is an infection caused by the invasion of bacteria into the subarachnoid space with subsequent inflammation of the pia mater, arachnoid, CSF, and ventricles.[45] Infecting bacteria usually reach the meninges by the hematogenous route but can also invade the meninges by direct spread from other intracranial foci or by direct inoculation of extradural bacteria. Bacteria are responsible for most cases of nosocomial acute meningitis[6] and will usually be recovered from CSF cultures.

Virtually any bacterium gaining access to the body can cause meningitis; however, the cause varies with the age group considered and the clinical setting in which the infection occurs.[45] The most common causes of meningitis in the United States for various age groups are listed in Table 18-1.

Predisposing conditions. The incidence of bacterial meningitis is higher for persons with certain predisposing conditions. Persons who have had splenectomies and persons with sickle cell disease appear to have a higher incidence of septicemia and meningitis than other persons.[31] The risk for pneumococcal meningitis for children with sickle cell disease has been reported to be 36 times greater than the risk for black children without sickle cell disease and 314 times greater than the risk for white children.[35] The risk associated with sickle cell disease is closely related to factors that predispose persons who have had splenectomies to a higher attack rate of meningitis. Bacterial infections in

TABLE 18-1. Frequent causes of meningitis in the United States in various age groups

Age group	Cause
Neonate	Group B streptococcus, *Escherichia coli*, and *Listeria monocytogenes*
1 month to 10 years	*Haemophilus influenzae*, *Neisseria meningitidis*, and *Streptococcus pneumoniae*
11 to 29 years	*Neisseria meningitidis* and *Streptococcus pneumoniae*
30 to 60 years	*Streptococcus pneumoniae*
Above 60 years	Gram-negative rods, *Streptococcus pneumoniae*, and other streptococci

From Fraser, D.W.: Post. Grad. Med. **62:**105-109, Aug. 1977.

patients without spleens are often unusually rapid and overwhelming. In the absence of specific bacterial antibody the spleen is thought to be an important site of bacteria entrapment and early antibody formation.[29,31] In patients with sickle cell disease the function of the spleen is abnormal.

Persons with hypogammaglobulinemia have an increased risk of bacterial meningitis.[29,31,34] Hypogammaglobulinemia is characterized by a marked deficiency in plasma globulins with a greatly decreased ability to synthesize humoral antibodies. This condition occurs in males as a sex-linked heredity defect and as an acquired illness in adults who have some other disease, such as lymphosarcoma, leukemia, multiple myeloma, sarcoidosis, extensive renal loss of protein catabolism, or decreased protein synthesis.[45]

Pathology. The pathological changes in acute bacterial meningitis are similar in all cases regardless of the causative organism.[6] Spread of infection through the subarachnoid space, involving the meninges, brain, and spinal cord, may be exceedingly rapid. In some patients 1 or 2 days may be required for meningitis to become fully developed. In others it may follow a fulminating course with only a few hours elapsing between onset of initial symptoms and death.[101]

Once bacteria gain access to the subarachnoid space, they seem to thrive in CSF.[94] The subarachnoid space becomes filled with a purulent exudate that may cover the whole cerebral cortex or may, occasionally, be confined to sulci.[6]

Phagocytes normally present in the meninges have been demonstrated to participate in the early stages of cellular response; however, Waggoner[94] recently presented evidence that phagocytes of hematogenous origin rapidly become the dominant component of the exudate. He describes the efforts of

meningeal cells (e.g., glial) as "feeble" in comparison with the ability of leukocytes to clear particulates from CSF.

Damage to neuronal tissue is usually associated with secondary infarction
caused by vasculitis and thrombosis.[94] The irritating effect of bacteria or their
toxins may induce vascular congestion, resulting in increased permeability of
venules and capillaries.

Hydrocephalus is caused by the collection of fibropurulent exudate that
blocks the subarachnoid space and interrupts the flow of CSF.[2] Fibrinogen
appears early in the course of the disease and is converted to fibrin in a few
days. This fibropurulent exudate may accumulate in the foramens of Magendie
and Luschka or in the subarachnoid space around the pons and midbrain. In
the later stages fibrous subarachnoid adhesions are an additional and sometimes more important factor interfering with CSF circulation.[2]

Ventriculitis may be present and is common in neonatal meningitis.[45] In the
later stages of meningitis the ependymal lining of the ventricles stretches and
breaks from the pressure of the developing hydrocephalus.[2] This offers an
avenue for bacteria to pass through to subependymal tissues and set up an
inflammatory reaction. The choroid plexus is also involved, initially becoming
congested and followed in a few days by infiltration with neutrophils and
lymphocytes.[2]

Later in the course of the disease pial cells are displaced into the toxic
exudate by neutrophils accumulating on the glial surface of the brain.[94] The
eventual disappearance of pial cells may be the result of their direct exposure
to the toxic exudate and the severe injury and necrosis that ensue. Conversely,
under usual circumstances, the outer membrane, the arachnoid, has been
shown to remain intact unless injury is sufficient to cause necrosis.[94] With
injury to the arachnoid, a subdural effusion or empyema may develop, which
happens more often in infants than in adults.[2,94] The arachnoid, unlike the pia
mater, has been shown to be capable of replenishing damaged areas and sealing
off the perforating defect.[94]

The underlying neuronal tissue apparently remains intact; however, tracer
studies have clearly outlined direct pathways from the subarachnoid space and
ventricles to the central extracellular spaces.[94] It has also been shown that
endotoxins can move from CSF to vital central ganglia and exert severe functional damage without causing perceptible histological damage.[2] It is impossible to say whether diffusion of toxins from the meninges, circulatory disturbances, or some other factor is responsible for the encephalopathy seen early in
the course of the disease (e.g., stupor, coma, seizures). It is known that these
changes are not caused by the presence of bacteria in the brain substance and
should therefore be regarded as noninfectious encephalopathy.[2]

Pathogens causing meningitis in adults and children. Although any bacterium gaining access to the body can cause meningitis, the three most common meningeal pathogens in a significant part of child and adult populations are inhabitants of the nasopharynx. In order of frequency in the United States meningitis is caused by *Haemophilus influenzae*, N. *meningitidis* (meningococcus), and *Streptococcus pneumoniae* (pneumococcus or diplococcus).[31,34] These pathogens cause 80% to 90% of the disease, with an estimated 10,000 to 15,000 cases per year.[38,46] Pneumococcal meningitis has the highest mortality rate (23% to 38%), followed by meningococcal meningitis (7% to 29%) and H. *influenzae* (5% to 14%) meningitis.[31]

Most studies report a higher incidence of meningitis in children than in adults.[31,34] Those most commonly affected are children from 1 month to 5 years of age, with a peak incidence at 6 to 8 months.[34] H. *influenzae* meningitis is a disease almost exclusively seen in young children.

There is also a higher incidence, caused by the three common meningeal pathogens, in males, blacks, and American Indians.[31,34,35]

Meningococcal, pneumococcal, and H. *influenzae* infections are endemic in all centers of the population and have a worldwide distribution.[45] Many persons are exposed to these meningeal pathogens, and many are carriers, yet few become sick.[31] This puzzling phenomenon has been the impetus of considerable research concerning host-organism interrelationships and environmental factors that might predispose to meningitis by these pathogens in the population.

The source of infection in H. *influenzae*, pneumococcal, and meningococcal meningitis must be a patient or a carrier; organisms reside in the nasopharynx of both. They leave the body in the nasal or buccal secretions; the mode of transfer is by close contact, and the portals of entry in the new host are the nose and mouth.[83] Invasion of the body is thought to occur in three steps: (1) implantation in the nasopharynx, (2) entrance into the bloodstream, and (3) localization in the meninges. For most persons invasion ends with implantation in the nasopharynx—the carrier state.[83]

The carrier state for typeable meningococcal infection begins in adolescence.[39] In ordinary situations about 25% to 38% of the population are carriers of meningococcal organisms, depending on the makeup of the population studied.[45] In patients who have recovered from meningococcal meningitis the carrier state lasts about 6 months; however, some authors[46,83] claim that convalescing patients do not play as much of a part in the spread of disease as do healthy carriers who have never had the disease. It is clear, however, that close contact with patients also increases the risk of infection, for the attack rate in household contacts is 500 to 800 times greater than that in the contemporaneous general population.[45]

The carrier rate for H. *influenzae* is generally higher in healthy young children than in adults.[65] The duration of carriage is unknown, but it is speculated that the organism may be present intermittently or may be present for months.[65] The increased risk of H. influenzae meningitis through close contact has only recently been demonstrated,[38] disproving traditional teaching in medical texts that H. influenzae is a sporadic disease of children and is not contagious.[38,84] A report by Glode et al.[38] suggests that young contacts of a child with H. influenzae are at significant risk of life-threatening secondary disease. They also report that the secondary attack rate in children 5 years or younger in the month after exposure to an index case is as high as 2.3%, or 800 times the endemic attack rate for H. influenzae meningitis.

A common property shared by H. influenzae, meningococcus, pneumococcus, and almost all bacteria that cause meningitis is the polysaccharide capsules they bear on their surfaces.[31,41,83] For each of these pathogens there is substantial evidence that the polysaccharide capsule is a virulence factor and that antibodies directed to the capsule confer protection from disease.[41]

The events stimulating production of bactericidal antibodies are unknown[31]; however, the age-specific incidence of meningitis caused by H. influenzae, N. meningitidis, and S. pneumoniae has been shown to be inversely correlated with the prevalence of antibodies against the bacteria.[33,39,40]

In 1932 Fothergill and Wright[33] reported that bactericidal antibody to H. influenzae could be detected in normal adults and in most newborns. Antibodies were found at birth, declined abruptly at about 2 months, and remained infrequent until about 3 years of age. An increasing number of older children had acquired antibodies such that after the age of 10 years all individuals tested had these antibodies. Although meningitis can develop at any age in the normal host, these findings are reported by some researchers[31,39] to explain, at least in part, the higher incidence of meningitis, by the three common meningeal pathogens, at the age when bactericidal antibodies are least prevalent.

Recent reports of H. influenzae meningitis in adults and the demonstration that adults may lack bactericidal antibodies to this organism have led some investigators to question whether there has been a decline in acquisition of immunity since the studies of Fothergill and Wright.[29,66]

In 1969 Goldschneider, Gotschlich and Artenstein[40] confirmed the role of humoral antibody in immunity to meningococcal meningitis, showing a direct correlation between susceptibility to this infection and the absence of detectable antibody.

Mechanisms reported to contribute to the development of bactericidal antibodies for the acquisition of natural immunity are (1) acquisition of the carrier state, (2) cross-reacting antibody, and (3) cross-reacting antigen.[39] To what extent each of these mechanisms actually contributes to natural immunity remains unsettled. Gold[39] suggests that the relative importance of each may vary with the time, place, and individual.

Meningitis caused by H. influenzae, N. meningitidis, and S. pneumoniae is seasonal, occurring mainly during the late fall, winter, or early spring.[31] In this respect these meningitides are similar to disease caused by other agents spread from person to person by the respiratory route. For example, H. influenzae meningitis is known for its importance as a secondary invader in influenza and other respiratory tract diseases,[83] whereas pneumococcal meningitis is frequently preceded by pneumonia.[2] The predilection among persons with dural defects for meningitis caused by these common pathogens is discussed elsewhere in this chapter.

Meningococcal meningitis is unique in that it may occur in epidemic form.[31,83] Until 1945, major epidemics, typically caused by group A organisms occurred approximately every 10 years in the United States, but for some unexplained reason there has not been one since.[34] Epidemics have occurred recently in Brazil,[31] Finland,[30] and several other countries in the so-called meningitis belt in Africa.[64] Recently there have also been outbreaks of group A meningitis in Manitoba and the skid row areas of Seattle, Washington; Portland, Oregon; and Anchorage, Alaska.[31,34]

Meningococcal meningitis has long been associated with overcrowded living conditions, particularly in barracks or dormitories.[45,83]

In a study of risk factors in Charleston County, South Carolina, Fraser et al.[35] reported that a low socioeconomic status, rather than overcrowded living conditions, was associated with a higher attack rate of H. influenzae meningitis in blacks. They suggested that the number of individuals per room may be less important than good nutrition or the prevention of complications of upper respiratory tract and ear infections through ready access to medical care. They also reported a higher rate for whites living in rural areas, suggesting a geographical barrier to medical therapy or a greater likelihood of exposure and antibody production in more crowded communities.

Pathogens causing meningitis in neonates. The neonatal period, the first 28 days of life, is a time of unprecedented risk for the development of bacterial septicemia and meningitis.[5] Meningitis in the neonate and premature infant accounts for between 7% and 10% of all meningitis and, in some series, up to 75% of the mortality of the disease.[46] The incidence of neonatal meningitis is approximately 1/2500 live births,[46] with about two thirds of the cases occurring in hospitals.[45]

The most frequent causes of meningitis in this group are Enterobacteriaceae, group B streptococci, and Listeria monocytogenes.[31,34] Enterobacteriaceae are responsible for 60% to 70% of the cases; Escherichia coli is isolated from approximately 40% of the patients overall.[45] Group B streptococci are second in frequency, accounting for 15% to 20%.[45]

The factors that facilitate the development of meningitis in the neonate can generally be placed into three groups: maternal, fetal, and environmental.

Maternal factors that facilitate the development of meningitis in the newborn are prolonged labor and traumatic delivery, premature rupture of fetal membranes,[1] and perinatal genitourinary tract infection.[1,8]

Genitourinary tract infection has been a significant finding in neonatal meningitis caused by *E. coli,* group B streptococci, and *Listeria monocytogenes.* Maternal urinary tract infection was the most frequent finding in a study by Berman and Banker.[8] In another study 85 out of 297 women in their third trimester had group B streptococci isolated from cervical and vaginal cultures; 71% of the infants born to these mothers became colonized.[1] In a recent outbreak of neonatal *Listeria* meningitis Felice and Fraser[31] found a high incidence of vaginitis among women of low socioeconomic status and concluded that the infection was vertically transmitted.

Group B streptococcal disease appears in two clinical and epidemiological forms.[31] In the early-onset form septicemia and, occasionally, meningitis occur within a few days of birth and are strongly associated with maternal complications.[1,5,8,31] In the late-onset form meningitis is most common and occurs from 1 week to several weeks after birth; it generally affects well infants whose mothers have not had complications. The distributions of serotypes of organisms causing early- and late-onset disease are different.[31] This clinical and epidemiological description of the early-onset and late-onset form is sometimes used to differentiate between maternally acquired infection and nosocomial infection. This description is used for other neonatal infections as well.

Although the majority of bacterial infections among neonates are the early-onset form and are the result of intrapartum exposure to maternal genital organisms,[1,5,8] an increasing percentage are the late-onset form and are caused by nosocomial pathogens.[5] Nosocomial septicemia and meningitis in newborns can result from their own compromised condition and/or from exposure within the environment (e.g., fetal monitoring).

Factors that place the neonate at high risk for septicemia and meningitis include prematurity and low birth weight (under 1500 g), with its concomitant immature immunological defense mechanisms,[5,45,101] and associated illness (e.g., hyaline membrane disease, congenital malformations, birth asphyxia).[5] Prior exposure to antimicrobial agents that select for resistance has also been implicated.[5,45]

Clinical manifestations—signs and symptoms. All forms of acute bacterial meningitis, whatever the cause, possess a number of symptoms in common.[6] Symptoms can generally be classified into four main categories: infection, meningeal inflammation, alterations in behavioral capacities and level of consciousness, and abnormal neurological findings.[21]

In adults and older children clinical signs of infection appear early in the course of disease and may be misdiagnosed as a severe respiratory tract infection or the "flu."[46] Fever, headache, chills, and malaise are common in almost all cases.[45] The temperature may exceed 101° F, and in some cases sinusitis, otitis, and other signs of focal infection mark the prodrome.

Fever and headache steadily worsen, followed by the major clinical features of meningeal inflammation. Headache is often described as severe beyond anything in the individual's prior experience, bursting in character, unremitting, diffuse, or mainly frontal and often radiating down the neck into the back and limbs.[6] Stiffness of the neck and back and pain on forced movement of the neck are common meningeal signs but may be absent in the very young, deeply stuporous, or comatose patient.[2]

Abnormal neurological findings may include a broad spectrum of symptoms. Alterations in levels of consciousness or behavioral capacities are frequently seen in persons with meningitis but are difficult to evaluate in the very young.

Delirium is common in the early stages, but it may be followed by drowsiness, then stupor, and eventually coma.[6] The presence of coma has been associated with a high mortality rate in meningitis.[46]

Signs of focal cerebral disease are seldom prominent early in the disease process.[2] Some of the more transitory focal cerebral signs may represent postictal phenomena, and others may be related to an unusually intense focal meningitis. Stable focal lesions develop most often in the second week of meningeal infection as a consequence of vasculitis, occlusion of cerebral veins, and infarction of cerebral vessels.[2]

Signs of increasing intracranial pressure may be present. Pupils are often unequal and react sluggishly, and in the later stages they tend to become dilated and fixed. The ocular fundi may be normal or show venous congestion or, rarely, papilledema.[45] Squint and diplopia are often present. Muscular power of the limbs is usually preserved, but some incoordination and tremor are common. Muscular hypertonia occurs quite regularly. A general, flaccid paralysis is a terminal event.

Acute bacterial meningitis in infants and newborns presents a number of special problems because signs and symptoms are largely behavioral and require individual interpretation. Infants cannot complain of headache, and a determinable stiff neck may be absent entirely. Fever, listlessness, and vomiting are by far the major symptoms in this age group and are referred to by Horenstein and Schreiber[46] as the *common triad*. Headache may be presumed if a small child constantly wipes or rubs his head. Vomiting occurs against a background of comparative well-being, without abdominal pain, cramping, diarrhea, or other enteric symptoms. Vomiting is often recurrent and forceful.[45,46]

The problems in the neonate are even more formidable. More often than not, the signs of meningeal irritation are absent, and one has only nonspecific signs and symptoms of systemic illness. Hyperirritability, lethargy, feeding difficulty, respiratory distress, and fever or hypothermia have all been reported in meningeal infection in the neonate.[6,46] Signs of meningeal irritation do occur but only late in the course of the illness. These symptoms may include focal or generalized seizures, bulging fontanels, and a range of consciousness from difficult to arouse to coma.

Since the pathological changes, morbidity, and mortality of acute bacterial meningitis are believed to be largely proportional to the duration of illness before the start of treatment, early recognition is imperative. Almost any other infection can cause fever and headache. If there is a history supported by physical or other findings consistent with otitis media, mastoiditis, sinusitis, or cavernous sinus thrombosis, secondary meningitis must be suspected.[45] Similarly, patients with pneumonia, osteomyelitis, bacteremia from any cause, or head trauma with or without rhinorrhea or otorrhea must be carefully studied for evidence of meningitis.[45]

Meningococcus meningitis should always be suspected in the following circumstances[2]: when the evolution is extremely rapid, when the onset is attended by a petechial or purpuric rash or by large ecchymoses and lividity of the skin of the lower parts of the body, and/or when circulatory collapse has occurred.

Diagnostic tests

CEREBROSPINAL FLUID EXAMINATION. Examination of CSF is the key to definitive diagnosis of acute bacterial meningitis. Most authors[2,45,96] recommend that CSF be examined in every patient in whom the clinical findings are consistent with the eventual possibility of meningitis, no matter how minimal the manifestation. This approach is necessary for the following reasons: (1) bacterial meningitis, untreated, is a lethal infection that may evolve with catastrophic speed, (2) bacterial meningitis treated early with appropriate antibacterial agents is curable, and (3) the selection of appropriate antimicrobial agents often requires etiological diagnosis and may depend on susceptibility testing in vitro.[45]

Normally, CSF is clear, colorless, odorless fluid that looks like water, has a specific gravity of 1.007, and contains an occasional lymphocyte (1 to 3 mm) and traces of minerals and organic materials of the blood, of which the total protein is the most significant. The normal pressure range for CSF is 60 to 180 mm in the lateral recumbent position.[21]

In acute bacterial meningitis pleocytosis of the spinal fluid is diagnostic. The fluid is usually turbid, containing 400 to 20,000 leukocytes per millimeter, of which 90% or more are polymorphonuclear.[45] Occasionally CSF may contain few leukocytes but many bacteria (water clear), and in some specimens there may be a large number of leukocytes and very few bacteria. Cell counts above 50,000/cu mm raise the possibility of a brain abscess that has ruptured into the ventricles.[2]

Gram stain of the spinal fluid may permit early identification of the causative agent.[2] In at least 75% of patients with bacterial meningitis, bacteria are readily found on microscopic examination of a Gram-stained smear of sediment collected by centrifuging CSF.[45] When the observed morphological and tinctorial properties of the bacteria are correlated with the epidemiological and clinical information, an informed guess concerning the specific cause can be made. Diagnostic errors in reading Gram-stained smears of CSF have been attributed to (1) misinterpretation of precipitated dye or debris as gram-positive cocci[2]; (2) confusion of pneumococci with *H. influenzae*[2]; (3) dismissal of organisms as contaminants, particularly those that are part of normal skin flora[28]; (4) contamination of prepackaged lumbar puncture equipment[95]; and (5) contaminated slide baths, which create a false-positive slide.[27] Following are some pitfalls regarding the procurement and bacteriological processing of CSF specimens and CNS abscess exudate, including exogenous and endogenous contaminations, errors in interpretation of Gram-stained smears, and inadequate transport and culture techniques*:

A. Exogenous and endogenous contamination
  1. Poor skin disinfection (lumbar puncture); contamination through bacteria of normal skin flora: staphylococci and *Propionibacterium acnes* (a)
  2. Contamination through aerosols from personnel; bacteria from normal flora of oropharynx and skin (b)
  3. Contamination of commercial lumbar puncture kits through non-viable bacteria, producing false-positive Gram stains (c)
  4. Faulty cleansing of glass slides; storage in contaminated ethanol (d).
B. Errors in interpretation
  1. Erroneous interpretation of stain precipitates and artifacts, such as use of stabilized commercial stain reagents (e)
  2. Gram stain variability of *N. meningitidis* in early stages of meningitis; differential diagnosis: staphylococci (f)
  3. Gram stain resemblance of *H. influenzae* to gram-positive diplococci (g)
  4. Dismissal of valid CSF culture findings as contamination from normal skin flora: *Propionibacterium* species (h)
C. Inadequate transport and processing techniques
  1. Specimen held for insufficient time for growth (anaerobic diphtheroids) (i)
  2. Transport and processing of specimen delayed (anaerobes) (j)
  3. Failure to culture adequately for strict anaerobes (culture media) (k)

*Modified from Traub, W.H.: Adv. Neurosurg. **9:**1-27, 1980. The letters in parentheses refer to references found in Traub's article.

A portion of the specimen of CSF must be cultured, and blood cultures should be obtained simultaneously, preferably before any chemotherapeutic agents are administered. Success in isolation of the etiological agent is more likely to be compromised by prior therapy in meningococcal and pneumococcal meningitis; however, neither smear, cellular response, nor concentration of protein or glucose is significantly affected.[45]

Cultures are best obtained by collecting the fluid in a sterile tube and immediately inoculating plates of blood, chocolate, and MacConkey agar for aerobes; tubes of thioglycolate for anaerobes; and at least one other broth.[2] CSF cultures are positive in 70% to 90% of cases of bacterial meningitis.

An exact etiological diagnosis can sometimes be made promptly by demonstrating capsular swelling on exposure of bacteria concentrated by centrifuging CSF to specific antiserums.[45]

Counterimmunoelectrophoresis has proven to be a valuable tool in diagnosing acute bacterial meningitis. This sensitive technique permits the detection of bacterial antigens in CSF in a matter of 30 to 60 minutes. It is particularly useful in patients with partially treated meningitis in whom CSF still contains bacterial antigen but in whom no organism can be detected on a smear or can be grown in culture.[2]

In acute bacterial meningitis the protein levels are higher than 45 mg/100 ml in 90% of the cases, and most fall in the range of 100 to 500 mg/100 ml.[26] The glucose content is depressed, usually to a level lower than 40 mg/100 ml, or less than 40% of the circulating blood glucose concentration (measured concomitantly).[46] Chloride levels in CSF are usually low—less than 700 mg/100 ml, reflecting dehydration and low serum chloride levels.[2]

Also of diagnostic and prognostic value is the measurement of CSF lactate dehydrogenase (LDH).[2] A rise in total LDH activity is consistently observed in patients with bacterial meningitis, most of this caused by fractions 4 and 5, which are derived from granulocytes. LDH fractions 1 and 2 are presumably derived from brain tissue and are only slightly elevated in bacterial meningitis; however, they rise sharply in patients who die or who develop neurological sequelae. Thus the test may be helpful in singling out the patient who is most at risk.[2]

CSF levels of lactic acid are also consistently elevated in bacterial and fungal meningitis.[2] A level above 35 mg/100 ml may be a helpful titer to distinguish bacterial and fungal disorders from viral meningitides in which lactic levels remain normal.

OTHER CULTURES. Blood cultures should be obtained concomitantly with CSF cultures before antimicrobial therapy is begun. Blood cultures are positive in 40% to 60% of patients with bacterial meningitis, and they may provide the only definite clue to the causative agent if CSF cultures are negative.

Large numbers of *N. meningitidis* may be recovered from developing petechiae.

Patients suspected of having meningitis should also have their nose, throat, urine, and ears cultured. In the case of ear infections any organisms removed should be typed for comparison with any others of the same species that might be retrieved from the blood or urine.[46]

Routine cultures of the pharynx may be misleading because pneumococci, *H. influenzae*, and meningococci are common inhabitants of healthy persons. However, such cultures may be helpful. Typeable encapsulated *H. influenzae* or groupable meningococci provide a clue to the cause of meningitis. The absence of such findings makes *H. influenzae* and meningococcus meningitis unlikely.[2]

Routes of bacterial invasion. There are essentially three primary routes of bacterial invasion of the CNS:

- Hematogenous
- Direct bacterial invasion
- Device- and procedure-related infections

HEMATOGENOUS. Very little is known regarding the hematogenous route of bacterial infection except that in some cases of meningitis a bacteremia is the only apparent forerunner of infection.[46,101] Theoretically, every patient with a bacteremia or septicemia is susceptible to meningitis or cerebral abscess; however, in most cases of blood infection the CNS does not seem to be infected.[2]

Invasion of the CNS by microorganisms secondary to bacteremia from primary infections elsewhere in the body is the most common basis for acute bacterial CNS infections.[101] Primary infections of the skin, lungs, intestinal tract, biliary system, and urinary tract are the most frequent sources of bacteremia resulting in meningitis, epidural or subdural abscesses of the spinal cord, or brain abscesses.

The predilection among persons with dural defects for bacterial meningitis is well known; however, patients with head injuries that do not disrupt the dura mater may be at risk for meningitis as well.[46] Contusions, infarctions, or subdural collections of blood may become secondarily infected if the patient has bacteremia.

DIRECT BACTERIAL INVASION. Patients with head injuries that transgress the skull and meninges are at risk for bacterial meningitis simply because of the nature of their wounds. The wound, however, is usually not sufficient by itself to produce CNS infection such as meningitis.[45] In these situations the onset of meningitis will usually depend on the presence of materials that provide a suitable culture medium for bacterial growth, such as blood clots, devitalized tissue,[45,46] or CSF fistula, which then serves as a persistent portal of entry for bacteria.[44,46]

Meningitis frequently complicates missile injuries (e.g., gunshot wounds of the head with indriven fragments that leave large amounts of dead tissue or blood clots).[45,46] *Staphylococcus aureus* or *Staphylococcus epidermidis* is most commonly identified when the organism has been implanted with foreign materials.[45] Missile injuries may also be complicated by basal or discontinuous fractures of the skull with subsequent development of CSF fistulas.[62]

A CSF fistula, an abnormal communication between the nasopharynx and the meninges, may develop when there has been a basal skull fracture in the region of the frontal or ethmoid sinuses or cribriform plate.[44] A CSF fistula may also develop in patients who appear to have a closed head injury.[46] In either case, if a fistula develops, the patient is particularly prone to pneumococcal, α streptococcal, and *S. epidermidis* meningitis. Patients may enter the hospital with wounds already contaminated through direct inoculation of bacteria at the time of injury. Mixed or unusual organisms may also indicate a nosocomial infection.

A CSF leak from the nose (rhinorrhea) is the most important indication of a CSF fistula but may be absent or difficult to detect in some patients.[44,62] A fracture through the petrous bone may also result in a CSF fistula and otorrhea (CSF from the ears), which may subsequently lead to meningitis. This avenue, however, is less common for posttraumatic meningitis than fractures involving the frontal bone.[44]

The clinical symptoms of bacterial meningitis may be the first and only indication of a CSF fistula. Two unique characteristics of an abnormal communication between the nasopharynx and the meninges are the delay from time of injury to onset of infection, which can vary from several hours to many years, and recurrent attacks of meningitis.[44,62] A CSF fistula is reported to be the most common cause of recurrent bacterial meningitis in the adult[2] and is usually attributed to failure to recognize the defect and close the dura mater primarily or by graft.[62]

The incidence of bacterial meningitis in association with CSF fistulas has been reported to be as high as 39% in one series.[62] In another study 16 adult patients developed 32 episodes of posttraumatic meningitis; 13 of the patients had a demonstrable skull fracture with CSF rhinorrhea documented in 12 patients.[44]

Early detection of CSF fistulas as a means of prevention of nosocomial meningitis is of primary importance.[44] Patients who enter the hospital with obvious head trauma or with meningitis possibly related to head trauma should be carefully evaluated for evidence of skull fracture and CSF rhinorrhea. On the nursing units nasal secretions can easily be tested for glucose with "sticks" containing glucose oxidase (Dextrostix). Because nasal secretions normally contain only small amounts of glucose, a positive reaction with Dextrostix offers evidence of the presence of CSF, which normally contains much higher concentrations of glucose. More sensitive glucose oxidase reagents (Tes-Tape and Clinistix) should not be used to test nasal secretions, since these have been reported to give positive reactions in the absence of CSF rhinorrhea.[44] Recognition of such a defect by radiographic means is difficult but may be facilitated by tomography or detection of the leak by the use of dye, a now obsolete method, or the instillation into the subarachnoid space of radioactive iodinated human serum albumin or radioactive indium.[46] If a CSF leak exists, scanning may show the appearance of the isotope in the nasal secretions.

External structural barriers may become the pathways for bacterial invasion of the CNS by extension of infection or by direct inoculation. Infection by extension occurs from structures such as the scalp, the bones of the skull (osteomyelitis), the paranasal sinus, the middle ear or mastoid, or the congenital sinus tracts.[2,6]

There are two common pathways from these sources: (1) infected thrombi may form in diploic veins and spread along these vessels into the dural sinuses (into which the CSF empties) and from there in retrograde fashion along the meningeal veins into the brain, and (2) an osteomyelitis focus may form with erosion of the inner table of bone and invasion of the dura mater, subdural space, pia mater and arachnoid, and even the brain substance.[2] Each of these pathways has been cited as a cause of leptomeningitis, epidural abscess, subdural empyema, and brain abscess.[22,100]

Direct bacterial invasion through cranial and spinal structures may occur with traumatic head injuries,[44] congenital malformations such as spina bifida,[45] neurodiagnostic procedures such as lumbar puncture,[23] and neurosurgical procedures involving the central or peripheral nervous system, contiguous bone, or other adjacent tissues.[42]

DEVICE- AND PROCEDURE-RELATED INFECTIONS

INTRACRANIAL PRESSURE MONITORING SYSTEMS. Increased intracranial pressure can cause permanent neurological damage, impaired cerebral circulation, and brain mass shift, leading to herniation of cranial contents and death. Clinical signs do not accurately allow for assessment of this life-threatening phenomenon; therefore intracranial pressure monitoring (ICPM) may be used for patients with either a head injury or craniotomy to assess, treat, and control the problem. ICPM allows a more rational approach to maintaining intracranial pressure within desired parameters through administration of drugs such as hyperosmotics and steroids and through controlled ventilation and CSF drainage from the ventricles.

The three types of ICPM devices commonly used are epidural, subdural, and intraventricular. The systems are prone to bacterial contamination and subsequent infection from several sources:

1. Direct inoculation during insertion of the sensing devices
2. Exogenous skin contamination and entry through the outside sensing wire

3. Contamination of the ICPM equipment, stopcocks, transducers, dome chambers, and pressure gauges
4. Contamination of CSF through subsequent leaks around the catheter

A brief description of the three systems and their placement follows:

Epidural. A burr hole is made, and a balloon with an extracranial transducer, a miniature intracranial transducer, or a fiberoptic transducer, is placed between the skull and the dura mater. The advantages to this placement and method is that it is less invasive and has no outside connections.[47] This system measures the pressure of the brain mass on the dura mater.[16] Sometimes the transducer is placed subdurally. When the dura mater is breached and because external wires are then required, the risk of infection is greater.[16]

Subdural. A twist drill burr hole is usually made over the right coronal suture 3 cm from the midline.[47] The dura mater is opened, and a small rubber catheter, a Scott cannula, or a hollow subarachnoid screw is inserted below the dura mater in the subarachnoid space. The other end of the catheter or screw is connected to an external electronic pressure transducer, a three-way stopcock, and fluid-filled pressure tubing. The transducer then converts fluid pressure into electric signals. When the system is calibrated, the electronic signals may be displayed on a bedside or nursing station monitor as a measurement of fluid pressure. Although this system offers access for volume-pressure determination, its invasive placement substantially increases the risk of infection.[37]

Intraventricular system. This system is also referred to as a ventriculostomy system and is frequently used for drainage of CSF from the ventricles. A twist drill burr hole is made at either the paramedian coronal suture or the forehead.[85] The dura mater is opened, and a small rubber or polyethylene catheter is inserted into the anterior horn of the lateral ventricle, usually on the nondominant side. The catheter is attached to the ICPM system in the same manner as in the subdural system, except when CSF drainage is anticipated or desirable. In the latter situation another three-way stopcock, intravenous tubing, and an intravenous transfer pack or sterile empty intravenous bag are usually added to the lines to allow for drainage collection and measurement of CSF. Patients with this system have a greater risk of infection because of the invasive presence in the ventricles, multiple stopcocks, and CSF drainage.

Lundberg's 1960 monograph[57] indicted a very low infection rate following ventricular pressure monitoring. However, in a recent series, Wyler and Kelly[99] reported an infection rate varying from 9% to 27% in 102 ventriculostomies. Poll, Waldhausen, and Brock[71] report an infection rate of 2% with no significant difference in the rate with or without CSF drainage. In these series S. aureus was the organism most frequently identified. However, in another study gram-negative organisms such as *Pseudomonas* and *Klebsiella* were identified as the predominant causative agents of meningitis.[85]

Infection from intraventricular pressure monitoring and CSF drainage is a risk usually regarded as acceptable considering the benefits of these procedures in diagnosis and treatment of patients with intracranial disease.[85] Smith and Alksne[85] recommend that when a ventriculostomy is placed primarily for pressure monitoring, the question of infection as a potential hazard must be carefully weighed against the value of the information gained.[85] In the meantime researchers continue to explore methods of placement and technique that will offer guidelines for prevention of sepsis and CNS infection.

The insertion technique for ICPM devices has been found to be important for prevention of wound infection and meningitis. It is best done in the operating room under routine or sterile conditions. Before insertion, a generous area of the scalp around the site of placement should be shaved and the scalp painted with tincture of iodine, followed by alcohol.[15,85] The area should be carefully draped with sterile plastic or cloth. The dural opening should be no larger than absolutely necessary to accommodate the ventricular catheter, so as to decrease the possibility of CSF egress along the catheter tract.[57,85] Leakage of CSF through the incision has been reported to be the cause of wound infection and meningitis.[85,99] For this reason some authors[85] have abandoned the use of the drill twist bit to perforate the dura mater. Smith and Alksne[85] report that they have had no further occurrence of CSF leak after modifying the procedure to penetration of the dura mater with a 15-gauge needle, which they feel allows a tighter fit around an 8-gauge French tube.

The catheter and connections must be well secured to prevent contamination from slippage or disconnection by a confused and restless patient. Some hospital procedures recommend purse-string sutures around the catheter.[47] In restless patients wrist restraints may be necessary for the time the system is in place. In the event that the system becomes disconnected the existing stopcocks and tubing should never be reconnected.[37] Instead, a new and sterile system must be immediately applied after covering the catheter with sterile dressings.

Recommendations for dressing changes vary with institution policy and physician preference. In some institutions the original dressing is not disturbed until the system is removed. Some procedures call for dressing changes every 24 hours beginning 48 hours after placement.[47] Dressings and manipulation of the line are done only by experienced personnel. In any case the dressing should be labeled with the date of insertion, and subsequent dressing changes and the nursing care plan should clearly state directions for care and maintenance of the system. Only personnel who have been certified in ICPM and care and maintenance of the system should have direct responsibility for the care of these patients.

Duration of the time the intraventricular system is in place has also been reported to be directly related to sepsis and meningitis.[99] (Ideally, placement should not exceed 72 hours.) In some series the duration has not been found to be significant in the incidence of infections.[85] Antibiotic prophylaxis has been reported to significantly reduce the rate of infection in patients who have ventriculostomies in place longer than 3 days.[99]

Intermittent obstruction of the tubing with subsequent irrigation to remove the blockage has been identified with a high infection rate.[99] For this reason some authors[85,100] recommend using an 8-gauge catheter instead of the standard small-bore shunt tubing. In the event that the tubing becomes obstructed the physician should be the only person allowed to irrigate the line. Unlike intravascular pressure monitoring systems, ICPM systems must never have continuous flush devices (Intraflo) attached to irrigate the system.[37]

Because the CNS is a sterile system, ICPM systems should be considered and maintained as a closed system.[15,85] Although this might be possible with epidural and subdural systems, the presence of multiple stopcocks for CSF drainage and sampling in the intraventricular system makes this goal more difficult. Closed systems can be achieved in part by avoiding air-vented collection bottles for CSF drainage.[72,85] Poppen[72] reported no infection in 500 ventriculostomies used for drainage in which he employed a closed system. Similarly, Smith and Alksne[85] reported no further occurrence of sepsis related to ventriculostomy after conversion from an air-vented bottle to the closed system. Prevention of exogenous contamination should be directed toward covering all stopcock outlets with sterile caps, keeping stopcocks on a sterile towel, and using aseptic technique when CSF samples are withdrawn.

Further recommendations and general guidelines for care and maintenance of invasive pressure monitoring equipment (e.g., domes, transducers) may be found in Chapter 13.

CEREBROSPINAL FLUID SHUNT SYSTEMS. CSF shunt is inserted primarily for the surgical treatment of hydrocephalus. The most commonly used shunts are ventriculoatrial (VA) and ventriculoperitoneal (VP). The one-way valve system shunts CSF from the ventricles to another body space. A shunt is generally placed in the ventricles through a burr hole and brought into the jugular venous system, the pleurae, and other areas.[92]

Bacterial infections associated with CSF shunts remain a major cause of morbidity and mortality.[79,80] The types of infections associated with CSF shunts include meningitis and ventriculitis,[68] endocarditis secondary to VA shunts, peritonitis secondary to VP shunts, and abscess formation along the shunt tubing tract.[92]

Clinical manifestations of meningitis or ventriculitis associated with shunt infections are usually related to the type of shunt system implanted, the virulence of the organism, and the inoculum size of the organism.[92] A shunt may initially occlude, leading to increased intracranial pressure. A valve in the peritoneal cavity may produce peritoneal signs if an abscess forms at the catheter site. An infected valve in the atrium may produce endocarditis. However, patients usually exhibit nonspecific complaints, such as stiff neck, nausea, vomiting, and malaise.[92] Fever appears to be associated with almost all shunt infections.[79,80] In patients with VP shunts erythema overlying the tubing may be the initial clinical sign.[79] Problems with feeding or activity are frequently seen in infants and small children.

In a recent 10-year series[79] of 289 hydrocephalic patients who had a total of 442 shunts placed and 743 operations, 27% of the patients had one or more shunt-related infections; 22% of the shunts became infected for an overall rate of 13.2% per surgical procedure. In this study the type of shunt placed made little difference in the infection rate. A similar rate of infection was reported in another series of patients with VA shunts: 15.7% of shunt insertions were followed by infection and 1.3% of the revisions for an overall rate of 14%.[81] In both series S. epidermidis was the most commonly identified organism.

The insertion of a shunt system poses several infection risks. First, the insertion technique may require several small cutaneous incisions to complete the system placement through a subcutaneous tunneling device, thus providing several sources for entry of organisms. Second, the shunt is a foreign body that may serve as a continuous source for infection. Third, shunt revisions for malfunctions may be frequent, requiring the insertion of a new shunt system each time.[92] Fourth, it is necessary to revise VA shunts to accommodate for growth and to relieve obstruction throughout the life of the patient.[81] A patient undergoing repetitive procedures would experience an increased patient case infection rate.

Shunt infections generally occur within 30 days of placement, and, as already mentioned, common skin flora are usually responsible. Although less common, infections caused by gram-negative organisms such as E. coli, Pseudomonas species and Klebsiella species have also been reported to be the result of perioperative contamination.[80]

Frequent errors in diagnosis of shunt infections have apparently been made by dismissal of organisms isolated as contaminants, particularly those that are part of normal skin flora.[28,79] Experts urge that all positive blood and CSF cultures in patients with shunts be considered presumptive evidence of infection rather than contamination.[79] The recent isolation of Propionibacterium species[28] as the causative agent of meningitis associated with shunt infection in six patients thoroughly supports this recommendation. These organisms grow slowly; therefore spinal fluid should be held for at least 14 days before being reported as negative.

In episodes of shunt infections multiple CSF and blood cultures should be obtained before antimicrobial therapy is begun. It has been suggested that pumping the shunt before blood cultures are taken may be helpful in express-ing organisms in the bloodstream.[79]

The exact pathogenesis of CSF shunt infection has not been elucidated. Bacteremia is frequently seen in patients with VA shunts[79] but is unusual in infected VP shunts.[81] Some authors[55,81] hypothesize that shunt infections occur when the distal catheter draining CSF causes local trauma and the formation of thrombi. These in turn may become infected from transient bacteremia, and ascending infection may result. Others argue that if shunt infections are usu-ally related to the occurrence of transient bacteremia, one would expect to see distribution of infection throughout the life of the shunt with no particular relationship to surgery.[79] The latter argument supports the theory that the most important factor is the introduction of organisms during the perioperative period.

Patients with shunts also appear to be at increased risk of infection by bacteria that commonly cause meningitis in the general population: *H. in-fluenzae*, *S. pneumoniae*, and *N. meningitidis*.[68,79,80] The reason for the in-creased risk is unknown, and the pathogenesis is poorly understood.

Preoperative diagnostic procedures that involve puncture of CNS mem-branes have been reported to predispose to indolent infection that does not become evident until after a subsequent shunt placement.[81] Although Shurtleff, Christie, and Foltz[81] report these procedures as responsible for infection in six children with shunts, the procedures are not defined. In another study lumbar puncture, ventricular taps, ventriculograms, and other diagnostic and thera-peutic procedures involving entry into the CNS were not found to be associated with a higher rate of infection in patients with shunts.[79] The authors attribute these results to a reflection of good technique rather than the absence of risk.

Treatment of shunt infections requires removal and replacement and/or systemic and intraventricular treatment with appropriate antibioics. In one study of 28 patients with VA shunt infections caused by *S. epidermidis* Shurt-leff et al.[82] reported a 100% cure rate with complete shunt replacement in a different site, combined with either systemic or systemic and intraventricular antibiotic therapy.

Patients entering the hospital for shunt placement or with a shunt already in place should be generally considered at high risk for nosocomial infections. Personnel caring for these patients should be aware of the potential for bac-teremic seeding of these foreign bodies, as well as the risks of wound infection. Predisposing factors to sepsis must be taken into consideration in medical and nursing therapies. The shunt must be sterile on insertion, and care must be taken to prevent local contamination.

SPINAL CORD PROCEDURES. Bacterial meningitis resulting from spinal procedures is apparently rare. Although the literature addresses the possibility of menin-gitis following spinal surgery as a result of extension of infection into deeper tissues, there are few definitive studies published. There have been a few cases of iatrogenic meningitis reported as a result of lumbar puncture and spinal anesthesia, but cases are infrequent.

The most important predisposing factor to nosocomial meningitis as a result of spinal surgery is the development of a wound infection.[92] Regional extension into deeper adjacent structures could produce meningitis, epidural abscess, subdural empyema, or vertebral osteomyelitis.

The incidence of nosocomial infection related to neurosurgical spinal procedures has been reported at 2.3%[42,78]; however, the type of infection is not described. Buckwold, Hand, and Hansebout[13] reported a single case in a 15-year period of bacterial meningitis as a result of laminectomy. In the latter study a pseudomonal organism was the causative agent.

Diagnostic or therapeutic procedures that involve puncture of CNS membranes predispose to meningitis by direct inoculation of bacteria into the subarachnoid space. In a recent series Corbett and Rosenstein[23] described three cases of *Pseudomonas* meningitis that resulted from lumbar puncture done on obstetrical patients at a small general hospital. The three patients were infected from a common reservoir, contaminated saline, and by a common mode, rinsing the sterile needle stylet in the unsterile saline.

The incidence of meningitis following spinal anesthesia has been reported as 1 in 22,000 cases.[23]

DEVICES AND PROCEDURES ASSOCIATED WITH THE NEONATE. Premature and low birth weight infants, as well as those with congenital illnesses, are frequently exposed to environmental risks through prolonged hospitalization in neonatal intensive care units. The risks for nosocomial septicemia and meningitis in this setting are associated with the use of potentially contaminated life-support equipment, such as intravenous catheters and solutions,[30] transducer devices,[15] and respiratory equipment.[25] Conditions that enhance infant contact with multiple antibiotic-resistant, gram-negative enteric bacteria, such as overcrowding, high nurse/infant ratios, and poor handwashing, also contribute to the high risk.[5]

Many of these factors are interrelated, and the precise contribution of a single determinant of risk in an individual is usually impossible to assess.

The source from which the nosocomial pathogen is introduced into the nursery is usually not known; however, introduction of gram-negative enteric bacilli commonly occurs from an individual infant contaminated by his own antibiotic-altered bowel flora or improperly sterilized life-support equipment.[5] Organisms may also be brought in from another hospital. Introduction by nursery personnel is common in infections caused by S. aureus and group A streptococcus.[5] A recent study by Aber et al.[1] implicates hospital personnel as reservoirs for group B streptococcus.

Baker[5] reports that the major reservoir for nosocomial microorganisms in the nursery environment is the colonized infants themselves. Once introduction of a particular strain has occurred, the major transmission of the agent is from colonized neonates to noncolonized infants by the hands of nursery personnel.

CRANIOTOMY. Hematogenous dissemination of organisms from intravenous and Foley catheter sites and other acute infections from remote sites in the body are the most likely pathogenesis in patients who develop meningitis more than 7 days after a neurosurgical procedure.[13] Buckwold, Hand, and Hansebout[13] reported that 80% of the cases of meningitis in neurosurgical patients were caused by gram-negative bacilli: *Klebsiella, Enterobacter,* and *Serratia* organisms. These findings were consistent with those of Mangi, Quintilani, and Andriole,[60] who reported gram-negative bacilli as the primary cause of nosocomial meningitis in neurosurgical patients. In the latter study the infecting organism was isolated from another site before or on the same day of the initial isolation from CSF in 79% of the patients: wound (12%), blood (9%), urine (7%), and upper respiratory tract (7%).

A patient with severe head injuries may require ventilatory assistance as a therapeutic measure to reduce cerebral edema. Controlled ventilation to reduce the plasma P_{CO_2} level to approximately 25 to 30 mm Hg results in constriction of cerebral blood vessels, thereby controlling, to some degree, the volume of blood that is delivered to the brain.

A patient with a head injury or craniotomy is subject to nosocomial pneumonia from other sources as well, including limited independent movement that may predispose to hypostatic pneumonia and frequent or continuous long-term tube feedings that may result in aspiration pneumonia. The patient may also require tracheal suctioning, compromising or circumventing the cilia and/or mucous membrane.

Obviously, careful attention to procedure regarding the use and maintenance of respiratory assistance devices and tracheostomy care is particularly vital to these patients, who frequently require long-term use. Equally important is adherence to correct tube feeding protocol to prevent aspiration pneumonia and repositioning of the patient at frequent intervals to prevent pulmonary and circulatory problems. Further recommendations for the prevention of hospital-acquired pneumonia may be found in Chapter 16.

Wound infection following craniotomy may result in meningitis, cerebritis, abscess formation, and death.[78] The most common causative agent in post-craniotomy wound infection is S. *aureus.*[42,58,78] Wound care using sterile technique is critical in reducing the incidence of meningitis secondary to a wound infection.

Overall, one of the most important points that needs to be emphasized by the ICP for prevention of postoperative wound infection is that the source of the infecting organism in nonoutbreak situations is usually the patient. Organisms from the environment can also cause disease if the patient becomes contaminated with them.

Subdural empyema. Subdural empyema is an intracranial suppurative process, usually involving one cerebral hemisphere, between the inner surface of the dura mater and the outer surface of the arachnoid. Subdural empyema accounts for about 20% of all cases of intracranial abscess[22] and is associated with a 40% mortality rate.[11,22]

Subdural empyema is most often associated with paranasal sinus infection[11,22,53] but also occurs with otitis,[22] head trauma,[11] facial infections,[53] intracranial surgery, and, rarely, hematogenous seeding of the subdural space.[22]

The usual route of infection of the subdural space is from the frontal and ethmoid sinuses or, less often, from the middle ear or mastoid cells.[2] Infection is thought to occur by extension through bony defects or osteomyelitis[11] or from sinuses through retrograde thrombophlebitis.[100]

In cases of sinus origin some authors[22,100] report aerobic nonhemolytic streptococci, α-hemolytic streptococci and S. epidermidis as the most frequently isolated organisms from cultures of subdural exudate. Others[11] report anaerobic streptococci and Bacteroides species as the predominant organisms. Subdural empyema following subdural surgery is likely to be caused by S. aureus, α-hemolytic streptococci, or gram-negative organisms.[22] In children under 5 years of age subdural empyema almost invariably follows bacterial meningitis, and the causative agent is the same as that causing the meningitis itself.

Subdural empyema is a rapidly fatal disease when it is not promptly recognized and treated with appropriate antibiotics and surgical drainage.[11,100] The collection of subdural pus causes pressure to be exerted on the underlying brain mass in the same manner as subdural hematoma and frequently creates an ipsilateral temporal lobe pressure cone.[2] The clinical picture is characteristic of and corresponds to a diffuse paralysis of the cortex, usually of one cerebral hemisphere, accompanied by signs and symptoms of focal neurological injury and increasing intracranial pressure.[100]

Subdural empyema secondary to otorrhinological disease can usually be recognized from the clinical course. Following acute sinusitis or, less often, otitis, severe headache appears with disturbance of consciousness, high temperature, chills, stiff neck, and, occasionally, frontal or orbital swelling and tenderness.[22] After a short period focal neurological signs appear, including homonymous hemianopsia (paralysis of lateral gaze), unilateral third nerve palsy, hemiplegia, hemianesthesia, aphasia, and focal unilateral seizures.[2,22]

In cases of subdural empyema secondary to subdural surgery or head trauma, clinical deterioration with signs of increased intracranial pressure, the appearance of new focal neurological signs, and fever with leukocytosis suggest superimposed subdural empyema.[22]

Lumbar puncture, in the presence of signs of increased intracranial pressure, can be extremely hazardous because of the potential for temporal lobe herniation.[11,22] However, when tested, the usual CSF findings are increased pressure and pleocytosis in the range of 50 to 1000/mm^3 with polymorphonuclear cells predominating.[2] The CSF protein is elevated, 75 to 300 mg/100 ml, and the glucose is normal. The fluid is usually sterile.[22]

Other diagnostic procedures are preferred to lumbar puncture in determining the presence of subdural empyema: roentgenograms of the skull or sinus, computerized axial tomography (CAT) scans, ventriculography, and arteriography. Arteriography is presently considered to be the most reliable method for detecting the presence of subdural empyema.[22]

Cultures of the pus recovered from the subdural space and from brain abscess have been reported to present major problems in accurate diagnosis of the causative agents.[11,32,100] In about half of the cases no organism can be isolated or seen on Gram stain.[2] Some authors[11,100] feel that inadequate specimen transport or culture technique accounts for the high incidence of sterile cultures and suggest that anaerobic bacteria may be more common in subdural empyema than previously reported.

Using sterile techniques for collection, transportation, and cultivation of anaerobic bacteria, Brook[11] isolated a total of 51 anaerobic and aerobic bacteria from 19 pediatric patients with subdural empyema or brain abscess. All 19 specimens yielded bacterial growth; anaerobic organisms alone were recovered in 63%; mixed aerobic and anaerobic bacteria were present in 26%; and aerobic bacteria alone were present in 11%. Brook's findings clearly demonstrate the need for meticulous collection of anaerobic cultures from pathological material at the time of surgery. Considerable care should be taken to ensure placement of the specimens in an adequate anaerobic environment with proper transport media and their rapid transportation to the laboratory. It is also important to use proper culture media in the processing and identification of anaerobic organisms.

Brain abscess. Brain abscesses may be single, multiple, or multilocular,[98] each consisting of a layer of pus surrounded by granulation tissue, with new vessels feeding the abscess and new hyperplastic tissue forming a thick, fibrous capsule.[94] The development of an abscess occurs in several stages, beginning with an acute inflammation of brain tissue and ending with an encapsulated, irregularly shaped mass containing approximately 5 to 10 ml of purulent exudate. This process is accompanied by an enormous amount of surrounding edema that is often of greater volume that that of the abscess and is responsible for much of the space-occupying effect.[94]

Brain abscesses almost always follow metastatic spread of infection from a chronic focus of suppuration elsewhere in the body.[2] The most common underlying condition predisposing to brain abscess is otitis media, with or without mastoiditis.[32] In order of frequency, other predisposing conditions are hematogenous spread from infections of the lungs or pleural spaces (e.g., chronic lung abscess, bronchiectasis, empyema, and necrotizing pneumonia[32]) and, less frequently, cardiac abnormalities, such as infected valves or congenital defects[10]; frontal or ethmoid sinusitis; and head injury or intracranial surgery.[10] In approximately 20% of the cases the source cannot be ascertained.[10] The site of primary infection or the underlying condition is a determinant of the cause of the abscess[11,32] Anaerobic organisms are the major etiological agents of brain abscess.[11,32]

Brain abscesses secondary to disease of the middle ear and mastoid or sinuses are usually solitary lesions[91] that result from extension of infection through cranial bones or that spread along vessel walls.[32] *Bacteroides* organisms are the most common anaerobic bacteria isolated in this setting.[32] *Fusobacterium* organisms, streptococci (anaerobic, microaerophilic, and aerobic), and Enterobacteriaceae have also been found.[10,11,32]

Hematogenous spread of infection from the lungs usually results in multiple abscesses and is believed to involve transport of infected material through the valve-free spinal venous system.[32] This source of brain abscess is rarely seen in children.[11] *Fusobacterium* species are the most common cause of anaerobic brain abscess related to the lungs and pleural spaces.[32]

With the exception of congenital heart disease, cardiac abnormalities, such as acute bacterial endocarditis, frequently give rise to small multiple brain abscesses.[2] About 5% of cases of congenital heart disease usually predispose to solitary brain abscess.[2,32]

Tetralogy of Fallot is by far the most common congenital cardiac defect; however, any right-to-left shunt that allows bypass of the filtering effect of the lungs may be implicated.[2] Anaerobic and microaerophilic streptococci, as well as α-hemolytic streptococci, are common isolates in abscesses associated with congenital heart disease.[11]

Brain abscesses resulting from head trauma and intracranial surgery evolve in much the same way as described for acute bacterial meningitis. *Staphylococci* remain the most common isolates in these situations[10]; however, Finegold[32] points out that anaerobic *Clostridium perfringens* and other clostridial organisms are also encountered in abscess secondary to trauma.

An intracerebral abscess may act as a rapidly expanding mass and compress the midbrain and brainstem structures, leading to coma and death.[14,76] Delayed and/or missed diagnosis, brain abscess ruptures into the ventricles,[76] multiple abscesses, and brainstem abscesses[10] have all been reported to account for the 40% to 50% mortality rate associated with brain abscess. Similarly, lumbar puncture has also been reported to contribute to the mortality in these patients.[2,10,14,76] In one study lumbar puncture accounted for 8% of the deaths in patients with brain abscess.[14] Postoperative deaths are reportedly caused by the failure to locate the abscess in surgery or untoward events such as cerebritis, edema, or hemorrhage.[14]

Patients with brain abscess who have intact midbrain structures are more likely to survive than those manifesting midbrain or brainstem compression.[76] When a brain abscess is suspected, close neurological observation is imperative while the patient is being treated with antibiotics and undergoing diagnostic tests. Any deterioration in the level of consciousness or significant increase in neurological deficit demands immediate surgical attention, usually excision and drainage of the abscess.[76]

Obviously, early recognition is essential; however, the clinical picture is often misleading. There is no stereotypical clinical course. For example, a brain abscess is frequently first seen as an expanding intracranial lesion with accompanying headache and neurological signs, rather than an infectious process.[10,14] Headache is the most frequent initial symptom of abscess[2] and is sometimes accompanied by nausea and vomiting.[14] Other presenting symptoms, roughly in order of frequency, are drowsiness, confusion, focal or generalized seizure, and focal, motor, sensory, or speech disorders. The nature of focal neurological signs will depend on the location of the abscess. Fever may or may not be present. Although fever is characteristic of the invasive phase of a cerebral abscess, the temperature may return to normal as the abscess becomes encapsulated. Papilledema is usually a late symptom. Early symptoms may improve with antimicrobial agents, but within a few days or weeks they may recur with increased intensity.[2]

Diagnosis of cerebral abscess is based on the patient's symptoms and also on results of CAT scan, arteriography, radioactive technetium scan, ventriculography, echoencephalography, electroencephalography (EEG), and x-ray studies of the skull and sinuses.[91]

Lumbar puncture as a diagnostic tool is not recommended in patients suspected of brain abscess because of the high mortality associated with this test, the lack of localizing infection, misleading laboratory results, and evidence of spinal fluid sterility.[14,76]

Viral etiology

Viral meningitis and encephalitis. CNS infections caused by viruses can be grouped into two categories: aseptic meningitis and encephalitis.

Aseptic viral meningitis involves an inflammatory process of the coverings of the brain and spinal cord. Encephalitis occurs when the inflammatory process involves parenchymal brain tissue. The prognosis for meningitis is favorable; however, significant morbidity and mortality accompany encephalitis.

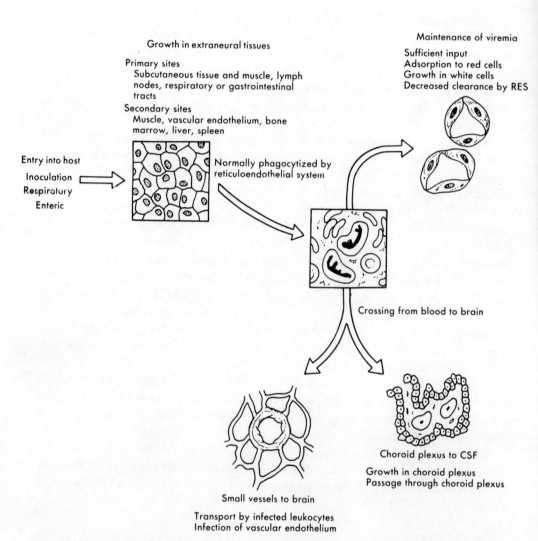

FIG. 18-3. Hematogenous spread of virus to central nervous system. (From Johnson, R.T.: Pathophysiology and epidemiology of acute viral infections of the nervous system, Adv. Neurol. **6**:27-40, 1974, Raven Press, New York.)

The hematogenous route is considered to be the most important pathway of viral spread to the CNS.[2,45,51] The steps in the hematogenous spread of viral infection are illustrated in Fig. 18-3.[2,48]

After entry into the body by one of several pathways (e.g., respiratory tract passages, oral route, genital route) the virus multiplies, probably at sites regional to the portal of entry, and gives rise to a viremia.[45] Extraneural target organs are infected as a consequence of primary viremia. Virus shed into the bloodstream from multiplications in extraneural tissue may prolong the viremia[51] or give rise to a secondary viremia.[45] The virus must then penetrate the blood-brain or blood-CSF barrier to infect susceptible cells within the brain or spinal cord.[45,51]

Hoeprich[45] offers the hypothesis that penetration of the blood-brain and blood-CSF barriers may be accomplished by means of virus-laden phagocytes migrating through blood vessels of the meninges or brain or by passage of virus particles through the choroid plexus or other areas of preferential permeability. Viral agents have been identified as the cause not only of inflammatory diseases but also malformations, tumors, and degenerative demyelinating and vascular diseases of the brain.[50]

According to Johnson,[50] one of the reasons that viral invasion of the CNS causes such diverse clinical and pathological effects is that different cell populations within the CNS vary in their susceptibility to infection with different viruses. For example, some infections are confined to the meninges, in which case the clinical manifestations will be those of aseptic meningitis. Others will involve parenchymal cells of the brain or spinal cord, causing more serious disorders, such as poliomyelitis and encephalitis. Some viruses are even more selective and involve only specific neural cell populations. For example, poliomyelitis is a disease that involves selective vulnerability of anterior horn cells, which leads to characteristic lower motor neuron paralysis. The exception to the selective involvement theory is thought to occur in the case of herpes simplex type 1 (HSV-1). Several theories have been postulated to explain the special characteristics of this virus (see p. 523).

Numerous viral agents can cause CNS infection, and, with the exception of certain types of herpes infections, almost all of the diseases are community acquired. Prevention of CNS viral infections as a complication of systemic illness is currently the focus of intensive research and special public health programs. Examples of these programs include development of vaccines and vaccination programs, pest control, and sanitation control. For this reason discussion of CNS viral infections will be limited to a broad description of the major viral infections and the responsible organisms. Herpesvirus infections will be discussed in more detail.

Aseptic meningitis. The term *aseptic meningitis* is used to describe a symptom complex that can be produced by any one of a number of infective agents, the majority of which are viral.[2] Viral infection is presumably confined to the meningeal coverings of the brain and spinal cord, producing a characteristic syndrome: fever, headache, stiff neck, and other signs of meningeal irritation, with a bacteriologically sterile mononuclear inflammatory response in CSF. The disease is described by most authors as being usually of short duration, benign, and relatively devoid of serious or persistent secondary complications.[2,101] Others[54] describe the disease as being more serious, particularly in children under 1 year of age. There is a growing incidence of enteroviral (aseptic) meningitis with potential serious consequences in this age group.

The viruses most frequently associated with the aseptic meningitis syndrome are the enteroviruses: ECHO virus, coxsackievirus, and nonparalytic poliomyelitis. Mumps virus is the next most common, followed by herpes simplex type 2 (HSV-2), lymphocytic choriomeningitis (LCM), and encephalomyocarditis (EMC) viruses.[2,45] Arboviruses are responsible for a small number of cases but are more frequently associated with encephalitis or meningoencephalitis.

The enteroviruses have a worldwide distribution, with most infections seen in children.[54] Viral infections are spread by direct person-to-person transfer of infected respiratory tract secretions or feces; thus family outbreaks are common. The LCM and EMC viruses are believed to be acquired by humans through contact with food or dust that is contaminated by infected mouse excretions.[45]

As previously described, viruses are thought to multiply in sites distant to the portal of entry, resulting in a primary viremia. Viral multiplication in extraneural targets creates a secondary viremia that eventually leads to CNS infection. This process may explain the involvement of other organs in aseptic meningitis,[45] orchitis during mumps, and enteroviral and herpesvirus infections. Pancreatitis, pleurodynia, grippe syndromes, and various types of exanthemas during similar viral infections are also common.

Because the infection (primary target) often precedes the onset of the CNS disease (secondary target), antibodies may already have developed to maximal titers in the first serum sample obtained when meningitis has become overt.[45] Three major test systems used to detect antibody response are complement fixation, hemagglutination inhibition, and serum neutralization.

The CSF findings consist of pleocytosis (mainly mononuclear), a small and variable increase in protein, no demonstrable microorganisms by smear and bacterial culture, and normal CSF glucose.[2,101]

Acute viral encephalitis. Acute viral encephalitis, a localized or diffuse inflammatory process involving parenchymal brain tissue,[101] can be conveniently separated into two descriptive forms: epidemic and sporadic.[63] The primary causes of epidemic encephalitis are members of the arbovirus or togavirus groups. The principal agent responsible for sporadic disease in the United States is herpesvirus.[63]

ARBOVIRUS (TOGAVIRUS). Arboviruses are a large group that are transferred to vertebrate hosts by a biting arthropod. Most arboviruses have been classified on the basis of structural and chemical properties as togaviruses.[73]

At the present time there are more than 350 distinct arboviruses[45] of which 50 or 60 are known to infect humans.[2,63] About a dozen cause severe illness, usually acute encephalitis, hemorrhagic fever, or arthralgia.[63] Of these, only five are known to be active in the United States.[45,63]

Eastern equine encephalitis is found chiefly along the eastern coast of the United States and appears predominantly in infants and children and adults over 55 years of age. Fortunately, the incidence of this disease is rare because nearly three fourths of the patients die.[63] In the most fulminant cases death occurs within 3 to 5 days. Patients who recover are usually left with severe impairments, such as mental deficiency, hemiplegia, convulsive disorders, aphasia, and cranial palsies.

Western equine encephalitis is uniformly distributed throughout the country,[2] inflicting mostly the very young and the very old. This disease is less severe than the eastern type, with a mortality of about 10%.[63] Severe and permanent sequelae are rare in adults, but more than half of the infants less than 1 month of age have recurrent seizures or marked motor and behavioral deficits.

St. Louis encephalitis is the most frequent kind of encephalitis and occurs in two types of epidemics: one is marked encephalitis in elderly persons in urban areas, and the other occurs in irrigated rural areas in the far west and southwest.[73] Although approximately 20% of the cases are fatal, significant permanent neurological sequelae are uncommon.

California encephalitis, which occurs throughout the United States, is the least serious of the infections. Children are usually affected, and complete recovery without significant neurological deficits can be expected.[63]

Venezuelan equine encephalitis occurs primarily in the southwestern part of the United States. Fatalities are rare and occur primarily in children.[63]

The neuropathological changes in the CNS in response to arbovirus infection vary in extent and severity, depending on the specific agent. The characteristic changes that are common to these infections include cellular infiltration, microglial hyperplasia and proliferation, and neuronal degeneration. Nerve cell changes range from slight swelling and hyalinization to total destruction. Neuronophagia is often observed. Although focal areas of severe changes are found, involvement tends to be widespread throughout the CNS affecting both gray and white matter. Perivascular cuffing by lymphocytes, mononuclear leukocytes, and plasma cells and a patchy infiltration of the meninges by similar cells are also characteristic.[2,63]

The clinical manifestations of the various arbovirus infections are similar, although they vary with age.[2] In infants there may be only an abrupt onset of fever and convulsions. In older children the onset is usually less abrupt, with complaints of headache, listlessness, nausea or vomiting, drowsiness, and fever for several days. Convulsions, confusion and stupor, and stiff neck then become prominent. Photophobia, diffuse myalgia, and tremor may be observed in children and adults. Reflex asymmetry, hemiparesis, Babinski's signs, and sucking and grasping reflexes may also occur.

CSF findings are similar to those of aseptic meningitis: elevated pressure, pleocytosis (predominantly polymorphonuclear), elevated protein content, and normal sugar. Isolation of arbovirus from the blood or CSF is rare.[63]

The diagnosis is usually made by serological means, using specimens obtained in acute and convalescent phases of the disease.[63]

HERPES SIMPLEX. Herpes simplex encephalitis is now recognized as the most common cause of sporadic fatal encephalitis and meningoencephalitis in the United States.[52] The mortality of this disease is approximately 50%[2] The disease may occur in all age groups and in all parts of the world. Persons over 15 years of age are most susceptible.[63]

Herpes simplex virus (HSV) consists of two antigenic types: HSV type 1 (HSV-1) and HSV type 2 (HSV-2).[45] Herpes simplex encephalitis is almost always caused by HSV-1.[2] HSV-2 may also cause acute encephalitis but only in the neonate.[12] HSV-2 infections in the adult may cause aseptic meningitis, usually in association with a genital herpes infection.[2]

In adults and children beyond the newborn age group primary HSV-1 infections usually involve nongenital sites, including the mouth, lips, skin above the waist, eyes, and brain.[45] HSV-1 is most often transmitted nonvenereally, but on occasion oral-genital contact or autoinoculation has been implicated as a source. HSV-2 is usually transmitted venereally in adolescents and adults, causing infection of the genitalia and skin below the waist. HSV-2, and occasionally HSV-1, can also be transmitted from the mother's genitalia to the newborn, in whom any site can be involved.[45]

HSV infections are uncommon in the newborn; however, when disseminated and local encephalitic infections occur, the outcomes are devastating. It is estimated that about 40% of neonates coming into contact with the infected maternal birth canal during delivery may acquire the infection in some form and that only about 30% of those will escape death or permanent brain damage.[12] There is also suggestive evidence that the virus may be transmitted to the fetus transplacentally. Congenital abnormalities, abortions, and stillbirths may be associated with this mode of infection.[12] Because the usual agent in neonatal encephalitis is HSV-2, postnatal acquisition from the mother or attendants should be suspected when HSV-1 is found to cause disease.

Primary herpetic infections are most commonly endemic. However, several reports of outbreaks in families, in institutions for children, and in hospitals have been reported.[45] HSV can be considered a cause of nosocomial infection in view of the many reports of herpetic paronychia occurring in hospital personnel, particularly in those attending neurosurgical patients.[45] Hoeprich[45] reports that the virus is acquired in such cases from the orotracheal cavities of patients or from contaminated tracheal catheters. Hospital personnel and patients have contracted herpetic infection from other patients, particularly those with eczema and herpeticum. Laboratory personnel are also reported to be at risk.[45]

A characteristic feature of the herpesviruses is their ability to establish latent infection in a susceptible host.[63] A generally accepted concept is that when persons who have no detectable antibodies to HSV develop a primary infection, antibodies to the virus appear in their serum.[45] Despite such circulating antibodies, many persons develop recurrent infection, usually at or close to the site of their initial infection, although at times it may be remote from the original site. Several theories have been postulated to explain the viral aspects of recurrent infection. One of these theories is based on the demonstration that HSV-1 is latent in the trigeminal ganglia in the majority of adults, suggesting that activation of the virus in the ganglia rather than primary infection may lead to herpetic encephalitis.[50] A second concept envisions a constant low-grade, chronic infection, with the virus persisting in sites such as the lacrimal glands in a sensitized but still infectious form.[45] The third concept is that of autoinfection, requiring transfer of the virus from a manifestly or subclinically infected site to a noninfected site.[45] Reinfection occurs when HSV, either of the homologous or heterologous type, is acquired from an exogenous source.

In addition to the usual abnormalities of acute encephalitis, the pathological lesions in the CNS caused by HSV include intense hemorrhagic necrosis of the inferior and medial parts of the temporal lobes and the orbital parts of the frontal lobes.[2]

In herpes simplex encephalitis the symptoms that evolve over several days are in most cases like those of any other acute encephalitis.[63] In some patients there are additional symptoms consistent with the propensity of this disease to involve the frontal and temporal lobes of the brain.[2] The latter manifestations include olfactory or gustatory hallucinations, anosmia, temporal lobe seizures, a brief period of bizzare psychotic behavior, aphasia, and hemiparesis. Swelling and herniation of one or both of the temporal lobes through the tentorium may occur.[2]

Information on the morbidity and mortality of herpes simplex CNS disease is difficult to evaluate because of the limitations of the available diagnostic methods. When recognized, the disease is described as severe, with an estimated mortality of 30% to 70%.[2] Many survivors are left with significant neurological deficits, either focal or generalized.

CSF findings are similar to those found in acute encephalitis caused by other agents. Red cells, sometimes numbering in the thousands, and xanthochromia are found in some cases, reflecting the hemorrhagic nature of the lesions. HSV has been isolated from CSF in only a few cases.[2,63]

Diagnosis of herpes simplex encephalitis is difficult. Serological means are considered unsatisfactory,[63] and presently the only certain way to establish a diagnosis is reported by fluorescent antibody study and by viral culture of cerebral tissue obtained by brain biopsy.[2]

Until recently there has been no specific treatment for herpes simplex encephalitis; however, the antiviral agent adenine arabinoside is reported to significantly reduce the mortality and morbidity.[2]

Prevention of viral meningitis and acute encephalitis. Widespread vaccination for mumps and poliomyelitis has decreased the incidence of meningitis from these viruses.[45] Unfortunately, there are no such means available to control coxsackievirus or ECHO virus. The diversity of the serotypes of these viruses precludes the development of vaccines.

The control of mice and other animal carriers and the maintenance of high standards of sanitation may help to secure abatement of infection from LCM and EMC viruses.[45] In recent epidemics of viral encephalitis control of the mosquito vector has been used with apparent success.

Because herpes simplex encephalitis is almost always caused by HSV-1, it seems reasonable to assume that adherence to infection control programs directed toward minimizing the transfer of infectious materials with secretion and discharge precautions between patients and/or hospital staff is sufficient to prevent spread of primary lesions. In addition, particular care should be taken to avoid inoculation of open areas or breaks in the skin with contaminated materials. Prevention of herpes simplex in newborns may, in part, be accomplished by cesarean section delivery in mothers with known infections.[12]

Slow viral infections. The term *slow virus* is relatively new to medical literature, having been coined only within the past decade, and its story is still evolving. Slow viruses are often described as unconventional agents because they differ both in nature and effect from conventional viruses.[49] One of the crucial differences is that although they are transmissible and capable of replication they produce no antibody response in affected individuals.[24,49] Another major difference is their insensitivity to the various forms of physiochemical treatment that inactivate conventional viruses.[24,36] These unconventional viruses are also referred to in the medical literature as subacute spongiform encephalopathy agents, as well as slow viruses, because of the slow degenerative diseases and histological changes that they produce in the CNS.

The subacute spongiform encephalopathies produced by slow virus in humans are known as kuru and Creutzfeldt-Jakob (C-J) disease. The precise nature of the transmissible agents of kuru and C-J disease or the agents of their animal prototypes scrapie (sheep) and mink encephalopathy is still not known.[49] Some authors[2] suggest that even though these agents are often grouped together as slow viruses because of their unconventional nature, it might be better to look at them as something new to microbiology.

Whatever the agents might prove to be, the histological changes they produce in humans (kuru and C-J disease) are reported as remarkably similar to scrapie and mink encephalopathy and to disease produced experimentally in other animals that have been inoculated with infected tissue.[24,49] The characteristic changes are a widespread neuronal loss and gliosis accompanied by a striking vacuolation or spongy state of the affected regions.[2]

Kuru. Kuru is the first slow viral infection documented in human beings.[2,49] The disease was first described in 1957 as a degenerative disease of the CNS endemic to the Fore natives in an isolated area of New Guinea.[36] The suspicion that this disease might be transmissible was confirmed when the brain tissue of a patient with kuru was injected into the brain of a chimpanzee, producing, within a couple of years, a similar noninflammatory, degenerative disease.

There has been no evidence to suggest person-to-person transmission of the disease except in association with the ritual of cannibalism.[36] Kuru occurs from ingestion of infected tissue or from direct contact with the infective agent, permitting absorption through conjunctivae, mucous membranes, and abrasions on the skin. Because of the long incubation period, 4½ to 8 years, some persons are still falling victim to the disease.[36]

Clinically, the disease takes the form of an afebrile, progressive cerebellar ataxia with abnormalities of extraocular movements, weakness progressing to immobility, incontinence in the late stages, and death within 3 to 6 months.[2] No abnormalities of clinical laboratory tests or spinal fluid are seen in the disease.[2,49]

The kuru virus has been found in high titers in the brain and sometimes in lower titers in the spleen, liver, and lymph nodes.[36]

Creutzfeldt-Jakob disease. Transmissible C-J disease is a rare, progressive, fatal disease of the CNS characterized by a rapidly progressing dementia, myoclonus, a characteristic EEG (with periodic paroxysmal bursts of spike-wave discharges against a slow background), and a variable amount of pyramidal, extrapyramidal, cerebellar, sensory, and lower motor neuron signs.[2,36,49] The disease is reported to be of 4 to 16 months' duration with dementia progressing to coma and death usually within 2 years of onset.

C-J disease occurs throughout the world at a rate of one to two cases per million with a few exceptions. Libyan Jews have a rate more than 30 times higher,[36] and in central Slovakia and Hungary the rate is also very high. Approximately 10% of the patients with the disease have a family history of dementia.[2,36]

The mode of transmission of C-J disease remains unknown; however, it is not believed to be contagious in the usual sense of the word.[24,36,90] Familial disease is thought to be transmitted from parents to their children.[75] Roos, Gajdusek, and Gibbs[75] suggest that if genetic factors do play a role, they may do so by influencing susceptibility to infection by permitting an otherwise latent agent to produce a slow pathogenic brain infection.

The disease has been transmitted experimentally to chimpanzees by inoculating the animal with brain tissue from infected patients.[36,75] The incubation period in animal experiments is reportedly 1 year.[2,36]

The only direct evidence that C-J disease can be transmitted from person to person (other than genetically) was reported in two separate episodes in 1974 and 1977.[9,24,36,90] In both episodes transmission was by iatrogenic mode through direct implantation of infected materials into the brains of patients during a surgical procedure. The first case involved a corneal transplant from a patient who was later found to have died of C-J disease.[24] In the other case the disease was transmitted to two persons by direct implantation of contaminated stereotactic electroencephalographic electrodes into brain tissue.[9]

Thus far there is no conclusive evidence to support the occurrence of natural transmission from one person to another other than on a genetic basis.[24,36,90] Some authors[24,36] report a growing concern among medical and laboratory personnel regarding the potential hazard involved in caring for these patients and handling their tissues that is out of proportion to the identified risks. The concern has apparently evolved from recent reports of accidental inoculation of patients previously mentioned and from the demonstration that the virus of the disease resists inactivation by boiling, ultraviolet radiation, 70% alcohol, and formaldehyde vapor and may remain active in pathological specimens fixed in 4% formaldehyde.[36] Gajdusek et al.[36] report that as a result of this anxiety, some patients have been refused admission to hospitals, medical and nursing personnel have refused to take part in biopsies and other surgical procedures, and pathologists have declined to do autopsies.

Most experts agree that although the route of transmission of the disease has not been determined, limited precautions should be developed, based entirely on prudent management, to prevent possible transmission of the disease:

1. Special precautions should be taken with blood and needles that are associated with brain tissue or CSF.
2. Thorough handwashing practices should be adhered to when brain tissue or CSF is being handled.

3. Should there be exposure to blood, brain tissue, and/or CSF percutaneously, the wound should be irrigated immediately with 0.5% sodium hypochlorite.
4. Specimens should be labeled "C-J" and "biohazard" to alert laboratory personnel of potential risk.
5. No organs and tissues from patients with C-J disease should be used for transplantation.[36]

The lack of evidence of clustering of cases in medical personnel concerned with the two episodes of accidental transmission or workers experimenting with the transmission of the disease[24] lends credence to the speculation that there is minimal risk attached either to day-to-day management of patients with C-J disease or to normal, domestic contact with them.

The virus of C-J disease has been found in the lymph nodes, liver, kidneys, spleen, lungs, cornea, and CSF, although less regularly and in far lower titers than in the brain and spinal cord.[36] Research with experimental animals has failed to produce infection within 8 months to several years after inoculation with high-titer virus by conjunctival, intranasal, oral, and intradental routes. The virus has been found in the leukocytes of guinea pigs.[36]

There is a risk of C-J virus being accidentally introduced from infected patient tissues through the broken skin of workers in operating rooms and laboratories.[36] Medical personnel should be aware of the safest ways to handle biopsy tissue, CSF, and blood.

Dental, surgical, and neurosurgical operations must be performed with particular regard to the methods of sterilization of instruments. Autoclaving for 1 hour at 121° C and 20 psi inactivates the virus completely. Also, 5% hypochlorite, 3% permanganate, phenolics, and iodine solution substantially inactivate the potency of the virus.[36]

Because the virus may remain active for a period of time after the patient's death, it is recommended that postmortem examination and preparation of tissues for microscopy should be done with caution, taking care that no fragment of infected tissue be allowed to penetrate skin surface and ensuring the sterility of any contaminated substance and equipment.[24,36]

Experts have published detailed recommendations for all persons who may care for or come in contact with the body fluids and tissues of patients with C-J disease. The first was published by Gajdusek et al.[36] in 1977, and the second is the recent report of the Howie Working Party.

Fungal etiology

CNS fungal infections can result in meningitis, meningoencephalitis, or brain abscess with pathological and clinical effects similar to those produced by bacterial infections.[2] Fungal infections are much less common than bacterial infections and are seen primarily in association with other disease processes.

Although they can occur in the absence of predisposing factors, the disease processes they are commonly associated with include lymphoma or other malignancies, diabetes, leukemia, collagen vascular disease, and organ transplantation operations.[7,56,89]

Fungal infection in conjunction with other disease processes is thought to be related to disturbances in normal flora as a result of prolonged antibiotic therapy,[7,17] lowering of the natural immunity with steroid therapy, cytotoxic drugs, and antimetabolites[67] or is secondary to diseases that cause leukopenia or interfere with normal immunological responses.[67,89]

Organisms that cause infection in the immunosuppressed patient are usually referred to as opportunistic. Opportunistic fungal infections of the CNS include cryptococcosis, nocardiosis, candidiasis (moniliasis), aspergillosis, and mucormycosis (phycomycosis).[89]

Cryptococcus neoformans is the most frequent cause of CNS fungal infection, occurring about half the time in patients with underlying disease.[2,89] This organism is a common soil fungus found in the roosting sites of pigeons and other birds.[45] Transmission to humans occurs most frequently by inhalation of particles containing the organism. Entry into the CNS is thought to occur by hematogenous dissemination from infected lungs.[45,56] In most cases both the brain and meningeal coverings are infected, resulting in meningoencephalitis.

Although a rare cause of CNS infection, *Candida* species has recently emerged as one of the most common pathogens to cause generalized infection in patients with underlying disease.[7] When the CNS is infected, the most frequent lesion is a parenchymal abscess, with *Candida* meningitis being identified as the etiological agent.[7,17]

Candida organisms are normal inhabitants of body surfaces that may overgrow and invade tissues when permitted by altered host defenses.[45] Overgrowth usually occurs in areas such as the mucous membranes of the oropharynx, the gastrointestinal tract, and the vagina.[45] The most likely route of CNS infection is hematogenous spread from a variety of peripheral sites of active candidal infection.[6]

Chronic indwelling urinary and central venous catheters have frequently been implicated as sources of systemic candidiasis.[17] *Candida* organisms may also be directly inoculated into the bloodstream during intravenous puncture[45] or into the CNS during neurological invasive procedures, such as a lumbar puncture.[7,86] Chadwick, Hartley, and Mackinnon[17] recently reported two cases of Candida meningitis in patients with CSF shunts. In both patients the infections were either preceded or acquired simultaneously with bacterial meningitis. A CSF leak into the oropharynx of one patient and a ventricular drain in another were thought to provide the portal of entry for candidal infection. However, intravenous cannulas and antimicrobial therapy were also considered by the authors to be possible predisposing factors.

Fungal infections of the CNS usually develop insidiously over a period of several days or weeks.[89] Although certain fungal infections have specific characteristics in their clinical and bacteriological patterns, as a group these infections tend to present a similar clinical picture. Clinical manifestations may include a low-grade fever; gradually developing headache, sweating, chills, tremor, and generalized weakness; nausea and vomiting; vertigo, blurred or double vision; and photophobia.[2,89] Signs of meningeal irritation and increased intracranial pressure are common.[7]

CSF analysis is the most important diagnostic tool for identifying CNS infections. A specific diagnosis can only be made from smears of the CSF sediment and from cultures. Special techniques are often necessary. Repeated examinations are often necessary because the results may be normal or nearly normal early in the disease.[45,89] The CSF pressure is usually elevated; there is a moderate pleocytosis (usually less than 1000 cells per cubic millimeter), and lymphocytes predominate. The CSF glucose is low (20% to 40%), and the protein is elevated but usually under 200 mg/100 ml.[101]

The mortality rate of CNS fungal infections is approximately 40%.[2] Before 1957, when antifungal therapy such as amphotericin B became available,[77] cryptococcal meningitis was almost always fatal. The use of amphotericin B has been reported to significantly improve the prognosis of this disease.[56] Amphotericin B is also recommended as the drug of choice for other CNS fungal infections.[7,89] A new drug, flucytosine, has been reported to be effective in reducing the mortality and the relapses that frequently occur with some CNS fungal infections.[2]

PREVENTION AND CONTROL

Intensive management of a patient with a severe head injury frequently includes therapies and diagnostic procedures that have been documented as predisposing to nosocomial infections and sepsis:

1. Insertion of peripheral and central venous catheters for administration of drugs and maintenance of fluid and electrolyte balance
2. Insertion of intraarterial catheter for blood pressure monitoring
3. Insertion of urinary catheters to monitor urine output, osmolality, and specific gravity
4. Insertion of ICPM devices to monitor for increasing intracranial pressure and, in some cases, ventricular CSF drainage
5. Intubation and use of mechanical ventilatory support equipment for controlled ventilation or respiratory assistance
6. Initiation of steroid therapy to reduce inflammation associated with injury (or cerebral edema)
7. Craniotomy for surgical correction of complications such as dural tears; CSF fistula; subdural, epidural, or intracerebral hematoma; or foreign bodies

TABLE 18-2. Prevention and control of CNS infections

Sources of infection	Preventive measures	Control measures
Direct inoculation Personal	Handwashing—single most important preventive measure to reduce risk of nosocomial infection in health care setting	Adequate handwashing facilities; appropriate soap for routine handwashing (one that does not cause skin irritation, chafing, or cracking); management expectations that handwashing is done by all personnel
Equipment	Use of properly sterilized and disinfected supplies and equipment	Establishment of quality control systems to assure proper sterilization and disinfection, including functional recall system
Contaminated wounds	Complete cleaning of contaminated wounds, when possible	Wound care as needed (see Chapter 17); wound and skin precautions as indicated by etiological agent
Device-procedure-related infections Invasive monitoring	Use of sterile equipment and supplies; inserted under operating room conditions; maintenance of *closed* system; only knowledgeable personnel will manipulate equipment; handwashing; daily care of catheter insertion site	Appropriate culturing of equipment when suspected as causing infection; recall system as above for suspected contamination of processed equipment and supplies; When system becomes disconnected and contaminated, new tubing and monitoring device should replace contaminated setup; routine staff education to ensure that they incorporate appropriate care in their daily practice; handwashing (as above); see Chapter 13 for specific catheter insertion site care
VP and VA shunts	Inserted under operating room conditions; use sterile equipment and shunt	Remove if shunt becomes infected; wound care as above

TABLE 18-2. Prevention and control of CNS infections—cont'd

Sources of infection	Preventive measures	Control measures
Additional sources of potential infection risks	*Respiratory tract* (intubation and tracheostomy; ventilator-assisted breathing): sterile suctioning, properly maintained equipment, and prevention of aspiration	See Chapter 16
	Urinary tract (indwelling Foley catheter): sterile equipment and aseptic insertion, properly maintained system, and removal of catheter as soon as possible	See Chapter 14
	Cardiovascular system (intravenous therapy): sterile equipment, sterile fluid, proper skin preparation, maintenance of system, daily catheter care, and insertion site care	See Chapter 13

Table 18-2 outlines the preventive and control measures to consider in the management of patients with different potential sources of CNS infections.

Following is a plan for control and prevention of nosocomial septicemia and meningitis in neonates that has been reported as effective in reducing the incidence at Jefferson Davis Hospital in Houston, Texas, from 8/1000 live births to 4/1000 live births*:

1. Surveillance data regarding disease rates per month as well as by site and pathogen should be reviewed by the hospital's infection control committee.
2. Periodic in-service programs to reinforce infection control policies such as handwashing should be provided. The mainstay of prevention of nosocomial infection in the newborn nursery is provision of conditions which minimize manual contact in the transmission of bacteria. Adequate and convenient handwashing facilities must be available, and a rigidly enforced policy for personnel to wash with one of several antiseptic skin cleansers immediately before handling an infant is mandatory.

*Modified from Baker, C.J.: Am. J. Med. **70:**698-701, 1981.

3. Nurseries must have adequate space as well as personnel. The American Academy of Pediatrics recommends one nurse for every one or two infants in intensive care, one for every three or four for immediate care and one for every six to eight for normal newborn nurseries.
4. Optimal procedures for disinfecting life-support equipment should be identified, publicized, enforced and monitored by periodic surveillance. Everything that comes in contact with the infant must be discarded or disinfected before use by another.
5. Nurseries should be cleaned with equipment not employed in other parts of the hospital.
6. When an increased incidence of infection is detected, information should be quickly gathered to ascertain whether there is a common etiologic agent and possible clues regarding its source and transmission.
7. Infants with known or suspected infection should be isolated, and their contacts within the nursery should be cohorted until the time of hospital discharge. In outbreaks due to enteric bacilli, cultures of specimens from equipment and environmental sources may be helpful and periodic cultures from throat and rectal sites in neonates for isolation of the epidemic agent may assist in cohorting of asymptomatically colonized infants.

Vaccines

Polysaccharide vaccines against serogroups A and C meningococcus have been licensed in the United States and are now available for three purposes: as a means to control epidemics, as prophylaxis for individuals planning to travel to areas with epidemics, and as prophylaxis for family contacts of persons with disease caused by meningococcal groups A or C.[34]

In 1976 polysaccharide vaccines for groups A and C meningococcus were used to control small outbreaks of meningococcal infection in Portland, Oregon; Seattle, Washington, and Anchorage, Alaska.[34] Blanket immunization in a limited population at the start of a possible outbreak is thought to offer an alternative to controlling epidemics by widespread vaccination, involving much less expense.[39]

Vaccine for group C meningococcus has become a routine vaccination for military recruits and has eradicated group C meningococcal disease from this population.[4,39] This vaccine affords no direct protection for children under 2 years of age.[87] The immunological tolerance it induces in this age group has been suggested to place them at a greater risk of disease.[39]

Vaccine for group A meningococcus is reported to protect children 3 months or older if booster immunizations are used at 18 and 24 months and again at 4 to 6 years of age.[70] Because there has been little disease caused by this serogroup in the United States for 30 years, routine immunization of children against the group A organism is thought to be inappropriate at this time.[39,97]

Some authors[39,64,96] believe that routine immunization of infants and children should be considered in those parts of the world where group A epidemics occur regularly, such as the meningitis belt of subsaharan Africa. There is a recent and promising report of the prevention of epidemics of meningococcal meningitis in the African meningitis belt by mass vaccination of children 3 to 15 years of age between 1977 and 1980.[64]

Some authors feel that vaccination should be offered to those persons who have an increased chance of contracting infection in a closed population, such as in a nursery or school,[39] household contacts of patients with the disease, or hospital personnel in regular contact with patients with meningococcal disease or with their laboratory samples.[96]

Pneumococcal vaccine became a licensed product in the United States in 1977.[41]

A potential vaccine against H. influenzae has been developed from the type B capsular polysaccharide and is currently available.[66]

Employee health

Current recommendations for prevention and control (also applicable to exposure) of H. influenzae, meningococcal, and pneumococcal meningitides generally fall into three categories: close observation, chemoprophylaxis, and vaccination.

Isolation of the affected individual is rarely mentioned in current studies of meningitis except in relationship to infection caused by meningococci and H. influenzae in the pediatric population. In these situations respiratory isolation—a private room and mask precautions—until 24 hours after initiation of antimicrobial therapy is recommended by the U.S. Public Health Service for patients suspected of having meningococcal infection.[93] Even more important than patient isolation is the need for careful handling and disposal of discharges from the patient's nose and throat and for meticulous handwashing by hospital personnel between treatment of patients.

In current literature chemoprophylaxis is advocated by some authors[20,31,61] for household contacts and all other individuals who have had "unusually close contact" with persons with meningococcal disease. Close contacts at high risk for disease have been defined as "individuals who frequently sleep and eat in the same dwelling with index cases,"[3] which in most studies have pertained to household contacts, individuals living in dormitories, and children in daycare centers. Hospital personnel who have had "unusually close contact" and are considered to be at risk are described as those who have performed mouth-to-mouth resuscitation on patients with N. meningitidis infection or those who have had accidental laboratory exposure to their samples.[3]

Other persons, including routine hospital contacts,[3,20,31] routine school contacts, and associations on buses and airplanes have not been found to be at increased risk.[3]

Three antimicrobial agents frequently mentioned in the literature as chemoprophylactic agents for close contacts of patients with N. meningitidis meningitis are sulfonamides, minocycline, and rifampin. Chemoprophylaxis reportedly prevents meningitis by interrupting the chain of person-to-person transmission.

Before 1963 sulfonamide drugs were widely used to terminate N. meningitidis carriage among military personnel and proved to be successful in prevention of outbreaks of meningococcal disease.[31] Wide-scale, routine use of this drug in military populations was discontinued during 1969 and 1970 because of the rapid emergence of sulfonamide-resistant strains, first of group B and then group C meningitides.[101] Although successfully used in 1975 and 1976 to control an outbreak of N. meningitidis meningitis type B in a civilian population,[18] wide-scale sulfonamide prophylaxis for populations at risk is not currently advocated for prevention of meningococcal disease.[31,46]

Although sulfonamide chemoprophylaxis is not recommended for large populations, some authors[3,31] agree that it may be useful for close contacts of patients with meningococcal meningitis in well-controlled situations. For example, Felice and Fraser[31] recommend that sulfonamides be used only if the prevalence of resistant organisms in a particular region is less than 10%. Artenstein[3] recommends sulfonamide chemoprophylaxis only if a physician has definitive knowledge of the serogroup and its sensitivity to sulfadiazine. In the absence of available data or if the organism is sulfadiazine resistant, Artenstein strongly advises a plan of close clinical observation of contacts to recognize and treat infection at its earliest stage. The exception to his plan for sulfonamide administration or close observation is in the case of hospital personnel who have been exposed to N. meningitidis through circumstances such as mouth-to-mouth resuscitation or exposure to laboratory samples. For these contacts Artenstein recommends intramuscular procaine penicillin, 500,000 units, three times daily for 2 days, followed by oral penicillin V, 500,000 mg, three times daily for 8 days.[3]

Minocycline and rifampin, licensed in the United States for treatment of the meningococcal carrier state, have been shown to be effective in eradicating meningococci from the nasopharynges of close contacts[3,31]; however, problems have been reported with each. Minocycline produces severe side effects, including nausea, vomiting, dizziness, and headaches.[3,31,45] Rifampin has been associated with the appearance of resistant strains, precluding the use of this drug in large populations at risk.[3]

Rifampin is currently recommended by some authors [31,102] to be the chemoprophylactic agent of choice for close contacts of patients with meningococcal meningitis. Rifampin has also been reported by some authors[38,84] to be effective in eradicating the *H. influenzae* carrier state; however, these authors and others recommend further trials with this drug to determine its effectiveness in prevention of *H. influenzae* infection.

Some authors[46] prefer a plan of close surveillance of contacts over the use of chemoprophylaxis. Close observation of contacts for early signs of illness and initiation of appropriate therapy without delay has been recommended for *H. influenzae* and meningococcal meningitis. This plan demands education of family and other close contacts regarding clinical signs and symptoms of meningitis and the importance of seeking medical attention at the earliest suspicion of disease.

SUMMARY

Because the morbidity and mortality resulting from CNS infections can result in devastating outcomes for patients, all health care workers should be knowledgeable about and skillful in working with equipment and performing procedures associated with the care of patients with CNS disease.

The anatomical and physiological mechanisms that protect the CNS from infections are effective when intact. However, once these have been violated through trauma, injury, or invasive procedures, the patient becomes at risk for developing infection.

The ICP should know and understand the causes of the major nosocomial CNS infections, especially meningitis and brain abscess. Special efforts should be made to monitor, to inform health care workers of appropriate infection control measures, and to evaluate specific invasive care practices that place the patient at risk, especially surgery, ICPM systems, and shunts.

REFERENCES

1. Aber, R.C., et al.: Nosocomial transmission of group B streptococci, Pediatrics **58:**346-353, 1976.
2. Adams, R.D., and Victor, M.: Principles of neurology, ed. 2, New York, 1981, McGraw-Hill, Inc.
3. Artenstein, M.S.: Prophylaxis for meningococcal disease, J.A.M.A. **231:**1035-1037, 1975.
4. Artenstein, M.S., et al.: Prevention of meningococcal disease by group C polysaccharide vaccine, N. Engl. J. Med. **282:**417-420, 1970.
5. Baker, C.J.: Nosocomial septicemia and meningitis in neonates, Am. J. Med. **70:**698-701, 1981.
6. Bannister, R.: Brain's clinical neurology, ed. 5, Oxford, 1978, Oxford University Press.
7. Bayer, A.S., et al.: *Candida* meningitis: report of seven cases and review of the English literature, Medicine **55:**477-486, 1976.
8. Berman, P.H., and Banker, B.: Neonatal meningitis: a clinical and pathological study of 29 cases, Pediatrics **38:**6-24, July 1966.
9. Bernoulli, C., et al.: Danger of accidental person-to-person transmission of Creutzfeldt-Jakob disease by surgery, Lancet **1:**478-479, 1977.
10. Brewer, N.S., MacCarty, C.S., and Wellman, W.E.: Brain abscess: a review of recent experience, Ann. Intern. Med. **82:**571-576, 1975.
11. Brook, I.: Bacteriology of intracranial abscess in children, J. Neurosurg. **54:**484-488, 1981.
12. Brown, R.S.: Herpes simplex virus encephalitis in the newborn, Dev. Med. Child Neurol. **19:**407-410, 1977.

13. Buckwold, F.J., Hand, R., and Hansebout, R.R.: Hospital-acquired bacterial meningitis in neurosurgical patients, J. Neurosurg. **46**:494-499, 1977.
14. Carey, M.E., Chou, S.N., and French, L.A.: Experience with brain abscess, J. Neurosurg. **36**: 1-9, Jan. 1972.
15. Centers for Disease Control: Recommendations for prevention of infection of patients with invasive pressure monitoring systems, reprinted from the National Nosocomial Infections Study Report, 1977; issued 1979 by the Hospital Infections Program; reprinted Feb. 1980 and June 1981, Atlanta, CDC.
16. Cervos-Navarro, J., et al.: A modifiied method for monitoring intra-cerebral pressure in brain edema, Adv. Neurol. **28**:27-38, 1980.
17. Chadwick, D.W., Hartley, E., and Mackinnon, M.: Meningitis caused by *Candida tropicalis*, Arch. Neurol. **37**:175-176, 1980.
18. Chester, T., et al.: House to house, community wide chemoprophylaxis for meningococcal disease: an aggressive approach to disease prevention, Am. J. Public Health **67**: 1058-1062, 1977.
19. Clark, R.G.: Manter and Gatz's essentials of clinical neuroanatomy and neurophysiology, ed. 5, Philadelphia, 1975, F.A. Davis Co.
20. Cohen, M.S., et al.: Possible nosocomial transmission of group Y *Neisseria meningitidis* among oncology patients, Ann. Intern. Med. **91**:7-12, 1979.
21. Conway, B.L.: Carini and Owens' neurological and neurosurgical nursing, ed. 8, St. Louis, 1982, The C.V. Mosby Co.
22. Coonrod, D., and Dans, P.E.: Subdural empyema, Am. J. Med. **53**:85-91, July 1972.
23. Corbett, J., and Rosenstein, B.: Pseudomonas meningitis related to spinal anesthesia, Neurology **21**:946-950, 1971.
24. Corsellis, J.A.N.: On the transmission of dementia: a personal view of the slow virus problem, Br. J. Psychiatr. **134**:553-559, 1979.
25. Cross, A.S., and Roup, B.: Role of respiratory assistance devices in endemic nosocomial pneumonia, Am. J. Med. **70**:681-685, 1981.
26. Cruse, P.J.E., and Foord, R.: A five-year prospective study of 23,649 surgical wounds, Arch. Surg. **107**:206-210, 1973.
27. Ericsson, C.D., et al.: Erroneous diagnosis of meningitis due to false-positive Gram stains, South Med. J. **71**:1524-1525, 1978.
28. Everett, E.D., Eickhoff, T.C., and Simon, R.H.: Cerebrospinal fluid shunt infections with anaerobic diphtheroids (*Proprionibacterium* species), J. Neurosurg. **44**:580-584, 1976.
29. Feigen, R.D., and Dodge, P.R.: Bacterial meningitis: newer concepts of pathophysiology and neurologic sequelae, Pediatr. Clin. North Am. **23**:541-556, 1976.
30. Fekety, P.R., and Murphy, J.F.: Factors responsible for development of infections in hospitalized patients, Surg. Clin. North Am. **52**:1385-1390, 1972.
31. Felice, G.A., and Fraser, D.W.: Epidemiology of bacterial meningitis: a review of selected aspects, Adv. Neurol. **19**:185-196, 1978.
32. Finegold, S.M.: Anaerobic bacteria in human disease, New York, 1977, Academic Press, Inc.
33. Fothergill, L.D., and Wright, J.: Influenzal meningitis: the relationship of age incidence to the bacterial power of blood against the causal organism, J. Immunol. **24**:273-284, 1933.
34. Fraser, D.W.: Vaccines against bacterial meningitis: an unfinished story, Post. Grad. Med. **62**:105-109, Aug. 1977.
35. Fraser, D.W., et al.: Risk factors in bacterial meningitis: Charleston County, South Carolina, J. Infect. Dis. **127**:271-277, 1973.
36. Gajdusek, C., et al.: Precautions in medical care of and in handling materials from patients with transmissible virus dementia (Creutzfeldt-Jakob disease), N. Engl. J. Med. **296**:1253-1258, 1977.
37. Gardner, D.: Intracranial pressure monitoring. In Borg, N., et al., editors: Core curriculum for critical care nursing, ed. 2, Philadelphia, 1981, W.B. Saunders Co.
38. Glode, M.P., et al.: *Haemophilus influenzae* type B meningitis: a contagious disease of children, Br. Med. J. **280**:899-901, 1980.

39. Gold, R.: Polysaccharide meningococcal vaccines: current status, Hosp. Pract., pp. 41-48, Dec. 1979.
40. Goldschneider, I., Gotschlich, E.C., and Artenstein, M.S.: Human immunity to the meningococcus, J. Exp. Med. **129**:1307-1326, 1969.
41. Gotschlich, E.C.: Bacterial meningitis: the beginning of the end, Am. J. Med. **65**:719-721, 1978.
42. Green, J.R., Kanshepolsky, J., and Turkian, B.: Incidence and significance of central nervous system infection in neurosurgical patients, Adv. Neurol. **6**:223-228, 1974.
43. Guyton, A.C.: Textbook of medical physiology, ed. 5, Philadelphia, 1976, W.B. Saunders Co.
44. Hand, W.L., and Sanford, J.P.: Posttraumatic bacterial meningitis, Ann. Intern. Med. **72**:869-874, 1970.
45. Hoeprich, P.D.: Infectious diseases, ed. 2, New York, 1977, Harper & Row, Publishers, Inc.
46. Horenstein, S., and Schreiber, D.J.: Clinical features of bacterial meningitis, Adv. Neurol. **6**:141-159, 1974.
47. Intracranial pressure monitoring: Procedure from San Francisco General Hospital, San Francisco, 1978.
48. Johnson, R.T.: Pathophysiology and epidemiology of acute viral infections of the nervous system, Adv. Neurol. **6**:27-40, 1974.
49. Johnson, R.T.: Slow infections of the nervous system and the subacute spongiform encephalopathies, Adv. Neurol. **6**:69-75, 1974.
50. Johnson, R.T.: Selective vulnerability of neural cells to viral infections, Brain **103**:417-442, 1980.
51. Johnson, R.T., and Mims, C.A.: Pathogenesis of viral infections of the nervous system, N. Engl. J. Med. **278**:23-30, 1968.
52. Johnson, R.T., Olson, L.C., and Buesher, E.L.: Herpes simplex virus infections in the nervous system, Arch. Neurol. **18**:260-264, 1968.
53. Le Beau, J., et al.: Surgical treatment of brain abscess and subdural empyema, J. Neurosurg. **38**:198-203, Feb. 1973.
54. Le Pow, M.L.: Enteroviral meningitis: a reappraisal, Pediatrics **62**:267-269, 1978.
55. Lerman, S.J.: *Haemophilus influenzae* infections of cerebrospinal fluid shunts: report of two cases, J. Neurosurg. **54**:261-263, Feb. 1981.
56. Lewis, J.L., and Rabinovich, S.: The wide spectrum of cryptococcal infections, Am. J. Med. **53**:315-322, 1972.
57. Lundberg, N.: Continuous recording and control of ventricular fluid pressure in neurosurgical practice, Acta Psychiatr. Scand. **36**(suppl. 149):1-193, 1960.
58. Majeda, C.: Postoperative infections on a neurosurgical service, J. Neurosurg. Nurs. **9**:84-86, June 1977.
59. Malis, L.I.: Control of neurosurgical infections by intraoperative antibiotics, Presented at a meeting of the American Association of Neurosurgical Surgeons, April 1976.
60. Mangi, R.J., Quintilani, R., and Andriole, V.T.: Gram-negative bacillary meningitis, Am. J. Med. **59**:829-836, 1975.
61. McCormick, J.B., and Bennett, J.V.: Public health considerations in the management of meningococcal disease, Ann. Intern. Med. **83**:883-886, 1975.
62. Meirowsky, A.M., et al.: Cerebrospinal fluid fistulas complicating missile wounds of the brain, J. Neurosurg. **54**:44-48, Jan. 1981.
63. Miller, J.R., and Harter, D.H.: Acute viral encephalitis, Med. Clin. North Am. **56**:1393-1404, 1972.
64. Mohammed, I., and Zaruba, K.: Control of epidemic meningococcal meningitis by mass vaccination, Lancet **2**:80-82, July 1981.
65. Norden, C.W.: *Haemophilus influenzae* infection in adults, Med. Clin. North Am. **62**:1037-1046, 1978.
66. Norden, C.W., Callerame, M.L., and Baum, J.: *Haemophilus influenzae* meningitis in an adult: a study of bactericidal antibodies and immunoglobulins, N. Engl. J. Med. **282**:190-194, Jan. 1979.

67. O'Laughlin, J.M.: Infections in the immunosuppressed patient, Med. Clin. North Am. **59:**495-501, 1975.
68. Patriarca, P.A., and Lauer, B.A.: Ventriculo peritoneal shunt–associated infection due to *haemophilus influnzae,* Pediatrics **65:**1007-1009, 1980.
69. Paulson, O.B., and Hertz, M.M.: Blood-brain barrier permeability during shortlasting intravascular hyperosmolarity, Eur. J. Clin. Invest. **8:**391-396, 1978.
70. Petola, H., et al.: Clinical efficacy of meningococcal group A capsular polysaccharide vaccine in children three months to five years of age, N. Engl. J. Med. **297:**686-691, 1977.
71. Poll, W., Waldhausen, W., and Brock, M.: Infection rate of continuous monitoring of ventricular fluid pressure with and without open cerebrospinal fluid drainage, Adv. Neurosurg. **9:**363-366, 1980.
72. Poppen, J.L.: Ventricular drainage as a valuable procedure in neurosurgery: report of a satisfactory method, Arch. Neurol. Psychiatr. **50:**587-589, 1943.
73. Powell, K.E., and Kappus, K.D.: Epidemiology of St. Louis encephalitis and other acute encephalitides, Adv. Neurol. **19:**197-215, 1978.
74. Rahol, J.J., et al.: Combined intrathecal and intramuscular gentamycin for gram-negative meningitis: pharmacology study of 21 patients, N. Engl. J. Med. **290:**1394-1398, 1974.
75. Roos, R., Gajdusek, C., and Gibbs, C.J.: The clinical characteristics of transmissable Creutzfeldt-Jakob disease, Brain **96:**1-20, 1973.
76. Sampson, D.S., and Clark, K.: A current review of brain abscess, Am. J. Med. **54:**201-210, 1973.
77. Sarosi, G.A., et al.: Amphotericin B in cryptococcal meningitis, Ann. Intern. Med. **71:**1079-1087, 1967.
78. Savitz, M.H., Malis, L.I., and Meyers, B.R.: Prophylactic antibiotics in neurosurgery, Surg. Neurol. **2:**95-100, Mar. 1974.
79. Schoenbaum, S.C., Gardner, P., and Shillito, J.: Infections of cerebrospinal fluid shunts: epidemiology, clinical manifestations and therapy, J. Infect. Dis. **131:**543-552, 1975.
80. Sells, C., Shurtleff, D.B., and Loeser, J.D.: Gram-negative cerebrospinal fluid shunt–associated infections, Pediatrics **59:**614-618, 1977.
81. Shurtleff, D.B., Christie, D., and Foltz, E.L.: Ventriculostomy associated infection: a 12 year study, J. Neurosurg. **35:**686-694, 1971.
82. Shurtleff, D.B., et al.: Therapy of *Staphylococcus epidermidis* infections associated with cerebrospinal fluid shunts, Pediatrics **53:**55-62, Jan. 1974.
83. Smith, A.L.: Microbiology, ed. 12, St. Louis, 1980, The C.V. Mosby Co.
84. Smith, A.L.: Is *Haemophilus influenzae* meningitis contagious? N. Engl. J. Med. **301:**155-156, 1979.
85. Smith, R.W., and Alksne, J.F.: Infections complicating the use of external ventriculostomy, J. Neurosurg. **44:**567-570, 1976.
86. Sugarman, B., and Massanar, M.R.: *Candida* meningitis in patients with CSF shunts, Arch. Neurol. **37:**180-181, Mar. 1980.
87. Taunay, A. de E., et al.: Disease prevention by meningococcal serogroup C polysaccharide vaccine in preschool children: results after eleven months in Sao Paulo, Brazil, Pediatr. Res. **8:**429, 1975.
88. Thoburn, R., et al.: Infections acquired by hospitalized patients: an analysis of the overall problem, Arch. Intern. Med. **121:**1-10, Jan. 1968.
89. Thompson, R.A.: Clinical features of central nervous system fungus infection, Adv. Neurol. **6:**93-100, 1974.
90. Transmission of Creutzfeldt-Jakob disease, Lancet, **2:**338-339, 1979.
91. Traub, W.H.: Brain abscess and acute purulent meningitis: recent developments in clinical microbiology, Adv. Neurosurg. **9:**1-27, 1980.
92. Tsinzo, M.: Nosocomial infections associated with neurosurgery, Infect. Control Urol. Care **6:**18-21, 1981.
93. U.S. Department of Health, Education, and Welfare: Isolation techniques for use in hospitals, Atlanta, 1975, Centers for Disease Control.

94. Waggoner, J.D.: The pathophysiology of bacterial meningitis and cerebral abscess: an anatomical interpretation, Adv. Neurol. **6**:1-17, 1974.
95. Weinstein, R.A., et al.: Factitious meningitis, J.A.M.A. **233**:878-879, 1975.
96. Who should be given meningococcal vaccine?: Lancet **2**:1185-1186, 1978.
97. Wille, R.L., et al.: Anatomy of the brain and skull, J. Neurosurg. Nurs. **9**:99-101, 1977.
98. Wing, S.: Brain abscess, J. Neurosurg. Nurs. **13**:123-126, June 1981.
99. Wyler, A.R., and Kelly, W.A.: Use of antibiotics with external ventriculostomies, J. Neurosurg. **37**:185-187, Aug. 1972.
100. Yoshikawa, T.T., Chow, A.W., and Guze, L.B.: Role of anaerobic bacteria in subdural empyema, Am. J. Med. **58**:99-103, Jan. 1975.
101. Youmans, G.P., Paterson, P.Y., and Sommers, H.M.: The biologic and clinical basis of infectious diseases, Philadelphia, 1975, W.B. Saunders Co.

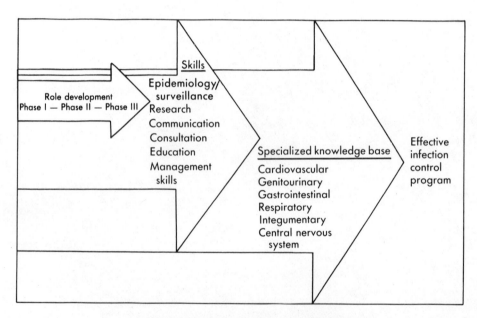

Model of integrated infection control practice

Stanford University Hospital Rubella Screening Program

INTRODUCTION

Rubella, usually a common, mild disease, poses a significant threat to the fetus of a susceptible woman who contracts the disease in early pregnancy, especially in the first trimester. Prevention of infection to the fetus and the consequent anomalies associated with congenital rubella syndrome is the major focus of the rubella screening/immunization program.

Twenty-five percent of adults, including medical personnel, are currently susceptible to rubella. Fifty percent of people with rubella have no rash. As a result, over 50 pregnant women have been exposed to rubella in each of seven hospitals during outbreaks that were inadvertently propagated by infected medical personnel. It is, therefore, necessary that all medical center personnel who have contact with pregnant women be immune to rubella.

SCOPE OF THE PROGRAM

Serological screening for rubella antibody (HI titer) is performed for medical center staff who are either at significant risk of personal exposure or who may, if they become infected, pose a serious threat to patients under their care.

Group I

Testing is performed for women in childbearing age groups who due to the nature of their responsibilities are at significant risk for exposure to patients with rubella or congenital rubella syndrome. This service is offered as an employee benefit, and participation in the program (including immunization) is optional.

Group II

Testing is performed for all staff members (regardless of age or gender) who due to the nature of their responsibilities may expose pregnant patients to rubella. Since this service is provided for both individual employee and *public health* benefits, serological screening and subsequent immunization of susceptible individuals is mandatory for continued employment in these high-risk areas.

IMPLEMENTATION PLAN

The primary goal of this program is to gain staff support and cooperation through education and understanding of the serious consequences of rubella infection.

Medical center employees

1. Serological testing

    All employees (including residents and interns) will have a blood sample obtained for serological screening as part of the preemployment physical examination. Employees who submit written documentation of prior testing will be exempted.

    Seropositive employees will be informed of their immune status via a memo from the Personnel Health Service (appended). Seronegative employees will be asked to report to Personnel Health Service to be given the results and their options dependent upon group I or II category of employment (memos appended).

2. Immunization

    Employees who elect to receive rubella immunization from their private physician must submit proof of immunization to Personnel Health Service within 2 months of notification of their seronegative status.

    Employees who desire immunization through the medical center are referred to:

    a. *GYN clinic*—Women will be seen by the nurse practitioner for contraceptive counseling and immunization.

    b. *Medical clinic*—Men will be seen by clinic staff.

    Informed consent (form appended) will be obtained from each employee prior to immunization. Time lost due to side effects of the immunization will be covered by worker's compensation.

3. Refusal to participate

    Participation of group I employees is optional.

    Since participation of group II employees is a condition of employment, a prospective employee who declines to participate will not be hired. Current employees who refuse to participate will be asked to sign a statement to this effect and will be counseled individually with an employee relations representative of the Personnel Department. Termination of employment will be considered only when all other avenues (including transfer to another work area) are exhausted.

Community/faculty physicians

The chairman of the department is responsible for ensuring that all physicians (including fellows) comply with the screening program. Records of immune status and immunization will be maintained in the department with an annual report submitted to the Infection Control Committee.

Disciplinary action for physicians refusing to participate in the program is left to the discretion of the departmental chairman.

Medical students

Students currently enrolled in the medical school will be screened (and immunized as necessary) through the student health service. Students who have not fulfilled this requirement will not be allowed to take clerkships in obstetrics and pediatrics.

Beginning in Fall 1979, all new students are required to show proof of seropositivity or immunization at the time of matriculation.

All visiting clerks in pediatrics and obstetrics must fulfill the same requirements before their applications are approved.

Other students

Health sciences students (nursing, respiratory therapy, radiology, etc.) must fulfill the requirements of this program. The responsibility for compliance and recordkeeping lies with the affiliating school.

SELECTED READINGS

Exposure of patients to rubella by medical personnel: Calif. Morbid., Berkeley, April 7, 1978, State of California, Department of Health Services.

Exposure of patients to rubella by medical personnel—California: Morbid. Mortal. Weekly Rep. **27**:123, 1978.

McLaughlin, M.C., and Gold, L.H.: The New York rubella incident: a case for changing hospital policy regarding rubella testing and immunization, Am. J. Public Health **69**:287-289, 1979.

Rubella testing and immunization of health personnel: Calif. Morbid., Berkeley, Sept. 22, 1978, State of California, Department of Health Services.

Public Health Service Advisory Committee on Immunization Practices: Rubella vaccine, Morbid. Mortal. Weekly Rep. **27**:451-454, 1978.

Weiss, K.E., et al.: Evaluation of employee health service as a setting for a rubella screening and immunization program, Am. J. Public Health **59**:281-283, 1979.

PROPOSAL: RUBELLA SCREENING PROGRAM

Group I: Females	Group II: Males and females
Testing being performed for individual employee benefit only	*Testing being performed for both public health and employee benefits*

1. Nursing service personnel—nurseries*

1. Obstetrical Service
   a. Faculty/community physicians
   b. Residents
   c. Fellows

2. Support services for pediatric unit/ nurseries
   a. Phlebotomists and lab technicians
   b. Blood gas technicians
   c. Respiratory therapists
   d. Physical therapists
   e. EEG technicians
   f. Sleep Apnea Study personnel
   g. Social service
   h. Dieticians

2. Radiology
   a. Faculty
   b. Residents
   c. Fellows
   d. Ultrasound technicians

3. Emergency service
   a. Nursing personnel
   b. Resident(s) in emergency medicine

3. Nursing service personnel*
   a. Labor and delivery room
   b. Postpartum unit
   c. Pediatric units
4. Obstetrical and pediatric clinical staff
   a. Nursing personnel*
   b. Dieticians
   c. Social service
   d. Outpatient registration*
   e. Outpatient phlebotomists
5. Pediatric service
   a. Faculty/community physicians
   b. Residents
   c. Interns
   d. Fellows
6. Transport service personnel

*Female personnel currently being done.

Rubella screening notification

To:

From:

Re: Rubella screening

The result of your blood test for rubella is *positive*. This means that you have had rubella (also known as *German measles* or *three-day measles*) in the past, even if you do not recall having had a rash.

These results indicate that you are protected against rubella. If you were to become pregnant and were exposed to rubella, your unborn child would also be protected. Consequently, there are no restrictions in caring for patients with rubella or congenital rubella syndrome.

Please contact either Personnel Health Service or the infection control staff if you have any questions or concerns.

Encl: Lab report

Rubella screening notification
Group I (optional)

To:

From:

Re: Rubella screening

The result of your blood test for rubella is *negative*. This means that you have never had rubella (also known as *German measles* or *three-day measles*) and are not protected against the disease.

Rubella is generally a mild childhood disease; however, if a pregnant woman develops rubella, there may be severe consequences to the unborn child. Since you currently work in a patient care area where there is a high probability of being exposed to children with rubella or congenital rubella syndrome, you are encouraged to seriously consider receiving rubella immunization. This is particularly important for women in childbearing age groups who may be inadvertently exposed to rubella during pregnancy.

Since there are some contraindications to and precautions for receiving the vaccine, you are urged to consult your private physician or you may contact Personnel Health Service to arrange for an appointment in the Stanford GYN Clinic.

Please give this recommendation careful thought. Until such time that you develop rubella or receive the immunization, it is recommended that you do not care for patients with documented or suspected rubella.

If you have additional questions or concerns please call Personnel Health Service or the infection control staff.

Encl: Lab report

Rubella screening notification
Group II (mandatory)

To:
From:
Re: Rubella screening

The result of your blood test for rubella is *negative*. This means that you have never had rubella (also known as *German measles* or three-day measles) and that you are *susceptible* to the disease.

Rubella, generally a mild disease, occurs in susceptible persons of all ages. If a susceptible pregnant woman develops rubella, there may be severe injury to her unborn child.

Twenty-five percent of adults, including medical personnel, are currently susceptible to rubella. Fifty percent of people with rubella have no rash. As a result, over 50 pregnant, susceptible women have been exposed in each of seven hospitals during epidemics that involved infected medical personnel. It is, therefore, necessary that all medical center personnel who have contact with pregnant women, as you do, be immune to rubella.

Please contact the Personnel Health Service nurse immediately to arrange the administration of the vaccine through the hospital or, if you choose, through your private physician. Proof of immunization must be on file with Personnel Health Service within 8 weeks of receipt of this notice.

Until you receive the vaccine, you should not care for patients with suspected or proven rubella. Should you inadvertently be exposed in the community or hospital, please report immediately to the infection control nurse.

Encl: Lab report

Consent for rubella (German measles) immunization

I hereby consent to the administration of rubella vaccine.

I have been informed that my rubella serology (blood test) is negative and that I am susceptible to rubella (German measles).

I understand that this screening/immunization procedure is part of an infection control program designed to prevent rubella among susceptible hospital staff. I understand that while rubella is a mild disease in children and adults, it can cause congenital defects in an infant whose mother becomes infected in the first and second trimesters of pregnancy. For this reason, I have been advised to receive the vaccine to prevent exposing pregnant susceptible patients I would contact within my duties at the medical center, as well as to protect my own child should I become pregnant in the future.

I understand that I may experience some side effects as a result of the immunization, including joint pain (arthralgia/arthritis), rash, and enlargement of lymph nodes. These symptoms, due to the vaccine virus, are the same symptoms which develop after exposure to the natural virus.

For women

I have been advised and understand that I should not become pregnant for three months following rubella immunization because the safety of the vaccine for a developing fetus is not known.

I have read and understand the above information.

_____   _____
          Employee signature   Witness signature

_____
                  Date

Refusal for rubella (German measles) immunization

I have been informed that my rubella serology (blood test) is negative and that I am susceptible to Rubella (German measles).

I understand that this screening procedure is part of an infection control program designed to prevent rubella among susceptible hospital staff. I understand that while rubella is a mild disease in children and adults, it can cause congenital defects in an infant whose mother becomes infected in the first and second trimesters of pregnancy. For this reason, I have been advised to receive the vaccine to prevent exposing pregnant susceptible patients I would contact within my duties at the medical center, as well as to protect my own child should I become pregnant in the future.

I also understand that my susceptible status prohibits my working in a high-risk area and will result in my reassignment or termination.

Despite this understanding, I refuse to participate in the immunization program.

_____   _____
        Employee signature   Witness signature

_____
            Date

INDEX

Demonstration of technique, 245
Denominator population, 90-91
    special procedure for, 102
    in surgical wound infection surveillance,
        477-479
Dental manipulation, 308
Dependency
    avoiding, 212
    client, 192
Dependent variable, 136
Depilatory, 314, 459
Dermatoglyphic abnormality, 455
Dermis, 440
Descartes, 55, 56
Descriptive epidemiology, 125
Detrusor muscle, 336, 338
Development of disease, incidence rate indicat-
        ing, 149
Device-related infection, 506-514
Dextrostix, 505
Diabetes mellitus, 407, 455, 463
Diagnosis
    of gastrointestinal infection, 377-378
    of respiratory infection, 427
Diagnostic errors in Gram staining, 502
Diagnostic tests
    for bacterial meningitis, 501-504
    for cardiovascular infection, 324
    for herpes simplex, 524
    preoperative, and shunt infection, 511
    for syphilis, 356-357
Diagraming of communication, 168-169
Dialdehydes, 431
Diapedesis, 298
Diarrhea
    epithelial, 369
    E. coli causing, 370
    secretory, 369
Digestion, 364-366
Dip slide culture method, 348
Diphtheroids, 338
Direct bacterial invasion, 504-506
Direct observation of practice, 230
Directing
    conflict in, 283-288
    delegation, 271-273
    leadership theories, 269-271
    motivational theory, 283
    planned change, 278-283
    time management, 273-278
Dirty wounds, 457
Disagreement, skills in, 171, 172
Discharge
    infection after, 95
    surveillance after, 481-482
Discharge diagnosis, 153
Disclosure in interviews, 19
Discussion section of written reports, 155
Disease
    chronic, 129
    defining particular, 125

Disease—cont'd
    rate calculation of, 149-152
    sexually transmitted, 352-361
Disinfection
    environmental, 462
    of respiratory equipment, 431-432
Disposable respiratory equipment, 432
Distension, bladder, 336
Distilled water, 324, 432
Distress, 59
Documentation, 46-47
Domain
    dominant, 243
    of objective, 237-238
Dome, transducer, 320
Dose relationship, 401
Double-blind technique, 133
Down's syndrome, 389
Drainage
    of operative site, 463
    postural, 423
Drainage bags, urinary, 342, 343
Drapes, sterile, 314, 319
Drawing conclusions, 152-154
Dressing
    for intracranial catheter, 508
    sterility of, 314-315
    for surgical wound, 462
Droplet nuclei, 403
Drowning, 410
Drug abuse
    and fungemia, 303
    and hepatitis, 389
    and infective endocarditis, 300
Drug administration; see Medications
Drying of respiratory equipment, 432
Duodenum, 366
Dura mater, 492
    defects of, 504
Duration and development of disease,
        149
Dynamic forces of change, 278
Dynamics of thinking, 256
Dyspareunia, 353
Dysuria, 341

E
e antigen; see HBeAg
Eastern equine encephalitis, 521
Ecchymoses, 501
ECHO virus
    and gastrointestinal infection, 375
    and meningitis, 520
    and respiratory infection, 415
Echoencephalography, 517
Ectoparasitic infestation, 474
Eczema, 523
Edema
    in brain abscess, 515
    bronchial, 410
    uterine, 360